Recent Progress in Hematologic Cancer Research

Recent Progress in Hematologic Cancer Research

Editor: Wesley Ortiz

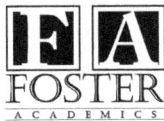

FA FOSTER
ACADEMICS

www.fosteracademics.com

www.fosteracademics.com

FA FOSTER
ACADEMICS

Cataloging-in-Publication Data

Recent progress in hematologic cancer research / edited by Wesley Ortiz.
     p. cm.
Includes bibliographical references and index.
ISBN 978-1-63242-894-3
1. Hematopoietic system--Cancer. 2. Hematopoietic system--Cancer--Research.
3. Lymphoproliferative disorders. 4. Cancer. 5. Hematology. I. Ortiz, Wesley.
RC280.H47 R43 2020
616.994 18--dc23

© Foster Academics, 2020

Foster Academics,
118-35 Queens Blvd., Suite 400,
Forest Hills, NY 11375, USA

ISBN 978-1-63242-894-3 (Hardback)

Contents

Preface

The purpose of the book is to provide a glimpse into the dynamics and to present opinions and studies of some of the scientists engaged in the development of new ideas in the field from very different standpoints. This book will prove useful to students and researchers owing to its high content quality.

Any malignancy of the blood, bone marrow, lymph or lymphatic system is called a hematologic cancer. These elements are closely connected through the immune and circulatory system. Therefore, a disease that affects one element affects others as well. This makes lymphoproliferation and myeloproliferation related and overlapping problems. Some hematologic cancers are lymphomas, leukemias, myelomas, myelogenous leukemia, lymphoid neoplasms, myeloid neoplasms, etc. A common cause of hematologic cancer is chromosomal translocations. As malignant cells are detected in light microscopy, a suspected hematological malignancy is usually analyzed using a complete blood count and blood film. The treatment of B-cell–derived hematologic malignancies, such as diffuse large B-cell lymphoma and follicular lymphoma, are treated using rituximab. Treatment may also involve immunotherapy, chemotherapy, radiotherapy, blood transfusions or bone marrow transplant. This book traces the progress in the field of hematologic cancer research and highlights some of the latest developments. It will also provide interesting topics for research, which interested readers can take up. With state-of-the-art inputs by acclaimed experts of this field, this book targets students and professionals.

At the end, I would like to appreciate all the efforts made by the authors in completing their chapters professionally. I express my deepest gratitude to all of them for contributing to this book by sharing their valuable works. A special thanks to my family and friends for their constant support in this journey.

Editor

Dasatinib Accelerates Valproic Acid-Induced Acute Myeloid Leukemia Cell Death by Regulation of Differentiation Capacity

Sook-Kyoung Heo[1], Eui-Kyu Noh[2], Dong-Joon Yoon[1], Jae-Cheol Jo[2], Jae-Hoo Park[2], Hawk Kim[1,2]*

[1] Biomedical Research Center, Ulsan University Hospital, University of Ulsan College of Medicine, Ulsan, Republic of Korea, [2] Division of Hematology and Hematological Malignancies, Department of Hematology and Oncology, Ulsan University Hospital, University of Ulsan College of Medicine, Ulsan, Republic of Korea

Abstract

Dasatinib is a compound developed for chronic myeloid leukemia as a multi-targeted kinase inhibitor against wild-type BCR-ABL and SRC family kinases. Valproic acid (VPA) is an anti-epileptic drug that also acts as a class I histone deacetylase inhibitor. The aim of this research was to determine the anti-leukemic effects of dasatinib and VPA in combination and to identify their mechanism of action in acute myeloid leukemia (AML) cells. Dasatinib was found to exert potent synergistic inhibitory effects on VPA-treated AML cells in association with G_1 phase cell cycle arrest and apoptosis induction involving the cleavage of poly (ADP-ribose) polymerase and caspase-3, -7 and -9. Dasatinib/VPA-induced cell death thus occurred via caspase-dependent apoptosis. Moreover, MEK/ERK and p38 MAPK inhibitors efficiently inhibited dasatinib/VPA-induced apoptosis. The combined effect of dasatinib and VPA on the differentiation capacity of AML cells was more powerful than the effect of each drug alone, being sufficiently strong to promote AML cell death through G_1 cell cycle arrest and caspase-dependent apoptosis. MEK/ERK and p38 MAPK were found to control dasatinib/VPA-induced apoptosis as upstream regulators, and co-treatment with dasatinib and VPA to contribute to AML cell death through the regulation of differentiation capacity. Taken together, these results indicate that combined dasatinib and VPA treatment has a potential role in anti-leukemic therapy.

Editor: Linda Bendall, Westmead Millennium Institute, University of Sydney, Australia

Funding: This work was supported by Priority Research Center Program through the National Research Foundation of Korea (NRF) funded by the Ministry of Education, Science and Technology (2009-0094050). The funders had no role in study design, data collection and analysis, decision to publish, or preparation of the manuscript.

Competing Interests: The authors have declared that no competing interests exist.

* E-mail: kimhawkmd@gmail.com

Introduction

Acute myeloid leukemia (AML) remains one of the most difficult hematologic malignancies to treat [1]. Efforts to improve standard cytotoxic chemotherapy, the current approach to AML treatment, have been unsuccessful, thus necessitating the development of new chemotherapeutic agents that can remove or diminish leukemic blasts in AML effectively.

Dasatinib (BMS-354825) is an FDA-approved small molecular compound that was developed primarily to treat chronic myeloid leukemia (CML) as a multi-targeted tyrosine kinase inhibitor against wild-type BCR-ABL and SRC family kinases [2]. To date, the compound has demonstrated promising anti-leukemic activity in both patients with imatinib-resistant or -intolerant CML and those with newly diagnosed CML [3–5]. The off-target effects of tyrosine kinase inhibitors, including dasatinib, on AML differentiation have attracted considerable research interest in the past few years. For example, imatinib, the first BCR/ABL inhibitor, was discovered to exert an effect on the potentiation of all-trans-retinoic acid (ATRA)-induced AML differentiation [6], and the epidermal growth factor receptor inhibitor gefitinib was later confirmed to enhance the ATRA-induced differentiation of AML

cells [7,8]. Dasatinib demonstrated similar effects on such differentiation in a separate study [2].

Valproic acid (VPA) is a well-known anti-epileptic drug that is also a class I histone deacetylase inhibitor [9]. Interest in the use of such inhibitors as anti-cancer agents was recently sparked by research showing them to strongly induce cell cycle arrest, differentiation and malignant cell apoptosis [10]. There were also earlier reports of VPA inducing cell cycle arrest and apoptosis in hepatoma [11], prostate carcinoma [12] and thyroid cancer cells [13]. Studies have also revealed the anti-leukemic activity of VPA in human Philadelphia chromosome-positive acute lymphatic and CML cells [14] and in AML cells expressing P-glycoprotein and multidrug resistance-associated protein 1 [15].

However, little is known about the anti-leukemic effects of dasatinib or whether its use in combination with VPA would have a synergistic treatment effect. The purpose of the research reported herein was thus to determine the anti-leukemic effects of both dasatinib and VPA and to identify their mechanism of action in acute myeloid leukemia (AML) cells. We hypothesized that dasatinib and VPA in combination would exert synergistic effects on the apoptotic activity and G_1 phase cell cycle arrest of AML cells.

Materials and Methods

Reagents

All of the reagents, including VPA, were obtained from Sigma-Aldrich (St. Louis, MO) unless otherwise indicated. The CellTiter 96 AQueous One Solution Cell Proliferation Assay (MTS) was purchased from Promega (Madison, WI), and RPMI 1640 medium and fetal bovine serum (FBS) from GibcoBRL (Grand Island, NY). Annexin V-FITC Apoptosis Detection Kit I, PI/RNase staining buffer, anti-human CD11b-PE, anti-human CD14-PE and mouse IgG_1-PE were purchased from BD Biosciences (San Diego, CA). DRAQ5 was purchased from Abcam (Cambridge, MA). The Apoptosis Antibody Sampler Kit, anti-p27[kip1], CDK4, CDK6 and cyclin D1 were purchased from Cell Signaling Technology (Beverly, MA). All of the inhibitors, including the mitogen-activated protein kinase (MAPK) inhibitors (U0126, PD98059, SB203580 and SP600125), caspase-3 inhibitor (Z-DEVD-FMK) and caspase-9 inhibitor (LEHD-CHO), were obtained from Merck Millipore (Billerica, MA). The ApoTarget Caspase-3 Protease Assay Kit for caspase-3 activity and Cas-GLOW Fluorescein Active Caspase-9 Staining Kit were purchased from Invitrogen (Camarillo, CA) and eBioscience (Atlanta, GA), respectively, and the Immun-star WesternC Kit was purchased from Bio-Rad (Hercules, CA). Finally, the Western antibodies, anti-p21[cip1], CDK2, cyclin E, β-actin and anti-rabbit IgG-HRP were purchased from Santa Cruz Biotechnology (Santa Cruz, CA).

Cells and Cell Culture

Human AML HL60, Kasumi-1 and NB4 cells were obtained from the American Type Culture Collection (ATCC, Manassas, VA). The HL60 and NB4 cells were grown as suspension cultures in 100-mm culture dishes in RPMI 1640 medium supplemented with 10% heat-inactivated FBS and 1% penicillin-streptomycin in a 5% CO_2 humidified atmosphere at 37°C. The Kasumi-1 cells were also grown as suspension cultures in RPMI 1640 medium, but were supplemented with 20% heat-inactivated FBS, 4.5 g/L glucose, 2 mM L-glutamine and 1% penicillin-streptomycin in the same condition. Human hepatoma cell lines Hep G2 and Hep 3B and breast cancer cell line MCF-7 were purchased from the ATCC, and were grown as adherent cultures in 100-mm culture dishes in RPMI 1640 medium and Eagle's Minimum Essential Medium supplemented with 10% heat-inactivated FBS and 1% penicillin-streptomycin in a 5% CO_2 humidified atmosphere at 37°C.

Patient Samples

Two patients recently diagnosed with AML (other diseases not specified) at Ulsan University Hospital, Ulsan, South Korea, participated in this study: patient AML-1, a 55-year-old woman, and patient AML-2, a 71-year-old woman. Blood and bone marrow samples were collected from both prior to their first round of chemotherapy.

Ethics Statement

Both subjects provided informed written consent before the study's commencement. The study protocol and patient consent form and information were approved by the Ulsan University Hospital Ethics Committee and Institutional Review Board (UUH-IRB-11-18).

Isolation of Patient Cells

The peripheral blood and bone marrow samples obtained from the two subjects were drawn into heparinized tubes, and separated via density gradient centrifugation at $400 \times g$ using Lymphoprep (Axis-Shield, Oslo, Norway). Peripheral blood mononuclear cells (PBMC) and bone marrow cells (BMC) were isolated and washed with RPMI 1640 medium, and then cultured in 24-well culture plates in the same medium with 10% FBS and 1% penicillin-streptomycin in a 5% CO_2 humidified atmosphere at 37°C. The cells were then subjected to a number of experiments, as described in the following.

Cell Viability Assay

Cell proliferation and cytotoxicity were assessed with the CellTiter 96 AQueous One Solution Cell Proliferation Assay. All cells were seeded in 96-well plates at a density of 2×10^4 cells/ml, with 100 μl of medium per well, and then incubated with 0.5 mM of VPA and 5 μM of dasatinib for 72 h at 37°C. In some of the experiments, the cells were cultured with various concentrations of VPA (0, 0.5, 1, 1.5 and 2 mM) and dasatinib (0, 1, 3, 5, 10 and 15 μM) for 72 h at 37°C. The CellTiter 96 solution (20 μl) was added directly to each well, and the plate was incubated for 4 h in a humidified 5% CO_2 atmosphere at 37°C. Absorbance was measured with a PowerWave XS2 Microplate Spectrophotometer (BioTek, Winooski, VT) at 490 nm, and the results were expressed as percentage changes from the base conditions using four to five culture wells for each experimental condition.

Cell Cycle Analysis

The HL60 cells (5×10^5 cells/ml) were seeded in 24-well plates, and treated with 0.5 mM of VPA and/or 5 μM of dasatinib for 24, 48 and 72 h at 37°C. They were washed twice with phosphate buffered saline (PBS), and fixed with 70% ethanol for 4 h at -4°C, and then washed again with PBS and incubated with 0.5 ml of PI/RNase stain buffer and incubated for 15 min at room temperature. The samples were then analyzed with a FACSCalibur flow cytometer and CellQuest Pro software (BD Biosciences).

Western Blotting of Cell Cycle- and Caspase-related Proteins

Samples of p21[Cip1], p27[Kip1], CDK2, CDK4, CDK6, cyclin D1 and cyclin E were cultured for 72 h, and samples of procaspase-3, -7, -9 and cleaved caspase-3, -7 and -9 for 96 h. Total cell extracts were prepared using RIPA buffer. Equal amounts of cell extract (40–80 μg) were resolved on sodium dodecyl sulfate polyacrylamide gel electrophoresis, and electro-transferred to nitrocellulose membranes for 1.5 h. The membranes were blocked with 4% nonfat dried milk in PBS-T (0.05% Tween-20) buffer for 1 h and blotted with their respective primary antibodies for 2 h. They were subsequently washed three times with PBS-T for 10 min each, and then incubated with their respective horseradish peroxidase (HRP)-conjugated secondary antibodies for 1 h. Finally, the membranes were developed using the Immun-star WesternC kit.

Annexin V and Propidium Iodide Staining

All of the cell types, including the HL60 cells, PBMC and BMC (5×10^5 cells/ml), were cultured with 0.5 mM of VPA and/or 5 μM of dasatinib for 72 h at 37°C. They were then washed twice with FACS buffer (PBS containing 0.3% BSA and 0.1% NaN_3), incubated with annexin V-FITC and propidium iodide (PI) from Apoptosis Detection Kit I, and finally analyzed using the FACSCalibur flow cytometer and CellQuest Pro software according to the manufacturer's protocol. In the experiments in which we used several inhibitors to prevent caspase or MAPK activation, the cells were pre-incubated with the caspase and

MAPK inhibitors for 1 h at 37°C before the addition of dasatinib/VPA.

DRAQ5 Nuclear Staining

Cells were incubated with 0.5 mM of VPA and/or 5 μM of dasatinib for 72 h at 37°C, and then harvested and washed twice with PBS buffer. For DNA content analysis of the nuclei, the cells were stained with 5 μM of DRAQ5 and incubated for 30 min at room temperature. The manufacturer describes DRAQ5 as a cell-permeable far-red fluorescent DNA dye that can be used in live and fixed cells. In our experiments, the stained cells were prepared using FlowSight and analyzed with IDEAS software (Merck Millipore).

Intracellular Staining of Cleaved Poly (ADP-ribose) Polymerase (PARP) and Cleaved Caspase-3

Cells were incubated with 0.5 mM of VPA and/or 5 μM of dasatinib for 72 h at 37°C, then harvested and washed twice with FACS buffer. Next, they were fixed with 4% paraformaldehyde in PBS, after which they were added to a solution of 0.1% Triton X-100 in PBS for permeabilization, as described in our previous report [16]. The cells were stained with anti-cleaved PARP, anti-cleaved caspase-3 mAb or isotype control mAb at 4°C for 30 min. The samples were then analyzed with the FACSCalibur flow cytometer and CellQuest Pro software. We also stained the cell nuclei with DRAQ5 (5 μM) and then analyzed the stained cells with FlowSight and IDEAS software.

Measurement of Caspase-3 and -9 Activity

Cells were incubated with 0.5 mM of VPA and/or 5 μM of dasatinib for 72 h at 37°C, then harvested and washed twice with PBS buffer. Caspase-3 activity was measured using the ApoTarget assay kit, and absorbance with the PowerWave spectrophotometer at 400 nm. Caspase-9 activity was measured using the CasGLOW staining kit. Finally, the cells were analyzed with the FACSCalibur flow cytometer and CellQuest Pro software, and the results were expressed as the percentage of positive cells.

Flow Cytometric Analysis

For flow cytometric analysis, cells were collected and treated in the same conditions as those described in the foregoing experiments. They were washed twice with FACS buffer and incubated with appropriate fluorochrome-labeled mAbs, such as anti-human CD11b-PE and CD14-PE or isotype control mAb, for 30 min at 4°C. The samples were then washed three times with FACS buffer and analyzed using the FACSCalibur flow cytometer and CellQuest Pro software, with the results again expressed as the percentage of positive cells.

Statistical Analysis

All data presented herein represent the means ± standard error of mean (SEM) of at least three independent experiments. All values were evaluated via one-way analysis of variance (ANOVA) followed by Tukey's range test using GraphPad Prism 6.0 software (San Diego, CA). Differences were considered significant at $p < 0.05$.

Results

Dasatinib and VPA Regulate Differentiation Capacity Differently

We examined the effects of dasatinib and VPA on differentiation markers and the cell surface expression of CD11b and CD14. The cells were treated with various concentrations of VPA and dasatinib for 72 h, with the differentiation markers then tested via flow cytometry. CD11b expression increased after exposure to dasatinib alone at days 3 and 5. However, combined dasatinib and VPA treatment led to a marked decrease on CD11b expression in HL60 cells, and the change occurred in a time-dependent manner (Figs. 1A and B). CD14 expression, in contrast, increased after exposure to VPA alone at day 3, whereas its combination with dasatinib resulted in a marked decrease in expression (down to the basal level) in HL60 cells (Fig. 1C).

VPA-dasatinib Combination Induces AML Cell Death

As noted previously, in some of the experiments the cells were treated with various concentrations of VPA (0, 0.5, 1, 1.5 and 2 mM) and dasatinib (0, 1, 3, 5, 10 and 15 μM). VPA and dasatinib significantly inhibited the viability of the HL60 cells in a dose-dependent manner (Figs. 2A and B). Interestingly, however, although 0.5 mM of VPA and 5 μM of dasatinib alone had little effect on the viability of these cells (over 85% and 90% cell viability, respectively), in combination these concentrations of VPA and dasatinib produced a significant inhibitory effect (46%; see Fig. 2C). Accordingly, we used these concentrations for the remainder of the experiments.

Our next task was to determine whether the aforementioned effects are AML-specific. We thus tested the combined effects of VPA and dasatinib on two additional AML cell lines with a different genetic phenotype, namely, NB4 and Kasumi-1, and on several non-AML cell lines, including hepatoma (HepG2 and Hep3B) and breast cancer (MCF-7) lines. NB4 cells belong to French-America-British (FAB) classification M3, and thus express the PML-RARA protein. Both Kasumi-1 and HL60 cells belong to FAB classification M2, but are different genetic phenotypes, with only the former expressing the AML1-ETO protein. We conducted an experiment to detect the effects of the VPA and dasatinib combination on the viability of all of these cell lines. As shown in Table 1, the combination exerted prominent effects on the viability of the AML cell lines, including Kasumi-1, NB4 and HL60, whereas both hepatoma cell lines died following treatment with dasatinib alone. Conversely, the MCF-7 cells proliferated following treatment with VPA, dasatinib or a combination of the two. These results indicate that the synergistic effects of the VPA and dasatinib combination do indeed appear to be AML-specific.

Dasatinib Accelerates G_1 Phase Cell Cycle Arrest in VPA-treated HL60 Cells

As shown in Figure 2, we observed the VPA-dasatinib combination to have a strong growth-inhibitory effect in the HL60 cells. Accordingly, we investigated the possible mechanism of this anti-proliferative activity, and also tested the effects of VPA (0.5 mM) and dasatinib (5 μM) on cell cycle progression in these cells. Figure 3 shows that the dasatinib-VPA combination resulted in a significantly higher percentage of G_0/G_1 phase cells in a time-dependent manner. In comparison with the control group, the percentage increase in cells in the G_0/G_1 phase was 13% at 24 h, 23% at 48 h and 24% at 72 h. The percentages of G_1 cells arrested were 63.5% (control), 71% (VPA), 70% (dasatinib) and 87% (combination) at 48 h (Fig. 3B) and 66% (control), 71.5% (VPA), 70.5% (dasatinib) and 90% (combination) at 72 h (control versus combination at 72 h, $p < 0.001$; Fig. 3C). Treatment with each drug alone also increased the number of arrested cells, but not to a statistically significant degree (less than 5% compared with the control group). The response to the combination treatment in terms of cell cycle progression was almost saturated at 48 h, and the signal patterns were very similar to those at 72 h. The results

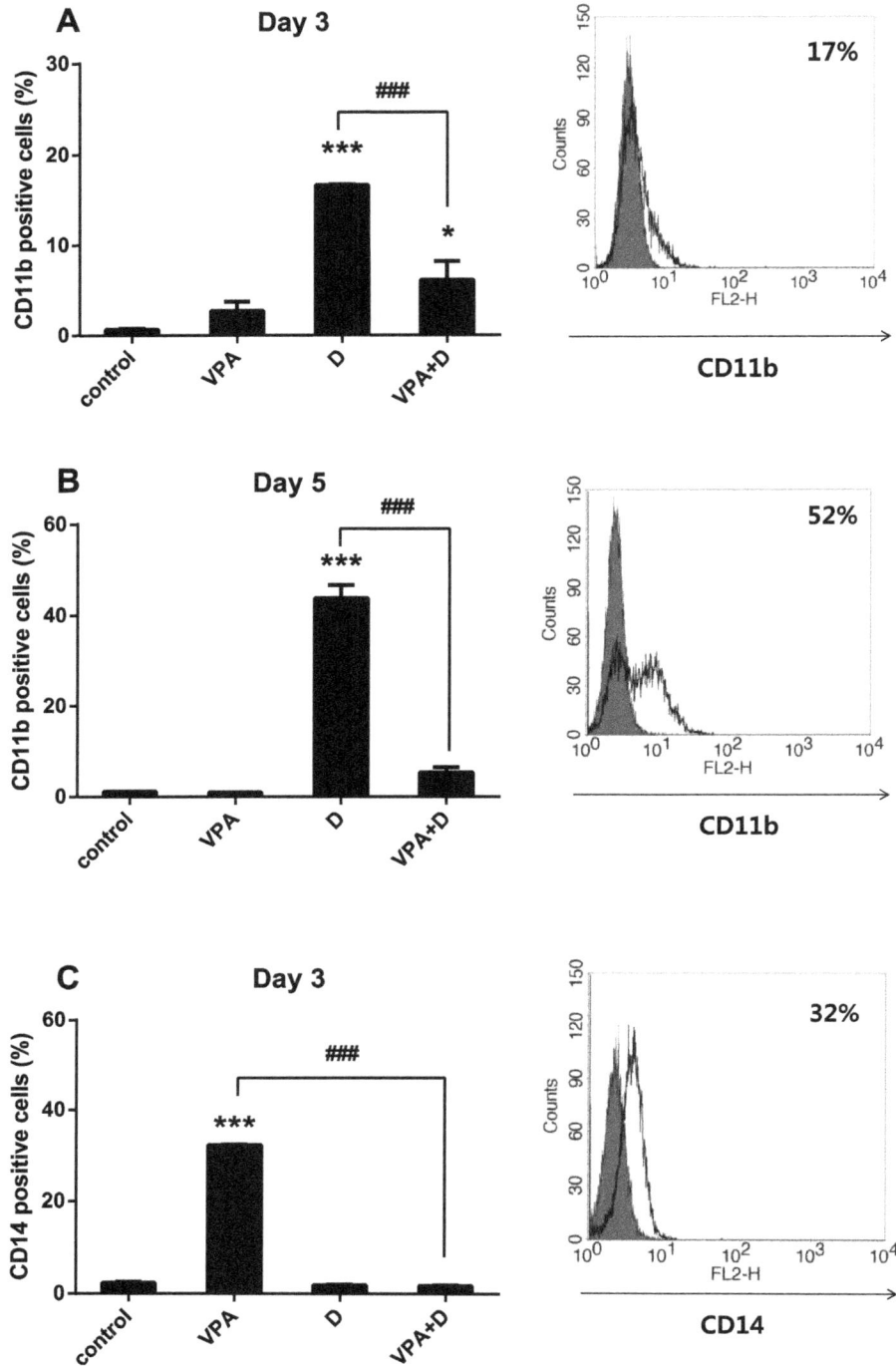

Figure 1. Effects of dasatinib and VPA on CD11b and CD14 expression in HL60 cells. Cells were incubated with 5 μM of dasatinib and 0.5 mM if VPA for 3 and 5 days. The cells were then harvested and immune stained with anti-human CD11b and CD14 mAb. The expression of CD11b and CD14 was then measured by flow cytometry. The filled histogram represents the isotype control, and the open histogram represents CD11b-positive cells treated with 5 μM if dasatinib alone at Day 3 (A) and Day 5 (B). The open histogram represents CD14-positive cells treated with 0.5 mM of VPA alone at Day 3 (C). These data represent the means ± SEM. Significantly different from the DMSO-treated control (*) or combination of VPA and dasatinib (#); ***, ###: $P<0.001$. VPA, valproic acid; D, dasatinib.

again revealed the level of G_0/G_1 arrest to be higher than 90% in the HL60 cells at 72 h (Fig. 3A–C).

VPA-dasatinib Combination Increases p21^{Cip1} and p27^{Kip1} Expression in HL60 Cells

Cyclin-dependent kinases (CDKs) are serine/threonine kinases whose catalytic activities are controlled by interactions with cyclins and CDK inhibitors (CKIs) [17]. CKIs also regulate cell

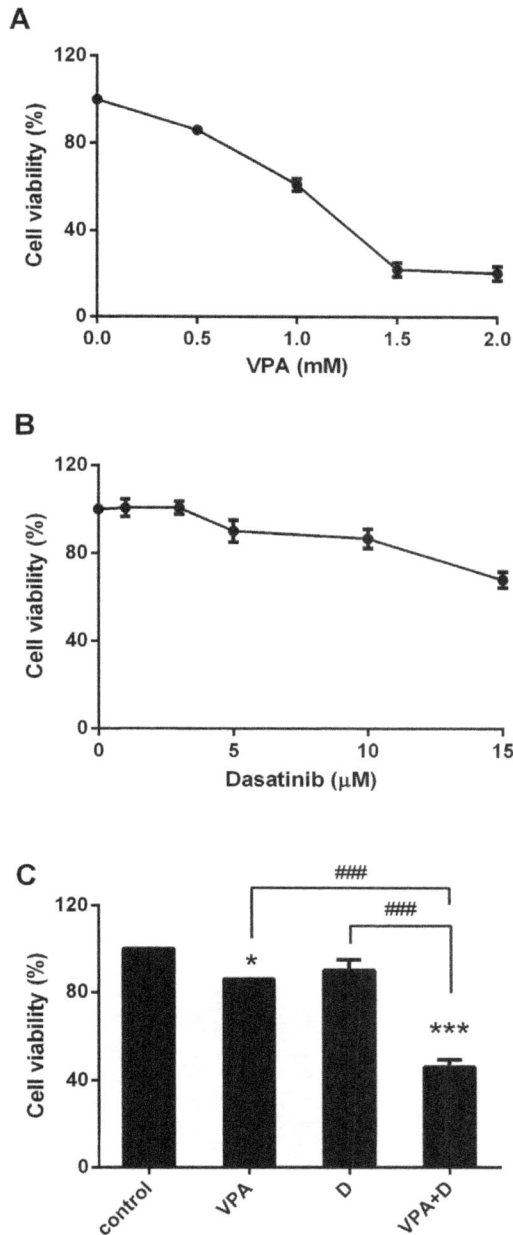

Figure 2. Combination of dasatinib and VPA inhibits HL60 cell proliferation. Cells were stimulated with various concentrations of 0, 0.5, 1, 1.5 and 2 mM VPA and 0, 1, 3, 5, 10 and 15 μM dasatinib for 72 hr. The cytotoxicity was then evaluated by an MTS assay. (A) Dose-dependent responses of VPA on cell viability. (B) Dose-dependent responses of dasatinib on cell viability. (C) Treatment of VPA and/or dasatinib at 72 hr. Representative data are shown for at least three independent experiments. These data represent the means ± SEM. Significantly different from the control (*) or combination of VPA and dasatinib (#); *: $P<0.05$; ***, ###: $P<0.001$.

progression, including CDKs, cyclins and CKIs. After stimulating the HL60 cells with 0.5 mM of VPA and/or 5 μM of dasatinib for 72 h, we determined the expression of $p21^{Cip1}$ and $p27^{Kip1}$ using Western blotting. Figure 3D shows the expression of the two following combination treatment to be 59- and 55-fold greater, respectively, than the control values, as we expected. However, the effect of dasatinib alone on $p21^{Cip1}$ expression was 18% higher than that of the combination treatment, and VPA seemed to reduce the dasatinib-induced $p21^{Cip1}$ levels (a 72-fold increase in $p21^{Cip1}$ band density with dasatinib alone versus a 59-fold increase with the combination). These results suggest that combined VPA-dasatinib treatment increases the expression of inhibitory proteins $p21^{Cip1}$ and $p27^{Kip1}$ in HL60 cells, consequently keeping those cells in the G_1 phase (Fig. 3D).

VPA-dasatinib Combination Decreases Expression of G_1 Phase Cell Cycle Regulatory Proteins, CDKs and Cyclins in HL60 Cells

Several studies have shown CDKs and cyclins to play important roles in the regulation of cell cycle progression [18,19]. In this research, we confirmed the effect of combined VPA-dasatinib treatment on the expression of CDKs and cyclins, which are negatively regulated by $p21^{Cip1}$ and $p27^{Kip1}$ during G_1 arrest in the cell cycle progression. We also assessed the effects of VPA and dasatinib on CDK2, CDK4 and CDK6 and cyclins D1 and E in the same conditions as those reported above. Figure 3E shows that the combination of the two led to a decrease in the expression of CDK2, CDK4 and CDK6, and the band density observed for CDK2 was 1/150-fold lower than that of the control. A similar marked reduction in cyclin D1 and E expression was observed at 72 h (Fig. 3F). The synergistic effects of VPA and dasatinib on the expression of G_1 phase cell cycle regulatory proteins thus appear to be regulated by the CKI-CDK-cyclin cascade in HL60 cells (Figs. 3D–F).

We also observed the expression of $p27^{Kip1}$ in the NB4, HepG2 and Hep3B cells. As shown in Figure 3G, VPA and dasatinib were found to exert synergistic effects on the AML and NB4 cells alone. The effects of the combination treatment appear to be dominant on AML cells.

Dasatinib Induces Apoptosis in VPA-treated AML Cells

Apoptosis was measured by the annexin V binding of phosphatidylserine following treatment with 0.5 mM of VPA and/or 5 μM of dasatinib, with combined treatment found to induce apoptosis in the HL60 cells (Figs. 4A and B). As shown in Figure 4C, the nuclei of the combination group cells were divided into several fragments. We further investigated the effects of dasatinib and VPA on the PBMC and BMC obtained from the two AML patients. The PBMC from patient AML-1 contained 60% blast cells, and the BMC from patient AML-2 contained 82%. Results similar to those in Figure 4B were found in primary culture cells from the two patients (Figs. 4D and E). However, the sensitivities of PBMC and BMC following VPA treatment were slightly higher than those of the HL60 cells.

We monitored the combined effects of VPA and dasatinib on apoptotic cells in the same conditions as those listed in Table 1. Table 2 shows the effects of the VPA and dasatinib combination on apoptosis to have been most prominent in the Kasumi-1, NB4 and HL60 AML cells. These effects were not observed in the solid cancer cells, i.e., HepG2, Hep3B or MCF-7. These results again confirm the synergistic effects of the VPA and dasatinib combination on AML cells.

progression in the G_1 phase of the cell cycle. The induction of $p21^{Cip1}$ and $p27^{Kip1}$, two well-known CKIs, is associated with blocking of the G_1 and S transition, which in turn results in G_0/G_1 phase arrest in the cell cycle [18]. Because the stimulation of HL60 cells with VPA and dasatinib induced G_0/G_1 arrest, as shown in Figure 3, we next analyzed the two drugs' effects on the cell cycle regulatory proteins involved in the G_1 phase of cell cycle

Table 1. Effects of VPA and dasatinib on the cell viability.

Cell lines	Control	VPA	D	VPA + D
Kasumi-1	100 ± 0.0	60 ± 1.5***, ###	37 ± 3.2***, ###	16 ± 3.6***
NB4	100 ± 0.0	46 ± 2.5***, ###	40 ± 2.2***, ###	24 ± 1.2***
HL60	100 ± 0.0	86 ± 0.5*, ###	90 ± 5.0###	46 ± 3.4***
HepG2	100 ± 0.0	95 ± 2.4	90 ± 2.5*	97 ± 2.0
Hep3B	100 ± 0.0	108 ± 3.0###	53.7 ± 2.5***	49 ± 2.9***
MCF-7	100 ± 0.0	132 ± 13	150 ± 2.8***	149 ± 4.8***

These data represent the means $\pm$ SEM. Significantly different from control (*) or combination of VPA and D (#); ***, ###: $P<0.001$. *: $P<0.05$. VPA, Valproic acid; D, dasatinib.

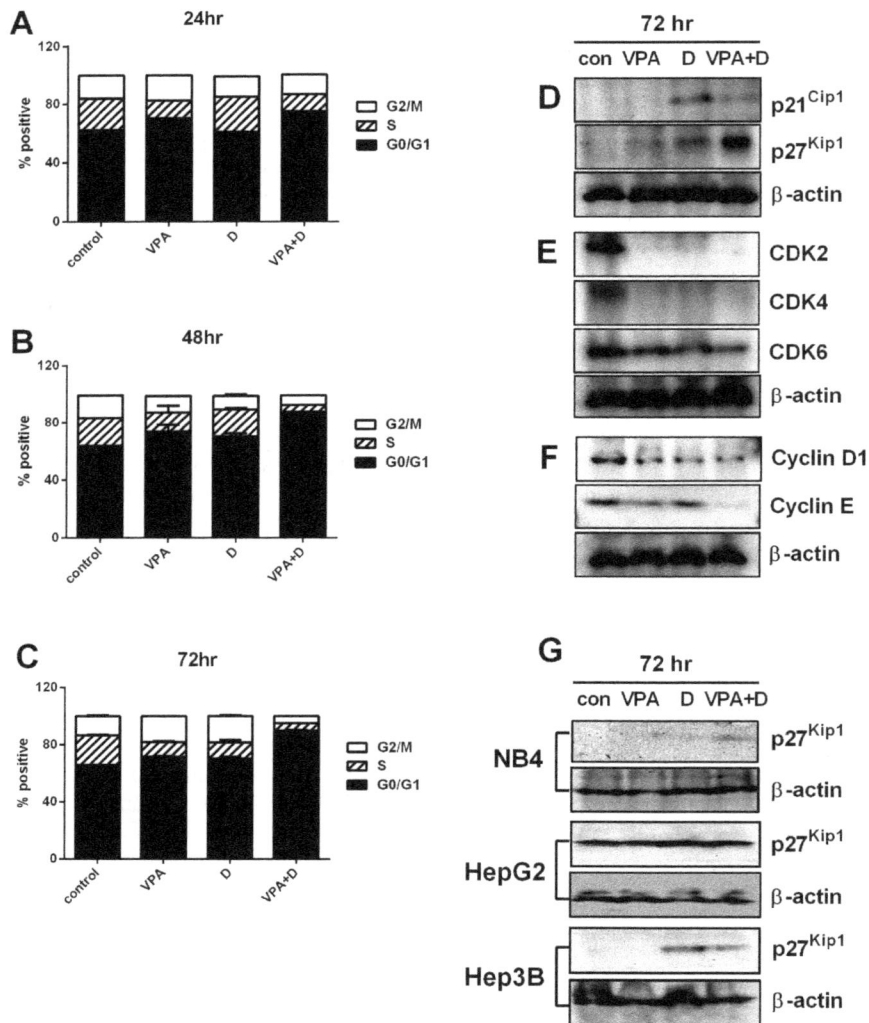

Figure 3. Synergistic effects of dasatinib and VPA on G$_1$ phase cell cycle arrest. Cells were incubated with 0.5 mM of VPA and 5 μM of dasatinib for 72 hr. The cells were harvested at 24 hr (A), 48 hr (B) and 72 hr (C) and then stained with PI/RNase staining buffer and analyzed by flow cytometry. The expression of G$_1$ phase cell cycle regulatory proteins was then measured by Western blot analysis. The membrane was stripped and reprobed with anti-β-actin mAb to confirm equal loading. (D) The expression of p21^{Cip1} and p27^{Kip1}. (E) The expression of CDK2, 4 and 6. (F) The expression of cyclin D1 and E. (G) The expression of p27^{Kip1} on NB4, HepG2, and Hep3B. Representative blots are shown from three independent experiments with similar pattern results.

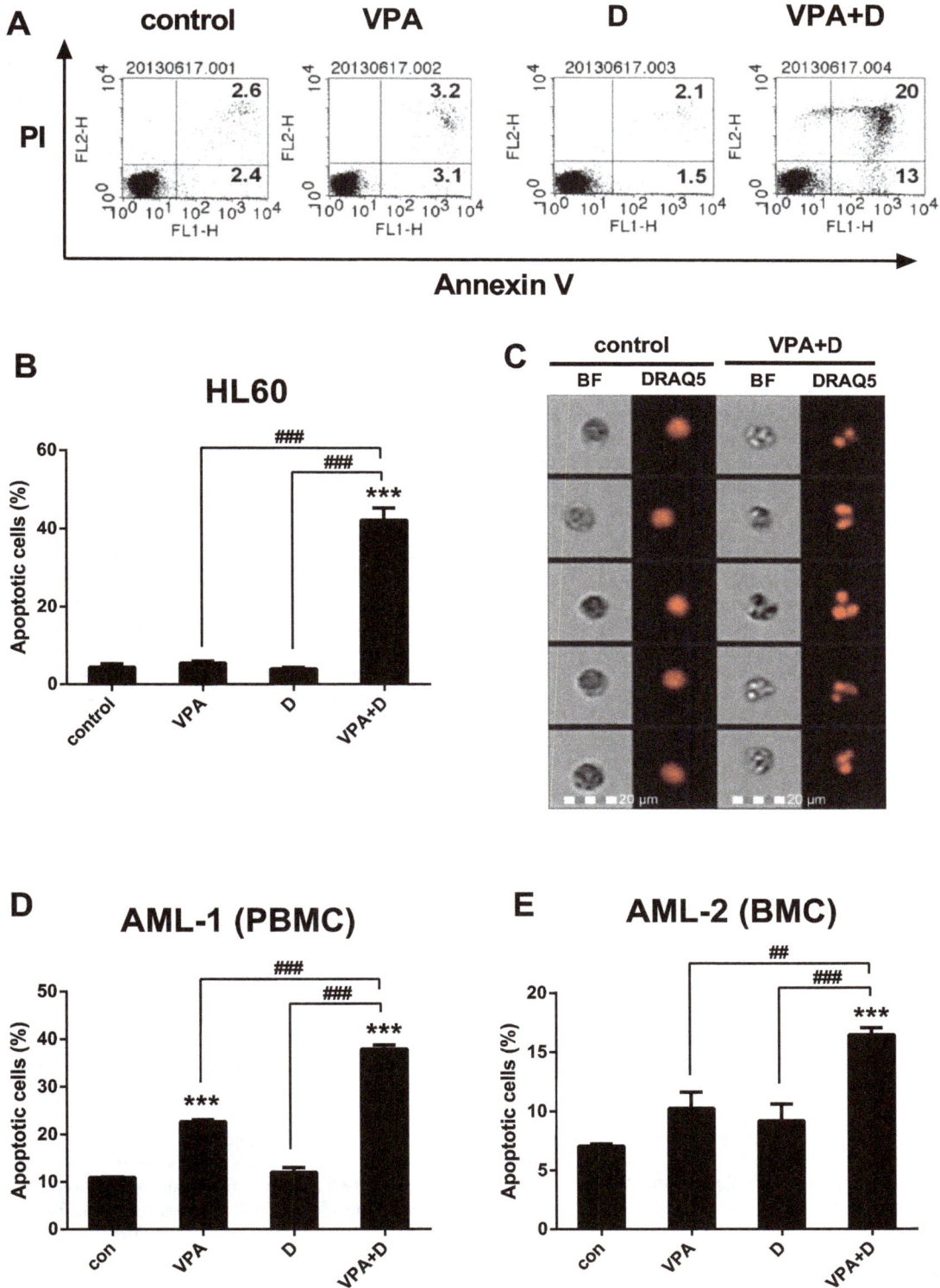

Figure 4. Dasatinib induces apoptosis in VPA-treated AML cells. The cells were also collected and treated under the same conditions described in Figure 3. Cells were stained with annexin V-FITC and/or propidium iodide (PI) followed by flow cytometry analysis. (A) Annexin V/PI staining of HL60 cells. (B) Data show the percentage of annexin V-positive cells (apoptotic cells) on (A). (C) DRAQ5 nuclear staining following combination treatment in HL60 cells. Data show the percentage of apoptotic cells of PBMC (D) and BMC (E) in the AML patients. These data represent the means ± SEM. Significantly different from the control (*) or combination of VPA and dasatinib (#); ##: $P<0.01$; ***, ###: $P<0.001$.

Table 2. Effects of VPA and dasatinib on the apoptotic cells.

Cell lines	Control	VPA	D	VPA + D
Kasumi-1	7.5±0.2	16.0±0.5***, ###	61.0±1.1***, ###	92.0±0.9***
NB4	6.5±0.9	24.8±4.1*, #	21.0±2.8**, ###	58.6±4.4***
HL60	4.3±0.9	5.4±0.5###	3.8±0.4###	42.2±3.1***
HepG2	10.0±0.4	13.7±1.2	20.2±3.9*	18.0±1.4
Hep3B	8.6±0.9	3.3±0.4***, ###	21.5±0.9***	18.5±1.0***
MCF-7	2.7±0.3	4.8±0.3*	2.8±0.2	3.1±0.2

These data represent the means ± SEM. Significantly different from control (*) or combination of VPA and D (#); ***, ###: $P<0.001$. **: $P<0.01$. *, #: $P<0.05$. VPA, Valproic acid; D, dasatinib.

Synergic Effects of Dasatinib and VPA on PARP and Caspase-9, -3 and -7 Activations in HL60 Cells

Caspase activation is a principal feature of apoptosis, with the key factors of this mechanism conserved throughout evolution [20]. Caspase-9 and -3 are known to play crucial roles in the terminal phase of apoptosis [16]. To determine the dasatinib-induced apoptosis pathway in VPA-activated HL60 cells, we examined the expression of intracellular cleaved PARP and cleaved caspase-3. As shown in Figures 5A and B, the expression of both was significantly induced by the combination of VPA and dasatinib. Intracellular cleaved PARP and cleaved caspase-3 expression was also monitored in the combination group with the FlowSight imaging system, with patterns similar to those in Figures 5A and B observed (Fig. 5C). The nuclei were then stained with DRAQ5 dye as a positive control, and we next confirmed the protein levels of both procaspase-9, -3 and -7 and cleaved caspase-9, -3 and -7. All of the cleaved caspases were activated via VPA and dasatinib stimulation in a time-dependent manner (Figs. 5D and E). The results indicate that activation of a series of caspases (caspase-9, -3, -7) and PARP is a necessary condition for dasatinib/VPA-induced apoptosis in HL60 cells (Fig. 5).

Caspase-9 and -3 are Essential to Dasatinib/VPA-induced Apoptosis Pathway in HL60 Cells

Caspase-9, an initiator caspase, forms a complex by binding to apoptotic protease-activating factor-1 (Apaf-1), and then recruits effector caspase-3 [20]. Dasatinib was found to induce the apoptosis of VPA-activated AML cells (Fig. 4) in this research, and thus appears to be associated with caspases. Accordingly, we set out to determine which apoptotic pathway is related to dasatinib/VPA-induced apoptosis. To do so, we pretreated HL60 cells with 10 μM of caspase-3 and -9 inhibitors prior to stimulation with VPA and dasatinib. The activity of each was then measured according to the manufacturer's protocol, with the combination drug found to markedly increase that of both, as shown in Figures 6A and B. Although the caspase-3 inhibitor did not reduce VPA/dasatinib-induced caspase-9 activity, the caspase-9 inhibitor did reduce combination-induced caspase-3 activity (down to the basal level), thus indicating that caspase-9 is the upstream caspase of caspase-3 (Figs. 6A and B).

Using annexin V staining, we also carried out an experiment to confirm whether caspase-9 and -3 would exert an influence on dasatinib/VPA-induced apoptosis in the same conditions. Both inhibitors were found to block such apoptosis, leading us to conclude that caspase-9 and -3 are essential to the dasatinib/VPA-induced apoptosis pathway in HL60 cells (Fig. 6C). This pathway thus appears to be caspase-dependent (Figs. 6A–C).

MEK/ERK and P38 MAPK Control Dasatinib/VPA-activated Apoptosis

Two recent studies demonstrated that MAPK is required for dasatinib-elicited AML cell differentiation [21,22]. To confirm whether MAPK also exerts an effect on dasatinib/VPA-treated HL60 cells, we pretreated these cells with MAPK inhibitors, including 5 μM of U0126, 10 μM of PD98059, 10 μM of SB203580 and 10 μM of SP600125, for 1 h, after which they were stimulated with 0.5 mM of VPA and/or 5 μM of dasatinib. We next measured such dasatinib/VPA-activated apoptotic signals as caspase-9 activity (Fig. 6D), caspase-3 activity (Fig. 6E) and the number of apoptotic cells (Fig. 6F), all three of which were observed to decrease significantly following treatment with MEK/ERK inhibitors U0126 and PD98059 and p38 MAPK inhibitor SB203580. The signals from MEK/ERK and p38 MAPK thus appear to be associated with the initiation of dasatinib/VPA-activated apoptosis (Figs. 6D–F).

Discussion

AML is characterized by increased leukemic blasts resulting from the deficient development of hematopoietic progenitor and stem cells in bone marrow [23]. The current primary treatment strategy for AML is an intensive course of cytotoxic chemotherapy consisting of induction and consolidation with the aim of achieving and maintaining complete remission (CR) [24,25]. There is no doubt that postremission therapy is important to helping AML patients to sustain CR [26]. Although CR has been achieved in younger AML patients, they still require hematopoietic cell transplantation as immunotherapy if their risk profile is unfavorable [27]. Timed-sequential induction therapy has been proposed to improve postremission therapy in AML, with all patients achieving remission receiving four cycles of such therapy [28]. Despite these trials and ongoing efforts to improve AML therapy, however, the high post-CR relapse rates and very poor post-relapse survival rates mean a gloomy long-term outlook for this patient group [24]. The development of more effective chemo-therapeutic agents is thus a matter of urgency.

Previous studies have shown dasatinib to exert an effect on the differentiation of megakaryocytes [29] and osteoblasts [30–32] and the adipogenic differentiation of human multipotent mesenchymal stromal cells [33] and of blasts to neutrophilic granulocytes [34]. It has also been found to induce myeloblast differentiation [22]. Moreover, dasatinib in combination with retinoic acid has been shown to promote AML differentiation [2,21] and to greatly increase the expression of differentiation marker CD11b. Accordingly, we believe dasatinib has the potential to induce cell differentiation. Recent research has also demonstrated the anti-

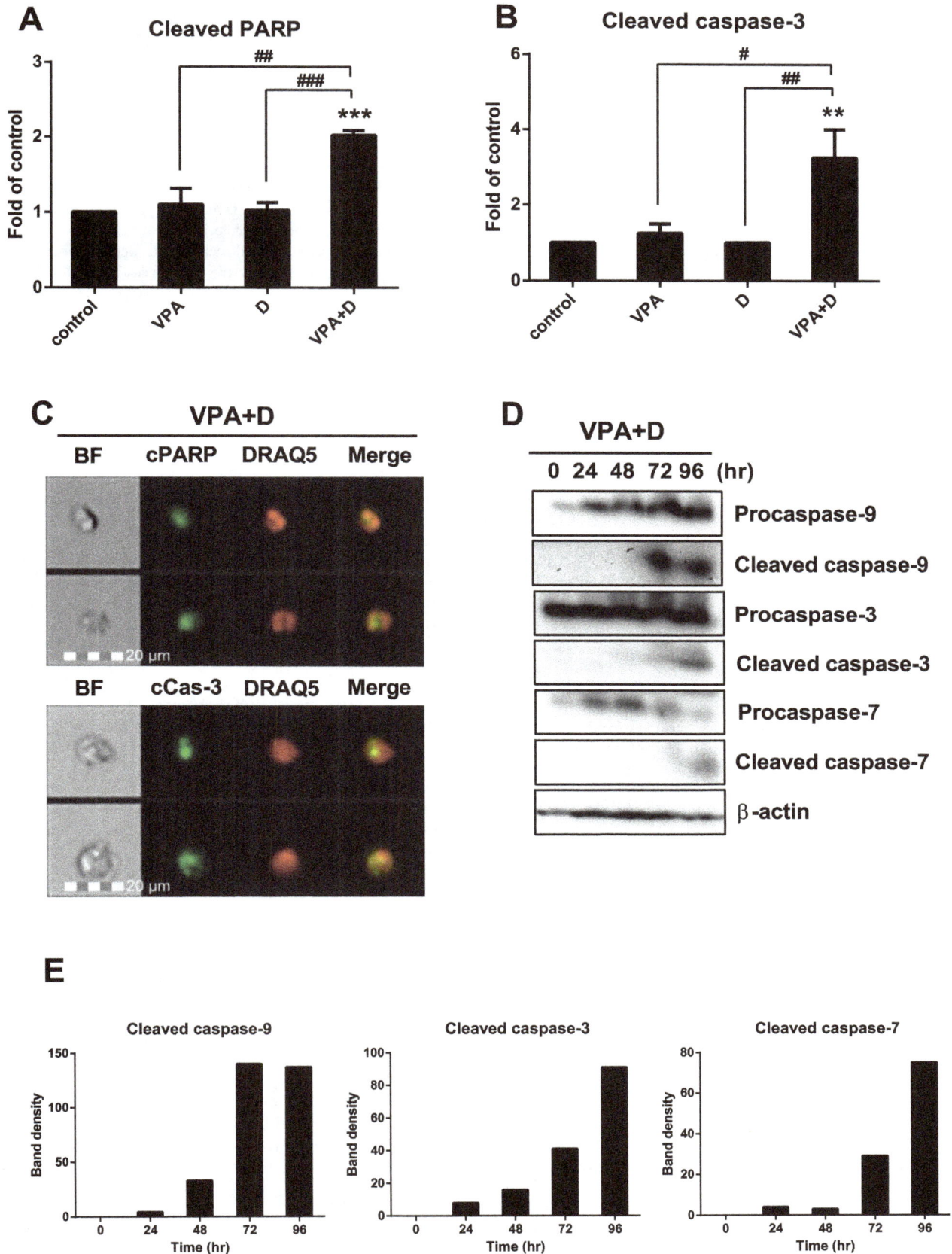

Figure 5. Dasatinib/VPA-induced apoptosis activates PARP and caspase-9, -3 and -7 in HL60 cells. Cells were collected and treated under the same conditions described in Figure 3. The cells were intracellular stained with anti-human cleaved PARP (cPARP), anti-human cleaved caspase-3

(cCas-3) and anti-rabbit IgG-FITC, followed by flow cytometry analysis. (A) The expression of intracellular cPARP. (B) The expression of intracellular cCas-3. (C) The intracellular expression of cPARP and cCas-3 in the combination group was monitored by FlowSight analysis. (D) The expression of capsase-9, -3 and -7 and procapsase-9, -3 and -7 was then measured by Western blot analysis. The membrane was stripped and reprobed with anti-β-actin mAb to confirm equal loading. (E) Data show the band density of (D). Representative blots are shown from three independent experiments with almost identical results. These data represent the means ± SEM. Significantly different from control (*) or combination of VPA and dasatinib (#); #: $P<0.05$; **, ##: $P<0.01$; ***, ###: $P<0.001$.

cancer effects of VPA in several types of cancer cells, although those effects have been found to be more powerful when the drug is combined with such agents as imatinib [14], bortezomib, the first therapeutic proteasome inhibitor [35], selective COX-2 inhibitor celecoxib [36] or radiation [37]. We thus chose VPA to investigate in conjunction with dasatinib in this research. We hypothesized that the differentiation capacity of dasatinib would potentiate VPA-induced apoptosis in AML cell line HL60.

First of all, we investigated the effects of dasatinib and VPA on the cell surface expression of differentiation markers CD11b and CD14 (Fig. 1), with both drugs found to have positive effects on such expression. Surprisingly, following the combined use of the two drugs, the differentiation signal completely disappeared in the AML cells, as shown in Figure 1. At first, the VPA-dasatinib combination seemed to down-regulate the differentiation capacity of each drug. The results presented in Figure 2 revealed 0.5 mM of VPA and 5 μM of dasatinib alone to produce little effect on cell viability in the HL60 cells, whereas their combination significantly inhibited cell proliferation, with cell viability falling below 50% (Fig. 2C). The observed decrease in differentiation markers following the combination treatment may thus have been the result of an increase in apoptosis.

We next searched for the possible mechanism linking apoptosis and differentiation. We stimulated the HL60 cells, with VPA and dasatinib for 48 h, and then monitored them for CD11b or CD14 and annexin V double-positive cells. As shown in Figure S1, the numbers of CD11b/annexin V and CD14/annexin V double-positive cells in the combination group were 1.5- and 1.6-fold higher, respectively, than those in the control group at 48 h, which was in line with our expectations. These cell populations disappeared rapidly thereafter, and we could find no double-positive cells at 72 h. The implication of these findings is that the cell differentiation following combined VPA and dasatinib treatment is the primary contributor to apoptosis initiation, thus confirming our hypothesis that differentiation capacity has an effect on AML cell death. More specifically, the differentiation of CD11b- and CD14-positive cells was accelerated by the combination of the two drugs, which ultimately contributed to apoptosis, thus allowing us to confirm that it was the differentiation capacity of dasatinib-potentiated VPA that induced AML cell apoptosis.

We also observed the VPA-dasatinib combination to exert a strong growth-inhibitory effect on the HL60 cells (Figure 2), and subsequently investigated the possible mechanism of such anti-proliferative activity on cell cycle progression and apoptosis. As shown in Figures 3 and 4, we observed the two drugs to have synergistic effects on both. More specifically, the VPA-dasatinib combination increased the expression of $p21^{Cip1}$ and $p27^{Kip1}$ in the HL60 cells (Fig. 3D), and decreased the expression of G_1 phase cell cycle regulatory proteins CDK2, 4 and 6 and cyclins D_1 and E (Figs. 3E and F). Although neither VPA nor dasatinib alone enhanced apoptosis in these cells, their combination produced a powerful apoptotic effect (Figs. 4A and B). We also confirmed the effects of dasatinib and VPA on PBMC and BMC taken from the two patients with AML, and found them to be very similar to those in the HL60 cells (Figs. 4D and E). These results again

demonstrate the synergistic effects of the VPA-dasatinib combination on cell viability in AML cells, as shown in Table 1.

Apoptosis, which is considered the ideal form of death for cancer cells, plays an important role in maintaining homeostasis [38]. This type of programmed cell death occurs when the activation of specific pathways results in a series of well-defined morphological events, such as nuclear and cytoplasmic condensation, DNA fragmentation, the exposure of phosphatidylserine residues in the outer plasma membrane leaflet and the release of apoptotic bodies [39,40]. Dasatinib/VPA-induced apoptosis is also related to nuclear condensation (Fig. 4C). Moreover, apoptotic cell death begins with the release of cytochrome c from the mitochondria to form a caspase-activating complex known as the Apaf-1 apoptosome [20]. This complex recruits and activates caspase-9, which then cleaves and activates such downstream caspases as caspase-3 and -7. Caspase-3 cleaves many substrates that respond to DNA strand breaks, such as PARP, eventually leading to apoptosis [41]. We confirmed in this research that the dasatinib-VPA combination evokes apoptosis not only via caspase-9, -3 and -7, but also via the PARP cleavage cascade (Figs. 5 and 6). The powerful combined effects of VPA and dasatinib on apoptosis in AML cells can be seen in the results presented in Table 2.

The most important finding in this research was that the dasatinib/VPA-activated apoptotic signal follows differentiation pathways, such as those of MEK/ERK and p38 MAPK (Figs. 6D and E). Dasatinib alone was found to promote MAPK-dependent cell differentiation and cell cycle arrest in a previous study [21]. We found about 40% of the AML cells in the combination group to have experienced apoptotic death. Differentiation of the cell population through combination treatment may thus hasten the apoptosis of AML cells. Our results also indicate that MEK/ERK and p38 MAPK may be associated with the initiation of such dasatinib/VPA-activated apoptosis (Fig. 6).

We also found the dasatinib-mediated induction of $p21^{Cip1}$ to be blocked by combination treatment with VPA, which is consistent with previous reports [42,43] indicating that $p21^{Cip1}$ induction decreases following co-treatment with dasatinib and such histone deacetylase inhibitors as sodium butyrate [42] and vorinostat [43]. We also observed the interruption of dasatinib-induced $p21^{Cip1}$ via VPA-potentiated apoptosis, as shown in Figure 4. The inhibitory effect of VPA on dasatinib-induced $p21^{Cip1}$ may contribute to the synergistic apoptotic effects of the combination treatment observed in the HL60 and primary AML cells. It remains unknown whether the inhibitory mechanism of Src and HDAC leads to AML cell death, although there is considerable evidence to suggest that HDAC interference with $p21^{CIP1}$ induction contributes to the potentiation of Src inhibitor-mediated apoptosis, at least in part. In contrast, the loss of $p21^{CIP1}$ has been found to sensitize cells to cytotoxic drugs [44], low doses of cytarabine [45] and various differentiation-inducing agents such as phorbol esters [44]. Given these findings, it is tempting to propose that the interruption of $p21^{CIP1}$ induction in Src inhibitor-treated cells may contribute to enhanced lethality. Direct evidence is lacking at present, however.

We also conducted numerous Western blot experiments on $p27^{kip}$ expression in NB4 and Kasumi-1 cells in an attempt to

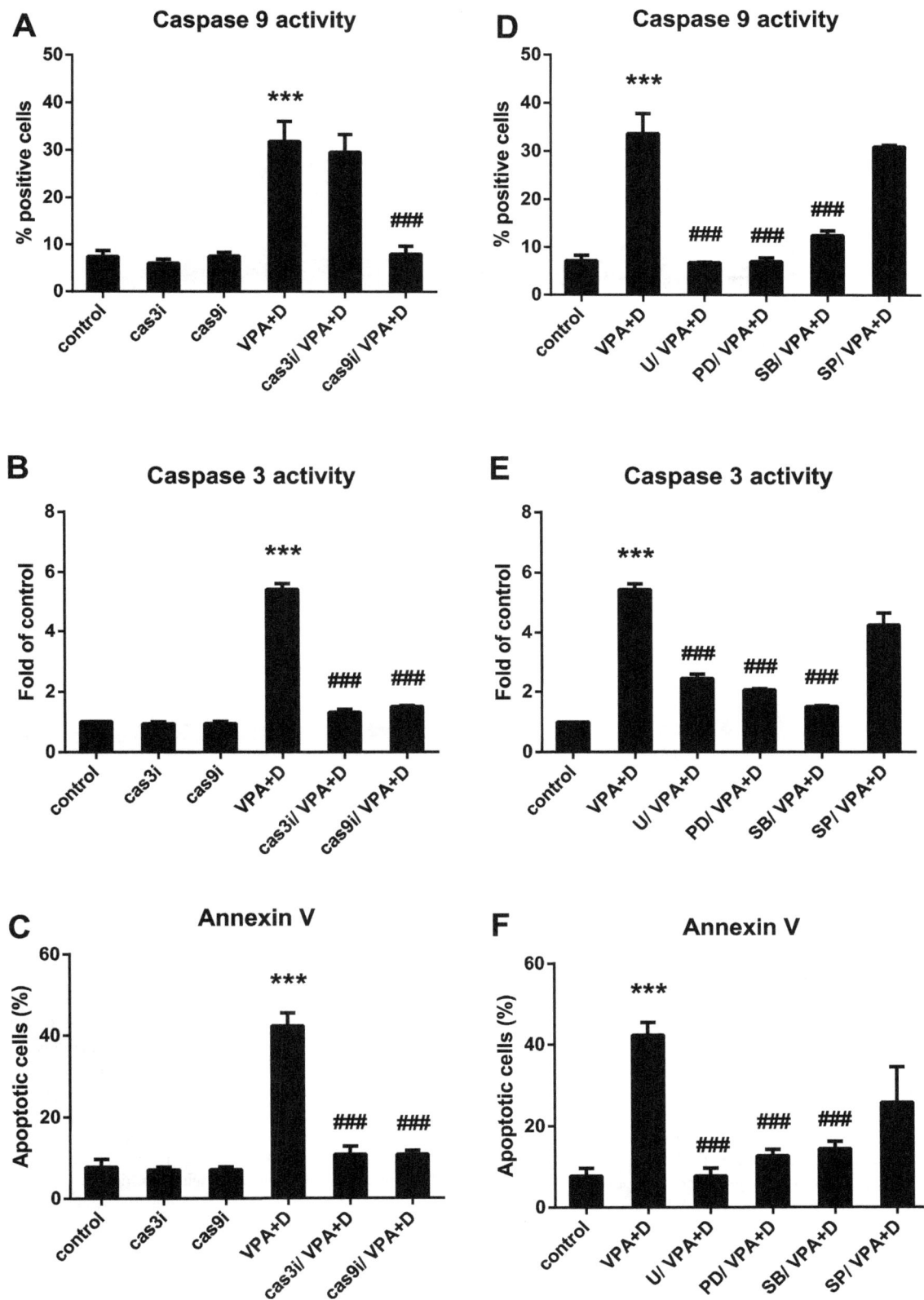

Figure 6. Dasatinib/VPA-induced apoptosis is via a caspase-dependent pathway and depends on MEK/ERK and p38 MAPK. Cells were preincubated with caspase-3 inhibitor (10 μM Z-DEVD-FMK), caspase-9 inhibitor (10 μM LEHD-CHO), MEK/ERK inhibitor (5 μM U0126 and 10 μM PD98059), p38 MAPK inhibitor (10 μM SB203580) and JNK inhibitor (10 μM SP600125) for 1 hr prior to treatment with 0.5 mM of VPA and 5 μM of dasatinib for 72 hr. (A, D) Caspase-9 activity; (B, E) caspase-3 activity (C, F); apoptotic cells. These data represent the means ± SEM. Significantly different from the control (*) or combination of VPA and dasatinib (#); ***, ###: P<0.001. Cas3i, caspase-3 inhibitor; cas9i, caspase-9 inhibitor; U,

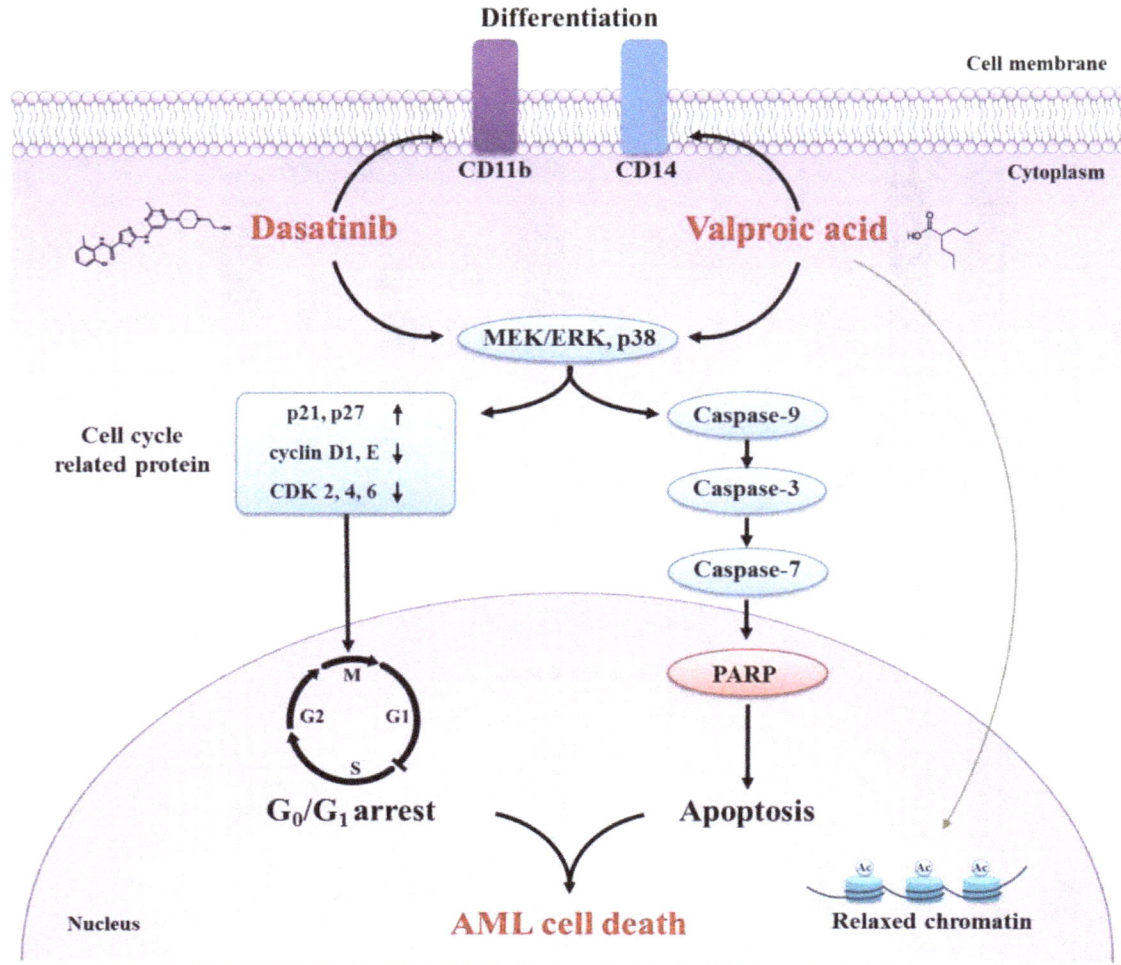

Figure 7. Mechanism by which dasatinib potentiates VPA-treated AML cell death. The combination of dasatinib and VPA on AML cell differentiation capacity is more potent than that of each drug alone. The combination is enough to promote intensive AML cell death through G_1 cell cycle arrest and caspase-dependent apoptosis. In addition, MEK/ERK and p38 MAPK control dasatinib/VPA-evoked apoptosis as upstream regulators. Eventually, the regulation of cell differentiation capacity contributes to AML cell death.

detect the combined effects of dasatinib and VPA in these cells, but were unable to obtain satisfactory results. Although we observed the poor induction of $p27^{kip}$ in dasatinib/VPA-treated Kasumi-1 cells (data not shown), and found the level of $p27^{kip}$ expression in the Kasumi-1 cells to be lower than that in the NB4 cells, we also observed $p27^{kip}$ expression to have synergistic effects in the Kasumi-1 cells. However, we found measurement of the effect on cell cycle arrest and $p27^{kip}$ expression in the Kasumi-1 cells to be very difficult, and thus omit the results from the paper, although we considered them to be reasonable. More than 92% of the Kasumi-1 cells and 60% of the NB4 cells experienced apoptotic death following treatment with the dasatinib and VPA combination, as shown in Table 2. Most cells were already dead, and thus it was impossible to detect the $p27^{kip}$ positive cells or G_1 phase arrest cells in these samples. That's why it had a poor induction of $p27^{kip}$ in combined treatment on NB4 cells, as shown in Figure 3G. In the case of the HL60 cells, in contrast, only 40% died via apoptosis, thus rendering the measurement of cell cycle regulatory proteins such as $p27^{kip}$ easier.

In conclusion, we found the effect of combined dasatinib-VPA treatment on the apoptotic activity of AML cells to be sufficiently

synergistic to promote intensive AML cell death through G_1 cell cycle arrest and caspase-dependent apoptosis. In addition, our results show MEK/ERK and p38 MAPK to control dasatinib/VPA-induced apoptosis as upstream regulators. Finally, we found that the regulation of cell differentiation capacity contributes to AML cell death. Taken together, our findings indicate that dasatinib accelerates VPA-induced AML cell death through G_1 arrest and caspase-dependent apoptosis via MEK/ERK and p38 MAPK (Fig. 7). To the best of our knowledge, this is the first study to report that AML cell death is involved in G_1 arrest and apoptosis following combined treatment with dasatinib and VPA. The results presented herein indicate that combined dasatinib-VPA therapy has a potential role in anti-leukemic treatment.

Supporting Information

Figure S1 The CD11b$^+$/Annexin V$^+$ or CD14$^+$/Annexin V$^+$ cells of combination group were 1.5-fold or 1.6-fold higher than that of control group at 48 hr. The cells were stimulated by VPA and dasatnib for 48 hr, and the CD11b$^+$/Annexin V$^+$ or CD14$^+$/ Annexin V$^+$ cells were monitored by flow cytometery analysis. These data represent the means ± SEM. Significantly different from control (*) or combination of VPA and dasatinib (#); **, ##: $P<0.01$; ***, ###: $P<0.001$.

Acknowledgments

We thank Bristol-Myers Squibb (New York, NY) for providing the dasatinib.

Author Contributions

Conceived and designed the experiments: SKH EKN HK. Performed the experiments: SKH EKN DJY JCJ JHP. Analyzed the data: SKH EKN DJY HK. Contributed reagents/materials/analysis tools: SKH EKN DJY. Wrote the paper: SKH EKN HK.

References

1. Guerrouahen BS, Futami M, Vaklavas C, Kanerva J, Whichard ZL, et al. (2010) Dasatinib inhibits the growth of molecularly heterogeneous myeloid leukemias. Clinical cancer research: an official journal of the American Association for Cancer Research 16: 1149–1158.
2. Kropf PL, Wang L, Zang Y, Redner RL, Johnson DE (2010) Dasatinib promotes ATRA-induced differentiation of AML cells. Leukemia 24: 663–665.
3. Luo FR, Yang Z, Camuso A, Smykla R, McGlinchey K, et al. (2006) Dasatinib (BMS-354825) pharmacokinetics and pharmacodynamic biomarkers in animal models predict optimal clinical exposure. Clinical cancer research: an official journal of the American Association for Cancer Research 12: 7180–7186.
4. Kantarjian HM, Shah NP, Cortes JE, Baccarani M, Agarwal MB, et al. (2012) Dasatinib or imatinib in newly diagnosed chronic-phase chronic myeloid leukemia: 2-year follow-up from a randomized phase 3 trial (DASISION). Blood 119: 1123–1129.
5. Kantarjian H, Shah NP, Hochhaus A, Cortes J, Shah S, et al. (2010) Dasatinib versus imatinib in newly diagnosed chronic-phase chronic myeloid leukemia. The New England journal of medicine 362: 2260–2270.
6. Gianni M, Kalac Y, Ponzanelli I, Rambaldi A, Terao M, et al. (2001) Tyrosine kinase inhibitor STI571 potentiates the pharmacologic activity of retinoic acid in acute promyelocytic leukemia cells: effects on the degradation of RARalpha and PML-RARalpha. Blood 97: 3234–3243.
7. Miranda MB, Duan R, Thomas SM, Grandis JR, Redner RL, et al. (2008) Gefitinib potentiates myeloid cell differentiation by ATRA. Leukemia 22: 1624–1627.
8. Noh EK, Kim H, Park MJ, Baek JH, Park JH, et al. (2010) Gefitinib enhances arsenic trioxide (AS$_2$O$_3$)-induced differentiation of acute promyelocytic leukemia cell line. Leukemia research 34: 1501–1505.
9. Leiva M, Moretti S, Soilihi H, Pallavicini I, Peres L, et al. (2012) Valproic acid induces differentiation and transient tumor regression, but spares leukemia-initiating activity in mouse models of APL. Leukemia 26: 1630–1637.
10. Torgersen ML, Engedal N, Boe SO, Hokland P, Simonsen A (2013) Targeting autophagy potentiates the apoptotic effect of histone deacetylase inhibitors in t(8; 21) AML cells. Blood 122: 2467–2476.
11. Schuchmann M, Schulze-Bergkamen H, Fleischer B, Schattenberg JM, Siebler J, et al. (2006) Histone deacetylase inhibition by valproic acid down-regulates c-FLIP/CASH and sensitizes hepatoma cells towards CD95- and TRAIL receptor-mediated apoptosis and chemotherapy. Oncology reports 15: 227–230.
12. Angelucci A, Valentini A, Millimaggi D, Gravina GL, Miano R, et al. (2006) Valproic acid induces apoptosis in prostate carcinoma cell lines by activation of multiple death pathways. Anti-cancer drugs 17: 1141–1150.
13. Shen WT, Wong TS, Chung WY, Wong MG, Kebebew E, et al. (2005) Valproic acid inhibits growth, induces apoptosis, and modulates apoptosis-regulatory and differentiation gene expression in human thyroid cancer cells. Surgery 138: 979–984; discussion 984–975.
14. Kircher B, Schumacher P, Petzer A, Hoflehner E, Haun M, et al. (2009) Anti-leukemic activity of valproic acid and imatinib mesylate on human Ph+ ALL and CML cells in vitro. European journal of haematology 83: 48–56.
15. Tang R, Faussat AM, Majdak P, Perrot JY, Chaoui D, et al. (2004) Valproic acid inhibits proliferation and induces apoptosis in acute myeloid leukemia cells expressing P-gp and MRP1. Leukemia 18: 1246–1251.
16. Heo SK, Yun HJ, Park WH, Park SD (2009) Rhein inhibits TNF-alpha-induced human aortic smooth muscle cell proliferation via mitochondrial-dependent apoptosis. Journal of vascular research 46: 375–386.
17. Lim S, Kaldis P (2013) Cdks, cyclins and CKIs: roles beyond cell cycle regulation. Development 140: 3079–3093.
18. Zurlo D, Leone C, Assante G, Salzano S, Renzone G, et al. (2013) Cladosporol a stimulates G1-phase arrest of the cell cycle by up-regulation of p21(waf1/cip1) expression in human colon carcinoma HT-29 cells. Molecular carcinogenesis 52: 1–17.
19. Mantena SK, Sharma SD, Katiyar SK (2006) Berberine inhibits growth, induces G1 arrest and apoptosis in human epidermoid carcinoma A431 cells by regulating Cdki-Cdk-cyclin cascade, disruption of mitochondrial membrane potential and cleavage of caspase 3 and PARP. Carcinogenesis 27: 2018–2027.
20. Cain K (2003) Chemical-induced apoptosis: formation of the Apaf-1 apoptosome. Drug metabolism reviews 35: 337–363.
21. Congleton J, MacDonald R, Yen A (2012) Src inhibitors, PP2 and dasatinib, increase retinoic acid-induced association of Lyn and c-Raf (S259) and enhance MAPK-dependent differentiation of myeloid leukemia cells. Leukemia 26: 1180–1188.
22. Fang Y, Zhong L, Lin M, Zhou X, Jing H, et al. (2013) MEK/ERK dependent activation of STAT1 mediates dasatinib-induced differentiation of acute myeloid leukemia. PLoS one 8: e66915.
23. Aurelius J, Thoren FB, Akhiani AA, Brune M, Palmqvist L, et al. (2012) Monocytic AML cells inactivate antileukemic lymphocytes: role of NADPH oxidase/gp91(phox) expression and the PARP-1/PAR pathway of apoptosis. Blood 119: 5832–5837.
24. Burnett A, Wetzler M, Lowenberg B (2011) Therapeutic advances in acute myeloid leukemia. Journal of clinical oncology: official journal of the American Society of Clinical Oncology 29: 487–494.
25. Tallman MS, Gilliland DG, Rowe JM (2005) Drug therapy for acute myeloid leukemia. Blood 106: 1154–1163.
26. Schiffer CA (2002) Postremission therapy in older adults with acute myeloid leukemia: an opportunity for new drug development. Leukemia 16: 745–747.
27. Appelbaum FR (2001) Haematopoietic cell transplantation as immunotherapy. Nature 411: 385–389.
28. Woods WG, Kobrinsky N, Buckley JD, Lee JW, Sanders J, et al. (1996) Timed-sequential induction therapy improves postremission outcome in acute myeloid leukemia: a report from the Children's Cancer Group. Blood 87: 4979–4989.
29. Mazharian A, Ghevaert C, Zhang L, Massberg S, Watson SP (2011) Dasatinib enhances megakaryocyte differentiation but inhibits platelet formation. Blood 117: 5198–5206.
30. Lee YC, Huang CF, Murshed M, Chu K, Araujo JC, et al. (2010) Src family kinase/abl inhibitor dasatinib suppresses proliferation and enhances differentiation of osteoblasts. Oncogene 29: 3196–3207.
31. Jonsson S, Hjorth-Hansen H, Olsson B, Wadenvik H, Sundan A, et al. (2010) Second-generation TKI dasatinib inhibits proliferation of mesenchymal stem cells and osteoblast differentiation in vitro. Leukemia 24: 1357–1359.
32. Id Boufker H, Lagneaux L, Najar M, Piccart M, Ghanem G, et al. (2010) The Src inhibitor dasatinib accelerates the differentiation of human bone marrow-derived mesenchymal stromal cells into osteoblasts. BMC cancer 10: 298.
33. Borriello A, Caldarelli I, Basile MA, Bencivenga D, Tramontano A, et al. (2011) The tyrosine kinase inhibitor dasatinib induces a marked adipogenic differentiation of human multipotent mesenchymal stromal cells. PloS one 6: e28555.
34. Chevalier N, Solari ML, Becker H, Pantic M, Gartner F, et al. (2010) Robust in vivo differentiation of t(8;21)-positive acute myeloid leukemia blasts to neutrophilic granulocytes induced by treatment with dasatinib. Leukemia 24: 1779–1781.
35. Wang AH, Wei L, Chen L, Zhao SQ, Wu WL, et al. (2011) Synergistic effect of bortezomib and valproic acid treatment on the proliferation and apoptosis of acute myeloid leukemia and myelodysplastic syndrome cells. Annals of hematology 90: 917–931.
36. Chen Y, Tsai YH, Tseng SH (2011) Combined valproic acid and celecoxib treatment induced synergistic cytotoxicity and apoptosis in neuroblastoma cells. Anticancer research 31: 2231–2239.
37. Chen X, Wong JY, Wong P, Radany EH (2011) Low-dose valproic acid enhances radiosensitivity of prostate cancer through acetylated p53-dependent modulation of mitochondrial membrane potential and apoptosis. Molecular cancer research: MCR 9: 448–461.
38. White E (1993) Death-defying acts: a meeting review on apoptosis. Genes & development 7: 2277–2284.
39. Deschesnes RG, Huot J, Valerie K, Landry J (2001) Involvement of p38 in apoptosis-associated membrane blebbing and nuclear condensation. Molecular biology of the cell 12: 1569–1582.
40. Peter ME (2011) Programmed cell death: Apoptosis meets necrosis. Nature 471: 310–312.
41. Thornberry NA, Lazebnik Y (1998) Caspases: enemies within. Science 281: 1312–1316.

42. Rosato RR, Almenara JA, Yu C, Grant S (2004) Evidence of a functional role for p21WAF1/CIP1 down-regulation in synergistic antileukemic interactions between the histone deacetylase inhibitor sodium butyrate and flavopiridol. Molecular pharmacology 65: 571–581.

43. Fiskus W, Pranpat M, Balasis M, Bali P, Estrella V, et al. (2006) Cotreatment with vorinostat (suberoylanilide hydroxamic acid) enhances activity of dasatinib (BMS-354825) against imatinib mesylate-sensitive or imatinib mesylate-resistant chronic myelogenous leukemia cells. Clinical cancer research: an official journal of the American Association for Cancer Research 12: 5869–5878.

44. Wang Z, Su ZZ, Fisher PB, Wang S, VanTuyle G, et al. (1998) Evidence of a functional role for the cyclin-dependent kinase inhibitor p21(WAF1/CIP1/MDA6) in the reciprocal regulation of PKC activator-induced apoptosis and differentation in human myelomonocytic leukemia cells. Experimental cell research 244: 105–116.

45. Wang Z, Van Tuyle G, Conrad D, Fisher PB, Dent P, et al. (1999) Dysregulation of the cyclin-dependent kinase inhibitor p21WAF1/CIP1/MDA6 increases the susceptibility of human leukemia cells (U937) to 1-beta-D-arabinofuranosylcytosine-mediated mitochondrial dysfunction and apoptosis. Cancer research 59: 1259–1267.

2

Integrative Genomic and Transcriptomic Analysis Identified Candidate Genes Implicated in the Pathogenesis of Hepatosplenic T-Cell Lymphoma

Julio Finalet Ferreiro[1], Leila Rouhigharabaei[1], Helena Urbankova[1], Jo-Anne van der Krogt[1], Lucienne Michaux[1], Shashirekha Shetty[2], Laszlo Krenacs[3], Thomas Tousseyn[4], Pascale De Paepe[5], Anne Uyttebroeck[6], Gregor Verhoef[7], Tom Taghon[8], Peter Vandenberghe[1], Jan Cools[1,9], Iwona Wlodarska[1]*

1 Center for Human Genetics, KU Leuven, Leuven, Belgium, 2 Molecular Pathology, Cleveland Clinic, Cleveland, Ohio, United States of America, 3 Laboratory of Tumor Pathology and Molecular Diagnostics, University of Szeged, Szeged, Hungary, 4 Translational Cell and Tissue Research KU Leuven, Department of Pathology UZ Leuven, Leuven, Belgium, 5 Department of Pathology, AZ St Jan AV, Brugge, Belgium, 6 Department of Pediatrics, UZ Leuven, Leuven, Belgium, 7 Department of Hematology, UZ Leuven, Leuven, Belgium, 8 Department of Clinical Chemistry, Microbiology and Immunology, Ghent University Hospital, Ghent University, Ghent, Belgium, 9 Center for the Biology of Disease, VIB, Leuven, Belgium

Abstract

Hepatosplenic T-cell lymphoma (HSTL) is an aggressive lymphoma cytogenetically characterized by isochromosome 7q [i(7)(q10)], of which the molecular consequences remain unknown. We report here results of an integrative genomic and transcriptomic (expression microarray and RNA-sequencing) study of six i(7)(q10)-positive HSTL cases, including HSTL-derived cell line (DERL-2), and three cases with ring 7 [r(7)], the recently identified rare variant aberration. Using high resolution array CGH, we profiled all cases and mapped the common deleted region (CDR) at 7p22.1p14.1 (34.88 Mb; 3506316–38406226 bp) and the common gained region (CGR) at 7q22.11q31.1 (38.77 Mb; 86259620–124892276 bp). Interestingly, CDR spans a smaller region of 13 Mb (86259620–99271246 bp) constantly amplified in cases with r(7). In addition, we found that TCRG (7p14.1) and TCRB (7q32) are involved in formation of r(7), which seems to be a byproduct of illegitimate somatic rearrangement of both loci. Further transcriptomic analysis has not identified any CDR-related candidate tumor suppressor gene. Instead, loss of 7p22.1p14.1 correlated with an enhanced expression of CHN2 (7p14.1) and the encoded β2-chimerin. Gain and amplification of 7q22.11q31.1 are associated with an increased expression of several genes postulated to be implicated in cancer, including RUNDC3B, PPP1R9A and ABCB1, a known multidrug resistance gene. RNA-sequencing did not identify any disease-defining mutation or gene fusion. Thus, chromosome 7 imbalances remain the only driver events detected in this tumor. We hypothesize that the Δ7p22.1p14.1-associated enhanced expression of CHN2/β2-chimerin leads to downmodulation of the NFAT pathway and a proliferative response, while upregulation of the CGR-related genes provides growth advantage for neoplastic δγT-cells and underlies their intrinsic chemoresistance. Finally, our study confirms the previously described gene expression profile of HSTL and identifies a set of 24 genes, including three located on chromosome 7 (CHN2, ABCB1 and PPP1R9A), distinguishing HSTL from other malignancies.

Editor: Jörg D. Hoheisel, Deutsches Krebsforschungszentrum, Germany

Funding: This study was supported by the concerted action grant from the K. U. Leuven no. 3M040406 (J-AvdK, TT, PV, JC and IW) (http://www.kuleuven.be/english), and a research grant from "Stichting tegen Kanker" (PV) (http://www.kanker.be/. PV is a senior clinical investigator of the FWO-Vlaanderen (http://www.fwo.be/en/). The funders had no role in study design, data collection and analysis, decision to publish, or preparation of the manuscript.

Competing Interests: The authors have declared that no competing interests exist.

* Email: iwona.wlodarska@uzleuven.be

Introduction

Hepatosplenic T-cell lymphoma (HSTL) is a rare and clinically aggressive subtype of peripheral T-cell lymphoma (PTCL) [1], recognized as a distinct clinico-pathological entity in the 2008 WHO classification [2]. Patients, predominantly young men, usually present with isolated hepatosplenomegaly and thrombocytopenia. Histologically, they show sinusoidal involvement of bone marrow, liver and spleen. HSTL is derived from the γδ

(occasionally αβ [3–5]) cytotoxic memory T-cells responsible for innate immunity. The disease shows a fulminant clinical course, therapy resistance and poor prognosis. The median survival of patients with HSTL is usually shorter than two years [6]. Cytogenetically, isochromosome 7q [i(7)(q10)] is a hallmark of HSTL [7–10], although sporadic cases with a ring chromosome 7 [r(7)] [11–13] or translocation involving chromosome 7 [14] have been published. The most common accompanying karyotype alteration is trisomy 8 [9]. Thus far, the functional and molecular

Table 1. Relevant clinical and genetic data.

Case	Sex/Age	Previous medical history	Histologically proven sites of involve-ment	Treatment	Outcome (months)	Cytogenetics Sample/status	Karyotype[b]	aCGH platform	PHF14 seq	GEP Affy 2.0	RNAseq	WB
1	M/26		S	splenectomy, allo BMTx	CR, alive (80)	S/D	46-48,XY,r(7),inc[2]	Agilent 244k	done	done		
2[a]	M/7	possible IgA nephropathy	S, L, BM	splenectomy, combined CT (POG 9404 induction protocol)	CR (12), lost to FU	BM/D	47,XY,r(7)(p22q36),+8[15]	Agilent 244k				
3[a]	F/62	ITP	S, L, BM	splenectomy, combined CT	DOD (2)	BM/D	47,XX,r(7),+8,der(19)t(?;19)t(?;p13)[10]	Agilent 244k				
4[a]	M/33	Budd-Chiari syndrome, liver Tx	S, L, BM	splenectomy	DOD (2)	S/D	45–46,X,-Y,-4,der(7)add(7)(p22)add(7)(q32), i(7)(q10),+i(7)(q10)[2],der(8)t(1;8)(q21;p23),-22,+mar1,+mar2(cp11],aCGH+8	Affymetrix CytoScan HD	done	done	done	done
5	M/52	Crohn's disease	S	splenectomy, combined CT, MAB	DOD (11.5)	S/D	46–47,XY,add(4)(p16),i(7)(q10),+8[4],-[20],+mar[2][cp6]	Agilent 244k		done	done	done
6	M/50		S, BM	splenectomy, combined CT	DOD (25)	S/D	43–45,X,-Y,i(7)(q10)[cp7],aCGH+8	Affymetrix CytoScan HD	done			
7	M/18	kidney Tx for dysplasia	S, Pe, BM	splenectomy, combined CT	DOD (8.5)	S/D	40–48,XY,+X [3],-5[4],i(7)(q10),+8[5],+10[2],add(11)(q22)[10],inc[cp12],aCGH+8	Affymetrix CytoScan HD		done	done	done
8	F/55		S, BM	splenectomy, combined CT	DOD (21)	BM/P	46–47,XX,i(7)(q10),+i(7)(q10)[4],+8,-10,add(15)(q26),add(22)(q13)[cp12]	Affymetrix CytoScan HD			done	done
9 DERL-2							46,XY,add(5)(q?),i(7)(q10),-10[5][cp15][c]. aCGH+8	Agilent 244k	done	done	done	done

a, previously published cases[10],[11,13].
b, karyotypes were described according to recommendations of ISCN (2013)[84]
c, karyotype according to Di Noto et al.(2001)[22].
abbreviations: ITP, idiopathic thrombocytopenic purpura; POG, Pediatric Oncology Group; MAB, Monoclonal Antibodies; Tx, transplantation; S, spleen; L, liver; BM, bone marrow; Pe, peritoneum; allo, allogeneic; CT, chemotherapy; FU, follow-up; D, diagnosis; P, progression; WB, Western blotting.

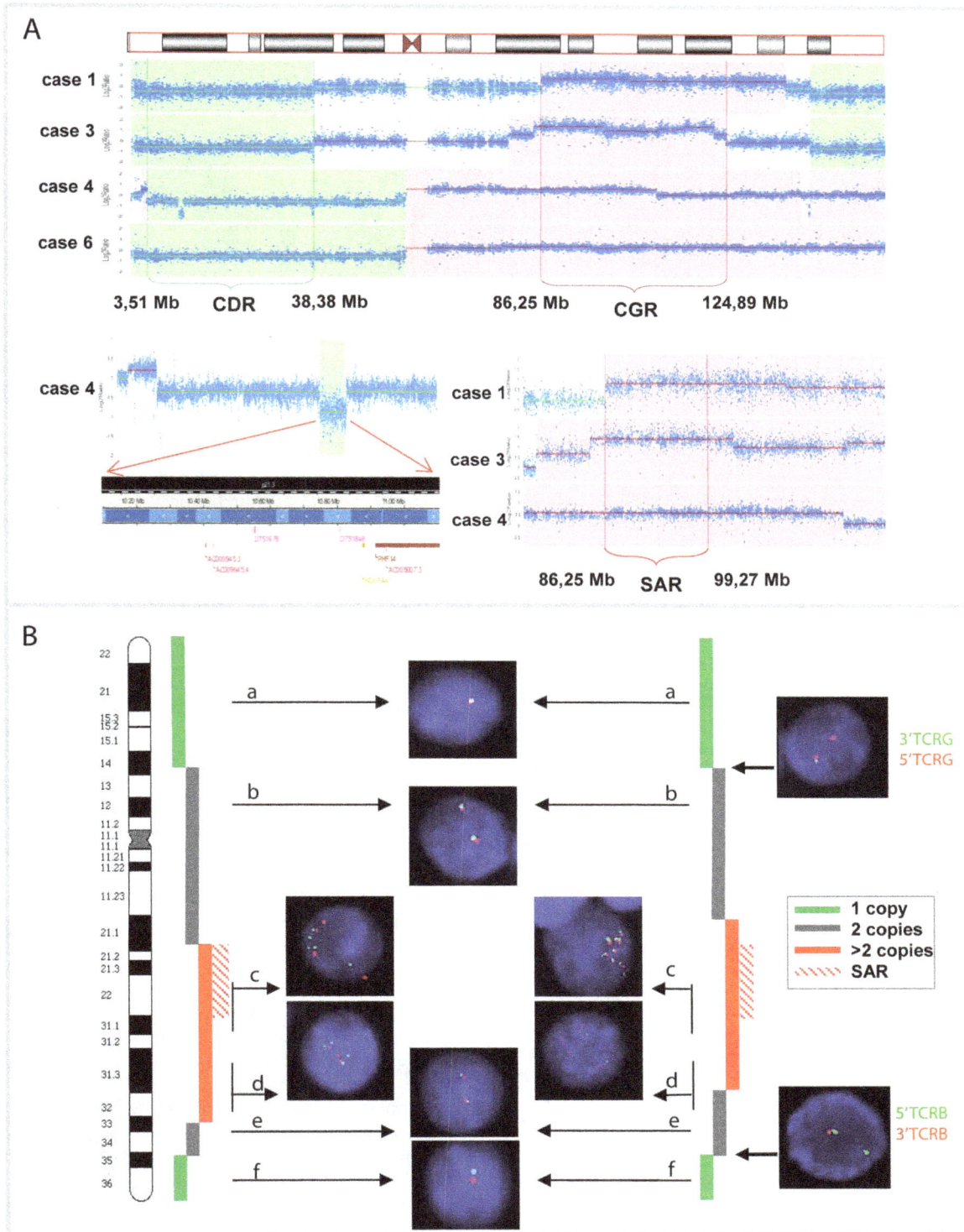

Figure 1. Examples of aCGH and FISH analysis. A) upper panel: genomic profile of chromosome 7 of four index cases with the indicated common deleted region (CDR) on 7p and common gained region (CGR) on 7q; lower left panel: gene content (Hg19) of the biallelically deleted 7p21 interval in case 4; lower right panel: zoomed CDR with the indicated selectively amplified region (SAR). B) Examples of interphase FISH validation of aCGH results performed in cases 1 (left panel) and 2 (right panel) with r(7). Applied probes: (a) RP11-99J06-SG/RP11-735O20-SO, (b) RP13-11C11-SG/RP11-807G04-SO, (c) RP11-513N08-SG/RP11-514N09-SO, (d) RP11-379L24-SO/RP11-16K22-SG,(e) RP11-269N18-SG/RP5-894A10-SO, (f) RP4-548K24-SG/RP11-135F23-SO.

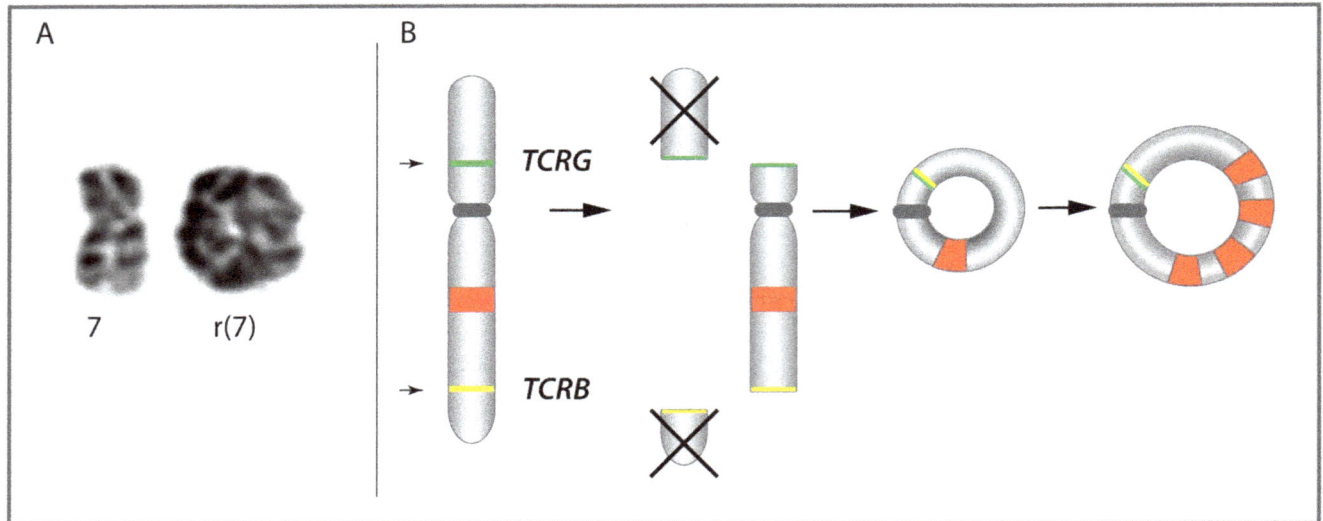

Figure 2. Mechanism underlying formation of r(7) in HSTL. A) Partial karyotype showing r(7). B) Proposed model of the r(7) formation. Illegitimate somatic rearrangement of *TCRB* and *TCRG* in δγT-cells leads to the aberrant *TCRB-TCRG* lesion and consequently to the formation of r(7) and loss of the terminal 7p and 7q regions, respectively. This process is followed by a subsequent gain/amplification of 7q sequences (shown in red).

genetic consequences of i(7)(q10) in HSTL remain largely unknown. As development of i(7)(q10) results in loss of one copy of the short arm of chromosome 7 (7p) and gain of the long arm of chromosome 7 (7q), neoplastic cells presumably suffer from an aberrant gene dosage effect. Some or all of these imbalances may represent the key event driving the development of HSTL. As HSTL tends to gain extra copies of i(7)(q10) [10,15] or selectively amplify 7q sequences [11–13], overrepresentation of 7q seems to have an important impact on the pathogenesis of this lymphoma. Combined gene expression profiling (GEP) and array-based comparative genomic hybridization (aCGH) of several HSTL cases recently reported by Travert *et al.* [5] showed downregulation of 7p genes, particularly *CYCS*, *IKZF1*, *HUS1* and *CBX3*, and upregulation of 7q genes, including the putative oncogene *PTPN12*. To gain further insight into the molecular pathogenesis of HSTL, we determined genomic profiles of six i(7)(q10)-positive HSTL cases, including DER-L2 cell line, and three cases with r(7), and significantly narrowed down the common deleted region on 7p and the common gained region on 7q. Subsequent transcriptomic studies using global microarray expression profiling and RNA-sequencing led to identification of candidate genes implicated in the pathogenesis of HSTL.

Materials and Methods

Patients

Six HSTL cases were collected from files of the Center for Human Genetics, KU Leuven, Leuven, Belgium. Two cases were provided by L. Krenacs (Laboratory of Tumor Pathology and Molecular Diagnostics, Szeged, Hungary) and S. Shetty (Department of Medical Genetics, Alberta Children's Hospital, Calgary, Canada). Diagnosis of HSTL was based on histopathology and immunophenotype, according to the WHO criteria [2]. The clinical, pathological and immunophenotypic features of the patients were reviewed. The study was approved by the institutional review board "Commissie Medische Ethiek" of the University Hospital. For this retrospective study the "Commissie Medische Ethiek" waived the need for written informed consent from the participants.

Cytogenetics and fluorescence *in situ* hybridization

R- and G-banding chromosomal analysis and fluorescence *in situ* hybridization (FISH) analysis followed standard procedures. Probes used for FISH analysis are listed in Table S1. Noncommercial probes were labeled with SpectrumOrange- and SpectrumGreen-d-UTP (Abbott Molecular, Ottigne, Belgium) using random priming. FISH experiments were evaluated using an Axioplan 2 fluorescence microscope equipped with a charge-coupled device Axiophot 2 camera (Carl Zeiss Microscopy, Jena, Germany) and a MetaSystems Isis imaging system (MetaSystems, Altlussheim, Germany). Two to 10 abnormal metaphases and/or 200 interphase cells were evaluated in each FISH experiment.

High resolution array CGH

Total genomic DNA was isolated from fresh frozen lymphoma samples or cytogenetic pellet (Table 1; case 2) using standard procedures. Genomic profiling, following the manufacturer's protocols, was performed using the Agilent 244k (www.agilent.com) (5 cases) and the Affymetrix CytoScan HD arrays (www.affymetrix.com) (4 cases). Array CGH data are available at GEO (Accession number: GSE57944).

Data analysis and visualization software

Downstream data analysis of the genomic profiling results was performed using the software ArrayStudio, version 6.2 (www.omicsoft.com). Unless otherwise specified, this software was also used for various analysis performed on the expression data retrieved from microarray and RNAseq technologies described below.

PHF14 sequencing

Mutation analysis of *PHF14* was performed on total genomic DNA from five index cases (Table 1) and four control PTCL cases without chromosome 7 abnormalities. PCR amplification and sequence analysis of genomic sequences spanning full exons of *PHF14* were performed using Sanger sequencing primers (Table S2) and conventional sequencing method.

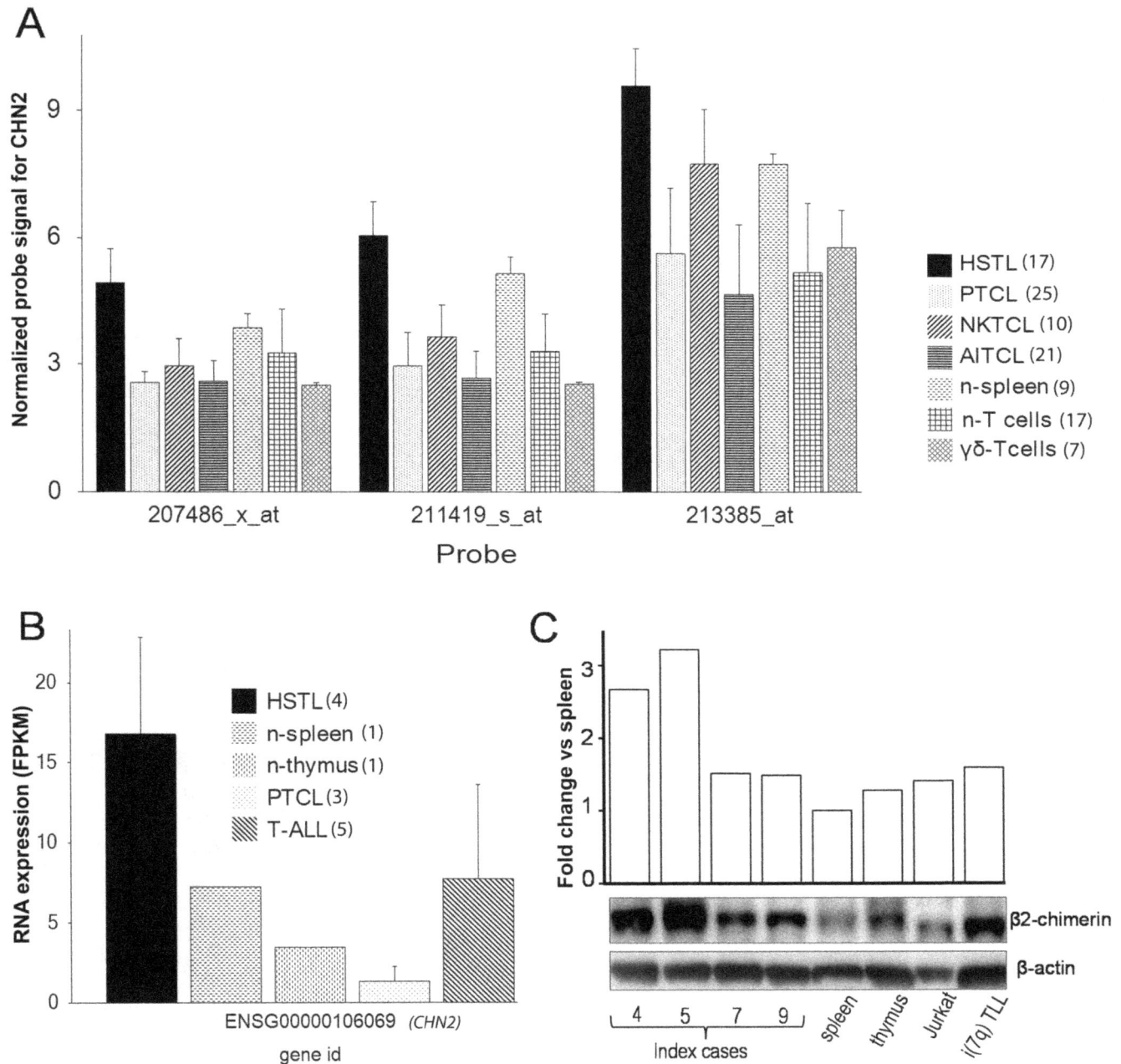

Figure 3. Expression of CHN2/β2-chimerin. A) Normalized values of all *CHN2* probes in the used U133 array for the analyzed malignancies and normal controls. The observed expression differences were statistically significant, with FDR_BH <0.05 (Table S6). B) Expression values of *CHN2* using the RNAseq data. FPKM (Fragments Per Kilobase of exon Model) is a measurement of transcript abundance in RNAseq experiments. C) Western blotting and densitometry of β2-chimerin. The bars represent the fold change of the normalized intensity of β2-chimerin (compared to β-actin) versus spleen. The number between parenthesis represent the number of samples.

454 sequencing

Custom designed Nimblegen sequence capture 385k Version 2.0 Arrays (Roche Applied Science, Mannheim, Germany) targeting sequences at 7p21.3/10106629-11176525 (hg18) were produced. Preparation of shot-gun DNA sequencing libraries and capturing of the target region was performed according to the manufacturer's instructions. Captured DNA was pyrosequenced on a GS FLX instrument (Roche Applied Science, Mannheim, Germany) according to the manufacturer's instructions.

Microarray gene expression analysis

Total RNA extraction from four frozen lymphoma samples (Table 1) and three nonmalignant spleens was performed using TRIzol LS Reagent (Life Technologies Europe B.V., Ghent, Belgium). For gene expression profiling, the Affymetrix platform HG-U133 Plus 2.0 was used. To increase the statistical significance of the study, data from 13 previously published HSTL cases, various T-cell malignancies [25 cases of PTCL (peripheral T-cell lymphoma), 10 cases of NK/TCL (Natural

Table 2. Ingenuity Pathway Analysis: Most significant networks, functions and pathways associated to the top 401 genes differentially expressed in HSTL.

Top Networks		
Associated Network Functions	**Score**	
Cellular Assembly and Organization, Hematological System Development and Function, Inflammatory Response	40	
Digestive System Development and Function, Embryonic Development, Organismal Development	40	
Cell Morphology, Cellular Assembly and Organization, Carbohydrate Metabolism	38	
Connective Tissue Disorders, Developmental Disorder, Skeletal and Muscular Disorders	37	
Cancer, Cell Morphology, Organ Morphology	33	
Top Diseases and Bio Functions		
Name	**p-value**	**No of molecules**
Cancer	3.08E-20 -3.87E-05	265
Reproductive System Disease	2.90E-16 -3.95E-05	104
Connective Tissue Disorders	3.43E-15 -1.54E-05	73
Inflammatory Disease	3.43E-15 -2.37E-05	95
Skeletal and Muscular Disorders	3.43E-15 -3.35E-05	83
Molecular and Cellular Functions		
Name	**p-value**	**No of molecules**
Cellular Development	1.98E-23 -2.92E-05	186
Cellular Growth and Proliferation	1.98E-23 -3.32E-05	180
Cellular Movement	6.53E-21 -3.62E-05	126
Cell Morphology	5.60E-19 -2.92E-05	129
Cell-To-Cell Signaling and Interaction	1.12E-15 -2.69E-05	148
Physiological System Development and Function		
Name	**p-value**	**No of molecules**
Tissue Morphology	2.19E-20 -2.00E-05	141
Hematological System Development and Function	5.86E-20 -3.62E-05	144
Immune Cell Trafficking	7.14E-16 -3.62E-05	95
Embryonic Development	6.66E-14 -2.35E-05	96
Lymphoid Tissue Structure and Development	6.66E-14 -2.84E-05	73
Top Canonical Pathways		
Name	**p-value**	**Ratio**
Natural Killer Cell Signaling	4.36E-07	13/118 (0.11)
Crosstalk between Dendritic Cells and Natural Killer Cells	1.73E-06	11/106 (0.104)
Granulocyte Adhesion and Diapedesis	4.54E-05	13/181 (0.072)
Agranulocyte Adhesion and Diapedesis	8.03E-05	13/191 (0.068)
Hepatic Fibrosis/Hepatic Stellate Cell Activation	4.38E-04	10/155 (0.065)

Killer/T-cell lymphoma), 21 cases of AITCL (angioimmunoblastic T-cell lymphoma) and nonmalignant samples (6 spleens, 26 samples of T-cells, including activated $\gamma\delta$T-cells] were retrieved from public sources (GEO and ArrayExpressed)) (Table S3). The raw data of all cases (CEL files) were normalized together using the GeneChip-Robust Multiarray Averaging (GC-RMA) algorithm. Principal component analysis (PCA), hierarchical clustering and a special application of Lewi's spectral mapping [16] to microarrays (Spectral Map Analysis, SMA) (www.vetstat.ugent.be/workshop/Nairobi2004/Bijnens/Bijnens2004.pdf) were used to detect relationship in the data and to identify outliers. To find differentially expressed genes, the General Linear Model (GLM) was used for inference analysis. The resulting Fold Change (FC) and False Discovery Rate (FDR) (using the Benjamini–Hochberg procedure, FDR_BH) were used to set differential expression cut-offs. The cut

offs values for FC ranged from an absolute value (Abs(FC)) of 2.0 (Abs(FC) $\geq$2.0) to 3.5 (Abs(FC)$\geq$3.5). The maximum FDR used as a cut off was 0.1 (FDR $\leq$0.1) and the minimum was 0.05 (FDR $\leq$ 0.05). The microarray data of four index cases and three nonmalignant spleens were deposited in GEO (Accession number: GSE57944).

Library preparation for paired-end RNA-sequencing and processing of RNAseq reads

Four samples of HSTL (Table 1) and one nonmalignant spleen sample were subjected to RNA-sequencing. The Illumina standard kit (Illumina TruSeq RNA Sample Preparation Kit, San Diego, CA, USA) was used for the mRNAseq sample preparation according to the manufacturer's protocol. Briefly, 1 μg of total

Table 3. List of genes comprising the HSTL signature.

Gene Symbol	Chromosome	Position	Name	Location*	Type molecules
Upregulated					
ABCB1	7	87133175	ATP-binding cassette, sub-family B (MDR/TAP), member 1	PM	transporter
CD200R1	3	112640056	CD200 receptor 1	PM	other
CD5L	1	157800704	CD5 molecule-like	PM	transmembrane receptor
ITGAD	16	31404633	integrin, alpha D	PM	other
PPP1R9A	7	94536948	protein phosphatase 1, regulatory subunit 9A	PM	other
S1PR5	19	10623623	sphingosine-1-phosphate receptor 5	PM	G-protein coupled receptor
TMEM178A	2	39892122	transmembrane protein 178A	PM	other
CHN2	7	29234120	chimerin (chimaerin) 2	C	other
CHSY3	5	129240165	chondroitin sulfate synthase 3	C	enzyme
FCRLB	1	161691353	Fc receptor-like B	C	other
PRDM16	1	2985732	PR domain containing 16	N	transcription regulator
Downregulated					
CCR7	17	38 710021	chemokine (C-C motif) receptor 7	PM	G-protein coupled receptor
CD200	3	112051915	CD200 molecule	PM	other
CD28	2	204571198	CD28 molecule	PM	transmembrane receptor
CD5	11	60869867	CD5 molecule	PM	transmembrane receptor
CD83	6	14117872	CD83 molecule	PM	other
CXCR3	X	70835766	chemokine (C-X-C motif) receptor 3	PM	G-protein coupled receptor
GPR183	13	99946784	G protein-coupled receptor 183	PM	G-protein coupled receptor
SLAMF1	1	160577890	signaling lymphocytic activation molecule family member 1	PM	transmembrane receptor
FAM134B	5	16473147	family with sequence similarity 134, member B	C	other
GZMK	5	54320081	granzyme K (granzyme 3; tryptase II)	C	peptidase
CAMK4	5	110559351	calcium/calmodulin-dependent protein kinase IV	Nucleus	kinase
PRRX1	1	170631869	paired related homeobox 1	Nucleus	transcription regulator
CCL19	9	34689564	chemokine (C-C motif) ligand 19	ES	cytokine

*PM, plasma membrane; C, cytoplasm; N, nucleus; ES, extracellular space.

RNA was used for polyA mRNA selection using poly-T oligo-attached magnetic beads, followed by thermal mRNA fragmentation. Using reverse transcriptase (Superscript II, Life Technologies Europe B.V.e, Ghent, Belgium) and random primers, cDNA was synthesized and subsequently double stranded, end-repaired (End Repair Mix) and ligated to the Illumina RNA Indexes Adaptor. The libraries were purified after enrichment using 15 cycles of PCR. The insert sizes of the libraries were checked by Agilent Technologies 2100 Bioanalyzer.

Processing of Illumina RNA-sequencing reads

Prepared libraries were sequenced using HiSeq 2000 (Illumina, San Diego, CA, USA) operated in paired-end 2×100 bp mode. Reads were quality-filtered using a standard Illumina process.

RNAseq bioinformatics analysis

For further analysis, we used additional RNAseq data of three cases of PTCL, five cases of T-ALL, the Jurkat T-cell line and one nonmalignant thymus available in our institution. The fastq files of all samples were mapped to the reference human genome (assembly GRCh37.68). The mapping was performed using OSA [17] with the default parameters allowing detection of insertions and deletions (indels). The mapped reads were used to calculate read counts and FPKM (Fragment Per Kilobase of exon model per Million of mapped read) per gene. The DESeq

algorithm [18] was applied to identify differentially expressed genes. Prediction of SNV followed the previously described approach [19] filtering out the variants found in normal spleen. The detection of indels was done independently using ArrayStudio. Fusion transcript discovery was performed using deFuse v.0.5.0 [20] with default parameters and a fusion detection algorithm provided by ArrayStudio [17,21]. Fusions with less than 8 spanning reads and less than 5 split reads were filtered out as well as those observed in adjacent genes.

Gene signature analysis

To find a gene signature of HSTL, at first we ran 10 different inference analyses (using both microarray and RNAseq data) comparing HSTL with PTCL-NOS, NK/TCL, AITCL, T-ALL, nonsorted normal T-cells, sorted activated γδT-cells, nonmalignant spleen and thymus. After selecting the differentially expressed genes in every comparison, the results (FC of the gene per comparison) were merged in a table. Then, we selected genes with a consistent expression pattern (either up- or downregulated) across the different comparisons and used these genes for unsupervised hierarchical clustering analyses. The resulting dendograms and heatmaps were visually inspected and the genes which were not essential to keep the integrity of the HSTL samples cluster were removed. This process was repeated until a minimal

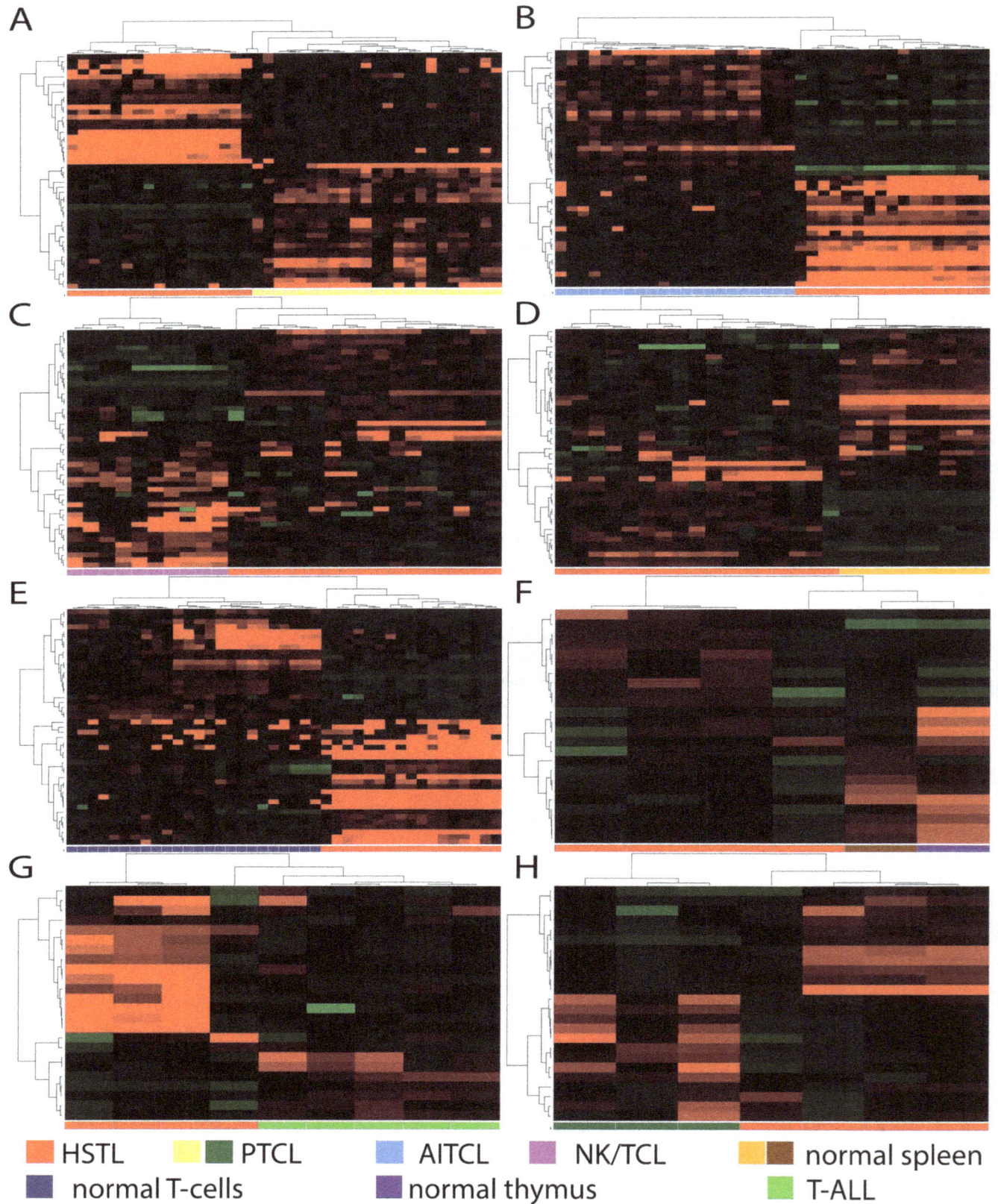

Figure 4. Hierarchical clustering using the 24 gene signature for HSTL. The MA data (A–E) and RNAseq data (F–H) show an accurate separation of the HSTL cluster from PTCL, AITCL, NK/TCL, nonmalignant spleen, normal T-cells, nonmalignant thymus and T-ALL.

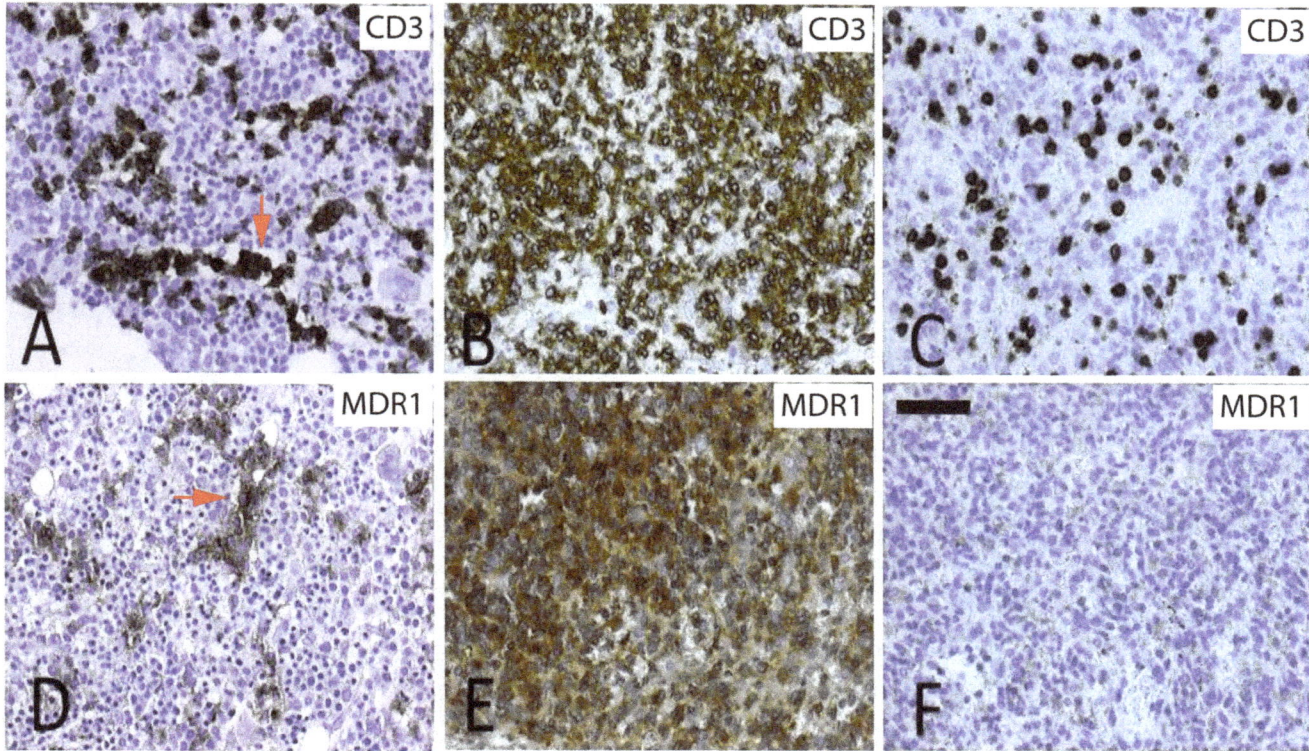

Figure 5. Morphology and ABCB1 expression in HSTL cases detected by IHC. Immunohistochemical stainings (A–C, anti-CD3; D-F, anti-MDR1/ABCB1) of the typical intrasinusoidal spread (red arrows) by HSTL cells in the bone marrow (A/D, case 4) and spleen (B/E, case 6), respectively, compared to staining pattern in normal spleen (C/F). Pictures captured by Leica DFC290HD camera at 400X. Scale bar = 50 μm.

number of genes was found, which keep the cluster formed by the HSTL samples intact.

Biological pathways analysis

To find significant enriched pathways and biological functions in HSTL, we uploaded the result of the inference analyses into the "Ingenuity Pathway Analysis" application (IPA, www.ingenuity.com). From the three confidence levels provided by the system, we used "Experimentally observed" and "Highly predicted" data. For details see: http://ingenuity.force.com/ipa/articles/Feature_Description/Canonical-Pathways-for-a-Dataset

QRT-PCR analysis

Quantitative RT-PCR was performed with the LightCycler 480 SYBR Green I master mix (Roche Diagnostics Belgium, Vilvoorde, Belgium) and the results were analyzed using the comparative dCt method. The analysis was done using 3 replicates and the two most similar values were used to calculate the mean. Primer sequences are shown in Table S2.

Western blot analysis

Sections from lymphoma frozen tissues and pellets of cultured DERL-2 cells were lysed and processed for Western blotting according to standard procedure using antibodies against β2-chimerin (2E3; Rat mAb nr. 4728, Cell Signaling Technology, Danvers, Massachusetts, USA) and β-actin (Sigma Aldrich, St. Louis, MO, USA). Protein detection was performed with Image Quant Las4000. Densitometric analysis of protein blots was performed using the ImageJ (1.45) software from the National Institutes of Health (http://rsb.info.nih.gov/ij/).

Immunohistochemistry

Expression of ABCB1 (MDR1) was analyzed by IHC with monoclonal MDR1 antibody (MAB4120, clone JSB-1, Millipore, Overijse, Belgium) used at dilution 1:200 with a high pretreatment. Results were visualized using the OptiView DAB IHC Detection Kit (Ventana, Oro Valley, Tucson, Arizona). Image acquisition was done through a Leica microscope at 200× and 100× magnification. Images were assembled using Adobe Photoshop CS5.

Results

Clinical characteristics of HSTL patients

The relevant clinical features of eight reported HSTL cases are shown in Table 1. There were six male and two female patients in age ranging from seven to 62 years (average 38.7). The cases displayed the common clinical, morphological and immunophenotypic features of HSTL, including γδT-cell origin [2]. Histologically, all patients showed spleen involvement. Liver and/or bone marrow (BM) involvement were histologically proven in three and six patients, respectively. Four patients (50%) had either a previous autoimmune disorder (i.e. idiopathic thrombocytopenic purpura, Crohn's disease) or underwent immunosuppressive treatment after solid organ transplantation. All patients underwent splenectomy, which was followed by allogenic BM transplantation (alloBMTX) (one case) or combined chemotherapy (CT) (six cases). One patient died two months after diagnosis, six patients treated with combined CT survived 2-25 months (average 11.7 months) and one patient was lost for follow-up after 12 months of

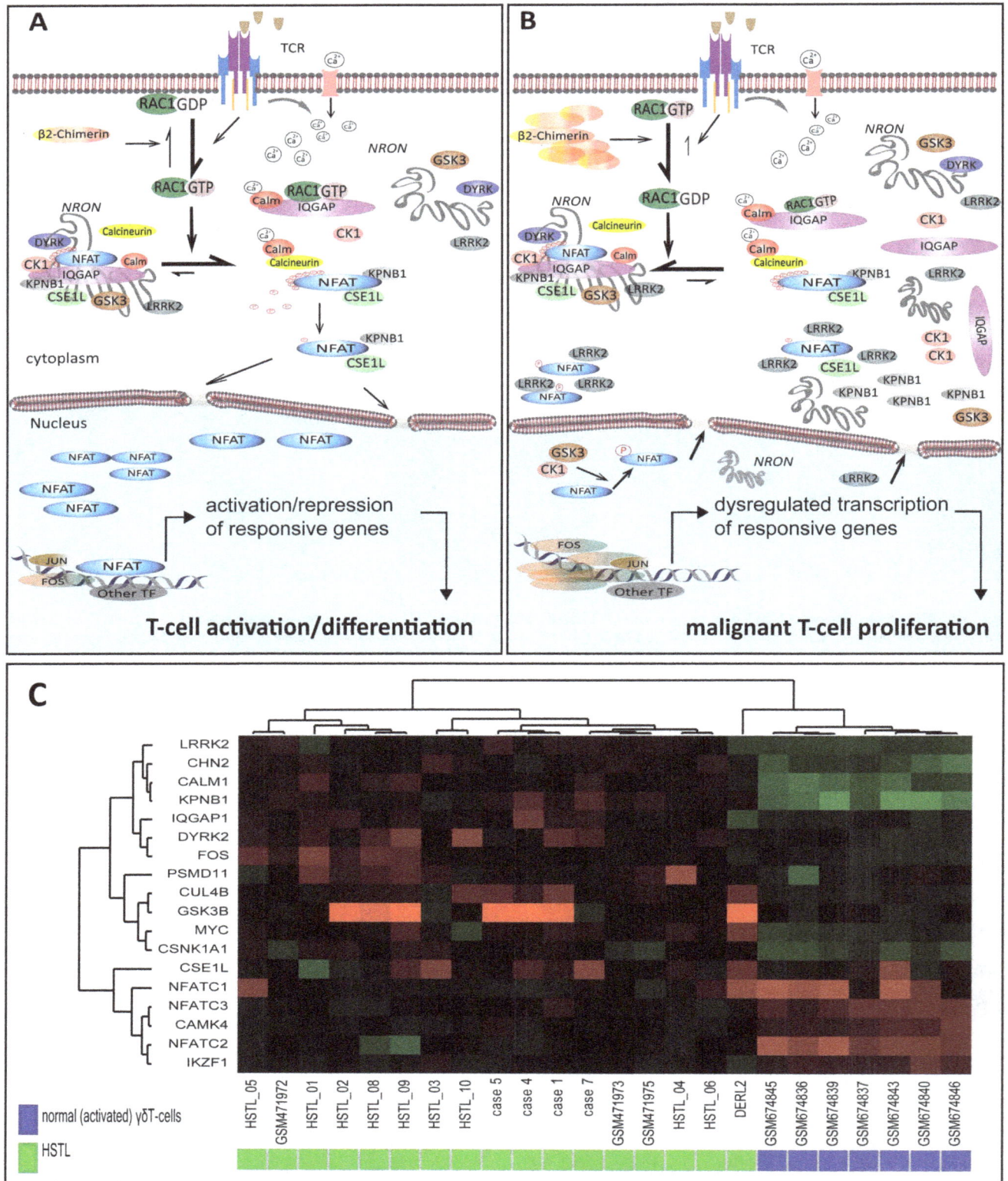

Figure 6. Postulated model for the pathogenesis of HSTL. (A) In resting T-cells, NFAT proteins are located in the cytoplasm and are associated with a large RNA-protein scaffold complex composed of the lincRNA NRON, a repressor of NFAT [30], and several additional proteins [31]. NFAT proteins are heavily phosphorylated through synergistic action of three different family of kinases, casein kinase 1 (CK1), glycogen synthase kinase 3 (GSK3), and dual specificity tyrosine phosphorylation regulated kinase (DYRK) [29]. When T-cells are stimulated, TCR engagement triggers a rapid increase in intracellular calcium (Ca^{2+}) and activation of RAC1, a GTPase which belongs to the RAS superfamily of small GTP-binding proteins [79]. The active, GTP-bound RAC1 binds to IQGAP (IQ-domain GTPase-activating protein) negatively regulating its binding affinity for other proteins and consequently, stimulating the disassembly of the NRON complex [31,82,83]. In parallel, the calcium increase leads to activation of calmodulin, a

calcium-binding messenger protein, which activates of the phosphatase calcineurin. This enzyme dephosphorylates NFAT and promotes nuclear transport of activated NFAT by importins (KPNB1, CSE1L). In the nucleus, NFAT, in synergy with a numbers of other transcriptional regulators (e.g. FOS and JUN), participates in a transcriptional regulation of a wide range of genes involved in immune system responses and organs development [29,66]. (B) We postulate that formation of i(7)(q10) or r(7) in γδT-cell triggers an aberrant expression of β2-chimerin which subsequently inactivates RAC1 by keeping it in a GDP-bound state. This prevents RAC1 binding with IQGAP resulting in a strengthening of the NRON complex and arrests the phosphorylated NFAT in the cytoplasm. Cytoplasmic retention of NFAT may be also attributed to the kinase LRRK2 (overexpressed in HSTL), which blocks the transport of NFAT to the nucleus [32,33]. The significantly reduced nuclear level of NFAT leads to dysregulated transcription of responsive genes controlling cell-cycle, cell death and proliferation, and eventually, to malignant transformation and clonal proliferation of i(7)(q10)/r(7)-positive γδT-cells. The candidate causative genes include the *MYC* oncogene (↑ in HSTL), known to be repressed by NFAT [62] and the *IKZF1* tumor suppressor gene (↓ in HSTL) which is activated by NFAT [66]. (C) Hierarchical clustering using NFAT-related genes, including components of the NRON complex. Note that all HSTL samples, except for DERL-2, form a distinct cluster apart from the activated γδT-cells.

complete remission (CR). Notably, patient 1 who received alloBMTX is alive and remaining in CR (80 months).

Molecular cytogenetic analysis

All eight patients and the included HSTL-derived DERL-2 cell line [22] displayed abnormal karyotypes with either i(7)(q10) (six cases) or r(7) (three cases) (Table 1). Of note, case 4 revealed additional aberrations of the other chromosome 7 and a subclonal duplication of i(7)(q10), which was also detected in case 8. Trisomy 8 was identified in five patients. The cases were further subjected to a high resolution aCGH analysis which detected genomic imbalances in all of them (Table S4).

Chromosome 7 profiles of cases 1 and 3 with r(7) were very similar. They were characterized by terminal losses of 7p/7q regions, with respective breakpoints at 7p14.1/*TCRG* (38406226 bp) and 7q32/*TCRB* (142502221 bp), and gain of 7q, which encompasses 7q21.12q33 (86259620–137506193 bp) in case 1 and 7q21.11q31.33 (79158260–124892276 bp) in case 3 (Figure 1A, upper panel). The profile of case 2 was less pronounced (<20% of abnormal cells), although loss of 7p22.3p22.1 and gain of 7q21.1q32.1 were evident. Five cases with i(7)(q10) revealed loss of the entire 7p and gain of 7q, as expected. Case 4 displayed complex imbalances, including duplication of the terminal 7p22.2p22.2 (2347596–3506315 bp) region, monoallelic loss of 7p22.1p11 (3506316–57883626 bp) and a biallelic microdeletion at 7p21.3 (10165499–11213632 bp) (Figure 1A, left lower panel). The long arm of chromosome 7 showed three copies of the 7q11q31.1 (61.831.840–110403720 bp) region and two copies of 7q31.1q36 (110413108–159118566 bp). Based on the aCGH data, we defined the common deleted region (CDR) at 7p22.1p14.1 (3506316–38406226 bp) (34.89 Mb) and the common gained region (CGR) at 7q21.22q31.1/(86259620–124892276 Mb) (38.78 Mb) (Figure 1A, upper panel). Cases 1 and 3 displayed a smaller amplified region (SAR)of 13 Mb (86259620–99271246 bp) at 7q21.22q22.1 (Figure 1A, right lower panel). To validate aCGH data, we analyzed two available cases with r(7) (cases 1 and 2) by interphase FISH with the selected 7p/7q BAC clones (Table S1). As illustrated in Figure 1B, FISH confirmed the localization of terminal 7p/7q breakpoints within *TCRG* and *TCRB*, respectively, and the associated loss of terminal sequences flanking both loci, suggesting their involvement in formation of r(7) (Figure 2). FISH also evidenced a different size of the gained 7q region and the level of 7q gain. For example, three SAR-related probes showed 4–5 signals in case 1 and 6–9 signals in case 2 (Figure 1B).

Other recurrent aCGH imbalances detected in at least two cases include a trisomy 8 (7 cases), duplication of 1q (3 cases; common gain of 1q31q34), loss of 4p (3 cases; common loss of 4p16.3p16.3), loss of 10p (2 cases; common loss of 10p14p13/10p12.2p11.22) and duplication of 17q (2 cases; common gain of 17q21.33q25.3) (Table S4). Of note, trisomy 8 was not detected in case 2 (low proportion of tumor cells) but it was identified in three

additional cases (no. 4, 6 and 9). Altogether, cytogenetics and aCGH detected trisomy 8 in eight out of nine (88.8%) studied cases.

Sequencing of the biallelically deleted 7p21 region

The 7p21.3 region biallelically deleted in case 4 harbors two protein-coding genes, *NDUFA4* and *PHF14*, a candidate tumor suppressor gene (TSG) [23–25]. To examine the mutational status of *PHF14* on the nondeleted 7p allele in other index cases, we sequenced the gene in cases 1, 5, 6, and 9 (DERL-2). No mutation, however, was identified. In the next step, the entire 10165499–11213632 bp region was sequenced using the 454 technology combined with region capturing. This analysis detected neither recurrent intergenic nor intragenic mutations in the four samples analyzed.

Quality of the RNAseq data

The average number of reads obtained was 98.7 million and the average percentage of uniquely mapped reads was 86.3%. No 3′ bias was detected. The full alignment report is in Table S5. The raw RNAseq data (fastq files) of all HSTL and PTCL-NOS cases analyzed plus the normal spleen are available at GEO (Accession number: GSE57944).

Gene expression and pathway analysis

Transcriptome of HSTL was studied using expression microarray (MA) [cases 1, 4, 5, 7 plus 100 publicly available samples, including HSTL (n = 13), various T/NK-cell malignancies (n = 54) and normal T-cell controls (n = 33); Table S3] and RNAseq approach [cases 4, 5, 7, DERL-2 plus 10 control samples including, PTCL-NOS (n = 3), T-ALL (n = 5), nonmalignant spleen (n = 1) and thymus (n = 1)] (see details in Materials and Methods). Given that the MA dataset included samples from five different laboratories, at first we performed data structure analysis including Spectral Map Analysis (SMA), hierarchical clustering and Principal Component Analysis (PCA). SMA showed that the MA samples selected for further bioinformatic analysis cluster according to their classification and there was no bias by their laboratory origin (Figure S1 A–B). PCA on the RNAseq expression data discriminated HSTL from other analyzed samples except for the nonmalignant thymus (Figure S2).

To identify critical genes targeted by chromosome 7 imbalances (presumably TSG located within CDR and/or oncogene(s) harbored by CGR) in HSTL, we ran 10 different inference analyses (using the MA and RNAseq data) comparing HSTL *vs* PTCL-NOS, NK/TCL, AITCL, T-ALL, nonsorted normal T-cells, sorted activated γδT-cells, nonmalignant spleen and thymus. Then, we focused on the CDR- and CGR-associated genes. Among the roughly 550 genes located within the CDR, only 17 genes were found dysregulated (Table S6). Of note, *PHF14*, our initial candidate TSG, was not dysregulated in any of the comparisons performed. Surprisingly, the comparison *vs* γδT-cells did not identify any downregulated gene in the CDR. Five genes (*TSPAN13, HDAC9, CHN2, EPDR1* and *TARP*), however, were frequently upregulated. Interestingly, *CHN2* was upregulated in all 10 comparisons (Figure 3A and 3B) with a 15 FC in the comparison *vs* γδT-cells (Table S6). The CGR comprises approximately 650 genes. Twenty nine of these genes were dysregulated, including 13 (44.8%) which were exclusively upregulated, four (13.8%) which were downregulated and 12 (41.3%) showing a heterogeneous pattern of expression. The 13 upregulated genes included *ABCB1, RUNDC3B, KRIT1, SAMD9, SGCE, PEG10, PPP1R9A, ZNF655, PILRB, NA-PEPLD, PUS7, PIK3CG* and *NRCAM*. Except for *NRCAM*, all these genes were upregulated in HSTL *vs* γδT-cells. Notably, *ABCB1, RUNDC3B* and *PPP1R9A* were upregulated in all 10 comparisons.

To unravel gene expression profile and gene signature of HSTL, we searched for dysregulated genes genomewide and focused on 401 genes which were up- or downregulated in at least four comparisons (Table S7). This 401 geneset, as well as genes found to be dysregulated in individual comparisons, were further explored using Ingenuity Pathway Analysis (IPA). As shown in Table 2, the 401 genes dysregulated in HSTL are implicated in important biological processes, pathways and diseases, including cancer (262 molecules) and inflammatory diseases (94 molecules). "Natural Killer Cell signaling" surfaced as the top canonical pathway dysregulated in HSTL. This pathway was also significantly dysregulated when HSTL was compared with activated γδT-cells, NK/TCL, AITCL, PTCL-NOS and spleen. Notably, the canonical pathway "Role of NFAT in regulation of the immune response" was the second and third top dysregulated pathway in HSTL *vs* activated γδT-cells (Figure S3) and *vs* nonmalignant spleen, respectively. Details of individual IPAs can be found in Figure S4.

Considering the important role of Nuclear factor of activated T cells (NFAT) transcription factors in T-cell biology and cancer [26–29], we additionally analyzed expression pattern of genes encoding proteins belonging to the large lincRNA-protein complex [also known as the Non-coding RNA Repressor Of NFAT (NRON) complex], recently found to be associated with NFAT [30,31], and the kinase LRRK2 which is linked to this complex as a negative regulator of NFATC2 [32,33]. Several of these genes were found dysregulated in HSTL *vs* γδT-cells (Table S7). Particularly interesting was the finding of *LRRK2* upregulation in 4 of 10 comparisons performed (FC = 31.25 in HSTL *vs* normal T-cells, FC = 22.77 in HSTL *vs* δγT-cells, FC = 9.22 in HSTL *vs* non-malignant thymus, and FC = 9.03, in HSTL *vs* T-ALL). In contrast, *CAMK4* was significantly downregulated in HSTL in 7 of the 10 inference analyses performed (Table S7, Figure S5). Calcium/calmodulin dependent kinase 4 (encoded by *CAMK4*) binds Ca2+/calmodulin in the cytoplasm [34]. In the nucleus, CAMK4 regulates, mainly by phosphorylation, the activity of several transcriptional activators, including NFATC2 [34,35]. Other interesting gene emerging in our study is *ITGAD*, found to be upregulated in HSTL. It encodes the integrin AlphaD, a member of a family of molecules implicated in immunological synapse formation, cell-matrix adhesion, integrin-mediated signaling pathway and proliferation of activated T-cells [36].

In addition, we analyzed expression pattern of chromosome 8-associated genes. Seven genes, *ANGPT1, CA1, CA2, SLC25A37, TOX,* and *MYBL1*, were found upregulated in at least four comparisons. The *MYC* oncogene was upregulated only in the comparison of HSTCL *vs* γδT-cells (FC = 7.01; FDR_BH = 0.0011).

To build the gene signature for HSTL several unsupervised hierarchical cluster analyses were performed to find the minimal number of genes that keep the integrity of the HSTL samples cluster in all the comparisons (see Materials and Methods). This yielded a list of 24 genes, including 11 upregulated and 13 downregulated (Table 3). IPA showed that the vast majority of these genes is involved in 'Cancer', 'Cellular growth and proliferation', 'Cell death and survival' and 'Cell-to cell signaling ' (Table S8). Using this geneset, HSTL was distinct from AITCL, NK/TCL, PTCL, nonmalignant spleen and T-cells in the MA data, and from PTCL, T-ALL, nonmalignant spleen and thymus in the RNAseq data (Figure 4, Figure S6).

Validation studies

Expression value of six genes, *CHN2, ITGAD, CAMK4, PEG10, PPP1R9A* and *NFATC2*, were validated by QRT-PCR performed on cases 4, 5, 7 and sorted γδT-cells (Figure S5). The analysis confirmed downregulation of *CAMK4* and *NFATC2* in all cases and showed upregulation of the remaining genes in at least two out of three cases analyzed, when compared with γδT-cells. Western blotting was applied to demonstrate expression of the *CHN2*-encoded β2-chimerin in four index cases (Table 1). As γδT-cells were not available, nonmalignant spleen was used as control. In addition, we analyzed Jurkat T-cells (positive control) [37] and i(7)(q10)-positive T-cell lymphoblastic lymphoma (Figure 3C). *B*2-chimerin was detected in all samples analyzed and its expression level in HSTL was higher than in spleen and ≥ than in Jurkat T-cells known to overexpress *CHN2*. The expression of the ABCB1 protein was demonstrated by IHC (Figure 5).

Mutation and fusion genes analysis

The obtained RNAseq data were subjected to mutation and gene fusion analysis. Three genes were found mutated in all 4 HSTL cases analyzed: *SEPT7* (7p14.2), *MAP4K5* (14q22.1) and *CYTH2* (19q13.33) (Table S9). However, all these mutations were predicted as benign or tolerated by VEP. Deleterious mutations were random (e.g. mutation of *ATM* in case 4). We did not detect any nonrandom indel except for Del-3'UTR (-/TCTC, chr7:29,550,568-29,550,571) in the *CHN2* gene. This deletion, however, was reported as SNP (rs71800296).

DeFuse revealed only four fusions, which were absent in nonmalignant spleen and thymus, and occurred in at least two cases (Table S10). Two of these fusions, LSP1->AC027612.6 and LL22NC03-80A10.6->RP11-236F9.4, involve either a gene with its pseudogene or two pseudogenes, respectively. The third fusion involves a sequence near an uncharacterized noncoding RNA (LOC402483) on chromosome 7q and a sequence (FLJ45340) on the telomere of chromosome 5q without gene annotation by UCSC or RefSeq. The fourth fusion, SEMA4D->RP11-156P1.3, was found in cases 4, 7 and DERL-2. An alternative fusion analysis performed with ArrayStudio did not reproduce the above mentioned fusions but identified four recurrent fusions (≥ two samples). Further analysis using the UCSC Blat tool suggested, however, that these fusions could be false positive predictions since at least one of the involved sequences align to the genome multiple times with 100 percent identity.

Discussion

Isochromosome 7q is a primary chromosomal aberration in HSTL detected in almost all affected individuals. The contribution of this aberration to the pathogenesis of disease is still unknown. Recent identification of r(7), a rare variant aberration in HSTL [11,13], provides an unique opportunity to narrow down the critical 7p/7q regions and identify the targeted genes. We set up a collaborative in-depth genomic study of six HSTL cases with i(7)(q10), including the DERL-2 cell line, and three cases with r(7). Using high resolution aCGH, we profiled all samples and defined a CDR (34.88 Mb) at 7p22.1p14.1 (3.48–38.36 Mb) and a CGR (38.77 Mb) at 7q22.11q31.1 (86.12–124.89 Mb) (Figure 1A). Interestingly, CGR encompasses a region of 13 Mb (86.25–99.27 Mb) selectively amplified in all three cases with r(7). In addition, aCGH mapped the r(7)-associated breakpoints within the *TCRG* (7p14.1) and *TCRB* (7q32) gene clusters, what suggests that r(7) is a byproduct of illegitimate somatic rearrangements of both loci. This defect results in an aberrant *TCRG-TCRB* lesion, formation of r(7) and a consequent loss of the distal 7p/7q regions (Figure 1B and Figure 2). Of note, similar inter-*TCR* rearrangements feature patients with chromosome instability syndromes [38]. We presume that formation of r(7) in γδT-cells was a primary event which was latter followed by a gradual gain of 7q sequences (Figure 2).

The compilation of all gained genomic data led us to hypothesize that loss of 7p22.1p14.1 is the critical pathogenetic event contributing to development of HSTL, while gain of 7q22.11q31.1 provides growth advantages and contributes to chemoresistance of the tumor. Significance of the former imbalance is supported by the cytogenetic finding of der(7)t(7;15)(p22;q21) associated with loss of 7p22pter (breakpoint not validated by FISH/aCGH) but not affecting 7q, in one case of i(7)(q10)-negative HSTL [14]. Chromosomal deletions, especially homozygous deletions, are considered as hallmarks of TSG localization in cancer cells [39]. Therefore, identification of a biallelic 7p21.3 microdeletion encompassing *PHF14*, a postulated TSG, in case 4 seemed to be the groundbreaking finding of the study. Particularly, that *PHF6*, other member of the PHF gene family, plays a role of tumor suppressor in T-ALL [40]. Subsequent investigations, including sequencing and MA/RNA-seq analysis, however, did not provide any evidence of inactivated mutation(s) or downregulated expression of *PHF14* in other HSTL cases.

To further attempt identification of genes targeted by i(7)(q10)/r(7), we performed an integrative genomic and transcriptomic analysis initially focusing on genes located within the common deleted (3.48–38.36 Mb) and gained (86.12–110.19 Mb) regions. Surprisingly, none of the CDR-associated genes was significantly and recurrently downregulated, however, one gene, *CHN2*, appeared to be commonly upregulated in HSTL. *CHN2* encodes β2-chimerin which displays GTPase-activating protein activity and is involved in small GTPase mediated signal transduction [41,42]. *B2*-chimerin is ubiquitously expressed in T-lymphocytes and engaged in the regulation of chemokine-modulated responses [41]. Recent studies implicate β2-chimerin in the downmodulation of RAC1 (ras-related C3 botulinum toxin substrate 1) activity during T-cell synapse formation and suggest its contribution to diacylglycerol-mediated regulation of cytoskeletal remodeling during T-cell activation [37,41,42]. Given the important role of β2-chimerin in T-cell biology, *CHN2* emerged as a candidate 7p gene targeted by i(7)(q10)/r(7) in HSTL. The molecular mechanism(s) underlying an enhanced expression of the nondeleted *CHN2* locus in HSTL is unclear, but either loss of 7p-associated negative regulators or gain/activation of 7q-associated positive regulators or deregulation of epigenetic effectors may contribute to this process. Interestingly, regulation data from the Encyclopedia of DNA Elements (ENCODE) (https://genome.ucsc.edu/ENCODE/) revealed several transcription factors regulating expression of *CHN2*, including EZH2, which targets the promotor region of *CHN2* (http://genome-euro.ucsc.edu/cgi-bin/

hgTracks?hgS_doOtherUser = submit&hgS_otherUserName = JulioFinalet&hgS_otherUserSessionName = regulation%20at%20 CHN2%20promotor_simple). EZH2, a catalytic subunit of the Polycomb Repressor Complex 2 [43], is involved in epigenetic transcriptional repression of genes through histone methylation and consequent chromatin condensation. As expression of *EZH2* is significantly downregulated in HSTL *vs* δγT-cells (FC = -3.012; FDR_BH = 0.0284), it may affect expression of *CHN2*. The *EZH2* gene (7q36.1) is not mutated in HSTL, but monoallelically deleted in all r(7)-positive cases.

Integrative analysis of chromosome 7q identified a set of 13 constantly upregulated genes, including *ABCB1, RUNDC3B* and *PPPAR9A*, found to be selectively amplified in cases with r(7). The top candidate is *ABCB1* (alias *MDR1*), already known to be overexpressed in HSTL [5,44]. *ABCB1* codes a multidrug transporter P-glycoprotein which belongs to the superfamily of ATP-binding cassette (ABC) transporters [45]. These molecules, which function in normal biology to protect cells from harmful toxins and xenobiotics, contribute to drug resistance of cancers by extruding a variety of chemotherapeutic agents from the tumor cells [46]. Amplification, rearrangement and/or overexpression of ABCB1 have been associated with chemotherapy failure in many cancers [47–51]. *RUNDC3B* is likely involved in multiple Ras-like GTPase signaling pathways [52,53] and is implicated in transformation and progression of breast cancer [54]. *PPP1R9A* encodes neurabin 1 which constitutes a regulatory subunit of protein phosphatase I [55]. Neurabin 1 is a multi-functional F-actin-binding protein, and like other phosphatases, is potentially implicated in tumorigenesis [56]. Although upregulation of *PEG10* was not constantly observed in HSTCL, it is worth note that this transcription factor is implicated in tumorigenesis [57–59]. *PEG10* is a postulated target of 7q21 amplification in hepatocellular carcinoma [59] and its overexpression in cancer correlates with disease progression, invasiveness and aggressiveness [57,60]. Altogether, these data support our hypothesis that the i(7)(q10)/r(7)-related duplication or amplification of 7q mainly activates genes which provide growth advantage of lymphoma cells and are responsible for an intrinsic drug resistance and aggressiveness of HSTL.

Gene expression profile of HSTL has been previously investigated by Miyazaki *et al.* (2009) [44] and Travert *et al.* [5]. The first group showed that the TCR-associated gene signature accurately classifies γδHSTL and distinguishes it from PTCL. The latter group demonstrated that HSTL is characterized by a distinct molecular signature, irrespective of the TCR-cell lineage. GEP revealed overexpression of multiple NK-cell-associated molecules and several cancer genes, including *FOS, VAV3, S1PR5* and *SYK*. Among the most downregulated genes was a tumor suppressor gene *AIM1*, found to be methylated in HSTL. Results of our transcriptomic analysis performed on altogether 17 HSTL cases (four index cases and 13 previously published cases [5,61]) are in line with the previous findings. Except for a few transcripts, we found the same differential expression of the vast majority of genes described by Travert *et al.* [5]. In addition, we significantly diminished a number of biomarkers discriminating HSTL from other malignancies to 24. Remarkably, the geneset comprises three chromosome 7 genes located either in CDR or CGR: *CHN2, ABCB1* and *PPP1R9A*.

Interestingly, IPA showed that the canonical pathway "Role of NFAT in regulation of the immune response" is one of the top dysregulated pathways in HSTL. NFAT is a family of transcription factors playing a crucial role in the development and function the immune system [29]. There are five NFAT family members and three of them, NFATC1, -C2 and -C3 are expressed by

T-cells and activated in response to TCR engagement. In resting T-cells, NFAT is located in the cytoplasm, in an inactive hyperphosphorylated form, associated with the NRON complex [31] Upon TCR engagement, NFAT disassociates from the complex and is rapidly dephosphorylated by the phosphatase calcineurin (Figure 6A). Activated NFAT translocates to the nucleus, where in cooperation with other transcriptional partners (e.g. FOS and JUN), it regulates transcription of a wide range of genes. NFAT responsive targets include numerous cytokine genes (IL2, IL3, IL4, IL5 and IFNG) and other genes involved in the control of the cell cycle and apoptosis (e.g. MYC, IKZF1, CDKN1A, CD40LG, FASLG, CDK4 and NR4A1) [26,62–66]. Recent studies strongly suggest an important role for the Ca^{2+}-calmodulin/calcineurin/NFAT signaling in tumor development and progression [27,28,63], and postulate that NFAT transcription factors may act either as oncogenes or TSG [67]. The latter function is assigned to NFATC2 (alias NFAT1 and NFATp), a postulated inhibitor of cell proliferation [63], which is significantly downregulated in HSTL (Table S7, Figure S5). Notably, mice deficient in NFATC2 showed hyperproliferation of lymphocytes, accompanied by a reduction in cell death and an increased cell cycle rate [64,68–71], whereas NFATC2-/NFATC3- double knock-out mice developed lymphoproliferative disorder with marked lymphadenopathy and splenomegaly, decreased activation-induced death and impaired Fas ligand induction [72]. Further studies demonstrated that NFATC2 suppresses neoplastic changes in chondrogenesis [73] and displays pro-apoptotic activity in Burkitt lymphoma [74]. Its ectopic expression in NIH3T3 cells results in cell cycle arrest, apoptosis and inhibition of Rasv12-mediated malignant transformation [67]. NFATC2 also controls the cell-cycle progression by repressing expression of the G0–G1 checkpoint kinase CDK4 and cyclins A2, BA, E and F [75–77], and induces apoptosis in NIH3T3 fibroblasts in cooperation with the Ras/Raf/MEK/ERK pathway [63]. Recently, it was reported that haploinsufficiency of NFATC2 contributes to the pathogenesis of essential thrombocythemia with del(20q) [78]. In this context, particularly interesting is the study of Caloca et al. (2008) linking the Ca^{2+}-calmodulin/calcineurin/NFAT pathway with β2-chimerin [37]. The authors showed that an experimental overexpression of β2-chimerin in Jurkat T-cells stimulated by anti-CD3 antibodies significantly inhibits the transcriptional activity of NFATC2. This is caused by β2-chimerin-mediated reduction in the levels of active, GTP-bound, RAC1. As demonstrated previously, activated RAC1 modulates calcineurin and consequently, regulates nuclear import and transcriptional function of NFAT [79].

Based on the published data summarized above, IPA (gene interactions and pathways) and our own data, we propose a hypothetical model for the molecular pathogenesis of HSTL (Figure 6A-B). We presume that defects in the NFAT pathway, reflected by the i(7)(q10)/r(7)-associated overexpression of CHN2/β2-chimerin, downregulation of NFATC2 and dysregulation of several NFAT/NRON-related genes (Figure 6C), may collectively lead to a downmodulation of the transcriptional activity of NFATC2. This ultimately results in a transcriptional dysregulation of NFATC2 targets, including genes controlling cell cycle, cell death and proliferation [e.g., MYC (↑) and IKZF1 (↓)], and likely NFATC2 itself, and eventually to malignant proliferation of γδT-cells.

In summary, our study provides further insight on the genetics and the pathogenic mechanisms of HSTL. We proved that HSTL cases harboring either a typical i(7)(q10) or variant r(7) are characterized by a constant loss of 7p22.1p14.1 and gain of 7q22.11q31.1. As RNAseq has not identified any disease-defining

mutations and/or gene fusions, chromosome 7 imbalances remain the only driver genetic events found in this tumor. Based on the integrated genomic and transcriptomic data, we hypothesize that loss of 7p sequences is critical for the development of HSTL. This aberration associates with an enhanced transcription of CHN2 and overexpression of β2-chimerin, what likely affects the NFATC2 related pathway and leads to a proliferative response. On the other hand, gain of 7q correlates with upregulation of several genes, including ABCB1, RUNDC3B and PPP1R9A, providing growth advantage to malignant cells and contributing to their intrinsic chemoresistance and aggressiveness. The latter process is probably also enhanced by genes activated by the frequently acquired trisomy 8, the set of dysregulated molecules previously discussed by Travert et al. (2012) [5] and by an impaired immune synapse formation in neoplastic δγT-cells caused by an overexpressed β2-chimerin and a downmodulated RAC1 [80]. The proposed here model of the pathogenesis of HSTL needs experimental validation. Further studies are also required to determine whether the mechanism(s) underlying the i(7q)/r(7)-driven pathogenesis of human HSTL are related to the id3-driven neoplastic transformation of murine γδT-cells [81].

Supporting Information

Figure S1   Unsupervised Spectral Map Analysis using the microarray data. Samples are separated according to their original classification (A) regardless of the lab of origin (B). The dots in grey ("variable") represent microarray probes. Note that HSTL separates from other T/NK cell malignancies and cluster near the spleen samples (reflecting the tissue of origin). The spreading across component one of some HSTL samples is related to the purity of the samples (C). Note that HSTL cases with sorted lymphoma cells cluster near the sorted normal T-cells. Interpretation of this analysis is similar to a principal component analysis (details in: www.vetstat.ugent.be/workshop/Nairobi2004/Bijnens/Bijnens2004.pdf). The values between parentheses in the axes mean the percentage of the total number of variables (here, microarrays probes) that contributes to the variance in a given direction (or component).

Figure S2   Principal Component Analysis (PCA) using the RNAseq data. The HSTL samples cluster separately from the T-ALL, PTCL and spleen samples. The values between parentheses in the axes mean the percentage of the total number of variables (here, microarrays probes) that contributes to the variance in a given direction (or component).

Figure S3   IPA canonical pathway "Role of NFAT in regulating the immune response": HSTL vs δγT-cells. The fold change values from the inference analysis of HSTL vs δγT-cells were overlaid in this pathway. The red color reflects a positive fold change (in this case, upregulation in HSTL as compared to δγT-cells) and green means negative fold change. Double circles represent a complex of molecules and a green to red gradient means that some components in the complex are downregulated while others are upregulated.

Figure S4   Top dysregulated canonical pathways resulting from individual analysis in IPA. The bold numbers mean the number of molecules involved in a given pathway. The percentage value on the top of the graph means the percentage of dysregulated molecules from the total number of molecules involved in the pathway. Pathways for a given analysis are ranked

from higher to lower statistical significance. The statistical significance (p-value) of a given pathway is calculated considering the percentage of dysregulated molecules in the pathways, as well as the fold change of dysregulation.
(PDF)

Figure S5 Expression of selected genes analyzed by QRT-PCR. The Y-axis represents the fold change of normalized mRNA expression compared to δγT-cells.

Figure S6 High resolution images of hierarchical clustering using the 24 gene signature for HSTL. The dendograms were generated using the Pearson correlation to calculate the distance and a complete link. The associated heatmap was normalized using a robust center scale.

Table S1 List of FISH probes.

Table S2 List of primers used for sequencing and QRT-PCR.

Table S3 List of cases included in the expression microarray analysis.

Table S4 Segment report from the aCGH data.

Table S5 Aligment report of RNAseq analysis of HSTL, PTCL, spleen and thymus.

Table S6 Dysregulated genes in CDR (7p) and CGR (7q).

Table S7 Genomewide dysregulated genes in 10 comparisons (XLSX).

Table S8 IPA functional annotation of genes included in the HSTL signature.

Table S9 Annotated mutations found in the index cases analyzed by RNAseq.

Table S10 Results of the gene fusion analysis.

Acknowledgments

The authors would like to thank Stein Aerts, Rekin's Janky and Luc Dehaspe for a bioinformatic support, Ursula Pluys and Emilie Bittoun for their excellent technical assistance, Dominik Selleslag, Vincent Maertens and Clément Huysentruyt for providing clinical data, Philippe Gaulard for providing the DERL-2 cell line, and Rita Logist for her editorial assistance.

Author Contributions

Conceived and designed the experiments: JFF JC IW. Performed the experiments: JFF LR HU J-AvdK T. Tousseyn. Analyzed the data: JFF LR LM T. Tousseyn JC IW. Contributed reagents/materials/analysis tools: SS LK T. Tousseyn PDP AU GV PV T. Tabhon. Contributed to the writing of the manuscript: JFF PV IW.

References

1. Tripodo C, Iannitto E, Florena AM, Pucillo CE, Piccaluga PP, et al. (2009) Gamma-delta T-cell lymphomas. Nat Rev Clin Oncol 6: 707–717.
2. Swerdlow SH, Campo E, Harris NL, Jaffe ES, Pileri SA, et al. (2008) WHO Classification of Tumours of Haematopoietic and Lymphoid Tissues. Lyon, France: IARC.
3. Macon WR, Levy NB, Kurtin PJ, Salhany KE, Elkhalifa MY, et al. (2001) Hepatosplenic alphabeta T-cell lymphomas: a report of 14 cases and comparison with hepatosplenic gammadelta T-cell lymphomas. Am J Surg Pathol 25: 285–296.
4. Suarez F, Wlodarska I, Rigal-Huguet F, Mempel M, Martin-Garcia N, et al. (2000) Hepatosplenic alphabeta T-cell lymphoma: an unusual case with clinical, histologic, and cytogenetic features of gammadelta hepatosplenic T-cell lymphoma. Am J Surg Pathol 24: 1027–1032.
5. Travert M, Huang Y, de Leval L, Martin-Garcia N, Delfau-Larue MH, et al. (2012) Molecular features of hepatosplenic T-cell lymphoma unravels potential novel therapeutic targets. Blood 119: 5795–5806.
6. Gaulard P, Jaffe E, Krenacs L, Macon WR (2008) Hepatosplenic T-cell lymphoma. In: Swerdlow SH, Campo E, Harris NL, Jaffe ES, Pileri SA, et al., editors. WHO Classification of Tumours of Haematopoietic and Lymphoid Tissues. Lyon, France: IARC. pp. 292–293.
7. Wang CC, Tien HF, Lin MT, Su IJ, Wang CH, et al. (1995) Consistent presence of isochromosome 7q in hepatosplenic T gamma/delta lymphoma: a new cytogenetic-clinicopathologic entity. Genes Chromosomes Cancer 12: 161–164.
8. Alonsozana EL, Stamberg J, Kumar D, Jaffe ES, Medeiros LJ, et al.(1997) Isochromosome 7q: the primary cytogenetic abnormality in hepatosplenic gammadelta T cell lymphoma. Leukemia 11: 1367–1372.
9. Jonveaux P, Daniel MT, Martel V, Maarek O, Berger R (1996) Isochromosome 7q and trisomy 8 are consistent primary, non-random chromosomal abnormalities associated with hepatosplenic T gamma/delta lymphoma. Leukemia 10: 1453–1455.
10. Wlodarska I, Martin-Garcia N, Achten R, De Wolf-Peeters C, Pauwels P, et al. (2002) Fluorescence in situ hybridization study of chromosome 7 aberrations in hepatosplenic T-cell lymphoma: isochromosome 7q as a common abnormality accumulating in forms with features of cytologic progression. Genes Chromosomes Cancer 33: 243–251.
11. Shetty S, Mansoor A, Roland B (2006) Ring chromosome 7 with amplification of 7q sequences in a pediatric case of hepatosplenic T-cell lymphoma. Cancer Genet Cytogenet 167: 161–163.
12. Patkar N, Nair S, Alex AA, Parihar M, Manipadam MT, et al. (2012) Clinicopathological features of hepatosplenic T cell lymphoma: a single centre experience from India. Leuk Lymphoma 53: 609–615.
13. Tamaska J, Adam E, Kozma A, Gopcsa L, Andrikovics H, et al. (2006) Hepatosplenic gammadelta T-cell lymphoma with ring chromosome 7, an isochromosome 7q equivalent clonal chromosomal aberration. Virchows Arch 449: 479–483.
14. Mandava S, Sonar R, Ahmad F, Yadav AK, Chheda P, et al. (2011) Cytogenetic and molecular characterization of a hepatosplenic T-cell lymphoma: report of a novel chromosomal aberration. Cancer Genet 204: 103–107.
15. Rossbach HC, Chamizo W, Dumont DP, Barbosa JL, Sutcliffe MJ (2002) Hepatosplenic gamma/delta T-cell lymphoma with isochromosome 7q, translocation t(7;21), and tetrasomy 8 in a 9-year-old girl. J Pediatr Hematol Oncol 24: 154–157.
16. Lewi PJ (1976) Spectral mapping, a technique for classifying biological activity profiles of chemical compounds. Arzneimittelforschung 26: 1295–1300.
17. Hu J, Ge H, Newman M, Liu K (2012) OSA: a fast and accurate alignment tool for RNA-Seq. Bioinformatics 28: 1933–1934.
18. Anders S, Huber W (2010) Differential expression analysis for sequence count data. Genome Biol 11: R106. gb-2010-11-10-r106 [pii];10.1186/gb-2010-11-10-r106 [doi].
19. Kalender AZ, Gianfelici V, Hulselmans G, De KK, Devasia AG, et al. (2013) Comprehensive analysis of transcriptome variation uncovers known and novel driver events in T-cell acute lymphoblastic leukemia. PLoS Genet 9: e1003997. 10.1371/journal.pgen.1003997 [doi];PGENETICS-D-13-01641 [pii].
20. McPherson A, Hormozdiari F, Zayed A, Giuliany R, Ha G, et al. (2011) deFuse: an algorithm for gene fusion discovery in tumor RNA-Seq data. PLoS Comput Biol 7: e1001138. 10.1371/journal.pcbi.1001138 [doi];10-PLCB-RA-2589R4 [pii].
21. Ge H, Liu K, Juan T, Fang F, Newman M, et al.(2011) FusionMap: detecting fusion genes from next-generation sequencing data at base-pair resolution. Bioinformatics 27: 1922–1928.
22. Di Noto R, Pane F, Camera A, Luciano L, Barone M, et al.(2001) Characterization of two novel cell lines, DERL-2 (CD56+/CD3+/Tcry5+) and DERL-7 (CD56+/CD3-/TCRgammadelta-), derived from a single patient with CD56+ non-Hodgkin's lymphoma. Leukemia 15: 1641–1649.
23. Ivanov I, Lo KC, Hawthorn L, Cowell JK, Ionov Y (2007) Identifying candidate colon cancer tumor suppressor genes using inhibition of nonsense-mediated mRNA decay in colon cancer cells. Oncogene 26: 2873–2884.

24. Akazawa T, Yasui K, Gen Y, Yamada N, Tomie A, et al. (2013) Aberrant expression of the gene in biliary tract cancer cells. Oncol Lett 5: 1849–1853.

25. Kitagawa M, Takebe A, Ono Y, Imai T, Nakao K, et al. (2012) Phf14, a novel regulator of mesenchyme growth via platelet-derived growth factor (PDGF) receptor-alpha1. J Biol Chem 287: 27983–27996.

26. Viola JP, Carvalho LD, Fonseca BP, Teixeira LK (2005) NFAT transcription factors: from cell cycle to tumor development. Braz J Med Biol Res 38: 335–344.

27. Muller MR, Rao A (2010) NFAT, immunity and cancer: a transcription factor comes of age. Nat Rev Immunol 10: 645–656.

28. Mancini M, Toker A (2009) NFAT proteins: emerging roles in cancer progression. Nat Rev Cancer 9: 810–820.

29. Macian F (2005) NFAT proteins: key regulators of T-cell development and function. Nat Rev Immunol 5: 472–484.

30. Willingham AT, Orth AP, Batalov S, Peters EC, Wen BG, et al. (2005) A strategy for probing the function of noncoding RNAs finds a repressor of NFAT. Science 309: 1570–1573.

31. Sharma S, Findlay GM, Bandukwala HS, Oberdoerffer S, Baust B, et al. (2011) Dephosphorylation of the nuclear factor of activated T cells (NFAT) transcription factor is regulated by an RNA-protein scaffold complex. Proc Natl Acad Sci U S A 108: 11381–11386.

32. Jabri B, Barreiro LB (2011) Don't move: LRRK2 arrests NFAT in the cytoplasm. Nat Immunol 12: 1029–1030.

33. Liu Z, Lee J, Krummey S, Lu W, Cai H, et al. (2011) The kinase LRRK2 is a regulator of the transcription factor NFAT that modulates the severity of inflammatory bowel disease. Nat Immunol 12: 1063–1070.

34. Racioppi L, Means AR (2008) Calcium/calmodulin-dependent kinase IV in immune and inflammatory responses: novel routes for an ancient traveller. Trends Immunol 29: 600–607.

35. Hanissian SH, Frangakis M, Bland MM, Jawahar S, Chatila TA (1993) Expression of a Ca2+/calmodulin-dependent protein kinase, CaM kinase-Gr, in human T lymphocytes. Regulation of kinase activity by T cell receptor signaling. J Biol Chem 268: 20055–20063.

36. Sims TN, Dustin ML (2002) The immunological synapse: integrins take the stage. Immunol Rev 186: 100–117.

37. Caloca MJ, Delgado P, Alarcon B, Bustelo XR (2008) Role of chimaerins, a group of Rac-specific GTPase activating proteins, in T-cell receptor signaling. Cell Signal 20: 758–770.

38. Taylor AM (2001) Chromosome instability syndromes. Best Pract Res Clin Haematol 14: 631–644.

39. Mestre-Escorihuela C, Rubio-Moscardo F, Richter JA, Siebert R, Climent J, et al. (2007) Homozygous deletions localize novel tumor suppressor genes in B-cell lymphomas. Blood 109: 271–280.

40. Van Vlierberghe P, Palomero T, Khiabanian H, Van der Meulen J, Castillo M, et al. (2010) PHF6 mutations in T-cell acute lymphoblastic leukemia. Nat Genet 42: 338–342.

41. Siliceo M, Garcia-Bernal D, Carrasco S, Diaz-Flores E, Coluccio LF, et al. (2006) Beta2-chimaerin provides a diacylglycerol-dependent mechanism for regulation of adhesion and chemotaxis of T cells. J Cell Sci 119: 141–152.

42. Siliceo M, Merida I (2009) T cell receptor-dependent tyrosine phosphorylation of beta2-chimaerin modulates its Rac-GAP function in T cells. J Biol Chem 284: 11354–11363.

43. Deb G, Singh AK, Gupta S (2014) EZH2: Not EZHY (Easy) to Deal. Mol Cancer Res e-pub ahead of print. 1541-7786.MCR-13-0546 [pii];10.1158/1541-7786.MCR-13-0546 [doi].

44. Miyazaki K, Yamaguchi M, Imai H, Kobayashi T, Tamaru S, et al.(2009) Gene expression profiling of peripheral T-cell lymphoma including gammadelta T-cell lymphoma. Blood 113: 1071–1074.

45. Gottesman MM, Pastan I, Ambudkar SV (1996) P-glycoprotein and multidrug resistance. Curr Opin Genet Dev 6: 610–617.

46. Szakacs G, Paterson JK, Ludwig JA, Booth-Genthe C, Gottesman MM (2006) Targeting multidrug resistance in cancer. Nat Rev Drug Discov 5: 219–234.

47. Holohan C, Van SS, Longley DB, Johnston PG (2013) Cancer drug resistance: an evolving paradigm. Nat Rev Cancer 13: 714–726.

48. Huff LM, Lee JS, Robey RW, Fojo T (2006) Characterization of gene rearrangements leading to activation of MDR-1. J Biol Chem 281: 36501–36509.

49. Knutsen T, Mickley LA, Ried T, Green ED, du MS, et al. (1998) Cytogenetic and molecular characterization of random chromosomal rearrangements activating the drug resistance gene, MDR1/P-glycoprotein, in drug-selected cell lines and patients with drug refractory ALL. Genes Chromosomes Cancer 23: 44–54.

50. Wang YC, Juric D, Francisco B, Yu RX, Duran GE, et al. (2006) Regional activation of chromosomal arm 7q with and without gene amplification in taxane-selected human ovarian cancer cell lines. Genes Chromosomes Cancer 45: 365–374.

51. Wang J, Tai LS, Tzang CH, Fong WF, Guan XY, et al. (2008) 1p31, 7q21 and 18q21 chromosomal aberrations and candidate genes in acquired vinblastine resistance of human cervical carcinoma KB cells. Oncol Rep 19: 1155–1164.

52. Balaguer TM, Gomez-Martinez A, Garcia-Morales P, Lacueva J, Calpena R, et al. (2012) Dual regulation of P-glycoprotein expression by trichostatin A in cancer cell lines. BMC Mol Biol 13: 25. 1471-2199-13-25 [pii];10.1186/1471-2199-13-25 [doi].

53. Wang S, Zhang Z, Ying K, Chen JZ, Meng XF, et al. (2003) Cloning, expression, and genomic structure of a novel human Rap2 interacting gene (RPIP9). Biochem Genet 41: 13–25.

54. Raguz S, De Bella MT, Slade MJ, Higgins CF, Coombes RC, et al. (2005) Expression of RPIP9 (Rap2 interacting protein 9) is activated in breast carcinoma and correlates with a poor prognosis. Int J Cancer 117: 934–941.

55. Nakabayashi K, Makino S, Minagawa S, Smith AC, Bamford JS, et al. (2004) Genomic imprinting of PPP1R9A encoding neurabin I in skeletal muscle and extra-embryonic tissues. J Med Genet 41: 601–608.

56. McCluskey A, Ackland SP, Gardiner E, Walkom CC, Sakoff JA (2001) The inhibition of protein phosphatases 1 and 2A: a new target for rational anti-cancer drug design? Anticancer Drug Des 16: 291–303.

57. Ip WK, Lai PB, Wong NL, Sy SM, Beheshti B, et al. (2007) Identification of PEG10 as a progression related biomarker for hepatocellular carcinoma. Cancer Lett 250: 284–291.

58. Tsou AP, Chuang YC, Su JY, Yang CW, Liao YL, et al. (2003) Overexpression of a novel imprinted gene, PEG10, in human hepatocellular carcinoma and in regenerating mouse livers. J Biomed Sci 10: 625–635.

59. Tsuji K, Yasui K, Gen Y, Endo M, Dohi O, et al. (2010) PEG10 is a probable target for the amplification at 7q21 detected in hepatocellular carcinoma. Cancer Genet Cytogenet 198: 118–125.

60. Kainz B, Shehata M, Bilban M, Kienle D, Heintel D, et al. (2007) Overexpression of the paternally expressed gene 10 (PEG10) from the imprinted locus on chromosome 7q21 in high-risk B-cell chronic lymphocytic leukemia. Int J Cancer 121: 1984–1993.

61. Iqbal J, Weisenburger DD, Chowdhury A, Tsai MY, Srivastava G, et al.(2011) Natural killer cell lymphoma shares strikingly similar molecular features with a group of non-hepatosplenic gammadelta T-cell lymphoma and is highly sensitive to a novel aurora kinase A inhibitor in vitro. Leukemia 25: 348–358.

62. Zheng J, Fang F, Zeng X, Medler TR, Fiorillo AA, et al. (2011) Negative cross talk between NFAT1 and Stat5 signaling in breast cancer. Mol Endocrinol 25: 2054–2064.

63. Robbs BK, Lucena PI, Viola JP (2013) The transcription factor NFAT1 induces apoptosis through cooperation with Ras/Raf/MEK/ERK pathway and upregulation of TNF-alpha expression. Biochim Biophys Acta 1833: 2016–2028.

64. Daniel C, Gerlach K, Vath M, Neurath MF, Weigmann B (2013) Nuclear factor of activated T cells-A transcription factor family as critical regulator in lung and colon cancer. Int J Cancer. 10.1002/ijc.28329 [doi].

65. Mognol GP, de Araujo-Souza PS, Robbs BK, Teixeira LK, Viola JP (2012) Transcriptional regulation of the c-Myc promoter by NFAT1 involves negative and positive NFAT-responsive elements. Cell Cycle 11: 1014–1028.

66. Macian F, Garcia-Cozar F, Im SH, Horton HF, Byrne MC, et al. (2002) Transcriptional mechanisms underlying lymphocyte tolerance. Cell 109: 719–731.

67. Robbs BK, Cruz AL, Werneck MB, Mognol GP, Viola JP (2008) Dual roles for NFAT transcription factor genes as oncogenes and tumor suppressors. Mol Cell Biol 28: 7168–7181.

68. Hodge MR, Ranger AM, Charles dlB, Hoey T, Grusby MJ, Glimcher LH (1996) Hyperproliferation and dysregulation of IL-4 expression in NF-ATp-deficient mice. Immunity 4: 397–405.

69. Caetano MS, Vieira-de-Abreu A, Teixeira LK, Werneck MB, Barcinski MA, et al. (2002) NFATC2 transcription factor regulates cell cycle progression during lymphocyte activation: evidence of its involvement in the control of cyclin gene expression. FASEB J 16: 1940–1942.

70. Schuh K, Kneitz B, Heyer J, Bommhardt U, Jankevics E, et al.(1998) Retarded thymic involution and massive germinal center formation in NF-ATp-deficient mice. Eur J Immunol 28: 2456–2466.

71. Xanthoudakis S, Viola JP, Shaw KT, Luo C, Wallace JD, et al.(1996) An enhanced immune response in mice lacking the transcription factor NFAT1. Science 272: 892–895.

72. Ranger AM, Oukka M, Rengarajan J, Glimcher LH (1998) Inhibitory function of two NFAT family members in lymphoid homeostasis and Th2 development. Immunity 9: 627–635.

73. Ranger AM, Gerstenfeld LC, Wang J, Kon T, Bae H, et al.(2000) The nuclear factor of activated T cells (NFAT) transcription factor NFATp (NFATc2) is a repressor of chondrogenesis. J Exp Med 191: 9–22.

74. Kondo E, Harashima A, Takabatake T, Takahashi H, Matsuo Y, et al. (2003) NF-ATc2 induces apoptosis in Burkitt's lymphoma cells through signaling via the B cell antigen receptor. Eur J Immunol 33: 1–11.

75. Baksh S, Widlund HR, Frazer-Abel AA, Du J, Fosmire S, et al. (2002) NFATc2-mediated repression of cyclin-dependent kinase 4 expression. Mol Cell 10: 1071–1081.

76. Carvalho LD, Teixeira LK, Carrossini N, Caldeira AT, Ansel KM, et al. (2007) The NFAT1 transcription factor is a repressor of cyclin A2 gene expression. Cell Cycle 6: 1789–1795.

77. Caetano MS, Vieira-de-Abreu A, Teixeira LK, Werneck MB, Barcinski MA, et al. (2002) NFATC2 transcription factor regulates cell cycle progression during lymphocyte activation: evidence of its involvement in the control of cyclin gene expression. FASEB J 16: 1940–1942.

78. Vieira L, Vaz A, Matos P, Ambrosio AP, Nogueira M, et al. (2012) Three-way translocation (X;20;16)(p11;q13;q23) in essential thrombocythemia implicates NFATC2 in dysregulation of CSF2 expression and megakaryocyte proliferation. Genes Chromosomes Cancer 51: 1093–1108.

79. Turner H, Gomez M, McKenzie E, Kirchem A, Lennard A, et al. (1998) Rac-1 regulates nuclear factor of activated T cells (NFAT) C1 nuclear translocation in response to Fcepsilon receptor type 1 stimulation of mast cells. J Exp Med 188: 527–537.

80. Ritter AT, Angus KL, Griffiths GM (2013) The role of the cytoskeleton at the immunological synapse. Immunol Rev 256: 107–117.

81. Li J, Maruyama T, Zhang P, Konkel JE, Hoffman V, et al.(2010) Mutation of inhibitory helix-loop-helix protein Id3 causes gammadelta T-cell lymphoma in mice. Blood 116: 5615–5621.

82. Jacquemet G, Morgan MR, Byron A, Humphries JD, Choi CK, et al. (2013) Rac1 is deactivated at integrin activation sites through an IQGAP1-filamin-A-RacGAP1 pathway. J Cell Sci 126: 4121–4135.

83. Fukata M, Kuroda S, Nakagawa M, Kawajiri A, Itoh N, et al. (1999) Cdc42 and Rac1 regulate the interaction of IQGAP1 with beta-catenin. J Biol Chem 274: 26044–26050.

84. Shaffer LG, MwGowan-Jordan J, Schmid M (2013) ISCN An International System for Human Cytogenetic Nomenclature (2013). Basel: S. Karger.

3

Characterization of Changes in Gene Expression and Biochemical Pathways at Low Levels of Benzene Exposure

Reuben Thomas[1]*, Alan E. Hubbard[1], Cliona M. McHale[1], Luoping Zhang[1], Stephen M. Rappaport[1], Qing Lan[2], Nathaniel Rothman[2], Roel Vermeulen[4], Kathryn Z. Guyton[3], Jennifer Jinot[3], Babasaheb R. Sonawane[3], Martyn T. Smith[1]

1 Superfund Research Program, School of Public Health, University of California, Berkeley, California, United States of America, 2 Division of Cancer Epidemiology and Genetics, National Cancer Institute, National Institutes of Health, Bethesda, Maryland, United States of America, 3 National Center for Environmental Assessment, Office of Research and Development, US EPA, Washington, DC, United States of America, 4 Institute of Risk assessment Sciences, Utrecht University, Utrecht, The Netherlands

Abstract

Benzene, a ubiquitous environmental pollutant, causes acute myeloid leukemia (AML). Recently, through transcriptome profiling of peripheral blood mononuclear cells (PBMC), we reported dose-dependent effects of benzene exposure on gene expression and biochemical pathways in 83 workers exposed across four airborne concentration ranges (from <1 ppm to > 10 ppm) compared with 42 subjects with non-workplace ambient exposure levels. Here, we further characterize these dose-dependent effects with continuous benzene exposure in all 125 study subjects. We estimated air benzene exposure levels in the 42 environmentally-exposed subjects from their unmetabolized urinary benzene levels. We used a novel non-parametric, data-adaptive model selection method to estimate the change with dose in the expression of each gene. We describe non-parametric approaches to model pathway responses and used these to estimate the dose responses of the AML pathway and 4 other pathways of interest. The response patterns of majority of genes as captured by mean estimates of the first and second principal components of the dose-response for the five pathways and the profiles of 6 AML pathway response-representative genes (identified by clustering) exhibited similar apparent supra-linear responses. Responses at or below 0.1 ppm benzene were observed for altered expression of AML pathway genes and *CYP2E1*. Together, these data show that benzene alters disease-relevant pathways and genes in a dose-dependent manner, with effects apparent at doses as low as 100 ppb in air. Studies with extensive exposure assessment of subjects exposed in the low-dose range between 10 ppb and 1 ppm are needed to confirm these findings.

Editor: Shyamal D. Peddada, National Institute of Environmental and Health Sciences, United States of America

Funding: Original data generated through funding from National Institutes of Health grants R01ES01896 and P42 ES004705 from the National Institute of Environmental Health Sciences with additional statistical analyses being funded in part by Environment Protection Agency contract number EP-11-001398. The funders had no role in study design, data collection and analysis, decision to publish, or preparation of the manuscript.

Competing Interests: S.M.R. has received consulting and expert testimony fees from law firms representing plaintiffs' cases involving exposure to benzene and has received research support from the American Petroleum Institute and the American Chemistry Council. M.T.S. has received consulting and expert testimony fees from law firms representing both plaintiffs and defendants in cases involving exposure to benzene. The other authors declare they have no actual or potential competing financial interests. Alan Hubbard is an Associate Editor of this journal.

* E-mail: reuben.thomas@berkeley.edu

Introduction

Benzene is a component of gasoline, and the starting ingredient in the production of plastics and polymers via styrene; of resins and adhesives via phenol; and, in the manufacture of nylon via cyclohexane. It is toxic to the bone marrow and is associated with various hematological cancers [1,2].

Multiple possible mechanisms of action are thought to be involved in benzene toxicity [3,4,5,6]. Benzene exposure has been shown to cause hematotoxicity [7], induce formation of protein adducts [8,9], and increase the risk of leukemia [10], in a dose-dependent manner. Linear or supra-linear dose-dependent effects on lymphocyte counts and colony formation from myeloid stem and progenitor cells and gene expression were reported at relatively low levels of occupational exposure (≤1 ppm to >

10 ppm) in exposed human populations [7,11,12]. Recently, through transcriptome profiling of peripheral blood mononuclear cells (PBMC), we reported dose-dependent effects of benzene on gene expression and biochemical pathways in 83 workers exposed to air benzene levels across four concentration ranges (from < 1 ppm to >10 ppm), compared with 42 subjects not occupationally exposed to benzene [13]. A 16-gene signature associated with all levels of benzene exposure exhibited an apparently supra-linear dose response. In addition, several immune response-related pathways and the pathway associated with AML were significantly modulated across several of the benzene dose ranges examined.

A deeper understanding of the dose-dependent, disease-relevant human biochemical responses resulting from benzene exposure, particularly at low doses, is important for next generation approaches to human health risk assessment. Therefore, the goal of the current study was to further characterize the dose-dependency of low-dose effects of benzene on genes and biochemical pathways identified in our recent benzene-related microarray analyses of PBMC [13]. Specifically, continuous data for individual benzene exposure across all dose groups was used to generate dose-response curves on a continuous scale. We used predicted measures of benzene exposure in the group of subjects with only ambient exposure to benzene. These subjects were regarded as controls in the previous study but were, in fact, non-occupationally exposed to benzene at varying, relatively low environmental concentrations. Inclusion of data from these individuals allowed us to examine more closely the responses in the low dose (environmental) region of exposure. Using data from all 125 study subjects, we applied non-parametric approaches, based on the SuperLearner [14], to fit the responses of individual gene expression as a function of benzene exposure. The use of non-parametric approaches is particularly relevant here and in epidemiological studies in general because it is impossible to know the exact functional relationships among the variables such as gene expression, dose from exposure, age, gender and smoking status of the subject, cell counts etc. Non-parametric approaches make minimal assumptions about these functional relationships and let the observed data guide the choice of the best models using rigorous statistical criteria (e.g., cross-validation [14]). The implication of making parametric assumptions is that if these assumptions are untrue (which is almost certainly the case), the results produced can be difficult to interpret. In the current study, we developed novel non-parametric approaches to model the responses in biochemical pathways of interest. We chose to model the responses in 5 pathways, including the AML pathway and two other pathways previously shown to be modified by benzene, and two pathways presumably unrelated to benzene exposure. We also employed the models to examine dose-response relationships in the expression of a set of candidate genes known to be associated with AML and with the metabolism of benzene.

The overall goals of this study were to estimate the benzene exposure-response patterns of relevant gene expression and biochemical pathways in a statistically rigorous, non-parametric manner. This approach allowed us to identify consistencies in the shapes of the resulting exposure-response curves and characterize responses particularly in the low-dose region of exposure. Since our original microarray data were generated from PBMCs which comprise various cell types [15], including T lymphocytes (CD4 and CD8 ~65%), B cells (~15%), natural Killer cells (~10%), and monocytes (~10%), we adjusted for changes in percentages of these subtypes after benzene exposure in our analyses.

Materials and Methods

A brief overview of the data and methods used is given in Figureô 1.

Data Sets

Ethics statement. This study complied with all applicable requirements of U.S. and Chinese regulations, including institutional review board approval at the National Cancer Institute, Bethesda, Maryland USA and the National Institute of Occupational Health and Poison Control, China CDC, Beijing. Participation was voluntary, and written informed consent was obtained.

Study population, hematotoxicity, and gene expression data. The overall molecular epidemiology studies investigating occupational exposure to benzene [7,16] and the gene expression data [13] upon which the analyses in the current study are based were previously described. The gene expression data were generated through transcriptome analysis by microarray of 125 subjects exposed to various levels of benzene. Among the 125 subjects, 42 were exposed to levels that were below the limit of detection of the benzene monitors (0.04 ppm) used; 29 were exposed to <<1 ppm (average <1 ppm and most individual measurements <1 ppm) benzene; 30 were exposed to <1 ppm (average <1 ppm); 11 were exposed to levels between 5 ppm and 10 ppm; and 13 were exposed to levels ≥10 ppm. For each of the exposed individuals in the study, benzene exposure was estimated in terms of the average air-benzene level (in units of parts-per-million). The exposure levels of the 42 subjects that were below the limit of detection were estimated using unmetabolized urinary benzene levels, as previously described [17]. Complete blood cell counts, including counts for CD4 and CD8 T lymphocytes, B lymphocytes, NK cells and monocytes, the major cell subsets of PBMCs, were available for all the individuals analyzed by microarray [7].

Biochemical Pathways

The biochemical pathways analyzed in this study were obtained from the Kyoto Encyclopedia of Genes and Genomes (KEGG) Pathway database [18,19,20]. The data for the set of genes within each pathway and their associated interactions were downloaded using the KEGG application programming interface (http://www.kegg.jp/kegg/soap/). Five pathways were analyzed, including three (AML, B-cell receptor signaling and Toll-like receptor signaling) previously shown to be differentially modulated with benzene exposure [13] and two (Steroid hormone biosynthesis and Maturity onset of diabetes) presumably unrelated to benzene exposure were not differentially modulated.

Linear Mixed Effect Models

We conducted variance components analysis using a linear mixed model [21] to assess the proportion of total variation due to differences between subjects, hybridizations, labels, and chips, both before and after normalization [quantile normalization in the Affy package [22] in R [23]]. For each probe, we estimated the association between exposure level and expression level using a mixed-effects model with random intercepts that accounted for clustering by subject, hybridization, and label. The fixed effects in our model included gender (1 = male, 0 = female), current smoking status (1 = yes, 0 = no), age (in years, linear term), B cells, Natural Killer (NK) cells, monocytes, and CD4 and CD8 cells (as counts and included as linear terms). These were potential confounders of associations (denoted by the vector of random variables, W) between logarithm to the base 2 of gene expression (denoted by the random variable, Y) and benzene exposure in five dose ranges (denoted by the random variable, A). The model is thus given by,

$$Y_{ijklm}^g = \beta_0^g a_i + \beta_1^g + \beta_2^g (sex_j) + \beta_3^g (smoke_j) + \beta_4^g (age_j)$$
$$+ \beta_5^g (\#B\,cells_j) + \beta_6^g (\#NK\,cells_j) + \beta_7^g (\#monocytes_j)$$
$$+ \beta_8^g (\#CD4\,cells_j) + \beta_9^g (\#CD8\,cells_j) + \mu_j^g (subject) \quad (1)$$
$$+ \mu_k^g (hybridization) + \mu_l^g (label) + \varepsilon_{ijklm}^g$$

Y_{ijklm}^g denotes the $\log_2$ of the gth gene expression, at the dose a_i, $a_i \in \{0,1,2,3,4\}$ obtained from the jth subject after the kth hybridization, l^{th} labeling step in the microarray sample preparation and the mth chip. The β^g parameters denote the fixed effects associated with the respective covariates; the μ parameters denote

Outcome (Y): Gene expression in PBMCs[a]

Predictor (A): Air borne benzene levels

Confounders (W): Gender, Smoking Status, Age, Counts of PBMCs

Data: Gene expression in PBMCs of 125 subjects exposed to a range of benzene levels

Parameter: Benzene-dose dependent expected fold change in $\log_2$ expression of each gene relative to the expression in control or very lowly exposed subjects (<0.11ppm) margining out the effects of the other confounders

Analyses:

	Parametric	Non-parametric
Dose	5 binned dose ranges	Continuous
Point estimation	Linear mixed models	SuperLearner
Gene parameter	Fixed effect corresponding to dose	Ψ_i^g (see equation 2)
Gene inference	Linear mixed models	SuperLearner + Bootstrapping
Biochemical pathway inference	Linear mixed models + SEPEA[d]	a. SuperLearner + Bootstrapping + PCA[b]
		b. SuperLearner + Bootstrapping + HOPACH[c]

[a]PBMC: Peripheral Blood Mononuclear Cells; [b]PCA: Principal Component Analyses; [c]HOPACH: Hierarchical Ordered Partitioning and Collapsing Hybrid; [d]SEPEA: Structurally Enhanced Pathway Enrichment Analyses

Figure 1. Overview of methods and analyses.

the random effects, and ε denotes the normally distributed error associated with the model. β_0^g, the fixed effect associated with benzene exposure, is the parameter of interest in the model. We

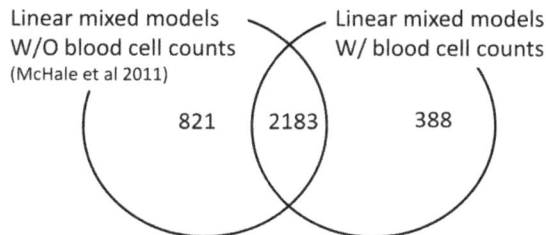

Figure 2. Overlapping sets of genes determined by two linear models. Two linear mixed models were used, a published model [13] (see Equation (2)) and a modified version including counts of different blood cell types as potential confounders of gene expression (see Equation (1)). Differential expression was determined based on altered fold changes in at least one of the four previously chosen dose ranges of benzene exposure, with an FDR-adjusted p-value<0.05.

fitted this mixed-effects model in R with the lmer function in the *lme4* package [24]. We also fit the mixed effects model without cell counts as potential confounders as given in Equation (2).

$$Y_{ijklm}^g = \beta_0^g a_i + \beta_1^g + \beta_2^g \left(sex_j\right) + \beta_3^g \left(smoke_j\right) + \beta_4^g \left(age_j\right) + \mu_j^g \left(subject\right) + \mu_k^g \left(hybridization\right) + \mu_l^g \left(label\right) + \varepsilon_{ijklm}^g \tag{2}$$

We identified differentially expressed probes as those with a statistically significant log-fold change (based on likelihood ratio tests). We computed p-values adjusted for multiple testing by controlling the false discovery rate (FDR) with the Benjamini-Hochberg procedure [25], using the *multtest* package in R. These FDR-adjusted p-values ≤0.05, the traditional experiment-wise type I error rate, were considered significant.

Pathway Enrichment Analysis

We used a method known as "structurally enhanced pathway enrichment analysis" (SEPEA_NT3) [26], which incorporates the

Scatter responses

Scatter responses

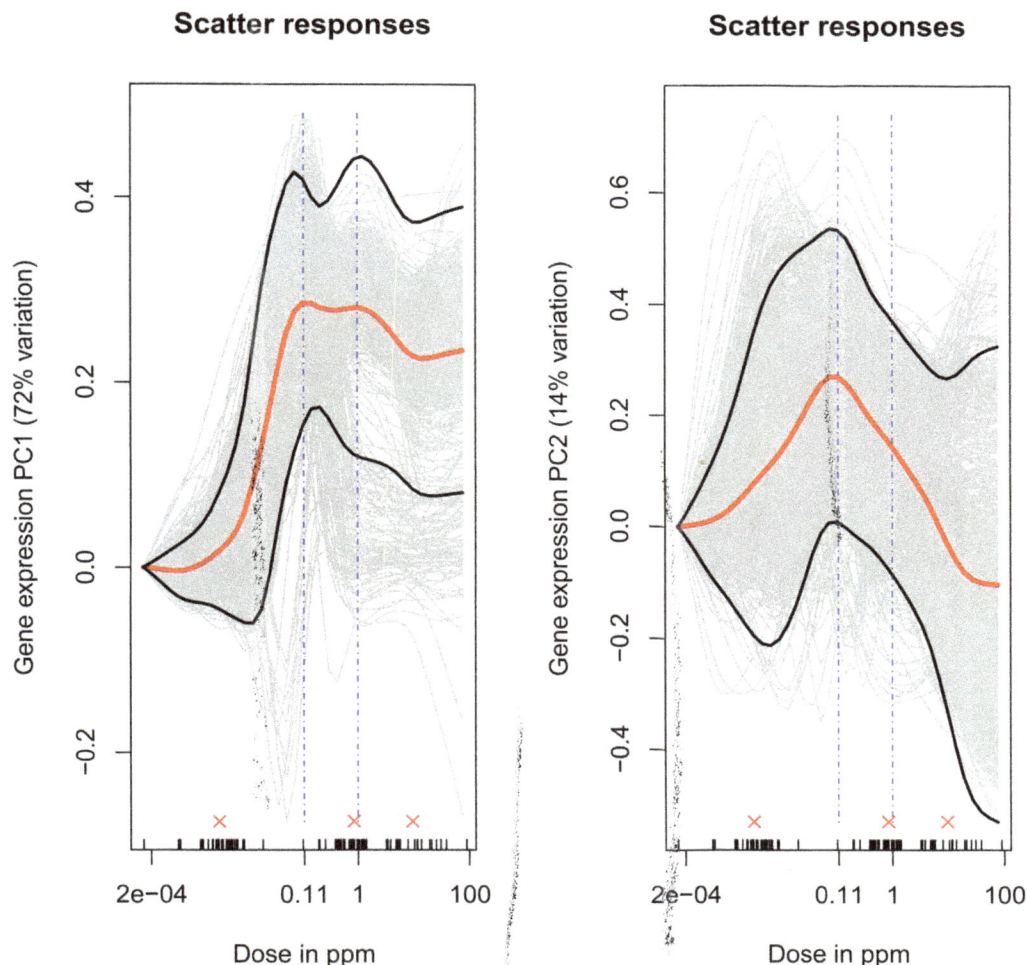

Figure 3. AML pathway-Principal Components-based response. The continuous fits in the two subplots use the first and second eigenvectors (that are slightly modified, see Material and Methods section) respectively from the eigenvector matrix, $Q^p_{s(n)}$ given in Equation (5). The elements of the individual eigenvectors are treated as the pathway response at the corresponding dose. The subscript p corresponds to the pathway under consideration and superscript s to a given bootstrap sample. The bold red line correspond the mean parameter estimates across the bootstrap samples and the bold black lines represent the corresponding 95% confidence intervals for the mean parameter estimates. The small vertical ticks on the x-axis denote doses to which one or more subjects in the study were exposed and consequently the doses for which data for all covariates under consideration were available. The three red 'x's above these ticks indicate the doses that there used to compare the rate of change of the marginal effect of benzene exposure from 0.001 to 1 ppm air benzene to the corresponding rate from 1 to 10 ppm air benzene.

associated network information of KEGG (Kyoto Encyclopedia of Genes and Genomes) human biochemical pathways [19,27,28]. Unlike traditional pathway enrichment methods that treat pathways as sets of genes, SEPEA treats pathways as networks of interacting proteins and/or enzymes. The genes corresponding to the proteins in the signaling network are given more weight according to whether they are at the receptor or the terminating end of the pathway that typically signals for transcription in a number of genes. Further, pathways where the perturbed genes are close relative to each other on the associated network are modeled as being more likely to be affected than pathways where he perturbed genes occur further apart over the network. The significance obtained by SEPEA_NT3 was based on 10000 randomizations.

Bootstrap-SuperLearner

The SuperLearner [14] method is a theoretically optimal (relative to the so-called Oracle estimator) approach to model

selection in a data adaptive manner. This method requires a set of different statistical learning algorithms that a user could consider as being appropriate models of the data. SuperLearner then uses a cross-validation-based loss function to estimate an optimal combination of predictions from the different input algorithms to produce model fits. The SuperLearner was used to fit $E\left[Y/_{A=a,W=w}\right]$ where Y, A and W have the same meaning as in the previous sections. Note in these analyses cell counts are included as additional confounders. The fits were computed in the SuperLearner package [29] implemented in the R statistical environment [23] with a choice of a 10-fold cross-validation-based loss function. The statistical learning algorithms used were random forests [30], multivariate adaptive regression splines [31],, bagging [32], Bayesian Generalized Linear Models [33], cforests [34,35,36], neural networks [37], loess regression [38] and support vector machines [39]. Different parameter settings for each of these algorithms in their respective R packages were used (see

Distance matrix for gene probes in pathway

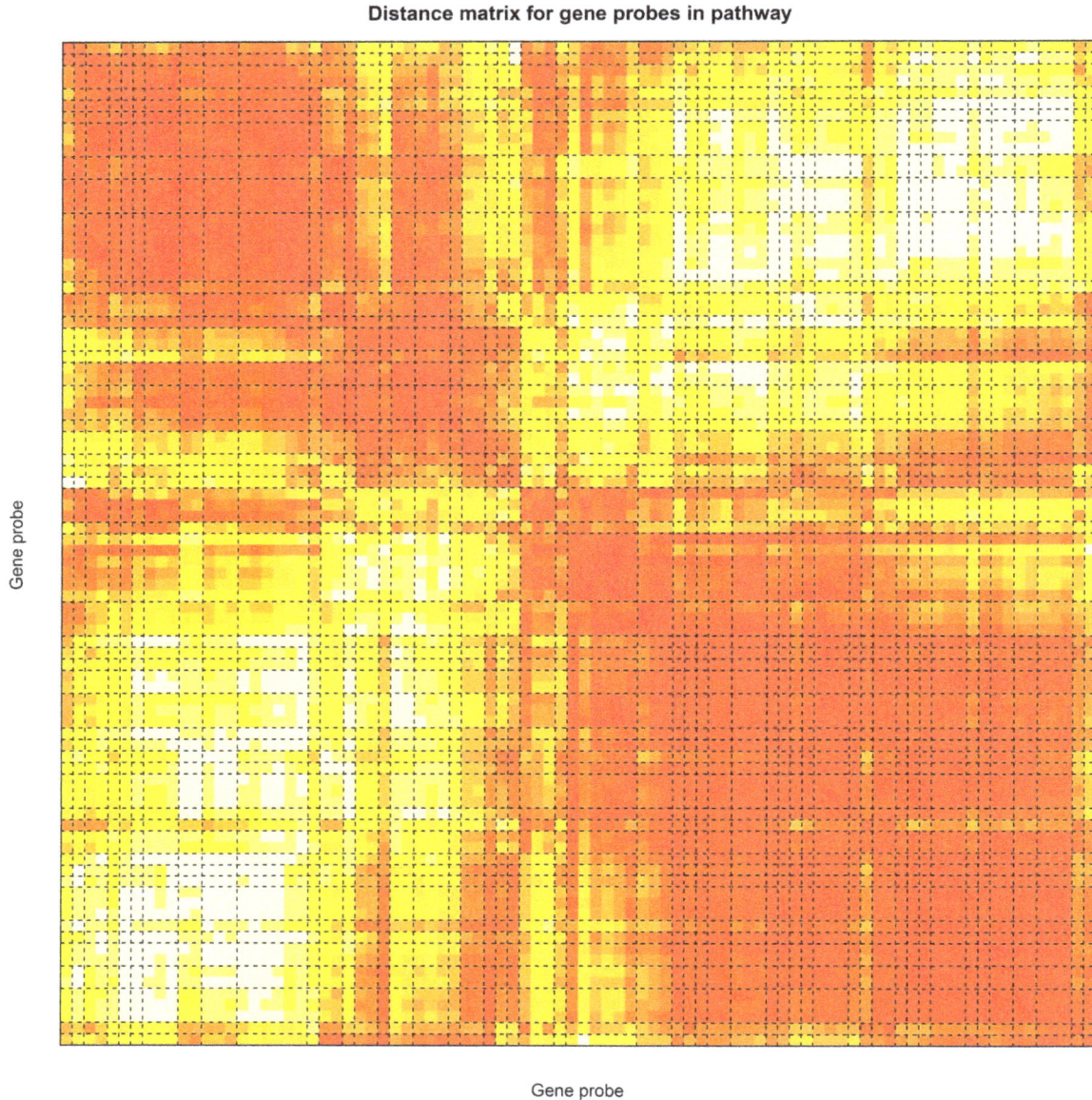

Figure 4. AML pathway-Clusters of probes/genes. Hierarchical cluster of the probes in the AML pathway. The probes are clustered based on the distance between the corresponding rows of the matrix, X_ℓ^p given in Equation (6). The figure is a visual representation of the distance matrix between all the probes/genes in the pathway. The color of the $(i,j)^{th}$ position of the distance matrix is a measure of how close probes i and j are to each other based on their response across the dose range. The color ranges from white to red. The closer the pair of probes is two each other, the greater the intensity of red at the corresponding position. The dashed black lines correspond to boundaries of clusters of probes as determined by the HOPACH algorithm [47].

Table S1)In total there were 32 learning algorithms. The reader interested in implementing the SuperLearner is referred to a vignette (http://cran.r-project.org/web/packages/SuperLearner/vignettes/SuperLearnerPresent.pdf) describing its implementation in R.

In order to determine the variability of the SuperLearner mean response estimates, a bootstrapping procedure was implemented. Let n denote the number of subjects and N_{BS} denote the number of bootstrap samples. 1000 bootstrap samples were chosen in all cases. Then for each bootstrap sample, n subjects are drawn randomly with replacement and the mean response is then estimated using the SuperLearner for each of the bootstrap samples.

The marginal association of a given response (expression of gene g) with the ith dose of benzene exposure (corresponding to $A = a$) was then estimated by,

$$
\begin{aligned}
\Psi_{s(n),i}^g = \Psi_{s(n)}^g(a) &= \Psi^g\left(P_{s(n)}\right)(a) \\
&= P_{s(n)}\left(Q_{s(n)}^g(a,W) - Q_{s(n)}^g(0,W)\right) \\
&= \frac{1}{n}\sum_{j\in s(n)} Q_{s(n)}^g(a,W_j) - Q_{s(n)}^g(0,W_j)
\end{aligned}
\tag{3}
$$

Where $s(n)$ represents a bootstrap sample, $P_{s(n)}$ represents the empirical distribution based on that sample, $Q_{s(n)}^g(a,W)$ the

Table 1. Median and 95% confidence interval (CI) estimates of the rate of change of marginal effect of benzene exposure below 1 ppm ($B^{i,1}/\beta^{g,1}$ – see equations (9) and (12)) and above 1 ppm ($B^{i,2}/\beta^{g,2}$ - see equations (10) and (13)) and the change in absolute rate of change of the marginal effects from below 1 ppm to above 1 ppm (D^{i}/δ^{g} – see equations (11) and (14)) for the first two principal components of the Acute Myeloid Leukemia pathway and six chosen genes of interest.

Pathway/Gene	$B^{i,1}/\beta^{g,1}$ Median	95% CI	$B^{i,2}/\beta^{g,2}$ Median	95% CI	Δ^{i}/δ^{g} Median	95% CI
Acute Myeloid Leukemia: Principal Component 1	0.333	(0.008, 0.394)	−0.006	(−0.016, 0.002)	0.328	(0.019, 0.380)
Acute Myeloid Leukemia: Principal Component 2	0.106	(−0.244, 0.349)	−0.024	(−0.040, 0.010)	0.108	(−0.012, 0.353)
RUNX1	0.07	(0.018, 0.158)	0.004	(−0.008, 0.025)	0.063	(0.010, 0.151)
FLT3	−0.079	(−0.204, −0.012)	0	(−0.005, 0.004)	0.078	(0.011, 0.202)
CEBPA	−0.877	(−1.11, −0.584)	0.03	(0.006, 0.069)	0.847	(0.561, 1.068)
LEF1	0.032	(−0.035, 0.120)	−0.009	(−0.019, −0.002)	0.025	(−0.008, 0.106)
CYP2E1	0.051	(−0.004, 0.147)	−0.002	(−0.007, 0.002)	0.049	(0.002, 0.146)
CYP2F1	0.002	(−0.033, 0.03)	−0.001	(−0.004, 0.001)	0.008	(−0.001, 0.038)

estimate of $E\left[Y^{g}/A=a,W=w\right]$ based on the SuperLearner applied to $s(n)$. $A=0$ represents doses ≤ 0.11 ppm. So for every $A=a$(at which we calculated $\Psi^{g}_{s(n)}(a)$, which were at points separated 0.5 units apart on the $\log_2$ dose range), we get the average difference of the predicted $\log_2$ gene expression value (averaged across the W) and the predicted $\log_2$ gene expression value if the sample represented very low to no exposure.

All the subjects with undetectable benzene exposure levels in this study had predicted air benzene exposures less than 0.11 ppm. Under certain assumptions [40,41], this parameter of interest in Equation (3) also has also a simple causal interpretation, i.e., it represents the mean log fold change of a given gene's expression due to exposure to a given dose relative to those with exposure less than 0.11 ppm air benzene levels.

Biochemical Pathway Response

The derivation of the non-parametric estimate of the mean response of a biochemical pathway with an outcome of interest in the presence of confounders to its constituent gene expressions is a statistical problem that does not appear to have been addressed before in the literature. Examples of model-based approaches include those in [42,43] who proposed generalized linear model-based approaches to test for pathway association with a binary clinical outcome and survival times. We propose two ideas to provide summary responses of the expression of all the genes in a biochemical pathway, both of which use non-parametric estimates from the previously described Bootstrap-SuperLearner approach. The first idea is based on using principal component analysis (PCA) on the estimates from the SuperLearner of the expressions of genes in the pathway. Principal component analysis has been used in the past to model the pathway response [44,45]. The change in expressions of the genes due to benzene exposure is potentially confounded by other covariates in the study. Hence it will not be correct to perform a direct analysis of the expressions of the genes in the pathway in order to get a summary response. Therefore, PCA is performed on the SuperLearner-based non-parametric estimates of changes in gene expressions due to benzene exposure. The second idea utilizes a clustering analysis of these SuperLearner estimates in order to identify clusters of gene expression responses and medoid genes or particular genes that

have responses that are representative of responses in the identified clusters. Clustering analysis of gene expression data [46] has been more or less standard for more than ten years.

Assume that the human biochemical pathways are identified by indices in the set $\{1,2,\ldots p,\ldots,N_{path}\}$ Let $\mathcal{N}_{p}$ denote the number of probes corresponding to genes involved in the given pathway identified by the index p. $\mathcal{N}_{d}$ is the number of points on the dose range of the exposed individuals where the SuperLearner [14] estimates are computed. Equally spaced points were chosen, 0.5 units apart on the logarithmic dose range.

In the first analysis, the dose-dependent responses were estimated by the first and second principal components (or first and second columns of the $Q^{p}_{s(n)}$ eigenvector matrix) of the covariance matrix, $\mathrm{cov}\left(\bar{X}^{p}_{s(n)}\right)$ created from the $N_{p} \times N_{d}$ matrix, $X^{p}_{s(n)}$ obtained for the SuperLearner [14] estimate of the parameters of interest (see Equations (4)-(6), where $\Lambda^{p}_{s(n)}$ represents diagonal matrix with the corresponding eigenvalues ordered in a decreasing manner). This was done for each bootstrap sample, s. Note, $\Psi^{\bullet}_{s(n),i}$ denotes the mean parameter of interest across all the probes at the ith dose level.

$$X^{p}_{s(n)} = \begin{pmatrix} \Psi^{1}_{s(n),1} & \cdots & \Psi^{1}_{s(n),N_d} \\ \vdots & \ddots & \vdots \\ \Psi^{N_p}_{s(n),1} & \cdots & \Psi^{N_p}_{s(n),N_d} \end{pmatrix} \quad (4)$$

$$\bar{X}^{p}_{s(n)} = \begin{pmatrix} \Psi^{1}_{s(n),1} - \Psi^{\bullet}_{s(n),1} & \cdots & \Psi^{1}_{s(n),N_d} - \Psi^{\bullet}_{s(n),N_d} \\ \vdots & \ddots & \vdots \\ \Psi^{N_p}_{s(n),1} - \Psi^{\bullet}_{s(n),1} & \cdots & \Psi^{N_p}_{s(n),N_d} - \Psi^{\bullet}_{s(n),N_d} \end{pmatrix} \quad (5)$$

RUNX1 (460341)

FLT3 (1230333)

CEBPA (2650148)

LEF1 (270102)

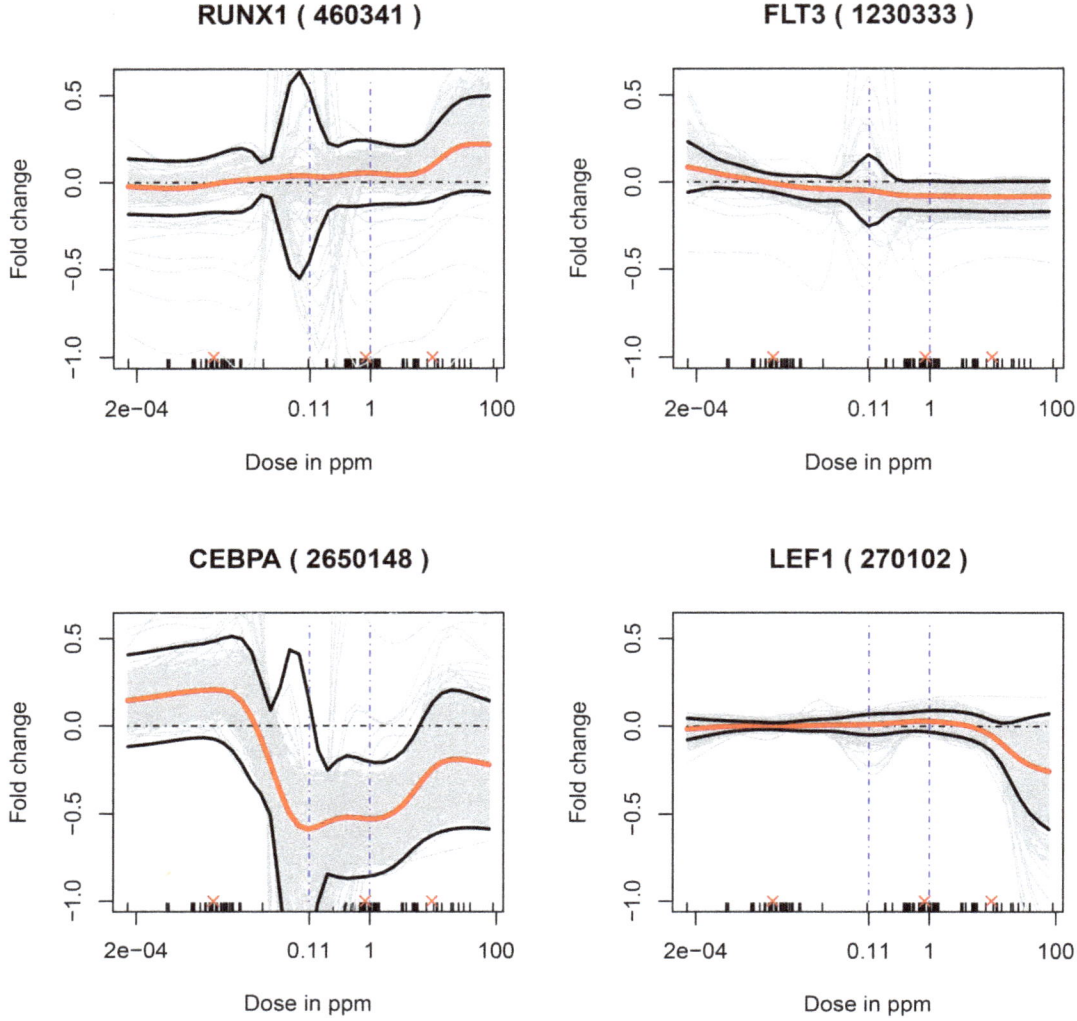

Figure 5. Responses of selected genes associated with the leukemia disease process. Non-parametric model fits to the expression response of the probes corresponding to six genes known to be associated with AML, with air-benzene concentrations in parts per million. Note the responses here are log fold-changes in expression. The dot-dashed horizontal line at a log fold change value equal to zero indicates the no-effect response. The gene names along with the corresponding probe id number on the microarray in parentheses are provided for each gene. The small vertical ticks on the x-axis denote doses to which one or more subjects in the study were exposed and consequently the doses for which data for all covariates under consideration were available. The three red 'x's above these ticks indicate the doses that there used to compare the rate of change of the marginal effect of benzene exposure from 0.001 to 1 ppm air benzene to the corresponding rate from 1 to 10 ppm air benzene.

$$\mathrm{cov}\left(\bar{X}_{s(n)}^{p}\right) = \bar{X}_{s(n)}^{p} T \bar{X}_{s(n)}^{p} = Q_{s(n)}^{p} T \Lambda_{s(n)}^{p} Q_{s(n)}^{p} \qquad (6)$$

Where

$$Q_{s(n)}^{p} = \left[q_{s(n)}^{1,p} \cdots q_{s(n)}^{Np,p} \right] \qquad (7)$$

And $q_{s(n)}^{1,p} \cdots q_{s(n)}^{Np,p}$ are the $\mathcal{N}_p$ eigenvectors corresponding to the eigenvalues in the matrix $\Lambda_{s(n)}^{p}$. Each of the $\mathcal{N}_d$ elements of the first and second eigenvector was taken to represent the pathway response at the corresponding dose. In order to make comparisons of these eigenvectors across all bootstrap samples, two modifications were made to these eigenvectors. First, the first element of the

(first or second) eigenvector for each of the bootstrap samples was normalized to zero. Second, if the sign of this normalized eigenvector responses at 0.1 ppm was negative, and then the negative of the elements of normalized eigenvector was plotted. This can be done because any scalar multiple of the reported eigenvector is an equally valid eigenvector for the given eigenvalue. We denote these modified eigenvectors by $\bar{q}_{s(n)}^{1,p}, \bar{q}_{s(n)}^{2,p}$ where for $i = 1,2$,

$$=$$

$$\bar{q}_{s(n)}^{1,p} = \left[\Phi_{s(n)}^{i,p}(a_1) \quad \cdots \quad \Phi_{s(n)}^{i,p}(a_{N_d}) \right] \qquad (8)$$

The pth pathway response at dose a_j is given by $\Phi_{s(n)}^{i,p}(a_j)$. Note by definition $\Phi_{s(n)}^{i,p}(a_1) = 0$.

CYP2E1 (5570228)   CYP2F1 (6580674)

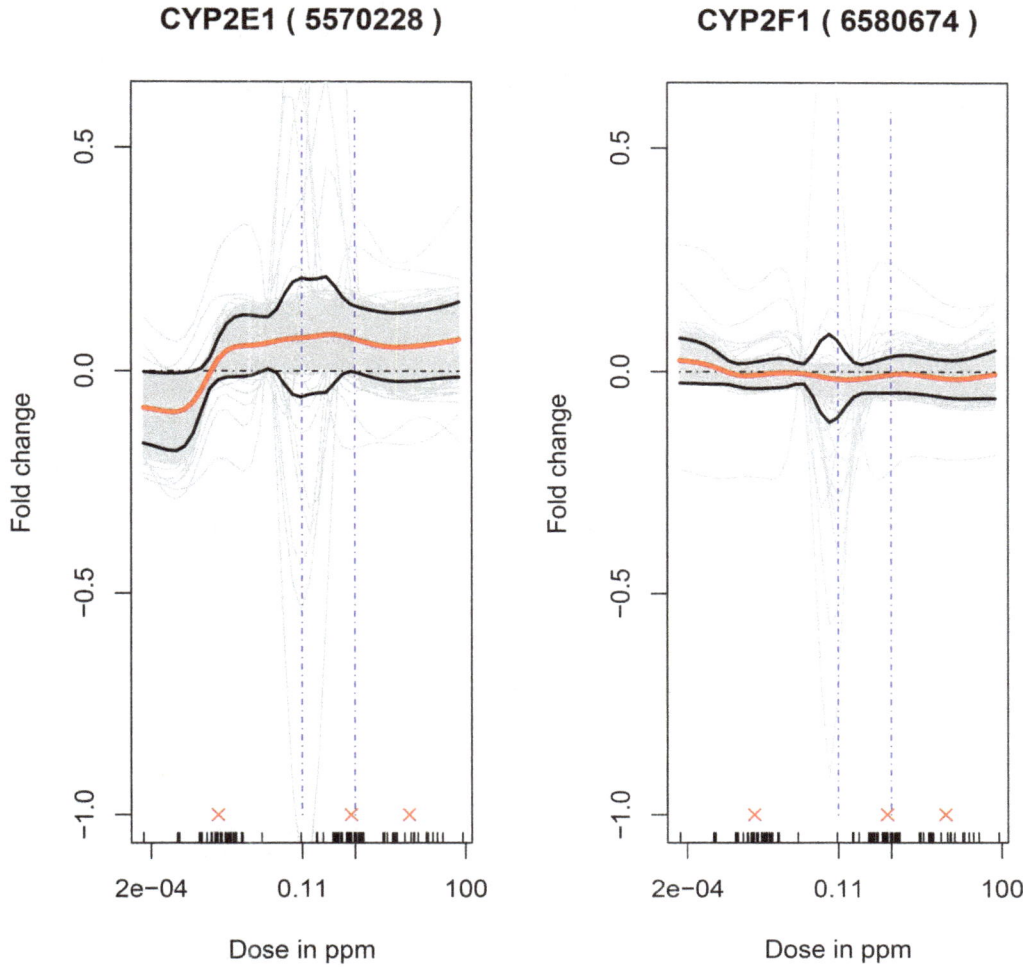

Figure 6. Response of two Cytochrome p450 genes associated with benzene metabolism. Non-parametric model fits to the expression response of the probes corresponding to two genes known to be associated with the metabolism of benzene, CYP2E1 and CYP2F1, with air-benzene concentrations in parts per million. Note the responses here are log fold-changes in expression. The dot-dashed horizontal line at a log fold change value equal of zero indicates the no-effect response. The gene names along with the corresponding probe id number on the microarray in parentheses are provided for each gene. The small vertical ticks on the x-axis denote doses to which one or more subjects in the study were exposed and consequently the doses for which data for all covariates under consideration were available. The three red 'x's above these ticks indicate the doses that there used to compare the rate of change of the marginal effect of benzene exposure from 0.001 to 1 ppm air benzene to the corresponding rate from 1 to 10 ppm air benzene.

For each bootstrap sample, these modified normalized eigen-vector-based pathway response with dose is plotted as a smoothed cubic spline using a smoothing parameter of 0.5. The plots were made in the R statistical environment [23].

In the second analysis, the dose-dependent responses were presented as a clustered $(N_p \times N_p)$ distance matrix between the probes associated with the genes involved in the pathway. The clustering was performed using the HOPACH algorithm [47] in the package *hopach* [48] in the R statistical environment [23] where the distance between the two $N_d \times 1$ vectors, $\underline{\Psi}^i_\bullet$ and $\underline{\Psi}^j_\bullet$ associated with a pair of probes, i and j is measured by the cosine distance metric. Using this distance metric, HOPACH builds a hierarchical cluster of trees by recursively partioning the data set. Note the analyses here were performed on the matrix $X^p_\bullet$ that represents the average of $X^p_{s(n)}$ over all the bootstrap samples.

$$X^p_\bullet = \begin{pmatrix} \Psi^1_{\bullet,1} & \cdots & \Psi^1_{\bullet,N_d} \\ \vdots & \ddots & \vdots \\ \Psi^{N_p}_{\bullet,1} & \cdots & \Psi^{N_p}_{\bullet,N_d} \end{pmatrix} \qquad (9)$$

From the clustering analyses, we also presented the responses of the genes identified as medoids for the six largest clusters as identified by the HOPACH algorithm [47].

The advantage of the principal component analyses of the pathway response is a one-picture summary response of the variability of the estimates of mean response of the pattern among a significant proportion of the genes in the pathway. However, this picture does not inform whether the genes are being over or under expressed at different levels of exposure. The plots of the medoid genes provide the sign of response of these chosen genes.

Estimates of the Change in the Rate of Change of Response

Characteristics of the shapes of the dose-response curves were obtained in terms of the change in the absolute rate of change of marginal effect of benzene exposure from below 1 ppm to above this level. For the two pathway responses $(i = 1,2)$, the rate of change of the marginal effect response below 1 ppm for the bootstrap sample $s(n)$ is estimated by,

$$B_{s(n)}^{i,1} = \frac{\Phi_{s(n)}^{i,p}(a_2) - \Phi_{s(n)}^{i,p}(a_1)}{a_2 - a_1} \qquad (10)$$

Where $a_2 = 1ppm$ and $a_1 = 0.001ppm$, $\Phi_{s(n)}^{i,p}(a_j)$ is as given in Equation (8). The rate of change of response above 1 ppm by,

$$B_{s(n)}^{i,2} = \frac{\Phi_{s(n)}^{i,p}(a_3) - \Phi_{s(n)}^{i,p}(a_2)}{a_3 - a_2} \qquad (11)$$

Where $a_3 = 10ppm$ and the estimate of the change in the absolute rate of change of response, $D_{s(n)}^i$ is chosen to be

$$D_{s(n)}^i = |B_{s(n)}^{i,1}| - |B_{s(n)}^{i,2}| \qquad (12)$$

Analogously the estimates of the change in the absolute rate of change of gene, g level responses, $\delta_{s(n)}^g$ are given by,

$$\beta_{s(n)}^{i,1} = \frac{\Psi_{s(n)}^{i,p}(a_2) - \Psi_{s(n)}^{i,p}(a_1)}{a_2 - a_1} \qquad (13)$$

$$\beta_{s(n)}^{i,2} = \frac{\Psi_{s(n)}^{i,p}(a_3) - \Psi_{s(n)}^{i,p}(a_2)}{a_3 - a_2} \qquad (14)$$

$$\delta_{s(n)}^i = |\beta_{s(n)}^{i,1}| - |\beta_{s(n)}^{i,2}| \qquad (15)$$

Where $\Psi_{s(n)}^{i,p}(a_j)$ is given by Equation (3). The bootstrap samples of $D_{s(n)}^i$ and $\delta_{s(n)}^g$ are used to estimate the 95% confidence intervals for D^i and δ^g. Significant positive values of these estimates suggest supralinearity of the marginal effects of benzene exposure while significant negative values suggests sublinearity of these effects between 0.001 ppm and 10 ppm benzene levels.

Results

Predicted Air Benzene Exposure Levels in Non-occupationally Exposed Subjects

The air benzene exposure levels for the 42 control subjects [13] were predicted from their urinary unmetabolized benzene levels [17]. For 8 of the control subjects, exposure predictions were unavailable and these subjects were excluded from the non-parametric analyses. The predicted benzene exposure levels ranged from 1.4×10^{-4} ppm to 0.11 ppm, with 32 subjects predicted to have levels below 0.009 ppm.

Peripheral Blood Cell Counts as Potential Confounders of Gene Expression

Two linear mixed models of gene expression as a function of air benzene exposure were fitted to the data from 125 subjects who had been exposed to benzene in four previously chosen concentration ranges, $<<1$ ppm, <1 ppm, >5 ppm and < 10 ppm, and ≥ 10 ppm, or were controls. One of the models was identical to that recently reported by us [13] and included the gender, age and smoking status of the subjects as potential confounders of gene expression. The second model was the same but also included the measured counts of different cell types present in the PBMC as additional confounders (see Equation (1)). The estimates of the fixed effects of this model are given in Table S2. The distribution of the estimates of the intra-class coefficients for each of the random effects do not change when moves from a model that does not include the PBMCs to one that does (see Figure S1). As shown in the Venn diagram in Figureô 2, there was a significant overlap (2183 genes) between the sets of genes identified as differentially expressed (FDR-adjusted p-value <0.05) by each linear model. Fisher's exact test estimated a p-value $< 2.2 \times 10^{-16}$ for the null hypothesis stating the independence between genes declared differentially expressed by the two linear models. When cell counts were incorporated as potential confounders, 821 out of 3004 genes identified as differentially expressed in the original model were no longer significant, while an additional 388 genes were found to be significant. There were also no major differences in the pathway enrichment values for all the KEGG human pathways using results from either model (Table S3). Pathway enrichment analyses were also done on the sets of genes that were commonly identified as differentially expressed genes (2183 genes) and uniquely by either of the models (821 or 388 genes) (see Table S3). The pearson correlation between the $\log_{10}$ transformed p-values across pathways for the set of genes uniquely identified by the model that did not incorporate cell count with the corresponding p-values for the set of genes commonly identified by both models is 0.06 (p-value = 0.32). The pearson correlation for the pathway p-values using the set of genes uniquely identified by the model that incorporated cell count with corresponding p-values for commonly identified set of genes is 0.22 (p-value = 0.0005).

Biochemical Pathway-based Responses

A dose-specific parameter of interest (defined in Equation (3)) was estimated non-parametrically for the expression of each probe/gene in the KEGG AML, B-cell receptor signaling, Toll-like receptor signaling, Steroid hormone biosynthesis, and Maturity onset of diabetes pathways, at points equally spaced 0.5 units apart on the logarithmic dose range. For a given gene at a chosen dose, this parameter is the expected log fold-change in the expression of the gene at that dose relative to the mean expression of subjects exposed to levels below 0.11 ppm. The parameters were estimated using the SuperLearner [14] that used 32 learning algorithms and the sampling distribution of these parameters was estimated via a bootstrapping procedure in which the parameters are re-estimated using random selection (with replacement) of the 125 subjects. The bootstrapping procedure was repeated 1000 times.

The first and second principal components of the estimated parameters for all genes in the AML pathway, evaluated across the entire study dose range, are shown in Figureô 3. Together, these two principal components captured 86% of the dose-dependent variation in expression of genes in the AML pathway. The first and second principal components of the dose-response parameters for all genes in the B-cell receptor signaling, Toll-like receptor signaling, Steroid hormone biosynthesis and Maturity onset of diabetes pathways are shown in figure S2, respectively. Visually, the mean estimates of the first principal components of the responses look similar across the five chosen pathways and suggest supra-linear responses. This is quantitatively reinforced by the fact that the estimates of the change in the absolute rate of change of marginal effect of benzene exposure from below 1 ppm to above 1 ppm for the first principal component of each of the five pathways (see Equation (12)) are significantly positive (p-value < 0.05) (see Table 1 and Table S4). There are suggestions of responses at doses below 0.1 ppm, and exposures of around 0.1 ppm and 1 ppm appear to be inflection points for at least three (AML, Toll-like receptor signaling and Maturity Onset of Diabetes) of the five pathways. The mean estimates of the second principal components are also similar across the five pathways, with exposures around 0.1 ppm appearing to represent inflection points for these responses. The responses of the probes in the pathway were clustered using HOPACH [49] (Figureô 4 and figure S3), and the results confirm that many sets of genes exhibit similar response patterns.

Expression-based Responses of Chosen Genes of Interest

A small set of genes was chosen based either on their known association with leukemogenesis or because they code for enzymes putatively associated with the metabolism of benzene to its toxic metabolites. In the first class, oncogenes (RUNX1, FLT3, LEF1) or tumor suppressors (RUNX1, CEBPA) implicated in leukemia [50,51,52,53,54,55] were selected. RUNX1 has been identified as both an oncogene and a tumor suppressor gene [56,57]. The responses (in terms of log-fold changes) of these genes are plotted in Figureô 5. Among these genes, RUNX1, LEF1 and CEBPA were differentially expressed (FDR<0.05) based on the linear model in Equation (1) across four binned dose ranges. Based on the position of the line corresponding to no change (i.e., log fold change equals zero) relative to the 95% confidence interval of the estimated fold change at a chosen dose, the expressions of FLT3 and CEBPAare all down regulated on exposure to levels of air benzene above around 0.1 ppm. RUNX1, FLT3 and CEBPA display profiles that are supralinear as captured by the significant positive values of the change in the absolute rate of change of marginal effect of benzene exposure from below 1 ppm to above 1 ppm (see Equation (15) and Tableô 1). The responses of the expression of two genes, CYP2E1 and CYP2F1 (enzymes putatively associated with the metabolism of benzene to its toxic metabolites), are shown in Figureô 6. CYP2E1 is known to be involved with the metabolism of benzene [58,59,60] and CYP2F1 has been hypothesized to be associated with benzene metabolism [3]. CYP2E1 expression was increased at levels of air benzene concentration as low as 0.01 ppm, while expression of CYP2F1 was largely unaltered.CYP2E1, but not CYP2F1, was found to be differentially expressed (FDR<0.05) based on the linear model in Equation (1) across four binned dose ranges. The dose-response of CYP2E1 is supralinear (see Equation (15) and Tableô 1).

Discussion

The analyses in this study sought to further characterize the dose-dependency of changes in gene expression associated with occupational exposure to benzene that we reported recently [13] and to extend them into the ambient environmental range by estimating exposures for the non-occupationally exposed 'controls'. We further extended the analyses to include PBMC subset cell counts as potential confounders of expression.

Significant overlap was seen for the majority of genes identified as differentially expressed using the parametric linear models, regardless of whether or not PBMC cell counts were incorporated as potential confounders. Genes that did not remain differentially expressed after incorporation of cell counts as confounders could

be indirectly related to benzene-induced cell count decrements. One plausible example is the CD44 gene; it encodes a marker for CD4 and CD8 cells, both of which were reduced in number in benzene-exposed individuals [7]. However, the estimation of additional parameters in the model to incorporate cell counts as confounders resulted in loss of statistical power to identify genes as differentially expressed. Conversely, the incorporation of cell counts in the model may improve the model fit and subsequently increase the ability of the model to detect true dose-specific changes in gene expression. This is partly suggested by the significant but relatively small correlation (0.22) of the pathway p-values using the set of genes uniquely identified by the model incorporating cell counts with the pathway p-values using the set of genes commonly identified by both models. In either case, the fact that a significant overlap was observed implies that the majority of the changes in gene expression are not directly mediated through the hematotoxicity of benzene.

We defined the dose-dependent effects on gene expressions as our parameters of interest as a marginal effect of benzene exposure. The definition of the parameter in dose-response studies of this kind is to the best of our knowledge novel in the toxicology literature – that is, as the marginally adjusted curve of the mean outcome versus exposure. This is extremely important in itself, because when measuring how dose-response affects a population, one should estimate a population level dose response parameter. However, what is typically done is to estimate the dose response in a parametric or semi-parametric model, where the resulting curve represents potentially a different curve for every covariate group. To avoid this problem, the predominant approach is to simply make the simplifying, but erroneous assumption, that all groups have the same dose response curve). We wanted to make no such bias inducing assumptions, and so we estimated these dose response curves in a nonparametric model, using optimal data-adaptive methods (SuperLeanrer [14]) for estimating the relationship of expression to exposure and the confounders. Thus, we have approached a problem typically approached using ad hoc methods, based on arbitrary statistical modeling assumptions, and used methods based on what is truly known about the relationship of expression to the covariates including exposure, that is nearly nothing, and derived optimal (the SuperLearner is not ad hoc, but based on the theorem of the Oracle Inequality [14]) estimators respecting the underlying knowledge. We use a bootstrapping approach in order to estimate the sampling variability of these estimates. Note that these estimates are essentially derived from data-adaptive methods in a very large (nearly non-parametric) model, where the number of assumptions made about the probability generating distributions is minimal, particularly as compared to standard approaches using parametric models.

The five pathways chosen for analyses were selected based on the results to our earlier analyses [13] with the same gene expression data on the same set of KEGG [19,27,28] human pathways. Ideally, we should have performed these analyses while being agnostic to the potential biochemical pathways being targeted. This would mean analyzing all 22177 probes on the microarray by the proposed non-parametric methodology. However, we chose to analyze the 5 pathways in part because the proposed non-parametric methodology requires significant computing power- one bootstrap sample run of the dose response of a given probe/gene using the SuperLearner [14] that ran 32 learning algorithms took around 20 seconds to run on a 4-core linux machine with around 1 GHz cpu and 16 GB RAM. We should note that the associations of benzene exposure are being made with biochemical pathways of diseases (AML and Maturity

Onset of Diabetes) and not with the diseases directly. These biochemical pathways represent a summary of the literature on the specific disease pathogenesis. Further the exact definition of a specific biochemical pathway in terms of its constituents and associated interactions will be consistent though not the same across different pathway databases. Therefore our choices of the pathways were from the same set of pathways analyzed before albeit with the same data – our goal here being a better characterization of the dose responses over the entire continuous range of exposures. The AML pathway was of particular interest because of the established association of benzene exposure with leukemia incidence [1,2]. The other two pathways (B-cell receptor and Toll-like receptor signaling) were randomly chosen from the set of pathways which displayed significant dose response over the range of benzene exposures. Similarly the Steroid Hormone Biosynthesis and Maturity onset of diabetes pathways were chosen from the list of pathways that did not display statistical significant responses.

The mean estimates of first and second principal components of the dose-response relationships determined by the our method method for all genes in the five chosen pathways (AML, B-cell receptor signaling, Toll-like receptor signaling, Steroid hormone biosynthesis and Maturity onset of diabetes) showed apparent similarities and similar inflection points were observed for several of the pathways. Since two of the analyzed pathways, Steroid hormone biosynthesis and Maturity onset of diabetes, are presumably unrelated to benzene, the noted similarities in response implies that the changes in expression of genes in these pathways are real effects though they were not large enough to provide statistical significance for modulation at the pathway level. Consistency of the shapes of the responses across the five chosen pathways may be a consequence of the correlation among gene expression levels on a system-wide basis through coordinated transcriptional regulation. However, analyses of the binding sites in the promoter regions of the differentially expressed genes (across doses, as determined by the linear model in Equation (1)) did not reveal enrichment of any transcription factor binding sites (data not shown).

Together, these similarities support the plausibility of the observed supra-linear dose-responses. In addition supralinearity is quantitatively supported by positive values of the parameter that captures the change in the absolute rate of change of marginal effect of benzene exposure from below 1 ppm to above 1 ppm (see Equations (12) and (15), Tableô 1). This adds to the literature of observed supra-linear responses associated with benzene exposure – see for example the response of benzene oxide-albumin adduct formation with benzene exposure [61], the dose related production of benzene metabolites [17] and the relative risk of leukemia with benzene exposure [10].

Our statistical tests for supralinearity are based on comparing the rate of change of the marginal effect of exposure below 1 ppm (0.001–1 ppm) benzene to the rate of change of this marginal effect above 1 ppm (1–10 ppm). We don't perform statistical tests for supra-linearity of the overall dose response curve. Testing for supra-linearity is a very subtle issue, since any data adaptive approach, compared to some model in a goodness of fit test, will always win out asymptotically (any null model will be not perfectly right, so as sample size grows, and the data-adaptive approach will favor more highly parameterized models to create a better fit, any improvement over the null becomes statistically significant). Thus, any conclusion made from a test in this context is dubious, since the asymptotic p-value will always go to 0. Therefore, we used an approach based on confidence intervals of the overall dose-response curve, which do not have this particular pathology.

Several genes of interest were chosen for examination based on their association with leukemogenesis or benzene metabolism. The observed significant decrease in CEBPA expression at benzene levels of around 0.1 ppm may be important in light of the fact that reduced CEBPA gene expression has been associated with increased risk of leukemia [55]. Changes in the expression of CYP2E1 were observed at levels of air benzene concentration as low as 0.01 ppm. As benzene metabolism occurs principally in the liver [62] and also in the lung [63,64], with secondary metabolism occurring in the bone marrow [65,66,67], the implication of altered expression of CYP2E1 in peripheral blood is not entirely clear.

In order to permit phenotypic anchoring of the observed dose-dependent changes in gene expression, the responses of counts of B-cells, white blood cells and the ratio of the counts of CD4 cells to CD8 cells, are estimated using the Bootstrap-SuperLearner approach (data not shown). The observed decreases in these cell counts have been previously reported [7]. Mean changes in gene expression can thus be associated with corresponding changes in mean cell counts. For example, a 0.75 expected fold change of CEBPA gene expression at 1 ppm of air benzene would be associated with a mean decrease of 600 white blood cells/μl or a decrease of 0.2 in the ratio of CD4 to CD8 cells.

In summary, this work presents a new approach, which is the combination of the choice of a statistical parameter to be estimated, the methods used to estimate the data generating distribution (our parameter is only a targeted part of that distribution), and rigorous and robust methods for deriving inference, applied to the scientific question of estimating the dose-dependent biological responses resulting from exposure to benzene in the air. This work extends our previous analyses of benzene-induced differential gene expression in occupationally exposed workers and demonstrates that the differential expression of the majority of genes is independent of changes in cell counts of various blood cell types; that many differentially expressed genes and disease-relevant pathways display an apparently supra-linear response; and, that benzene alters these pathways and genes at exposure levels as low as 0.1 ppm. However, limitations in the statistical models and in the interpretation of some of these findings suggest that studies with a larger number of samples from individuals exposed to benzene in the low-dose range between 0.01 and 1 ppm are needed to clarify and confirm our interpretations. More precise exposure measurement and/or estimation in the low-dose region are needed to clarify the nature of the dose-response relationship of gene alteration in the low-dose range.

Supporting Information

Figure S1 Distribution of intra-class coefficients of the chip, subject, labeling and hybridization random effects.

Figure S2 Pathways-Principal Components-based Response. Non-parametric model fits to the marginal association of the expression of the probes corresponding to the genes involved in the a. B-cell receptor signaling, b.Toll-like receptor signaling, c. Steroid Hormone bio-synthesis and d.Maturity onset of diabetes pathways with air-benzene concentrations in parts per million. The continuous fits in the two subplots use the first and second eigenvectors (that are slightly modified, see Material and Methods section) respectively from the eigenvector matrix, $Q^p_{s(n)}$ given in Equation (5). The elements of the individual eigenvectors are treated as the pathway response at the corresponding dose. The subscript p corresponds to the pathway under consideration and superscript s to a given bootstrap sample. The bold red line correspond the mean parameter estimates across the bootstrap samples and the bold black lines represent the corresponding 95% confidence intervals for the mean parameter estimates. The small vertical ticks on the x-axis denote doses to which one or more subjects in the study were exposed and consequently the doses for which data for all covariates under consideration were available. The three red 'x's above these ticks indicate the doses that there used to compare the rate of change of the marginal effect of benzene exposure from 0.001 to 1 ppm air benzene to the corresponding rate from 1 to 10 ppm air benzene.

Figure S3 Pathways-Clusters of probes/genes. Non-parametric model fits to the marginal association of the expression of the probes corresponding to the genes involved in the a. B-cell receptor signaling, b.Toll-like receptor signaling, c. Steroid Hormone bio-synthesis and d.Maturity onset of diabetes pathways with air-benzene concentrations in parts per million. The probes are clustered based on the distance between the corresponding rows of the matrix, $X_\bullet^p$ given in Equation (6). The figure is a visual representation of the distance matrix between all the probes/genes in the pathway. The color of the $(i,j)^{th}$ position of the distance matrix is a measure of how close probes i and j are to each other based on their response across the dose range. The color ranges from white to red. The closer the pair of probes is two each other, the greater the intensity of red at the corresponding position. The dashed black lines correspond to boundaries of clusters of probes as determined by the HOPACH algorithm [47].

Table S1 List of supervised learning algorithms.

Table S2 Fixed effects estimates for the mixed model in Equation (1).

Table S3 p-Values for KEGG pathways. The p-values were computed using the *SEPEA_NT3* procedure [26] based on results of differential from expression (in at least one of the four benzene exposure groups) from the linear mixed models with (L1) and without (L0) using the blood cell counts as potential confounders of gene expression. Also listed are the p-values obtained the KEGG pathway enrichment using genes commonly identified by both models, unique to the model (L0) and unique to the model (L1).

Table S4 Median and 95% confidence interval (CI) estimates of the rate of change of marginal effect of benzene exposure below 1 ppm ($B^{i,1}$ / $\beta^{g,1}$ – see equations (10) and (13)) and above 1 ppm ($B^{i,2}$ / $\beta^{g,2}$ - see equations (11) and (14)) and the change in absolute rate of change of the marginal effects from below 1 ppm to above 1 ppm (D^i / δ^g – see equations (12) and (15)) for the first two principal components of the for the B-cell receptor signaling, Toll-like receptor signaling, Steroid hormone synthesis and Maturity onset of diabetes pathways.

Acknowledgments

Disclaimer: The views expressed in this manuscript are those of the authors and do not necessarily represent opinion or policy of the US Environmental Protection Agency.

Author Contributions

Analyzed the data: RT AEH. Designed the study: MTS NR LZ QL. Developed the statistical methods: RT AEH. Performed the microarray experiments: CMM. Performed the exposure assessment: RV SMR. Prepared the manuscript draft: RT. Provided important intellectual and editorial input: CMM AEH LZ MTS AEH NR QL RV SMR JJ KZG BRS. All authors Approved the final manuscript: RT AEH CMM LZ SMR QL NR RV KZG JJ BRS MTS.

References

1. Khalade A, Jaakkola MS, Pukkala E, Jaakkola JJK (2010) Exposure to benzene at work and the risk of leukemia: a systematic review and meta-analysis. Environmental Health 9: 31.
2. Steinmaus C, Smith AH, Jones RM, Smith MT (2008) Meta-analysis of benzene exposure and non-Hodgkin lymphoma: biases could mask an important association. Occupational and environmental medicine 65: 371.
3. Rappaport SM, Kim S, Lan Q, Vermeulen R, Waidyanatha S, et al. (2009) Evidence that humans metabolize benzene via two pathways. Environmental health perspectives 117: 946.
4. Smith MT, Zhang L, McHale CM, Skibola CF, Rappaport SM (2011) Benzene, the Exposome and Future Investigations of Leukemia Etiology. Chemico-Biological Interactions.
5. Zhang L, McHale CM, Rothman N, Li G, Ji Z, et al. (2010) Systems biology of human benzene exposure. Chem Biol Interact 184: 86–93.
6. McHale CM, Zhang L, Smith MT (2012) Current understanding of the mechanism of benzene-induced leukemia in humans: implications for risk assessment. Carcinogenesis 33: 240–252.
7. Lan Q, Zhang L, Li G, Vermeulen R, Weinberg RS, et al. (2004) Hematotoxicity in workers exposed to low levels of benzene. Science 306: 1774.
8. Rappaport SM, Waidyanatha S, Yeowell-O'Connell K, Rothman N, Smith MT, et al. (2005) Protein adducts as biomarkers of human benzene metabolism. Chemico-Biological Interactions 153: 103–109.
9. Rappaport SM, Yeowell-O'Connell K, Smith MT, Dosemeci M, Hayes RB, et al. (2002) Non-linear production of benzene oxide-albumin adducts with human exposure to benzene. Journal of Chromatographyô B 778: 367–374.
10. Vlaanderen J, Portengen L, Rothman N, Lan Q, Kromhout H, et al. (2010) Flexible meta-regression to assess the shape of the benzene-leukemia exposure-response curve. Environ Health Perspect 118: 526–532.
11. Lan Q, Vermeulen R, Zhang L, Li G, Rosenberg PS, et al. (2006) Benzene Exposure and Hematotoxicity: Response. Science 312: 998–998.
12. Qu Q, Shore R, Li G, Jin X, Chen LC, et al. (2002) Hematological changes among Chinese workers with a broad range of benzene exposures. Amô Jô Ind Med 42: 275–285.
13. McHale CM, Zhang L, Lan Q, Vermeulen R, Li G, et al. (2011) Global Gene Expression Profiling of a Population Exposed to a Range of Benzene Levels. Environmental Health Perspectives 119: 628–640.
14. van Der Laan MJ, Polley EC, Hubbard AE (2007) Super learner. Statistical applications in genetics and molecular biology 6: 25.
15. Bolen CR, Uduman M, Kleinstein SH (2011) Cell subset prediction for blood genomic studies. BMC bioinformatics 12: 258.
16. Vermeulen R, Li G, Lan Q, Dosemeci M, Rappaport SM, et al. (2004) Detailed exposure assessment for a molecular epidemiology study of benzene in two shoe factories in China. Annals of Occupational Hygiene 48: 105.
17. Kim S, Vermeulen R, Waidyanatha S, Johnson BA, Lan Q, et al. (2006) Using urinary biomarkers to elucidate dose-related patterns of human benzene metabolism. Carcinogenesis 27: 772.
18. Kanehisa M, Araki M, Goto S, Hattori M, Hirakawa M, et al. (2008) KEGG for linking genomes to life and the environment. Nucleic acids research 36: D480.
19. Kanehisa M, Goto S (2000) KEGG: Kyoto encyclopedia of genes and genomes. Nucleic acids research 28: 27.
20. Kanehisa M, Goto S, Hattori M, Aoki-Kinoshita KF, Itoh M, et al. (2006) From genomics to chemical genomics: new developments in KEGG. Nucleic acids research 34: D354.
21. Laird NM, Ware JH (1982) Random-effects models for longitudinal data. Biometrics: 963–974.
22. Gautier L, Cope L, Bolstad BM, Irizarry RA (2004) affy–analysis of Affymetrix GeneChip data at the probe level. Bioinformatics 20: 307.
23. Team RDC (2004) R: a language and environment for statistical computing. Rô foundation for Statistical Computing.
24. Bates D, Maechler M, Dai B (2008) lme4: linear mixed-effects models using S4 classes. R package version 0.999375–33. R Foundation for Statistical Computing. Vienna, Austria. lme4 r-forge r-project org/i.
25. Benjamini Y, Hochberg Y (1995) Controlling the false discovery rate: a practical and powerful approach to multiple testing. Journal of the Royal Statistical Society Seriesô Bô (Methodological): 289–300.

26. Thomas R, Gohlke J, Stopper G, Parham F, Portier C (2009) Choosing the right path: enhancement of biologically relevant sets of genes or proteins using pathway structure. Genome Biology 10: R44.

27. Kanehisa M, Araki M, Goto S, Hattori M, Hirakawa M, et al. (2008) KEGG for linking genomes to life and the environment. Nucleic acids research 36: D480.

28. Kanehisa M, Goto S, Hattori M, Aoki-Kinoshita K, Itoh M, et al. (2006) From genomics to chemical genomics: new developments in KEGG. Nucleic acids research 34: D354.

29. Polley EC (2010) SuperLearner: Super Learner Prediction. Rô package version 11–18. Available: http://wwwstatberkeleyedu/~ecpolley/SL/.

30. Breiman L (2001) Random forests. Machine learning 45: 5–32.

31. Friedman JH (1991) Multivariate adaptive regression splines. The annals of statistics: 1–67.

32. Breiman L (1996) Bagging predictors. Machine learning 24: 123–140.

33. Gelman A, Su YS, Yajima M, Hill J, Pittau MG, et al. (2010) arm: Data analysis using regression and multilevel/hierarchical models. Rô package version: 1.3–02.

34. Hothorn T, Bühlmann P, Dudoit S, Molinaro A, Van Der Laan MJ (2006) Survival ensembles. Biostatistics 7: 355.

35. Strobl C, Boulesteix AL, Kneib T, Augustin T, Zeileis A (2008) Conditional variable importance for random forests. BMC bioinformatics 9: 307.

36. Strobl C, Boulesteix AL, Zeileis A, Hothorn T (2007) Bias in random forest variable importance measures: Illustrations, sources and a solution. BMC bioinformatics 8: 25.

37. Haykin S (1999) Neural networks: a comprehensive foundation: Prentice hall.

38. Cleveland W, Grosse E, Shyu W, Chambers J, Hastie T (1991) Statistical models in S. Wadsworth and Brooks/Cole, Pacific Grove, Ch Local regression models: 309–376.

39. Hearst MA, Dumais S, Osman E, Platt J, Scholkopf B (1998) Support vector machines. Intelligent Systems and their Applications, IEEE 13: 18–28.

40. Gill RD, Robins JM (2001) Causal inference for complex longitudinal data: the continuous case. Annals of Statistics: 1785–1811.

41. van Der Laan MJ, Rose S (2011) Targeted Learning: Causal Inference for Observational and Experimental Data: Springer Verlag.

42. Goeman JJ, Oosting J, Cleton-Jansen AM, Anninga JK, Van Houwelingen HC (2005) Testing association of a pathway with survival using gene expression data. Bioinformatics 21: 1950–1957.

43. Goeman JJ, Van De Geer SA, De Kort F, Van Houwelingen HC (2004) A global test for groups of genes: testing association with a clinical outcome. Bioinformatics 20: 93–99.

44. Chen X, Wang L, Smith JD, Zhang B (2008) Supervised principal component analysis for gene set enrichment of microarray data with continuous or survival outcomes. Bioinformatics 24: 2474–2481.

45. Ma S, Kosorok MR (2009) Identification of differential gene pathways with principal component analysis. Bioinformatics 25: 882–889.

46. Eisen MB, Spellman PT, Brown PO, Botstein D (1998) Cluster analysis and display of genome-wide expression patterns. Proceedings of the National Academy of Sciences 95: 14863.

47. van der Laan MJ, Pollard KS (2003) A new algorithm for hybrid hierarchical clustering with visualization and the bootstrap. Journal of Statistical Planning and Inference 117: 275–303.

48. Pollard KS, Wall G, van der Laan MJ (2010) hopach: Hierarchical Ordered Partitioning and Collapsing Hybrid (HOPACH). Rô package version 2100. Available: http://CRANR-projectorg/package = hopach.

49. van der Laan M, Pollard K (2003) A new algorithm for hybrid hierarchical clustering with visualization and the bootstrap. Journal of Statistical Planning and Inference 117: 275–303.

50. Choudhary C, Müller-Tidow C, Berdel WE, Serve H (2005) Signal transduction of oncogenic Flt3. International journal of hematology 82: 93–99.

51. Lorsbach RB, Downing JR (2001) The role of the AML1 transcription factor in leukemogenesis. International journal of hematology 74: 258–265.

52. Metzeler KH, Heilmeier B, Edmaier KE, Rawat VP, Dufour A, et al. (2012) High expression of lymphoid enhancer-binding factor-1 (LEF1) is a novel favorable prognostic factor in cytogenetically normal acute myeloid leukemia. Blood 120: 2118–2126.

53. Mizuki M, Schwäble J, Steur C, Choudhary C, Agrawal S, et al. (2003) Suppression of myeloid transcription factors and induction of STAT response genes by AML-specific Flt3 mutations. Blood 101: 3164–3173.

54. Steffen B, Muller-Tidow C, Schwable J, Berdel WE, Serve H (2005) The molecular pathogenesis of acute myeloid leukemia. Critical reviews in oncology/hematology 56: 195–221.

55. Van Doorn SBVW, Khosrovani CE, Meijer J, Van Oosterhoud S, Van Putten W, et al. (2003) Biallelic mutations in the CEBPA gene and low CEBPA expression levels as prognostic markers in intermediate-risk AML. Hematolô J 4: 31–41.

56. Silva FP, Morolli B, Storlazzi CT, Anelli L, Wessels H, et al. (2003) Identification of RUNX1/AML1 as a classical tumor suppressor gene. Oncogene 22: 538–547.

57. Wotton S, Stewart M, Blyth K, Vaillant F, Kilbey A, et al. (2002) Proviral insertion indicates a dominant oncogenic role for Runx1/AML-1 in T-cell lymphoma. Cancer research 62: 7181–7185.

58. Koop DR, Laethem CL, Schnier GG (1989) Identification of ethanol-inducible P450 isozyme 3a (P450IIE1) as a benzene and phenol hydroxylase. Toxicology and applied pharmacology 98: 278–288.

59. Nedelcheva V, Gut I, Souček P, Tichavska B, Týnkova L, et al. (1999) Metabolism of benzene in human liver microsomes: individual variations in relation to CYP2E1 expression. Archives of toxicology 73: 33–40.

60. Powley MW, Carlson GP (2000) Cytochromes P450 involved with benzene metabolism in hepatic and pulmonary microsomes. Journal of Biochemical and Molecular Toxicology 14: 303–309.

61. Rappaport SM, Yeowell-O'Connell K, Smith MT, Dosemeci M, Hayes RB, et al. (2002) Non-linear production of benzene oxide–albumin adducts with human exposure to benzene. Journal of Chromatographyô B 778: 367–374.

62. Sammett D, Lee EW, Kocsis JJ, Snyder R (1979) Partial hepatectomy reduces both metabolism and toxicity of benzene. Jô Toxicol Environ Health 5: 785–792.

63. Powley MW, Carlson GP (2002) Benzene metabolism by the isolated perfused lung. Inhal Toxicol 14: 569–584.

64. Sheets PL, Yost GS, Carlson GP (2004) Benzene metabolism in human lung cell lines BEAS-2B and A549 and cells overexpressing CYP2F1. Jô Biochem Mol Toxicol 18: 92–99.

65. Andrews LS, Sasame H, Gillette JR (1979) 3H-Benzene metabolism in rabbit bone marrow. Life sciences 25: 567–572.

66. Subrahmanyam VV, Doane-Setzer P, Steinmetz KL, Ross D, Smith MT (1990) Phenol-induced stimulation of hydroquinone bioactivation in mouse bone marrow in vivo: possible implications in benzene myelotoxicity. Toxicology 62: 107–116.

67. Subrahmanyam VV, Kolachana P, Smith MT (1991) Hydroxylation of phenol to hydroquinone catalyzed by a human myeloperoxidase-superoxide complex: possible implications in benzene-induced myelotoxicity. Free radical research communications 15: 285–296.

4

C-MYC Aberrations as Prognostic Factors in Diffuse Large B-cell Lymphoma

Kuangguo Zhou, Danmei Xu, Yang Cao, Jue Wang, Yunfan Yang, Mei Huang*

Department of Hematology, Tongji Hospital, Tongji Medical College, Huazhong University of Science and Technology, Wuhan, Hubei, P. R. China

Abstract

Objectives: Various studies have investigated the prognostic value of C-MYC aberrations in diffuse large B-cell lymphoma (DLBCL). However, the role of C-MYC as an independent prognostic factor in clinical practice remains controversial. A systematic review and meta-analysis were performed to clarify the clinical significance of C-MYC aberrations in DLBCL patients.

Methods: The pooled hazard ratios (HRs) for overall survival (OS) and event-free survival (EFS) were calculated as the main effect size estimates. The procedure was conducted according to the Cochrane handbook and PRISMA guidelines, including the use of a heterogeneity test, publication bias assessment, and meta-regression, as well as subgroup analyses.

Results: Twenty-four eligible studies enrolling 4662 patients were included in this meta-analysis. According to the nature of C-MYC aberrations (gene, protein, and mRNA), studies were divided into several subgroups. For DLBCL patients with C-MYC gene abnormalities, the combined HR was 2.22 (95% confidence interval, 1.89 to 2.61) for OS and 2.29 (95% confidence interval, 1.81 to 2.90) for EFS, compared to patients without C-MYC gene abnormalities. For DLBCL patients with overexpression of C-MYC protein and C-MYC mRNA, pooled HRs for OS were 2.13 and 1.62, respectively. C-MYC aberrations appeared to play an independent role among other well-known prognostic factors in DLBCL. Addition of rituximab could not overcome the inferior prognosis conferred by C-MYC.

Conclusion: The present systematic review and meta-analysis confirm the prognostic value of C-MYC aberrations. Screening of C-MYC should have definite prognostic meaning for DLBCL stratification, thus guaranteeing a more tailored therapy.

Editor: Hiroyoshi Ariga, Hokkaido University, Japan

Funding: This study was sponsored by the Program of the National Natural Science Foundation of China (Grant No. 81270599). The funder had no role in study design, data collection and analysis, decision to publish, or preparation of the manuscript.

Competing Interests: The authors have declared that no competing interests exist.

* E-mail: huangmei@medmail.com.cn

Introduction

Non-Hodgkin lymphoma (NHL) is the fifth most frequent cancer worldwide, in which diffuse large B-cell lymphoma (DLBCL) ranks the most common histologic subtype. DLBCL comprises a heterogeneous group with varied clinical and molecular features and different prognoses, despite uniform treatment. Recognition of the biological heterogeneity of DLBCL is thus of clinical importance [1]. The International Prognostic Index (IPI) is currently the most well-established index for risk stratification of DLBCL patients [2]. However, this prognostic index has limitations in reflecting the biologic or genetic features of DLBCL. Even within the same IPI risk group, substantial variability in clinical outcome has been observed. A significant improvement in overall survival of DLBCL has been achieved since rituximab (R) was used in combination with cyclophosphamide, doxorubicin, vincristine, and prednisone (CHOP) as the first-line chemotherapy regimen [3]. However, the prognosis in high-risk DLBCL patients remains dismal. Identification and

validation of novel prognostic biomarkers may contribute to better stratification of DLBCL and guide optimal treatment.

To date, several prognostic biomarkers of lymphoma have been investigated, in which C-MYC is one of the most prominent factors [4]. The nature of the C-MYC aberrations included gene translocation, gene amplification, and C-MYC mRNA or C-MYC protein overexpression. C-MYC gene translocation is a hallmark of Burkitt lymphoma and can be detected in 5–17% of DLBCL patients [5]. Despite the advances achieved in the assessing prognostic significance of C-MYC in DLBCL, recent studies have implied the prognostic value of C-MYC was complicated by other factors and is far from straightforward. For example, C-MYC gene translocation was frequently found in DLBCL with concurrent translocations of BCL2 and/or BCL6, referred to as ''double-hit'' or ''triple-hit'' lymphomas, and has a dismal prognosis [6]. Although some studies have shown that the presence of C-MYC aberrations was significantly associated with shorter survival in DLBCL [7,8,9,10,11,12,13,14,15,16,17,18,19,20,21,22,23,24], other studies failed to show such an association between C-

MYC and worse prognosis [25,26,27,28,29,30]. Therefore, the role of C-MYC as independent prognostic factors needs to be further addressed in well-designed clinical trials. On the other hand, although numerous studies had been conducted to explore the prognostic values of C-MYC, no meta-analysis has assessed the predictive role of C-MYC aberrations in DLBCL. In the present study, we have conducted the first comprehensive systematic review and meta-analysis regarding the impact of C-MYC aberrations on DLBCL patients.

Materials and Methods

Selection criteria

A literature search was conducted in PUBMED, EMBASE, and COCHRANE databases. All the studies published before 31 January 2014 were included. Search criteria used synonyms of the following terms variably combined: C-MYC, prognosis and diffuse large B-cell lymphoma. The search was restricted to human studies with no language limitations.

According to the PRISMA guidelines [31], studies included in this meta-analysis should meet the following criteria: (i) C-MYC aberrations in adult patients with primary DLBCL had been examined by fluorescent in situ hybridization (FISH), immuno-histochemistry (IHC) or other techniques; (ii) detailed survival information was available; and (iii) the median follow-up time exceeded one year. In the screening and eligibility stage, patients with evidence of an indolent lymphoma, human immunodeficien-cy virus infection, or primary central nervous system disease were excluded. Because compared to other DLBCL patients, patients with evidence of these factors mentioned above had some distinct features. Moreover, all studies were carefully evaluated to identify duplicate patient populations. Criteria used to determine duplicate populations included the study period, hospital, treatment information, and any additional inclusion items. However, subsequent reports containing new data on prognostic factors or survival were also incorporated into pooled analyses of the specific point.

Quality assessment

Two investigators (KGZ and DMX) independently evaluated the methodological quality of the studies twice, applying the Newcastle-Ottawa Quality Assessment scale for case-control and cohort studies [32]. According to the quality scales, if a study met a requirement, then it gained a score of 1; otherwise, it gained a score of 0. REMARK guidelines, which provide a useful start for assessing tumor prognostic markers, were used to help identify study bias [33]. When discrepancies between investigators occurred, a third investigator (MH) conducted an additional evaluation.

Data extraction

Baseline characteristics of the included studies, such as follow-up time, were independently recorded on a spreadsheet. In each

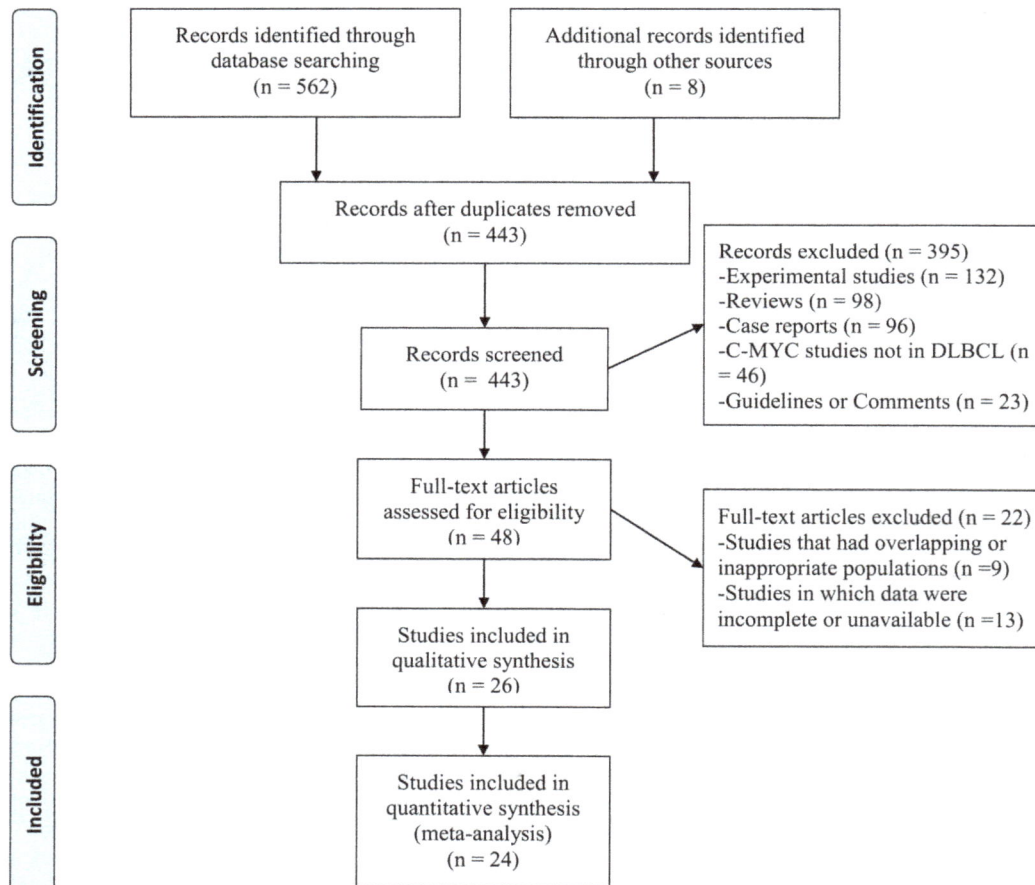

Figure 1. PRISMA flow chart of study selection.

Table 1. Features summary of the eligible studies in the meta-analysis.

Study	Year	Region	Number of patients	Detection rate	Detection method	Main treatment	Outcome	Median follow-up months (minimum, maximum)	HR	Study quality
Klapper	2008	Germany	177	7.9%	FISH	CHOP-like	EFS, OS	29 (1, 71)	Reported in text	9
Yoon	2008	Korea	156	16.1%	FISH	Mainly CHOP-like	OS	42 (3, 76)	Reported in text	7
Niitsu	2009	Japan	252	11%	Conventional G-banding technique	CyclOBEAP or CHOP-like	EFS, OS	64 (18-90)	Reported in text	7
Savage	2009	Canada	135	8.8%	FISH	R-CHOP	EFS, OS	36 (0.8, 84)	Reported in text	8
Barrans	2010	Britain	245	14%	FISH	R-CHOP	OS	24 (1, 41)	Reported in text	7
Zhang	2011	China	106	12.3%	FISH	Mainly CHOP-like	OS	35 (4, 104)	Reported in text	6
Hummel	2006	Germany	146	16.6%	FISH	Mix treatment	OS	60 (0.1, 209)	Reported in text	8
Cuccuini	2012	France	161	17%	FISH	R-DHAP or R-ICE	EFS, OS	30 (2, 76)	Reported in text	8
Green	2012	Denmark	193	11%	FISH	R-CHOP	OS	47 (1, 102)	Reported in text	8
Kramer	1998	Netherlands	151	7%	Southern blot	CHOP-like	OS	40 (1, 96)	Data-extrapolated	7
Akasaka	2000	Japan	203	11.8%	LD-PCR	CHOP-like	OS	49 (29, 118)	Data-extrapolated	8
Akyurek	2012	Turkey	239	6%	FISH	R-CHOP	OS	26 (2, 96)	Data-extrapolated	7
Kawasaki	2001	Japan	137	10.2%	Southern blot	CHOP-like	OS	25 (0.1, 99)	Data-extrapolated	8
McClure	2005	America	76	5%	FISH	Mix treatment	OS	32 (1, 219)	Reported in text	7
Saez	2003	Spain	48	27%	RT-PCR	CHOP	EFS, OS	62 (12, 110)	Reported in text	7
Rimsza	2008	Mix	208	NA	qNPA	R-CHOP and CHOP analyzed separately	OS	26 (0.6, 70)	Reported in text	8
Kojima	2013	Japan	100	10%	FISH	R-CHOP	OS	49 (2, 118)	Reported in text	8
Horn	2013	Germany	442	31.8%/8.8%	IHC/FISH	Mix treatment	EFS, OS	29 (4, 64)	Reported in text	8
Johnson	2012	Mix	307	33%/NA	IHC/Microarray	R-CHOP	OS	49 (6, 136)	Reported in text	8
Aukema	2013	Germany	562	11.5%	FISH	Mix treatment	OS	63 (3, 120)	Data-extrapolated	8
Perry	2014	Mix	106	65%	IHC	Mix treatment	OS	54 (7, 145)	Data-extrapolated	7
Tzankovet	2013	America	432	9%	FISH	R-CHOP	EFS	50 (10, 95)	Data-extrapolated	8
Kluk	2012	America	56	17.8%	IHC	R-CHOP	OS	42 (2, 87)	Data-extrapolated	9
Gupta	2012	America	24	29%/10.4%	IHC/FISH	R-CHOP/epratuzumab	EFS	24 (3, 55)	Data-extrapolated	7

Abbreviations: HR, hazard ratio; OS, overall survival; EFS, event-free survival; IHC, immunohistochemistry; FISH, interphase fluorescent *in situ* hybridization; RT-PCR, reverse transcription-polymerase chain reaction; qNPA, quantitative nuclease protection assay; LD-PCR, long-distance polymerase chain reaction; CHOP, cyclophosphamide, doxorubicin, vincristine, and prednisone; R-CHOP, rituximab, cyclophosphamide, doxorubicin, vincristine, and prednisone; CyclOBEAP, cyclophosphamide, vincristine, bleomycin, etoposide, doxorubicin, and prednisone; R-DHAP, rituximab, dexamethasone, aracytine, and cisplatin; R-ICE, rituximab, ifosfamide, etoposide, and carboplatin; NA, not available.

study, both overall survival (OS) and event-free survival (EFS) were considered endpoints for survival analysis. We assessed the prognostic impact of C-MYC using hazard ratios (HRs) and their 95% confidence intervals (95%CIs) as the main effect size estimate. For each study, HR was estimated by a method depending on the data provided in the publication. For those studies that reported the value of HR and its standard error straightforward, these data would be extracted directly. For those studies that did not report the HR but provided sufficient data on survival, the log HRs and variances were estimated based on the methodology published previously [34]. An HR greater than 1 implied a worse survival for those patients with C-MYC. Otherwise, if the value of HR was smaller than 1, a better prognosis was indicated for the group with C-MYC. Additionally, if a 95% CI for the hazard ratio included the null value of 1, then this estimate of HR was not statistically significant. If the value of HR could be obtained from both multivariate and univariate analyses, we extracted the HR from multivariate analyses.

The secondary effect size estimate was odds ratio (OR), which reflects the possible association between the previously well-known prognostic factors with C-MYC status in DLBCL, and $P < 0.05$ was considered statistically significant.

Statistical analysis

The procedure was conducted according to the Cochrane handbook, including a sensitivity test, heterogeneity test, publication bias test, and meta-regression, as well as subgroup analyses. Heterogeneity among studies was evaluated using the Cochran's Q test as well as the I^2 index. If the heterogeneity was substantial (I^2 ≥50%), the random effects model was performed. Otherwise, the fixed effects model was used. Meta-regression analysis of multiple covariates was also performed to examine the sources of heterogeneity, particularly the differences in the length of follow-up time [35,36]. Begg's and Egger's test were used to reveal possible publication bias [37,38]. A sensitivity analysis was performed to assess the stability. The inverse of the estimates' variance was used as study weight, such that larger studies tended to contribute more than smaller studies to the weighted average. The weighting factor was 1/(standard error)^2 in our study. All calculations were performed using Stata 12.0 (StataCorp, College Station, TX).

Results

Characteristics of the included studies

The selection procedure of eligible studies was shown as a flow chart (Figure 1). Twenty-four articles finally met the inclusion criteria, and their data were summarized in Table 1. The sample size in each study varied from 24 to 562, with a median follow-up time ranging from 24 to 64 months. Eight studies had reported the effect of C-MYC on EFS endpoints, and twenty-two studies on OS endpoints. Among these publications, the nature of the C-MYC aberrations included gene translocation, gene amplification, and C-MYC mRNA or C-MYC protein overexpression. The HRs and 95%CIs were therefore calculated according to the manifestation of C-MYC aberrations (gene, protein, and mRNA). In particular, Gupta et al. and Horn et al. evaluated the association of survival endpoints with both C-MYC gene translocation and C-MYC protein overexpression in DLBCL [11,26]. In Johnson et al. study, high levels of both C-MYC mRNA and C-MYC protein were both investigated [27]. Based on the nature of C-MYC aberrations, the prognostic values of C-MYC aberrations were analyzed in corresponding subgroups. The hazard ratios were carefully retrieved. Fifteen studies had the direct data for HR. For the other nine studies, the hazard ratios were extrapolated from the graphical survival distributions.

Meta-analysis for the associations between previously well-known prognostic factors with C-MYC aberrations

Six studies investigated the correlation of C-MYC with the cell-of-origin classified subgroups, including the germinal center B-cell-like (GCB) and non-GCB groups [39]. Meta-analysis revealed C-MYC were significantly more prevalent in the GCB type than in the non-GCB type ($P = 0.0002$). The correlations of the previously well-known prognostic factors with C-MYC aberrations are summarized in Table 2. Patients with C-MYC presented more frequently with poor performance status (PS), an elevated level of lactate dehydrogenase (LDH), a high Ki-67 proliferation index and poor IPI. However, the frequencies of extranodal lesion, Ann Arbor stages III~IV or bone marrow involvement were not significantly different between DLBCL patients with and without C-MYC aberrations ($P > 0.05$).

Meta-analysis for the prognostic effects of C-MYC aberrations in DLBCL patients

The forest plots of HRs and 95%CIs for OS or EFS endpoints in DLBCL patients are shown in Figure 2 and Figure 3. In particular, subgroup analyses were performed according to the subtypes of C-MYC aberrations (gene, protein, and mRNA) and treatment.

Initially, the prognostic value of C-MYC gene abnormalities was analyzed. Nineteen selected studies had investigated C-MYC gene abnormalities [7,8,9,10,11,12,13,15,16,17,20,21,22,23,25,26, 28,29,30]. Among them, seventeen studies focused on only C-MYC gene translocation, whereas the other two studies examined

Table 2. Associations between the previously well-known prognostic factors with C-MYC aberrations.

	Studies	Pooled ORs	95% CI	P-value	I^2 value
Ann Arbor stage (III~IV)	10	1.15	[0.82, 1.63]	0.4137	23.8%
Bone marrow involvement	4	1.36	[0.73, 2.52]	0.3349	45.9%
IPI (3~5)	10	1.74	[1.21, 2.51]	0.0028	23.5%
Ki-67 index (> 80~90%)	4	2.49	[1.13, 5.47]	0.0236	46.2%
LDH level (> Normal)	7	2.61	[1.63, 4.19]	0.0001	0%
Extranodal lesion (> 1)	9	1.07	[0.71, 1.63]	0.7300	36.8%
Performance status (score > 1)	7	2.17	[1.38, 3.41]	0.0008	0%

Abbreviations: IPI, international prognostic index; LDH, lactate dehydrogenase; OR, odd ratio; CI, confidence interval.

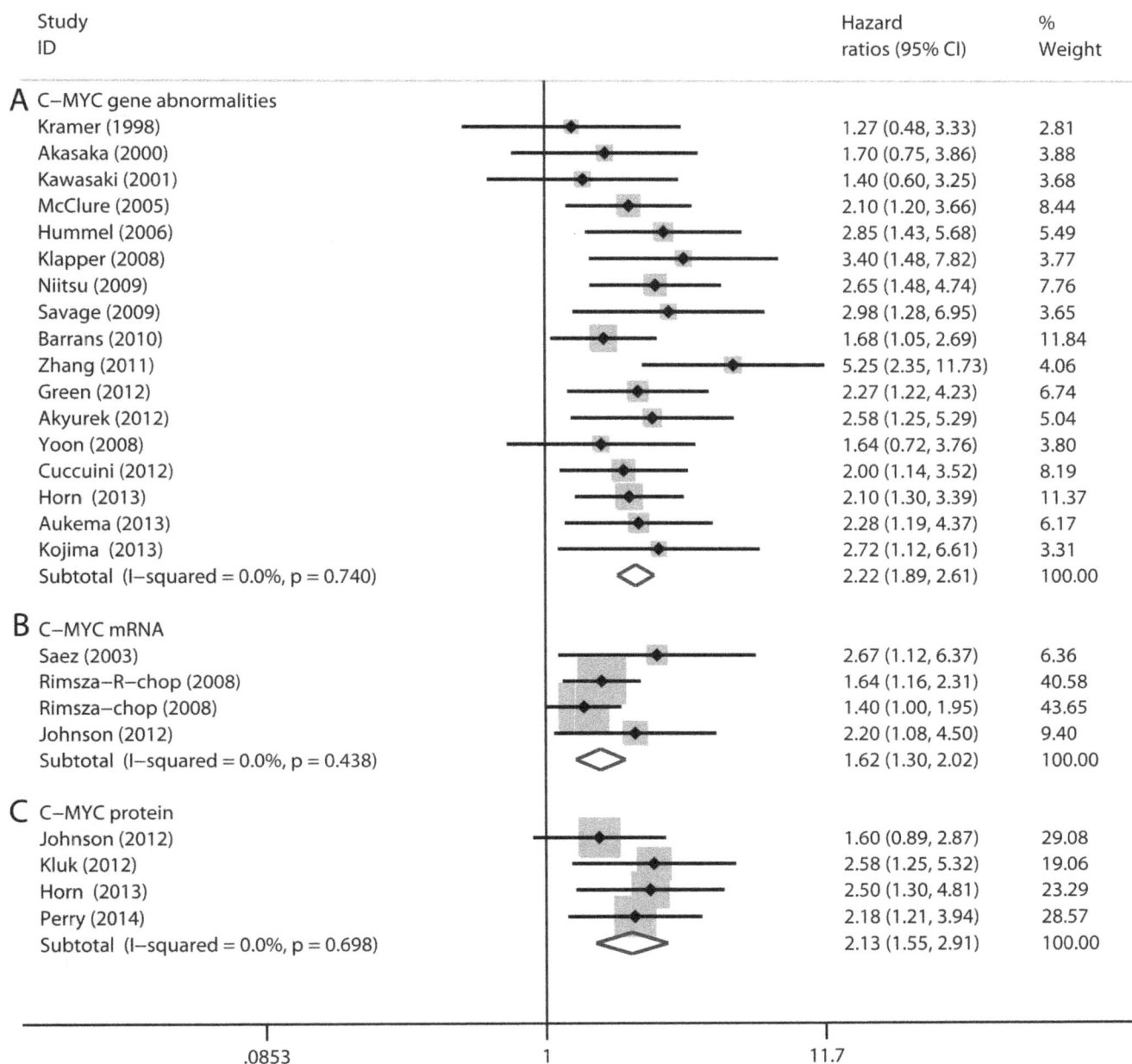

Figure 2. Forest plots of hazard ratios (HRs) and 95% confidence intervals (95% CIs) for overall survival endpoints in DLBCL patients with C-MYC gene abnormalities (A), overexpression of C-MYC mRNA (B) and C-MYC protein (C). Squares represent the HR of each study, and the area of each square was proportional to the weight of each study in the meta-analysis; Horizontal lines, 95% CIs; Closed diamond, pooled HRs with their 95% CIs.

both C-MYC gene amplification and translocation [9,30]. For C-MYC gene abnormalities, the overall HRs for OS were 2.22 (95% CI, 1.89 to 2.61) and for EFS were 2.29 (95% CI, 1.81 to 2.90) compared with the patients without C-MYC gene abnormalities. Among the studies that investigated the prognostic value of C-MYC gene translocation, five studies had further explored whether the addition of rituximab to CHOP could reduce the prognostic value of C-MYC [7,8,10,15,20]. Our study revealed that the overall HR for OS in the R-CHOP subgroup was 2.17 (95% CI, 1.62 to 2.91), similar with the overall HR for OS in the patients who were not treated with rituximab-containing regimen (detailed results were shown in Table 3), indicating that the

inferior OS conferred by C-MYC gene translocation could not be overcome by rituximab.

Among the eligible studies, nine studies [8,9,13,15,17,20, 21,26,30] that comprised 1774 patients altogether evaluated the prognostic effects of C-MYC among multivariate risk factors, such as age, IPI, and LDH. They used multivariable regression analysis to determine the independent prognostic value of C-MYC gene abnormalities. The conclusion of an 'independent effect' was based on the multivariate analysis. If the coefficient of a factor in a regression model did not change substantially after including other factors, it was defined as an independent factor. For this subgroup that used multivariable analysis, the pooled HR for OS was 2.31

Study ID		Hazard ratios (95% CI)	% Weight
A C–MYC gene abnormalities			
Klapper (2008)		2.50 (1.19, 5.23)	10.19
Niitsu (2009)		2.71 (1.50, 4.91)	15.75
Savage (2009)		3.28 (1.49, 7.22)	8.94
Gupta (2012)		2.70 (0.86, 8.51)	4.21
Cuccuini (2012)		1.80 (1.08, 3.01)	21.09
Horn (2013)		1.50 (0.90, 2.50)	21.30
Kojima (2013)		4.87 (2.03, 11.71)	7.22
Tzankovet (2013)		2.52 (1.25, 5.08)	11.30
Subtotal (I–squared = 8.3%, p = 0.366)		2.29 (1.81, 2.90)	100.00
B C–MYC mRNA			
Saez (2003)		2.94 (1.22, 7.07)	100.00
Subtotal (I–squared = .%, p = .)		2.94 (1.22, 7.07)	100.00
C C–MYC protein			
Gupta (2012)		2.10 (0.68, 6.53)	18.70
Horn (2013)		2.24 (1.30, 3.86)	81.30
Subtotal (I–squared = 0.0%, p = 0.920)		2.21 (1.36, 3.61)	100.00

.0854   1   11.7

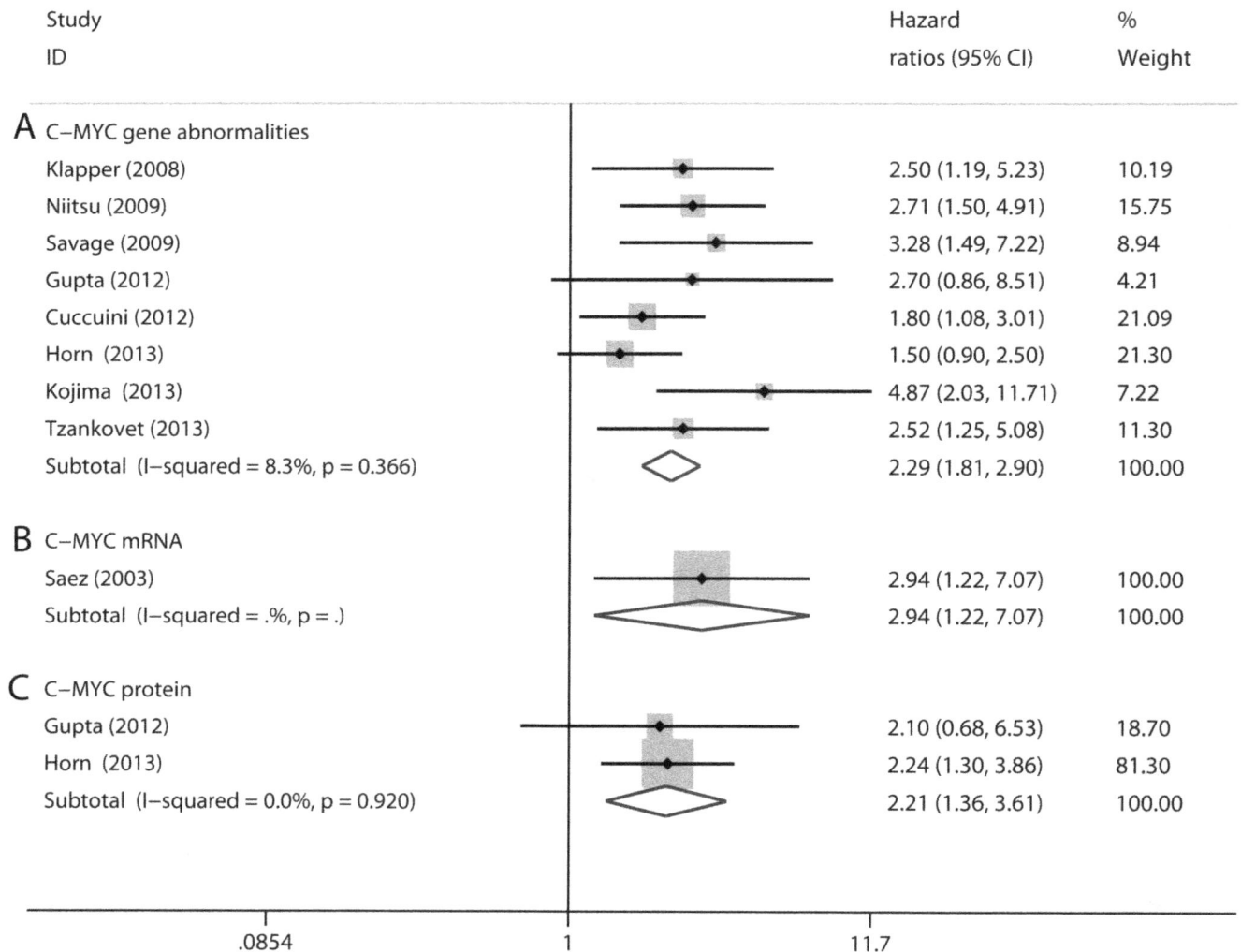

Figure 3. Forest plots of hazard ratios (HRs) and 95% confidence intervals (95% CIs) for event-free survival endpoints in DLBCL patients with C-MYC gene abnormalities (A), overexpression of C-MYC mRNA (B) and C-MYC protein (C). Squares represent the HR of each study, and the area of each square was proportional to the weight of each study in the meta-analysis; Horizontal lines, 95% CIs; Closed diamond, pooled HRs with their 95% CIs.

(95% CI, 1.87 to 2.86) compared with that for the C-MYC negative patients.

Next, the prognostic value of C-MYC overexpression was analyzed. Five studies had analyzed the prognostic value of C-MYC protein overexpression [11,14,24,26,27], and three studies had investigated that of overexpression of C-MYC mRNA [18,19,27]. For C-MYC protein overexpression, the pooled HR for OS was 2.13 (95% CI, 1.55 to 2.91) and that for EFS was 2.21 (95% CI, 1.36 to 3.61). For C-MYC mRNA overexpression, the pooled HR for OS was 1.62 with a 95% CI from 1.30 to 2.02. Meta-analysis for EFS endpoints of C-MYC mRNA could not be performed because only one study was available. In the R-CHOP subgroup, C-MYC overexpression remained to a poor prognostic factor because the pooled HR for OS was 1.93 for protein overexpression [14,27] and 1.73 for mRNA overexpression [18,27].

Detailed results of subgroup analyses for C-MYC aberrations are listed in Table 3. An additional meta-regression analysis also confirmed the worse survival of C-MYC was not influenced by the difference in follow-up time ($P > 0.05$). Taken together, our study

demonstrated that there was no significant heterogeneity for either EFS or OS (I^2 value < 50%). Publication bias tests showed no bias ($P > 0.05$). Exclusion of any single study did not alter the overall findings in the sensitivity test.

Systematic review of the prognostic role of C-MYC amplification and the isolated C-MYC aberrations (single-hit lymphoma) in DLBCL

Apart from chromosome translocation, gene amplification was another mechanism for C-MYC overexpression that had not been widely investigated. With respect to the role of C-MYC amplification, only a few studies with diverse designs were performed. Therefore, a qualitative systematic review, rather than a quantitative meta-analysis, was performed. Only three studies with a small sample size singled out the prognosis value of C-MYC amplification in DLBCL. In the two studies that evaluated the copy-number changes by FISH, C-MYC amplification appeared to be associated with a similarly poor prognosis as C-MYC translocation [9,30]. However, in another study that detected C-

Table 3. Subgroup analyses for the prognostic values of C-MYC aberrations in DLBCL patients.

Endpoints	Studies	Pooled HRs	95% CI	I^2 value	Publication bias
C-MYC gene abnormalities					
OS	17	2.22	[1.89, 2.61]	0%	PBegg = 0.56; PEgger = 0.45
OS (translocation)	15	2.27	[1.91, 2.70]	0%	PBegg = 0.43; PEgger = 0.38
OS (translocation and amplification)	2	1.88	[1.18, 3.00]	0%	PBegg = 0.32; PEgger = 1.00
OS (R-CHOP)	5	2.17	[1.62, 2.91]	0%	PBegg = 0.09; PEgger = 0.06
OS (without R)	5	2.09	[1.48, 2.95]	2.2%	PBegg = 0.14; PEgger = 0.29
OS (adjusted)	9	2.31	[1.87, 2.86]	4.3%	PBegg = 0.25; PEgger = 0.08
EFS	8	2.29	[1.81, 2.90]	8.3%	PBegg = 0.07; PEgger = 0.06
EFS (translocation)	7	2.44	[1.87, 3.18]	8.7%	PBegg = 0.23; PEgger = 0.08
EFS (translocation and amplification)	1	1.80	[1.08, 3.01]	NA	NA
EFS (R-CHOP)	4	3.18	[2.09, 4.84]	0%	PBegg = 0.63; PEgger = 0.77
EFS (without R)	2	2.63	[1.65, 4.17]	0%	PBegg = 0.32; PEgger = 1.00
C-MYC mRNA overexpression					
OS	3	1.62	[1.30, 2.02]	0%	PBegg = 0.09; PEgger = 0.07
OS (R-CHOP)	2	1.73	[1.27, 2.36]	0%	PBegg = 0.32; PEgger = 1.00
EFS	1	2.94	[1.22, 7.07]	NA	NA
C-MYC protein overexpression					
OS	4	2.13	[1.55, 2.91]	0%	PBegg = 0.09; PEgger = 0.24
OS (R-CHOP)	2	1.93	[1.23, 3.05]	2.2%	PBegg = 0.32; PEgger = 1.00
EFS	2	2.21	[1.36, 3.61]	0%	PBegg = 0.32; PEgger = 1.00

Abbreviations: HR, hazard ratio; OS, overall survival; EFS, event-free survival; CI, confidence interval; R-CHOP, rituximab, cyclophosphamide, doxorubicin, vincristine, and prednisone; without R, treatment without rituximab; NA, not available.

MYC amplification by array-based comparative genomic hybridization, extra copies of C-MYC were associated with poor OS and progression-free survival only in the present of concomitant del(8p), but not in all DLBCL patients [40].

Similarly, to find whether presence of double or triple hits might influence the outcome, a qualitative systematic review was performed to investigate the prognostic effects of isolated C-MYC aberrations (single-hit lymphoma). Generally, two comparison methods were applied to demonstrate the role of isolated C-MYC aberrations in DLBCL. Six studies compared single-hit patients with complex-hit cases. Among them, one study showed the complex-hit group had a worse prognosis than the single-hit group [17]; however, other studies found no difference between the two subgroups [9,12,22,26,30]. Furthermore, another three studies directly compared single-hit patients with C-MYC-negative patients. Two of them found the presence of C-MYC alone retained unfavorable prognostic significance [12,20], but another study did not [41]. Comparisons among different studies were hampered by only a few studies available, with the diverse study designs as well as the small-size cases.

Discussion

Thus far, the present study is the first systematic review and meta-analysis about the prognostic value of C-MYC in DLBCL. The current meta-analysis integrated 4662 DLBCL cases and strongly confirmed the role of C-MYC as a prognostic factor in DLBCL. To increase accuracy, studies were divided into several subgroups according to the nature of C-MYC aberrations and treatment. Based on this meta-analysis, several critical issues had been addressed. First, DLBCL patients with C-MYC were proven to be associated with several adverse clinical features. Second, the

addition of rituximab did not seem to overcome the inferior outcome conferred by C-MYC. Moreover, after pooling the HRs adjusted by multivariate Cox models from nine studies, C-MYC appeared to maintain its independent prognostic value, regardless of other well-established factors. In light of meta-regression and subgroup analysis, the pooled results appeared not to be influenced by the length of follow-up time. In addition, the median follow-up time in all the included studies exceeded 24 months. C-MYC aberrations represented the most reproducible biomarker with unfavorable prognosis regardless of the biological test used. Screening of C-MYC should have definite prognostic meaning for DLBCL stratification, thus guaranteeing more tailored therapy.

Some questions remain uncertain regarding the prognostic role of C-MYC aberrations in DLBCL. First, a qualitative systematic review was performed on the role of C-MYC amplification due to the rarity and heterogeneity of the selected studies. It had been postulated that overexpression of C-MYC by amplification had a similar effect to up-regulation by C-MYC translocation in DLBCL [42,43,44]. However, different studies with small-size cases appeared to be inconsistent. Similarly, the prognostic effects of isolated C-MYC aberrations (single-hit lymphoma) also remained controversial due to the limited studies with inconsistent conclusion. In the future, prospective studies with large sample size or a patient-level meta-analysis need to be conducted to address these issues.

Second, assessment of C-MYC aberrations in pathology specimens is becoming increasingly important in the routine clinical practice. Statistical analysis has demonstrated there is a significant correlation between deregulation of C-MYC protein and mRNA with C-MYC gene abnormalities [43,44,45]. Unfortunately, in contrast to the ease in detecting C-MYC gene translocation, it is not so straightforward to define DLBCL patients with C-MYC mRNA or protein overexpression because markedly different cut-off values and methods were apparent between centers. Some studies established cut-off values (50% or 70%) for classifying tumors as the lowest C-MYC IHC score that captured all cases with a confirmed C-MYC translocation [14,45], while others used a lower threshold (40%) which was set based on the relationship between C-MYC protein and survival, not the presence of a translocation [27]. The difference in tissue processing, inter-observer variability and cut-off values contributes to poor reproducible results of the mRNA/protein expression levels among different institutions. Therefore, at this point, it is difficult to make definitive recommendations regarding the optimal cut-off points for C-MYC for general use, as these needs to be validated in large prospective cohorts of DLBCL patients. Nevertheless, the conclusion of this meta-analysis is still valid. Standardization and validation of current assays and agreement upon the techniques to quantitate C-MYC mRNA or protein are at urgent need for its widespread application in clinical practice.

In conclusion, this systematic review and meta-analysis underscores the prognostic value of C-MYC in DLBCL. Screening of C-MYC aberrations could enable the early identification of DLBCL patients with poor prognosis and guide a more tailored therapy. Further well-designed clinical trials should be warranted to address the uncertain problems due to the current limited studies.

Acknowledgments

We thank for all the patients and clinical investigators who are involved in the studies selected in this systematic review and meta-analysis.

Author Contributions

Conceived and designed the experiments: KGZ MH. Performed the experiments: KGZ DMX MH. Analyzed the data: KGZ YC JW YFY. Contributed reagents/materials/analysis tools: DMX. Wrote the paper: KGZ MH.

References

1. Sehn LH (2012) Paramount prognostic factors that guide therapeutic strategies in diffuse large B-cell lymphoma. Hematology Am Soc Hematol Educ Program 2012: 402-409.
2. The International Non-Hodgkin's Lymphoma Prognostic Factors Project (1993) A predictive model for aggressive non-Hodgkin's lymphoma. N Engl J Med 329: 987–994.
3. Coiffier B, Lepage E, Briere J, Herbrecht R, Tilly H, et al. (2002) CHOP chemotherapy plus rituximab compared with CHOP alone in elderly patients with diffuse large-B-cell lymphoma. N Engl J Med 346: 235–242.
4. Perry AM, Mitrovic Z, Chan WC (2012) Biological prognostic markers in diffuse large B-cell lymphoma. Cancer Control 19: 214–226.
5. Slack GW, Gascoyne RD (2011) MYC and aggressive B-cell lymphomas. Adv Anat Pathol 18: 219–228.
6. Pfreundschuh M (2012) Growing importance of MYC/BCL2 immunohistochemistry in diffuse large B-cell lymphomas. J Clin Oncol 30: 3433–3435.
7. Akyurek N, Uner A, Benekli M, Barista I (2012) Prognostic significance of MYC, BCL2, and BCL6 rearrangements in patients with diffuse large B-cell lymphoma treated with cyclophosphamide, doxorubicin, vincristine, and prednisone plus rituximab. Cancer 118: 4173–4183.
8. Barrans S, Crouch S, Smith A, Turner K, Owen R, et al. (2010) Rearrangement of MYC is associated with poor prognosis in patients with diffuse large B-cell lymphoma treated in the era of rituximab. J Clin Oncol 28: 3360–3365.
9. Cuccuini W, Briere J, Mounier N, Voelker HU, Rosenwald A, et al. (2012) MYC+ diffuse large B-cell lymphoma is not salvaged by classical R-ICE or R-DHAP followed by BEAM plus autologous stem cell transplantation. Blood 119: 4619–4624.
10. Green TM, Young KH, Visco C, Xu-Monette ZY, Orazi A, et al. (2012) Immunohistochemical double-hit score is a strong predictor of outcome in patients with diffuse large B-cell lymphoma treated with rituximab plus cyclophosphamide, Doxorubicin, vincristine, and prednisone. J Clin Oncol 30: 3460–3467.
11. Gupta M, Maurer MJ, Wellik LE, Law ME, Han JJ, et al. (2012) Expression of Myc but not pSTAT3, is an adverse prognostic factor for diffuse large cell lymphoma treated with epratuzumab/R-CHOP. Blood 119:4400–4406.
12. Hummel M, Bentink S, Berger H, Klapper W, Wessendorf S, et al. (2006) A biologic definition of Burkitt's lymphoma from transcriptional and genomic profiling. N Engl J Med 354: 2419–2430.
13. Klapper W, Stoecklein H, Zeynalova S, Ott G, Kosari F, et al. (2008) Structural aberrations affecting the MYC locus indicate a poor prognosis independent of clinical risk factors in diffuse large B-cell lymphomas treated within randomized trials of the German High-Grade Non-Hodgkin's Lymphoma Study Group (DSHNHL). Leukemia 22: 2226–2229.
14. Kluk MJ, Chapuy B, Sinha P, Roy A, Dal Cin P, et al. (2012) Immunohistochemical detection of MYC-driven diffuse large B-cell lymphomas. PLoS One 7: e33813.
15. Kojima M, Nishikii H, Takizawa J, Aoki S, Noguchi M, et al. (2013) MYC rearrangements are useful for predicting outcomes following rituximab and chemotherapy: multicenter analysis of Japanese patients with diffuse large B-cell lymphoma. Leuk Lymphoma 54: 2149–2154.
16. McClure RF, Remstein ED, Macon WR, Dewald GW, Habermann TM, et al. (2005) Adult B-cell lymphomas with burkitt-like morphology are phenotypically and genotypically heterogeneous with aggressive clinical behavior. Am J Surg Pathol 29: 1652–1660.
17. Nitsu N, Okamoto M, Miura I, Hirano M (2009) Clinical significance of 8q24/c-MYC translocation in diffuse large B-cell lymphoma. Cancer Sci 100: 233–237.
18. Rimsza LM, Leblanc ML, Unger JM, Miller TP, Grogan TM, et al. (2008) Gene expression predicts overall survival in paraffin-embedded tissues of diffuse large B-cell lymphoma treated with R-CHOP. Blood 112: 3425–3433.
19. Saez AI, Artiga MJ, Romero C, Rodriguez S, Cigudosa JC, et al. (2003) Development of a real-time reverse transcription polymerase chain reaction assay for c-myc expression that allows the identification of a subset of c-myc+ diffuse large B-cell lymphoma. Lab Invest 83: 143–152.
20. Savage KJ, Johnson NA, Ben-Neriah S, Connors JM, Sehn LH, et al. (2009) MYC gene rearrangements are associated with a poor prognosis in diffuse large B-cell lymphoma patients treated with R-CHOP chemotherapy. Blood 114: 3533–3537.
21. Zhang HW, Chen ZW, Li SH, Bai W, Cheng NL, et al. (2011) Clinical significance and prognosis of MYC translocation in diffuse large B-cell lymphoma. Hematol Oncol 29: 185–189.
22. Aukema SM, Kreuz M, Kohler CW, Rosolowski M, Hasenclever D, et al. (2013) Biologic characterization of adult MYC-translocation positive mature B-cell lymphomas other than molecular Burkitt lymphoma. Haematologica Epub ahead of print.
23. Tzankov A, Xu-Monette ZY, Gerhard M, Visco C, Dirnhofer S, et al. (2013) Rearrangements of MYC gene facilitate risk stratification in diffuse large B-cell lymphoma patients treated with rituximab-CHOP. Mod Pathol [Epub ahead of print].
24. Perry AM, Alvarado-Bernal Y, Laurini JA, Smith LM, Slack GW, et al. (2014) MYC and BCL2 protein expression predicts survival in patients with diffuse large B-cell lymphoma treated with rituximab. Br J Haematol [Epub ahead of print].
25. Akasaka T, Akasaka H, Ueda C, Yonetani N, Maesako Y, et al. (2000) Molecular and clinical features of non-Burkitt's, diffuse large-cell lymphoma of B-cell type associated with the c-MYC/immunoglobulin heavy-chain fusion gene. J Clin Oncol 18: 510–518.
26. Horn H, Ziepert M, Becher C, Barth TF, Bernd HW, et al. (2013) MYC status in concert with BCL2 and BCL6 expression predicts outcome in diffuse large B-cell lymphoma. Blood 121:2253–2263.
27. Johnson NA, Slack GW, Savage KJ, Connors JM, Ben-Neriah S, et al. (2012) Concurrent Expression of MYC and BCL2 in Diffuse Large B-Cell Lymphoma Treated With Rituximab Plus Cyclophosphamide, Doxorubicin, Vincristine, and Prednisone. J Clin Oncol 30: 3452–3459.
28. Kawasaki C, Ohshim K, Suzumiya J, Kanda M, Tsuchiya T, et al. (2001) Rearrangements of bcl-1, bcl-2, bcl-6, and c-myc in diffuse large B-cell lymphomas. Leuk Lymphoma 42: 1099–1106.
29. Kramer MH, Hermans J, Wijburg E, Philippo K, Geelen E, et al. (1998) Clinical relevance of BCL2, BCL6, and MYC rearrangements in diffuse large B-cell lymphoma. Blood 92: 3152–3162.
30. Yoon SO, Jeon YK, Paik JH, Kim WY, Kim YA, et al. (2008) MYC translocation and an increased copy number predict poor prognosis in adult diffuse large B-cell lymphoma (DLBCL), especially in germinal centre-like B cell (GCB) type. Histopathology 53: 205–217.

31. Moher D, Liberati A, Tetzlaff J, Altman DG (2009) Preferred reporting items for systematic reviews and meta-analyses: the PRISMA statement. PLoS Med 6: e1000097.

32. Stang A (2010) Critical evaluation of the Newcastle-Ottawa scale for the assessment of the quality of nonrandomized studies in meta-analyses. Eur J Epidemiol 25: 603–605.

33. McShane LM, Altman DG, Sauerbrei W, Taube SE, Gion M, et al. (2005) Reporting recommendations for tumor marker prognostic studies. J Clin Oncol 23: 9067–9072.

34. Parmar MK, Torri V, Stewart L (1998) Extracting summary statistics to perform meta-analyses of the published literature for survival endpoints. Stat Med 17: 2815–2834.

35. Zhang LQ, Wang J, Jiang F, Xu L, Liu FY, et al. (2012) Prognostic value of survivin in patients with non-small cell lung carcinoma: a systematic review with meta-analysis. PLoS One 7: e34100.

36. Moja L, Piatti A, Pecoraro V, Ricci C, Virgili G, et al. (2012) Timing matters in hip fracture surgery: patients operated within 48 hours have better outcomes. A meta-analysis and meta-regression of over 190,000 patients. PLoS One 7: e46175.

37. Begg CB, Mazumdar M (1994) Operating characteristics of a rank correlation test for publication bias. Biometrics 50: 1088–1101.

38. Egger M, Davey Smith G, Schneider M, Minder C (1997) Bias in meta-analysis detected by a simple, graphical test. BMJ 315: 629–634.

39. Hans CP, Weisenburger DD, Greiner TC, Gascoyne RD, Delabie J, et al. (2004) Confirmation of the molecular classification of diffuse large B-cell lymphoma by immunohistochemistry using a tissue microarray. Blood 103: 275–282.

40. Testoni M, Kwee I, Greiner TC, Montes-Moreno S, Vose J, et al. (2011) Gains of MYC locus and outcome in patients with diffuse large B-cell lymphoma treated with R-CHOP. Br J Haematol 155: 274–277.

41. Visco C, Tzankov A, Xu-Monette ZY, Miranda RN, Tai YC, et al. (2013) Patients with diffuse large B cell lymphoma of germinal center origin with BCL2 translocations have poor outcome, irrespective of MYC status: a report from an International DLBCL rituximab-CHOP Consortium Program Study. Haematologica 98:255–263.

42. Mossafa H, Damotte D, Jenabian A, Delarue R, Vincenneau A, et al. (2006) Non-Hodgkin's lymphomas with Burkitt-like cells are associated with c-Myc amplification and poor prognosis. Leuk Lymphoma 47: 1885–1893.

43. Stasik CJ, Nitta H, Zhang W, Mosher CH, Cook JR, et al. (2010) Increased MYC gene copy number correlates with increased mRNA levels in diffuse large B-cell lymphoma. Haematologica 95: 597–603.

44. Valentino C, Kendrick S, Johnson N, Gascoyne R, Chan WC, et al. (2013) Colorimetric in situ hybridization identifies MYC gene signal clusters correlating with increased copy number, mRNA, and protein in diffuse large B-cell lymphoma. Am J Clin Pathol 139: 242–254.

45. Green TM, Nielsen O, de Stricker K, Xu-Monette ZY, Young KH, et al. (2012) High levels of nuclear MYC protein predict the presence of MYC rearrangement in diffuse large B-cell lymphoma. Am J Surg Pathol 36: 612–619.

5

NF-Kappa B Modulation is Involved in Celastrol Induced Human Multiple Myeloma Cell Apoptosis

Haiwen Ni[1], Wanzhou Zhao[2], Xiangtu Kong[1], Haitao Li[3], Jian Ouyang[4]*

1 Affiliated Hospital of Nanjing University of TCM, Nanjing, China, **2** Sino-EU Biomedical Innovation Center (SEBIC), OG Pharma Corporation, Nanjing, China, **3** Nanjing University of Chinese Medicine, Nanjing,China, **4** Department of Hematology, Nanjing Drum Tower Hospital, the Affiliated Hospital of Nanjing University Medical School, Nanjing, China

Abstract

Celastrol is an active compound extracted from the root bark of the traditional Chinese medicine *Tripterygium wilfordii Hook F*. To investigate the effect of celastrol on human multiple myeloma cell cycle arrest and apoptosis and explore its molecular mechanism of action. The activity of celastrol on LP-1 cell proliferation was detected by WST-8 assay. The celastrol-induced cell cycle arrest was analyzed by flow cytometry after propidium iodide staining. Nuclear translocation of the nuclear factor kappa B (NF-κB) was observed by fluorescence microscope. Celastrol inhibited cell proliferation of LP-1 myeloma cell in a dose-dependent manner with IC50 values of 0.8817 μM, which was mediated through G1 cell cycle arrest and p27 induction. Celastrol induced apoptosis in LP-1 and RPMI 8226 myeloma cells in a time and dose dependent manner, and it involved Caspase-3 activation and NF-κB pathway. Celastrol down-modulated antiapoptotic proteins including Bcl-2 and survivin expression. The expression of NF-κB and IKKa were decreased after celastrol treatment. Celastrol effectively blocked the nuclear translocation of the p65 subunit and induced human multiple myeloma cell cycle arrest and apoptosis by p27 upregulation and NF-kB modulation. It has been demonstrated that the effect of celastrol on NF-kB was HO-1-independent by using zinc protoporphyrin-9 (ZnPPIX), a selective heme oxygenase inhibitor. From the results, it could be inferred that celastrol may be used as a NF-kB inhibitor to inhibit myeloma cell proliferation.

Editor: Salvatore V. Pizzo, Duke University Medical Center, United States of America

Funding: The authors have no support or funding to report.

Competing Interests: Wanzhou Zhao is employed by Sino-EU Biomedical Innovation Center (SEBIC), OG Pharma Corporation.

* E-mail: ouyangjiangulou@gmail.com

Introduction

Multiple myeloma (MM) is still an incurable hematological malignancy with a median survival of 4 years despite the use of various treatment options including thalidomide, lenalidomide, bortezomib, and hematopoietic stem cell transplantation [1,2]. The findings in molecular mechanisms that lead to MM and its progression have lead to the clarification of molecular targets of this disease and may contribute to the development of new biological targeted therapies for MM [3].

MM is a fatal plasma cell malignancy arising from the mature plasma cells in the bone marrow characterized by bone destruction, hypercalcemia, anemia, immunodeficiency, and renal damage [4]. The patients suffering from MM often result in recurrent or increased susceptibility to bacterial, fungal, and viral infections which remain a major cause of their deaths [5,6].

For the past 30 years, many natural products derived from plants and marine have provided leading structures for developing new agents with enhanced biological properties and less toxicity than chemotherapeutic agents [7,8].

Many natural products induced apoptosis of human cancer cells through the basic molecular mechanisms that take place in cancer [9,10]. It has been reported that the cancer and inflammation may have common signal pathways [11–14]. It is our hypothesis that the novel therapeutic agents with anti-inflammatory activity may prolong MM progression and overcome drug resistance.

Celastrol is an active compound extracted from the root bark of the traditional Chinese medicine Tripterygium wilfordii Hook F [15–18]. It has been effectively used in the treatment of chronic inflammation and autoimmune diseases such as arthritis, lupus erythematosus, and lateral sclerosis [19,20]. Although celastrol was reported to inhibit multiple cancer cell proliferation and induce cell death such as breast cancer [21], colon cancer [22], prostate cancer [23,24], oral squamous cell carcinoma [25], glioma [26], melanoma [27], and leukemia [28], the direct targets and molecular mechanisms of celastrol-induced apoptosis in cancer cells remain unknown. In present the study, an attempt to investigate the effect of celastrol on LP-1 human myeloma cell apoptosis and its molecular mechanism of action was made.

Material and Methods

2.1. Reagents

A 100 mM solution of celastrol (from Sigma) was prepared in dimethyl sulfoxide (DMSO) and stored as small aliquots at −20°C. Subsequent dilutions were made in a cell culture medium. The same proportion of DMSO/culture medium was added to the controls. The final DMSO content was less than 0.1%. Penicillin, streptomycin, Dulbecco's modified Eagle's medium, Rosewell Park Memorial Institute (shortly RPMI-1640) medium, and fetal bovine serum were obtained from Invitrogen. Propidium Iodide/Ribonuclease (shortly PI/RNase) Staining Buffer and Annexin V-

Fluorescein Isothiocyanate (FITC) Apoptosis Detection Kit I were purchased from BD Pharmingen (USA).

2.2. Cell line and culture conditions

Human MM cell line LP-1 (Deutsche Sammlung von Mikroorganismen und Zellkulturen GmbH, Germany) was cultured in Iscove's modified Dulbecco's medium (Gibco), and RPMI 8226 (ATCC) was cultured in RPMI 1640 medium (Gibco) containing 10% fetal calf serum, 2 mmol/L l-glutamine, and 100 U/mL penicillin, and 100 mg/mL streptomycin. All cell lines were maintained at 37°C in a fully humidified atmosphere of 5% carbondioxide in air.

2.3. Cell viability assay [29]

The antiproliferative effects of celastrol on MM cells were determined by the WST-8 dye uptake method. The cells were plated into a 96-well plate at a density of 1×10^4/well and treated with the indicated dose of celastrol for 72 hours of incubation. For the cell viability assay, 20 μL of WST-8 solution (EnoGene) was added to each well. The plates were further incubated for 4 hours. The absorbance of each well was measured using an enzyme-linked immunosorbent assay reader at 450 nm.

2.4. Deoxyribonucleic acid (DNA) content and cell cycle analysis [30]

The celastrol-treated cells were fixed in 70% ethanol at 4°C overnight. After twice washed with phosphate buffer solution (PBS), the cells were suspended in hypotonic solution containing 0.1% Triton X-100, 1 mM Tris-hydrochloride (pH 8.0), 3.4 mM sodium citrate, 0.1 mM EDTA; and the cells were stained with PI (50 μg/mL) and RNase A (1 mg/mL) for 30 min. A total of 10,000 events were analyzed by flow cytometry using an excitation wavelength set at 488 nm and emission set at 610 nm. The DNA content was analyzed by flow cytometry (FACScalibur, BD Biosciences). The population of cells in each cycle phase was analyzed using WinMDI 2.8 software (Purdue University Cytometry Laboratory).

2.5. Annexin V apoptosis assay [31]

The cells were treated with celastrol (0.25 and 0.5 μM) for the indicated times (0–48 h). The apoptotic cells were determined by double staining with Annexin V-FITC and PI according to the instructions of kit's manufacturer (EnoGene). The cells were analyzed on a flow cytometer (FACSCalibur, Becton-Dickinson, San Jose, CA) using CellQuest software. The cells that were Annexin V (−) and PI (−) were considered viable cells; Annexin V (+) and PI (−) were considered early-stage apoptotic cells; Annexin V (+) and PI (+) were considered late-stage apoptotic cells; and Annexin V (−) and PI (+) were considered necrotic cells.

2.6. Caspase activation assay [32]

Caspase-3 activity was determined by using a caspase-3 assay kit (PharMingen, San Diego, CA) according to the manufacturer's instructions. The cells (1×10^5) were homogenized in a lysis buffer containing 0.1% CHAPS, 50 mM HEPES (pH 8.0), 12.5 mM NaCl, 0.1 mM EDTA, and 5 mM DTT freshly added. The whole cell lysates (40 mg) were incubated with 20 mM of colorimetric substrate acetyl-Asp-Glu-Val-Asp p-nitroanilide (Ac-DEVD-pNA) in a reaction buffer (BioVision) containing 5 mM DTT at 37°C for 1 h. pNA was released from the substrate upon cleavage by DEVDase. The yellow color produced by free pNA was monitored by a spectrophotometer at 405 nm. The amount of yellow color produced upon cleavage was proportional to the amount of DEVDase activity.

2.7. Western blotting [33]

The celastrol-treated cells were lysed in a lysis buffer containing 20 mM Tris (pH 7.4), 250 mM NaCl, 2 mM EDTA (pH 8.0), 0.1% Triton X-100, 0.01 mg·mL-1 aprotinin, 0.005 mg·mL-1 leupeptin, 0.4 mM PMSF, and 4 mM NaVO4. The proteins were separated by SDS-polyacrylamidegel electrophoresis. After electrophoresis, the proteins were electrotransferred onto nitrocellulose membranes and blotted with various primary antibodies (1:1000). Antibodies against Cyclin D1, P21, P27, Bcl-2, Bax, survivin, NF-kappa B p65, and internal control antibody GAPDH were obtained from EnoGene. The blot was washed, exposed to horseradish peroxidase-conjugated secondary antibodies for 1 h, and finally detected by ECL reagent (GE Healthcare). The band densitometric analysis of the scanned blots was performed using Image J software, and the results are expressed as fold change relative to the internal control.

2.8. Immunofluorescence [34]

The cells were grown on coverslips and cultured for 24 hours. After treatment with the indicated doses of celastrol, the cells were fixed in 4% paraformaldehyde for 15 minutes, washed in PBS, and treated for 15 minutes with PBS containing 0.1% Triton X-100. The cells were then washed, blocked with 10% bovine serum albumin (BSA) for 1 hour at room temperature, and incubated at 4°C overnight with NF-kappa B p65 antibody (1:100) diluted in 0.1% BSA. After extensive washing, a 1:200 dilution of FITC-conjugated goat anti-mouse immunoglobulin was applied as the secondary antibody for 1 hour at room temperature. Nuclear staining was achieved by incubating cells in DAPI for 5 minutes. The slides were then washed and photographed with an OLYMPUS 1X71 fluorescence microscope. Zinc Protoporphyrin-9 (ZnPPIX) is a potent, selective heme oxygenase inhibitor. In this study, 24 hrs before celastrol treatment, cells were treated with 1 μM Zinc Protoporphyrin-9 (Santa Cruz Biotechnology) to study if the effect of Celatrol on NF-kB is heme oxygenase-dependent.

2.9. Statistical analysis

All assays were repeated thrice to ensure reproducibility. The results are expressed as mean ± standard deviation (SD). The significance of results obtained from the control and treated groups was performed by Student's unpaired t-test and one way analysis of variance. Means and standard deviations were calculated. A probability (P) value less than 0.05 was considered statistically significant.

Results

3.1. Celastrol induced proliferation inhibition in LP-1 MM cell

The effects of celastrol was examined with triterpenoid quinone methide structure (Figure 1) on the cellular proliferation of human MM cell line LP-1. Celastrol inhibited cell proliferation of LP-1 MM cell in a dose-dependent manner with IC50 values of 0.8817 μM (Figure 2). At the concentration of 50 μM, the cell proliferation inhibitory rate was over 80%. Significant morphological changes such as shrinkage of cell and detachment of cell from the surrounding of LP-1 myeloma cell were observed at a concentration of 0.78125 μM.

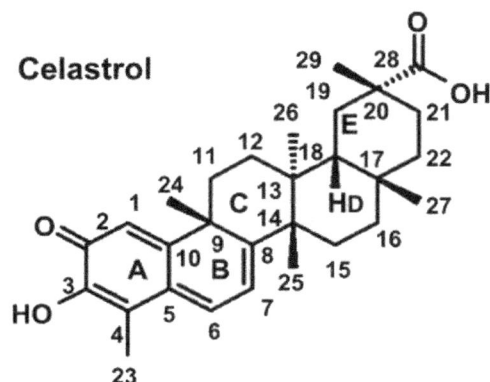

Figure 1. Chemical structures of Celastrol. Celastrol is a natural triterpenoid quinone methide isolated from the Chinese plant genuses of celastrus, maytenus, and tripterygium.

3.2. Celastrol-induced cell proliferation inhibition was mediated through G1 cell-cycle arrest in LP-1 myeloma cells

To investigate if the proliferation inhibition by celastrol was caused by cell cycle arrest of LP-1 myeloma cell, the cell cycle distribution of LP-1 cell treated with 0.5 μM of celastrol for 12 and 24 h was analyzed using flow cytometry. There was an increase in the cells in the G1 phase (Fig. 3), which suggested that celastrol induced G1 phase arrest.

3.3. p27 induction was essential for Celastrol induced cell cycle arrest in LP-1 MM cell

The cell division relies on the activation of cyclins, which bind to the cyclin-dependent kinases (CDKs) to induce cell-cycle progression towards S phase and later to initiate mitosis. Since the uncontrolled CDK activity is often the cause of human cancer, their function is tightly regulated by cell-cycle inhibitors such as the p21 and p27 Cip/Kip proteins. Therefore, the cyclin D1, p21, and p27 Cip/Kip expression was investigated in LP-1 cell treated with 0.25, 0.5, and 1 μM of celastrol for 24 h. The study findings convincingly showed that an up-regulation of p27 but not p21 and down-regulation of cyclin D1 were the most important and central event in celastrol-induced G1 arrest in human myeloma cells (Figure 4).

3.4. Induction of apoptosis by celastrol in myeloma cells

To investigate the mechanism of cytotoxic effect of celastrol, the apoptosis using Annexin-V and PI-double staining was measured in both LP-1 and RPMI 8226 cells to investigate that the apoptotic effect of celastrol is not specific to only LP-1 cells. An early indicator of apoptosis is the rapid translocation and accumulation of the membrane phospholipid phosphatidylserine from the cytoplasmic interface to the extracellular surface. This membrane asymmetry loss could be detected by utilizing the binding properties of Annexin V. Staining was tested by both fluorescence microscope (Figure 5) and flow cytometry (Figure 6). After treatment with 1 μM celastrol for 0 h, 12 h, 24 h, 36 h, and 48 h, the apoptotic LP-1 cell percentage was 7.8±0.4%, 16.1±1.2% (p<0.05 vs 0 h), 18.0±3.1% (p<0.05 vs 0 h), 39.5±5.8% (p<0.01 vs 0 h), and 71.2±8.6% (p<0.01 vs 0 h), respectively.

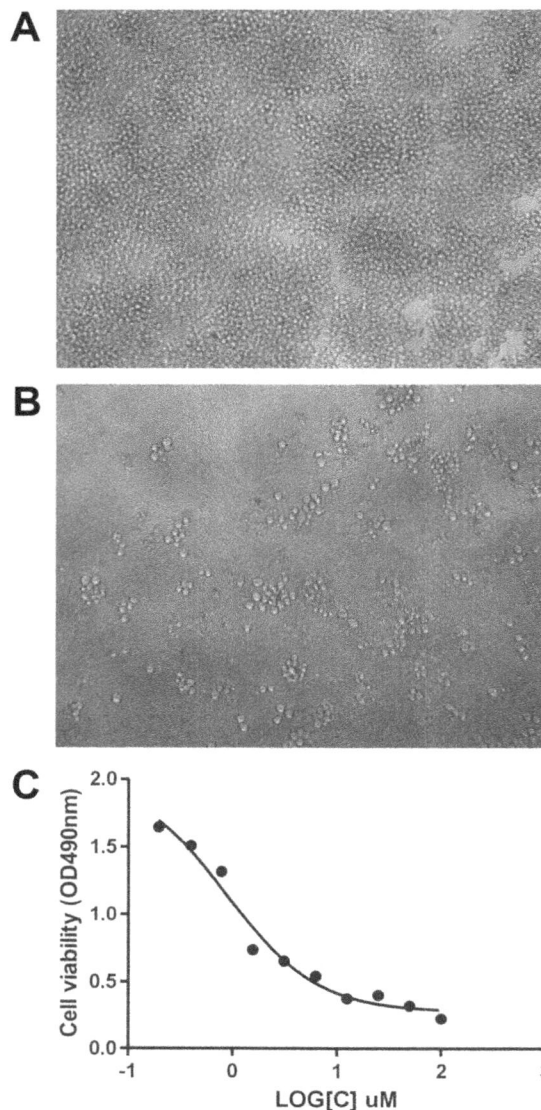

Figure 2. Celastrol inhibited LP-1 human multiple myeloma cell proliferation. Morphological signatures of celastrol growth inhibitory effects. Cells were treated with various doses of celastrol and cell viability was determined by MTT assay. Computer-assisted phase-contrast microscopy illustrations of control LP-1 human multiple myeloma cells (A) and treated with celastrol at concentration 0.78125 μM for 72 h (B). IC50 was shown as calculated by Prism 5.0. The IC50 growth inhibitory concentration for 72 h is 0.8817 μM (C).

3.5. Caspase-3 activation was involved in celastrol induced apoptosis

Caspase-3 is a crucial mediator of apoptosis and it catalyzes the specific cleavage of many key cellular proteins. Therefore, the activity of caspase-3 in LP-1 cell treated with 1 μM, 2 μM, and 4 μM of celastrol for 0 h, 12 h, 24 h and 48 h were investigated. After 24 h treatment with 4 μM of celastrol, the caspase-3 activation fold was 8.7 times than that at 0 h. The activity of caspase-3 increased in a time-dependent and dosage-dependent manner (Figure. 7), suggesting that the caspase-3 pathway might play an essential role in celastrol-induced apoptosis in LP-1 MM cell.

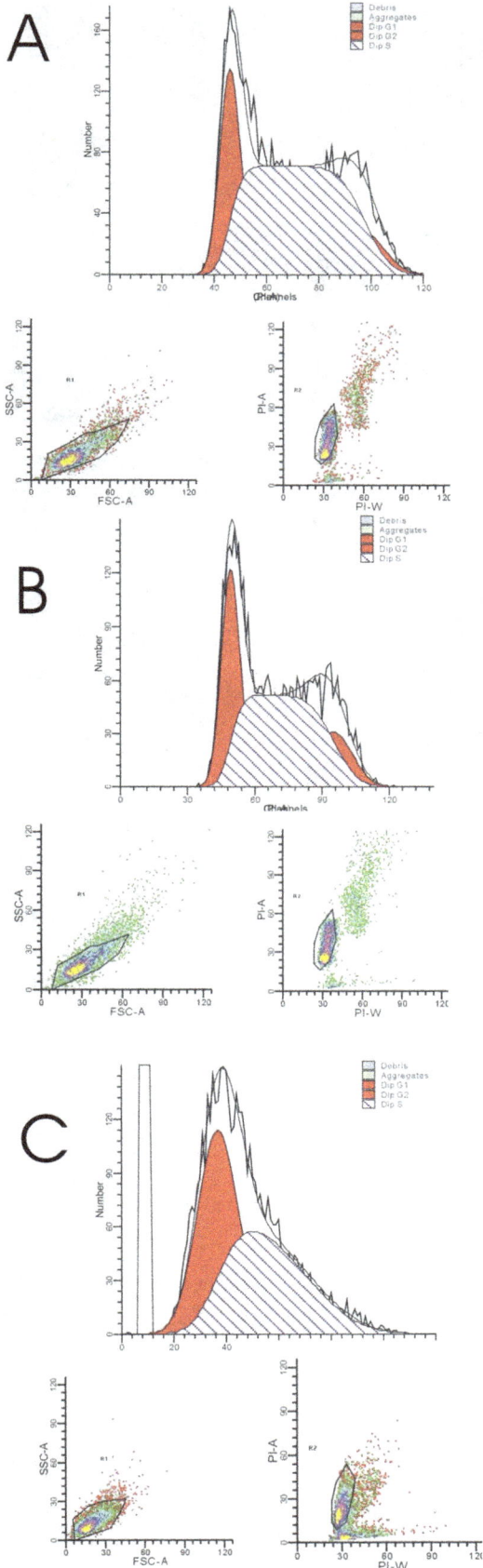

Figure 3. Celastrol causes accumulation of LP-1 human multiple myeloma cells in the G1 phase. LP-1 cells (2×10^6 mL-1) were treated with 0.5 µM celastrol for 0 (A), 12 (B) or 24 h (C), after which the cells were washed, fixed, stained with PI, and analyzed for DNA content by flow cytometry. Cell population in each cell cycle phase was numerically depicted. The G1 phase cell population was 24.15%, 29.79% and 49.20%, respectively. Data represent one of three independent experiments.

3.6. Celastrol Down-modulated the Expression of Antiapoptotic Proteins

The mechanism of celastrol induced apoptosis was investigated. LP-1 cells were treated with different concentrations of celastrol for 24 h and then examined for the expression of antiapoptotic proteins using relevant antibodies. The results indicated that celastrol down-regulated the expression of Bcl-2 and survivin (Figure 8A), whereas the down-regulation of Bax was less pronounced. The down-regulation of Bcl-2 was quite dramatic and was dose-dependent (Figure 8A).

3.7. NF-κB pathway is crucial in celastrol-induced apoptosis

The NF-κB pathway is a key regulator of cytokine stimulation, cell cycle, apoptosis, and angiogenesis [35]. It is also critical in the progression and apoptosis of cancer cells including MM. Recently, the inhibition of NF-κB pathway using the proteasome inhibitor bortezomib was found to be pivotal in the treatment of untreated and relapse/refractory myeloma [36,37]. Hence, the NF-κB pathway was examined in this study by Western blotting. The expression of NF-κB and IKKa were decreased after celastrol treatment (Figure 8A) and this effect was HO-1-independent by using ZnPPIX, a potent heme oxygenase inhibitor (Figure 8B). Nuclear translocation of the NF-kappa B p65 subunit was examined by immunofluorescence after treatment with celastrol. As shown in Figures 9A, 9B, celastrol effectively blocked nuclear translocation of the p65 subunit as well as IκB-α cleavage in a time-dependent manner, and this effect was also HO-1-independent by using ZnPPIX (Figure 9C, 9D).

Discussion

MM is a clonal plasma cell malignancy with a clinical median overall survival of 3–5 years. The existing treatment modalities included thalidomide, lenalidomide, bortezomib, and autologous transplantation. All these target myeloma cells and their microenvironments and have shown remarkable activity against refractory prolonged the progression-free and overall survival of MM patients. However, the majority of patients eventually experiences a relapse and chemoresistance, and ultimately dies due to the disease.

The plants used in traditional Chinese medicine are rich sources of biologically active substances with potential therapeutic effects towards many human diseases. In this study, celastrol was found to inhibit the growth of human myeloma cell line LP-1 cells with an IC50 of <1 µM. In addition, celastrol induced G1 cell cycle arrest followed by cell apoptosis.

The cell division relies on the activation of cyclins, which bind to CDKs to induce cell-cycle progression towards S phase and later to initiate mitosis. Since the uncontrolled CDK activity is often the cause of human cancer, their function is tightly regulated by cell-cycle inhibitors such as the p21 and p27 Cip/Kip proteins. Following anti-mitogenic signals or DNA damage, p21, and p27 bind to cyclin-CDK complexes to inhibit their catalytic activity and induce cell-cycle arrest.

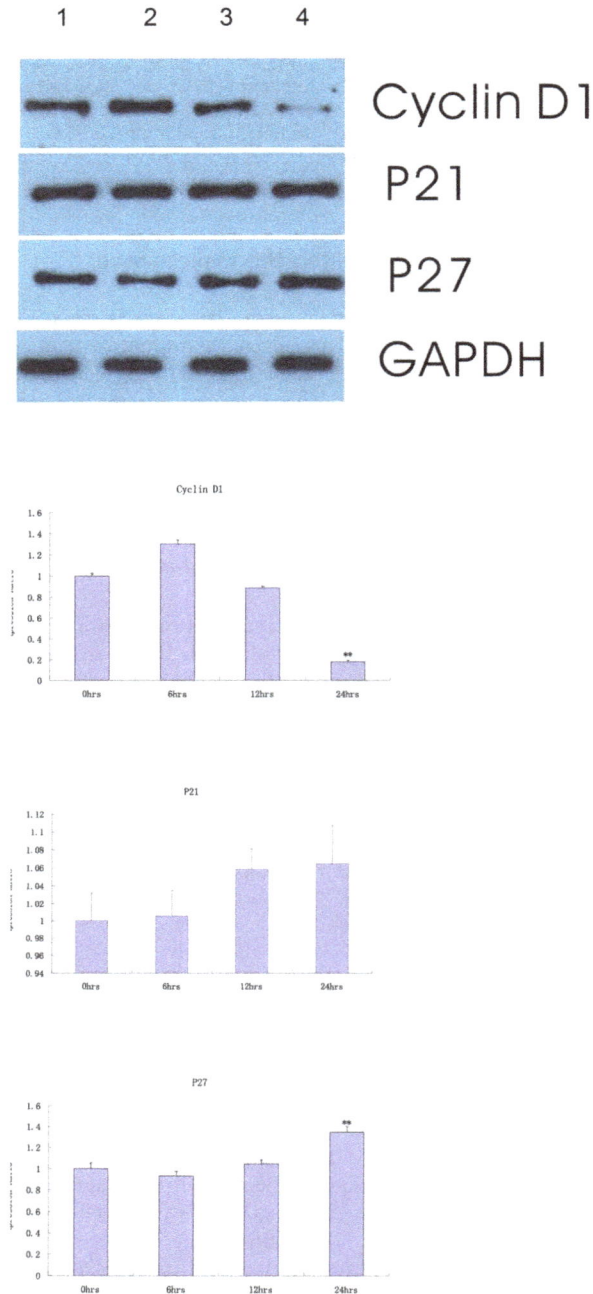

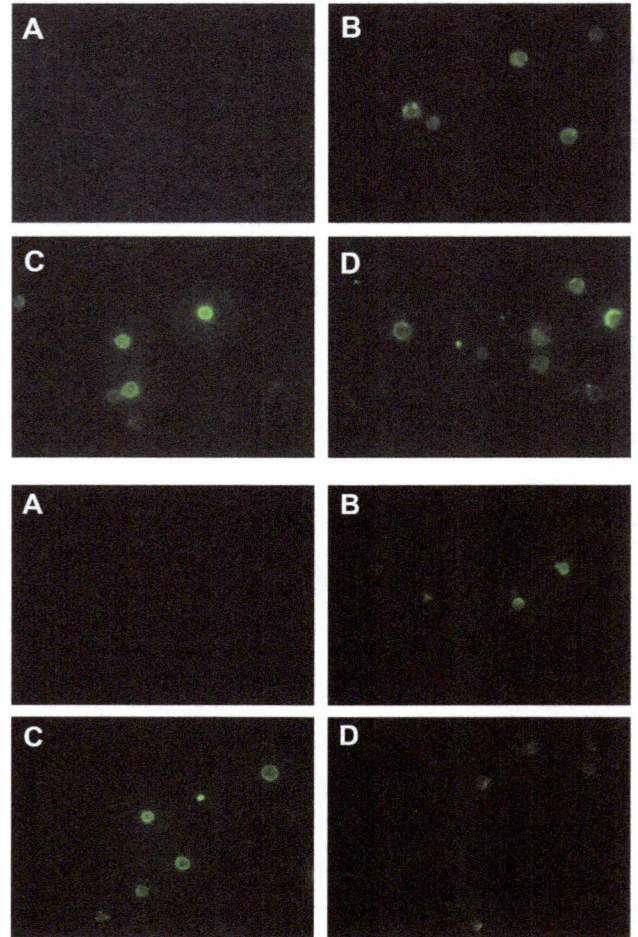

Figure 4. Celastrol up-modulated p27 protein expression in LP-1 cells. LP-1 cells were treated with 0.5 μM celastrol for 0 h (lane 1), 6 h (lane 2), 12 h (lane 3), and 24 h (lane 4), respectively. Whole cell lysates were prepared, separated on SDS-PAGE, and subjected to Western blot using antibodies against Cyclin D1, p27, and p21. The same blots were stripped and reprobed with GAPDH antibody to show equal protein loading. Expression fold was the ratio of protein expression in the celastrol-treated group to 0 h. Columns, mean; bars, SD (n = 3). *, p < 0.05; **, p < 0.01.

In the present study, the protein level of Cyclin D1 started decreasing at 0.5 μM celastrol for 24 h, and there was a significant Cyclin D1 decreased expression (p < 0.01). On the other hand, the celastrol treatment of cells for 24 h showed a strong increase in p27 protein level (p < 0.01), which further suggested a possible role

Figure 5. Celastrol induced apoptosis in LP-1 cells (up) and RPMI 8226 cells (down). Cells were treated with 1 μM celastrol for 0 h (A), 12 h (B), 24 (C), and 36 h (D) incubated with Annexin V conjugated with EGFP and analyzed with a fluorescence microscope for early apoptotic effects.

of p27 in celastrol to cause G1 arrest. In the case of p21, its protein level remained sustained until 24 h. After an up-regulation, p27 negatively regulate the kinase activity of the CDKs that alters the phosphorylation of Rb protein, keeping it in hypophosphorylated form and bound to transcription factor E2Fs [38]. The Rb-bound E2Fs are inactive and therefore fail to activate their downstream target genes involved in the cell cycle progression and DNA replication.

Activation of NF-κB is initiated by the signal-induced degradation of IκB proteins [39]. This occurs primarily through the activation of IκB kinase (IKK). When activated by signals usually come from the outside of the cell, the IκB kinase phosphorylates two serine residues located in an IκB regulatory domain [40]. When phosphorylated on these serines (e.g., serines 32 and 36 in human IκBα), the IκB inhibitor molecules are modified by ubiquitination, which then leads them to be degraded by proteasome. The NF-κB pathway is a potential therapeutic target for cancer [39]. Proteasome inhibitor bortezomib, which inhibits NF-κB activation, has been widely been used to treat MM patients worldwide [41]. Therefore, the natural products that inhibit NF-κB activation could be the novel potential agents for the treatment of MM [42].

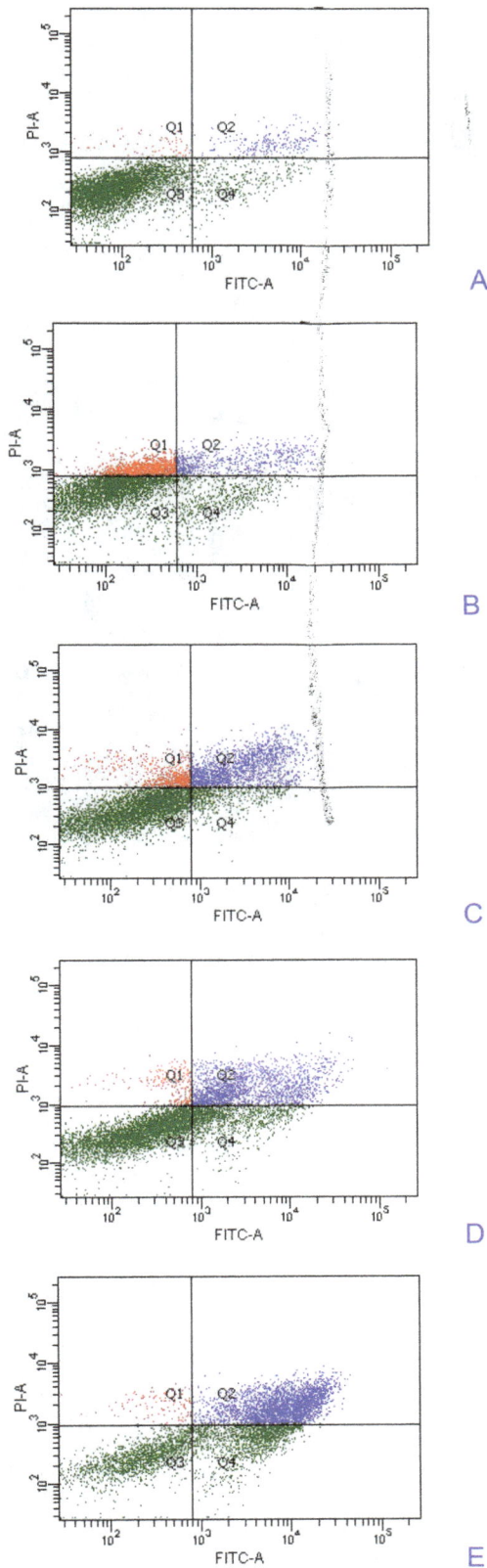

Figure 6. Celastrol induced apoptosis in a LP-1 cells. LP-1 cells were treated with 1 μM celastrol for 0 h (A), 12 h (B), 24 h (C), 36 h (D), and 48 h (E) incubated with Annexin V conjugated with EGFP and analyzed with a flow cytometer for apoptotic effects. The apoptotic cell

percentage was 7.8±0.4%, 16.1±1.2% (p<0.05 vs 0 h), 18.0±3.1% (p<0.05 vs 0 h), 39.5±5.8% (p<0.01 vs 0 h), and 71.2±8.6% (p<0.01 vs 0 h), respectively. The results shown are representative of three independent experiments.

Celastrol functions as an active natural proteasome inhibitor, and the celastro-induced myeloma cell apoptosis is associated with NF-kB attenuation in vitro [43]. The present study finding suggests that the suppression of NF-kB by targeting proteasome in myeloma may be applicable in disrupting myeloma progression including its primary growth and metastasis. Although more evidence is needed to delineate the role of NF-kB in the celastrol-mediated myeloma regression, the current study reveals that celastrol inhibits multiple NF-kB-driven protein expression that is involved in myeloma proliferation.

In accordance with the previous reports, it was found that the MM cell lines expressed the constitutively activated NF-kB, and that celastrol suppressed this activation and nuclear translocation of NF-kappa B p65. Although celastrol has been shown to inhibit NF-kB activation in various tumour cell lines, how celastrol can inhibit the constitutively activated NF-kB in MM cell lines has not been previously studied. It was observed that celastrol suppressed constitutively p65 and IKK, which may led to the inhibition of phosphorylation of p65 and IkBa, respectively [44].

In the recent years, NF-kappa B activation has been linked to many aspects of tumorigenesis including the control of apoptosis, cell cycle, differentiation, cell adhesion, cell migration, and angiogenesis [45]. NF-kappa B regulates the expression of several genes whose products are involved in anti-apoptosis such as Bcl-xL, cIAP, and TRAF. Bcl-2 [46]. The finding that residual tumors at the completion of chemotherapy express increased levels of Bcl-2 compared with pretreatment specimens suggests that Bcl-2 expression might be one mechanism for tumor resistance [47]. In the present study, the levels of Bcl-2 were significantly decreased after exposure to celastrol, although there was little change in Bax in response to celastrol. In comparison, the activation of caspase-3 could easily be detected. It has been found that many chemo-therapeutic agents (including taxol, doxorubicin, and etoposide) can activate NF-kappa B, which can prevent apoptosis, block the ability of therapeutic agents to induce cell death, and lead to

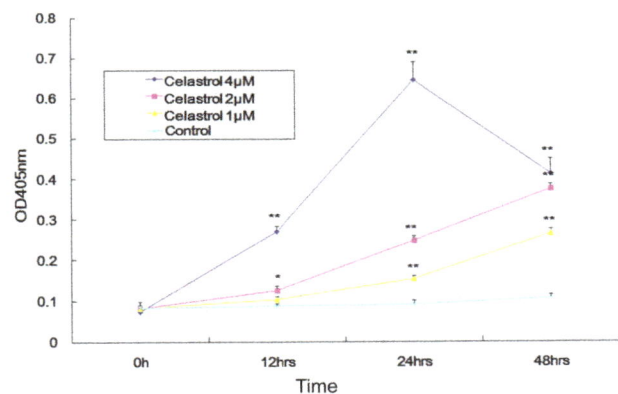

Figure 7. Celastrol induced caspase-3 activation. The cells were treated with 0 μM, 1 μM, 2 μM, and 4 μM celastrol for the indicated times. The whole cell extracts were prepared and subjected to enzymatic activity of caspase-3 by colorimetric substrate Ac-DEVD-pNA. The amount of yellow color at 405 nm indicating Caspase-3 activation fold was compared in the celastrol treated group to 0 h. point, mean; bars, SD (n = 3). *, p<0.05; **, p<0.01.

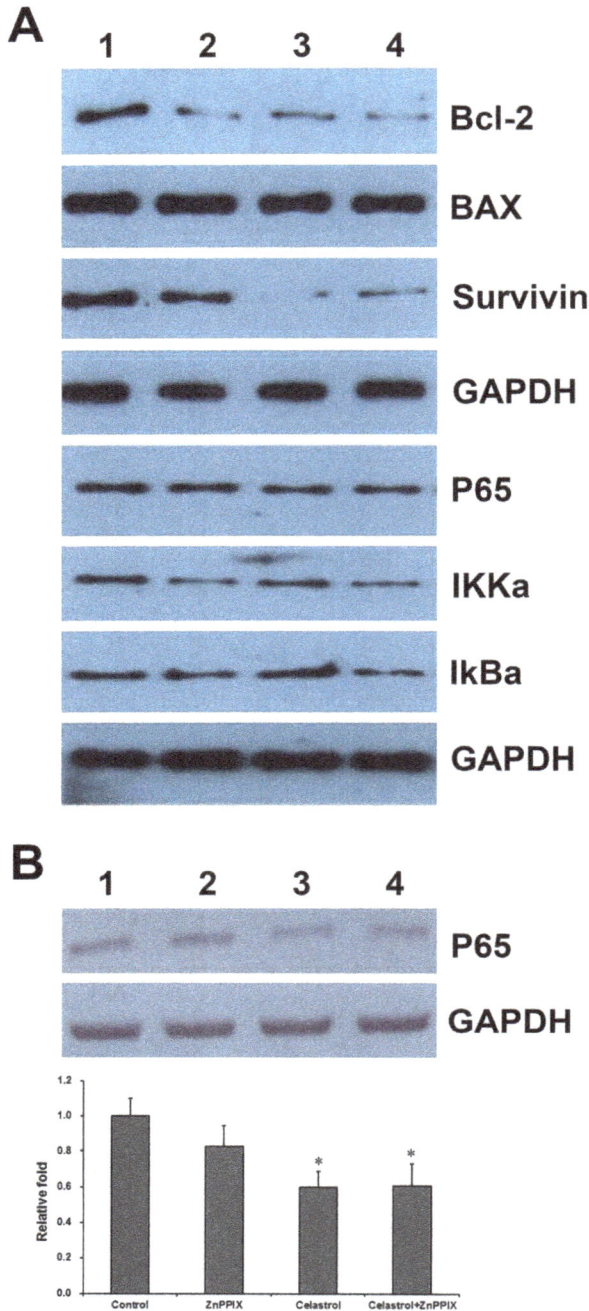

Figure 8. Celastrol down-modulated antiapoptotic proteins expression in LP-1 cells. (A). LP-1 cells were treated with 1 μM celastrol for 0 h (lane 1), 12 h (lane 2), 24 h (lane 3), and 48 h (lane 4), respectively. The whole cell lysates were prepared, separated on SDS-PAGE, and subjected to Western blot using antibodies against Bcl-2, Bax, Survivin, P65, IKKa, and IkBa. (B). LP-1 cells were treated with medium (lane 1), 1 μM ZnPPIX (lane 2), 1 μM celastrol (lane 3), and 1 μM celastrol combined with 1 μM ZnPPIX (lane 4) for 24 h, respectively. The same blots were stripped and reprobed with GAPDH antibody to show equal protein loading. Relative expression fold was first normalized by GADPH and then the ratio of protein expression in the celastrol/ZnPPIX -treated group was compared to control. Columns, mean; bars, SD (n = 3). *, p<0.05. No significance was observed from cells treated with Celastrol combined with ZnPPIX and those treated with only Celastrol (p>0.05).

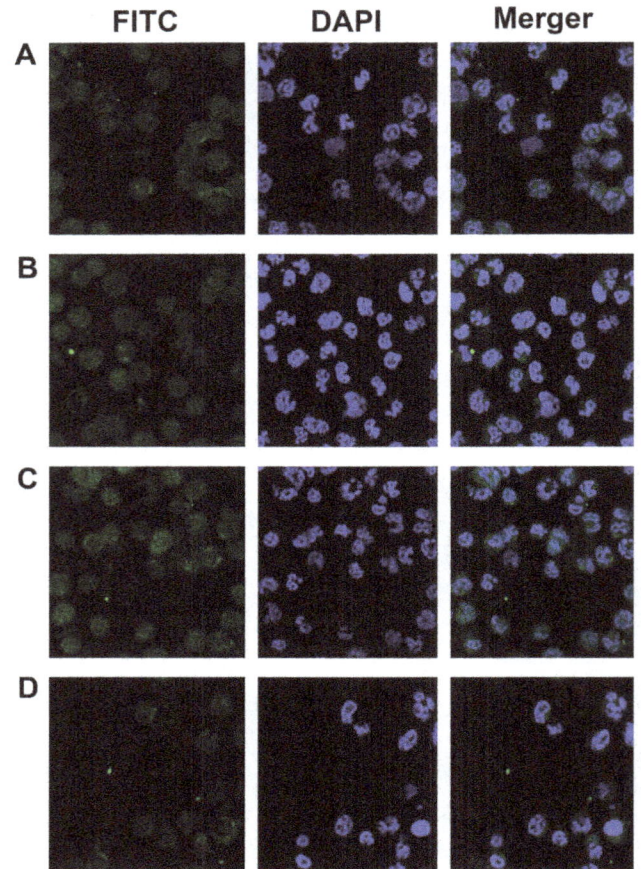

Figure 9. Celastrol inhibited constitutively active NF-kB in LP-1 MM cells. An altered subcellular distribution of NF-κb was observed. LP-1 cells were incubated with medium (A), 1 μM celastrol for 30 min (B), 1 μM Zinc Protoporphyrin-9 (ZnPPIX) (C), 1 μM celastrol combined with 1 μM ZnPPIX (D) and then analysed for the intracellular distribution of p65 by fluorescence microscope. Green indicates p65, and blue indicates nuclei (original magnification ×400). The results shown are representative of three independent experiments.

resistance to apoptosis induced by chemotherapeutic agents.

It has been reported that in AML-derived cells, but not primary cells, Heme oxygenase-1 (HO-1) is upregulated in response to TNF stimulation in conjunction with NFκB inhibition [48]. Heme oxygenase-1 (HO-1) is an Nrf2 transcription factor-regulated gene that is commonly induced following oxidative stress and cellular injury, functioning to decrease oxidative stress and inflammatory responses, protecting against apoptosis and altering the cell cycle [49]. It has been reported that bortezomib increases HO-1 expression in a time- and concentration- dependent manner. Moreover, we also observe that HO-1 is increased in lenalido-mide-resistant multiple myeloma cell lines [50].

The pivotal role of the NF-kappa B pathway in the inhibition of cell apoptosis strongly suggests that NF-kappa B inhibitors would be useful in cancer therapy. Our study has identified that the effect of Celatrol on NF-kB is HO-1-independent. It is highly possible that celastrol could overcome the apoptosis resistance of multiple myelome chemotherapy caused HO-1 and Nrf2 induction. Work is ongoing to study whether celastrol induced NF-kB inhibitory effect is through Nrf2-HO-1 pathway.

Conclusion

The present study results show that celastrol may be used as a NF-kappa B inhibitor to inhibit myeloma cell proliferation.

Author Contributions

Conceived and designed the experiments: JO. Performed the experiments: WZ. Analyzed the data: XK. Contributed reagents/materials/analysis tools: HL. Wrote the paper: HN.

References

1. Richardson PG, Mitsiades C, Schlossman R, Ghobrial I, Hideshima T, et al. (2008) Bortezomib in the front-line treatment of multiple myeloma. Expert Rev Anticancer Ther 8: 1053–1072.
2. Hideshima T, Chauhan D, Shima Y, Raje N, Davies FE, et al. (2000) Thalidomide and its analogs overcome drug resistance of human multiple myeloma cells to conventional therapy. Blood 96: 2943–2950.
3. Glasmacher A, Hahn C, Hoffmann F, Naumann R, Goldschmidt H, et al. (2006) A systematic review of phase-II trials of thalidomide monotherapy in patients with relapsed or refractory multiple myeloma. Br J Haematol 132: 584–593.
4. Raab MS, Podar K, Breitkreutz I, Richardson PG, Anderson KC (2009) Multiple myeloma. Lancet 374: 324–339.
5. Kumar S, Rajkumar SV (2006) Thalidomide and lenalidomide in the treatment of multiple myeloma. Eur J Cancer 42: 1612–1622.
6. Kyle RA, Rajkumar SV (2008) Multiple myeloma. Blood 111: 2962–2972.
7. Gupta SC, Kim JH, Prasad S, Aggarwal BB (2010) Regulation of survival, proliferation, invasion, angiogenesis, and metastasis of tumor cells through modulation of inflammatory pathways by nutraceuticals. Cancer Metastasis Rev 29: 405–434.
8. Bharti AC, Donato N, Singh S, Aggarwal BB (2003) Curcumin (diferuloyl-methane) down-regulates the constitutive activation of nuclear factor-kappa B and IkappaBalpha kinase in human multiple myeloma cells, leading to suppression of proliferation and induction of apoptosis. Blood 101: 1053–1062.
9. Zhao W, Entschladen F, Liu H, Niggemann B, Fang Q, et al. (2003) Boswellic acid acetate induces differentiation and apoptosis in highly metastatic melanoma and fibrosarcoma cells. Cancer Detect Prev 27: 67–75.
10. Liu JJ, Nilsson A, Oredsson S, Badmaev V, Zhao WZ, Duan RD (2002) Boswellic acids trigger apoptosis via a pathway dependent on caspase-8 activation but independent on Fas/Fas ligand interaction in colon cancer HT-29 cells. Carcinogenesis 23: 2087–2093.
11. Aggarwal BB, Vijayalekshmi RV, Sung B (2009) Targeting inflammatory pathways for prevention and therapy of cancer: short-term friend, long-term foe. Clin Cancer Res 15: 425–430.
12. Feinman R, Siegel DS, Berenson J (2004) Regulation of NF-kB in multiple myeloma: therapeutic implications. Clin Adv Hematol Oncol 2: 162–166.
13. Karin M (2009) NF-kappaB as a critical link between inflammation and cancer. Cold Spring Harb Perspect Biol 1: a000141.
14. Kannaiyan R, Shanmugam MK, Sethi G (2011) Molecular targets of celastrol derived from Thunder of God Vine: potential role in the treatment of inflammatory disorders and cancer. Cancer Lett 303: 9–20.
15. Wong KF, Yuan Y, Luk JM (2012) Tripterygium wilfordii bioactive compounds as anticancer and anti-inflammatory agents. Clin Exp Pharmacol Physiol 39: 311–320.
16. Allison AC, Cacabelos R, Lombardi VR, Alvarez XA, Vigo C (2001) Celastrol, a potent antioxidant and anti-inflammatory drug, as a possible treatment for Alzheimer's disease. Prog Neuropsychopharmacol Biol Psychiatry 25: 1341–1357.
17. Morita T (2010) Celastrol: a new therapeutic potential of traditional Chinese medicine. Am J Hypertens 23: 821.
18. Salminen A, Lehtonen M, Paimela T, Kaarniranta K (2010) Celastrol: Molecular targets of Thunder God Vine. Biochem Biophys Res Commun 394: 439–442.
19. Huang S, Tang Y, Cai X, Peng X, Liu X, et al. (2012) Celastrol inhibits vasculogenesis by suppressing the VEGF-induced functional activity of bone marrow-derived endothelial progenitor cells. Biochem Biophys Res Commun 423: 467–472.
20. Paris D, Ganey NJ, Laporte V, Patel NS, Beaulieu-Abdelahad D, et al. (2010) Reduction of beta-amyloid pathology by celastrol in a transgenic mouse model of Alzheimer's disease. J Neuroinflammation 7: 17.
21. Yang HS, Kim JY, Lee JH, Lee BW, Park KH, et al. (2011) Celastrol isolated from Tripterygium regelii induces apoptosis through both caspase-dependent and -independent pathways in human breast cancer cells. Food Chem Toxicol 49: 527–532.
22. Yadav VR, Sung B, Prasad S, Kannappan R, Cho SG, et al. (2010) Celastrol suppresses invasion of colon and pancreatic cancer cells through the downregulation of expression of CXCR4 chemokine receptor. J Mol Med (Berl) 88: 1243–1253.
23. Dai Y, Desano J, Tang W, Meng X, Meng Y, et al. (2010) Natural proteasome inhibitor celastrol suppresses androgen-independent prostate cancer progression by modulating apoptotic proteins and NF-kappaB. PLoS One 5: e14153.
24. Yang H, Chen D, Cui QC, Yuan X, Dou QP (2006) Celastrol, a triterpene extracted from the Chinese "Thunder of God Vine," is a potent proteasome inhibitor and suppresses human prostate cancer growth in nude mice. Cancer Res 66: 4758–4765.
25. He D, Xu Q, Yan M, Zhang P, Zhou X, et al. (2009) The NF-kappa B inhibitor, celastrol, could enhance the anti-cancer effect of gambogic acid on oral squamous cell carcinoma. BMC Cancer 9: 343.
26. Huang Y, Zhou Y, Fan Y, Zhou D (2008) Celastrol inhibits the growth of human glioma xenografts in nude mice through suppressing VEGFR expression. Cancer Lett 264: 101–106.
27. Chen M, Rose AE, Doudican N, Osman I, Orlow SJ (2009) Celastrol synergistically enhances temozolomide cytotoxicity in melanoma cells. Mol Cancer Res 7: 1946–1953.
28. Nagase M, Oto J, Sugiyama S, Yube K, Takaishi Y, Sakato N (2003) Apoptosis induction in HL-60 cells and inhibition of topoisomerase II by triterpene celastrol. Biosci Biotechnol Biochem 67: 1883–1887.
29. Yamai H, Sawada N, Yoshida T, Seike J, Takizawa H, et al. (2009) Triterpenes augment the inhibitory effects of anticancer drugs on growth of human esophageal carcinoma cells in vitro and suppress experimental metastasis in vivo. Int J Cancer 125: 952–960.
30. Li F, Rajendran P, Sethi G (2010) Thymoquinone inhibits proliferation, induces apoptosis and chemosensitizes human multiple myeloma cells through suppression of signal transducer and activator of transcription 3 activation pathway. Br J Pharmacol 161: 541–554.
31. Berda-Haddad Y, Robert S, Salers P, Zekraoui L, Farnarier C, et al. (2011) Sterile inflammation of endothelial cell-derived apoptotic bodies is mediated by interleukin-1alpha. Proc Natl Acad Sci U S A 108: 20684–20689.
32. Zorn JA, Wolan DW, Agard NJ, Wells JA (2012) Fibrils colocalize caspase-3 with procaspase-3 to foster maturation. J Biol Chem 287: 33781–33795.
33. Zorn JA, Wolan DW, Agard NJ, Wells JA (2012) Fibrils colocalize caspase-3 with procaspase-3 to foster maturation. J Biol Chem 287: 33781–33795.
34. Hubackova S, Krejcikova K, Bartek J, Hodny Z (2012) Interleukin 6 signaling regulates promyelocytic leukemia protein gene expression in human normal and cancer cells. J Biol Chem 287: 26702–26714.
35. Nishikori M (2005) Classical and Alternative NF-kB Activation Pathways and Their Roles in Lymphoid Malignancies. Journal of Clinical and Experimental Hematopathology 45:15–24.
36. Ni H, Ergin M, Huang Q, Qin JZ, Amin HM, et al. (2001) Analysis of expression of nuclear factor kappa B (NF-kappa B) in multiple myeloma: downregulation of NF-kappa B induces apoptosis. Br J Haematol 115: 279–286.
37. Nakanishi C, Toi M (2005) Nuclear factor-kappaB inhibitors as sensitizers to anticancer drugs. Nat Rev Cancer 5: 297–309.
38. Alessandrini A, Chiaur DS, Pagano M (1997) Regulation of the cyclin-dependent kinase inhibitor p27 by degradation and phosphorylation. Leukemia 11: 342–345.
39. Dai Y, Lawrence TS, Xu L (2009) Overcoming cancer therapy resistance by targeting inhibitors of apoptosis proteins and nuclear factor-kappa B. Am J Transl Res 1: 1–15.
40. Sethi G, Tergaonkar V (2009) Potential pharmacological control of the NF-kappaB pathway. Trends Pharmacol Sci 30: 313–321.
41. Ganten TM, Koschny R, Haas TL, Sykora J, Li-Weber M, et al. (2005) Proteasome inhibition sensitizes hepatocellular carcinoma cells, but not human hepatocytes, to TRAIL. Hepatology 42: 588–597.
42. Shah JJ, Orlowski RZ (2009) Proteasome inhibitors in the treatment of multiple myeloma. Leukemia 23: 1964–1979.
43. Adams J (2004) The proteasome: a suitable antineoplastic target. Nat Rev Cancer 4: 349–360.
44. Gasparian AV, Yao YJ, Kowalczyk D, Lyakh LA, Karseladze A, et al. (2002) The role of IKK in constitutive activation of NF-kappaB transcription factor in prostate carcinoma cells. J Cell Sci 115: 141–151.
45. Li F, Sethi G (2010) Targeting transcription factor NF-kappaB to overcome chemoresistance and radioresistance in cancer therapy. Biochim Biophys Acta 1805: 167–180.
46. Catz SD, Johnson JL (2001) Transcriptional regulation of bcl-2 by nuclear factor kappa B and its significance in prostate cancer. Oncogene 20: 7342–7351.
47. Arumugam TV, Cheng YL, Choi Y, Choi YH, Yang S, et al. (2011) Evidence that gamma-secretase-mediated Notch signaling induces neuronal cell death via the nuclear factor-kappaB-Bcl-2-interacting mediator of cell death pathway in ischemic stroke. Mol Pharmacol 80: 23–31.
48. Rushworth SA, MacEwan DJ (2008) HO-1 underlies resistance of AML cells to TNF-induced apoptosis. Blood 111: 3793–3801.
49. Alam J, Stewart D, Touchard C, Boinapally S, Choi AM, Cook JL (1999) Nrf2, a Cap'n'Collar transcription factor, regulates induction of the heme oxygenase-1 gene. J Biol Chem 274: 26071–26078.
50. Barrera LN, Rushworth SA, Bowles KM, MacEwan DJ (2012) Bortezomib induces heme oxygenase-1 expression in multiple myeloma. Cell Cycle 11: 2248–2252.

6

Inherited Polymorphisms in Hyaluronan Synthase 1 Predict Risk of Systemic B-Cell Malignancies but not of Breast Cancer

Hemalatha Kuppusamy[1], Helga M. Ogmundsdottir[2], Eva Baigorri[1], Amanda Warkentin[1], Hlif Steingrimsdottir[3], Vilhelmina Haraldsdottir[3], Michael J. Mant[1], John Mackey[1], James B. Johnston[4], Sophia Adamia[5], Andrew R. Belch[1], Linda M. Pilarski[1]*

1 University of Alberta and Cross Cancer Institute, Edmonton, Alberta, Canada, 2 University of Iceland, Reykjavik, Iceland, 3 Landspitali University Hospital, Reykjavik, Iceland, 4 Dept. of Hematology, Cancer Care Manitoba and the University of Manitoba, Winnipeg, Manitoba, Canada, 5 Medical Oncology, Dana-Farber Cancer Institute, Harvard Medical School, Boston, Massachusetts, United States of America

Abstract

Genetic variations in the hyaluronan synthase 1 gene (HAS1) influence HAS1 aberrant splicing. HAS1 is aberrantly spliced in malignant cells from multiple myeloma (MM) and Waldenstrom macroglobulinemia (WM), but not in their counterparts from healthy donors. The presence of aberrant HAS1 splice variants predicts for poor survival in multiple myeloma (MM). We evaluated the influence of inherited HAS1 single nucleotide polymorphisms (SNP) on the risk of having a systemic B cell malignancy in 1414 individuals compromising 832 patients and 582 healthy controls, including familial analysis of an Icelandic kindred. We sequenced *HAS1* gene segments from 181 patients with MM, 98 with monoclonal gammopathy of undetermined significance (MGUS), 72 with Waldenstrom macroglobulinemia (WM), 169 with chronic lymphocytic leukemia (CLL), as well as 34 members of a monoclonal gammopathy-prone Icelandic family, 212 age-matched healthy donors and a case-control cohort of 295 breast cancer patients with 353 healthy controls. Three linked single nucleotide polymorphisms (SNP) in *HAS1* intron3 are significantly associated with B-cell malignancies (range $p = 0.007$ to $p = 10^{-5}$), but not MGUS or breast cancer, and predict risk in a 34 member Icelandic family ($p = 0.005$, Odds Ratio = 5.8 (OR)), a relatively homogeneous cohort. In contrast, exon3 SNPs were not significantly different among the study groups. Pooled analyses showed a strong association between the linked *HAS1* intron3 SNPs and B-cell malignancies (OR = 1.78), but not for sporadic MGUS or for breast cancer (OR<1.0). The minor allele genotypes of HAS1 SNPs are significantly more frequent in MM, WM, CLL and in affected members of a monoclonal gammopathy-prone family than they are in breast cancer, sporadic MGUS or healthy donors. These inherited changes may increase the risk for systemic B-cell malignancies but not for solid tumors.

Editor: Klaus Roemer, University of Saarland Medical School, Germany

Funding: This work was funded by grants to LMP and ARB from Myeloma Alberta, the Alberta Cancer Foundation and the Canadian Institutes of Health Research (www.cihr-irsc.gc.ca). The funders had no role in study design, data collection and analysis, decision to publish, or preparation of the manuscript.

Competing Interests: The authors have declared that no competing interests exist.

* Email: lpilarsk@ualberta.ca

Introduction

Hyaluronan synthase 1 (HAS1) produces hyaluronan (HA), a polysaccharide with complex biological effects [1]. Here, we evaluated the influence of inherited HAS1 single nucleotide polymorphisms (SNP) on the risk of having a systemic B cell malignancy in 832 patients and 582 controls. Using targeted sequencing of HAS1 SNPs to unequivocally genotype patient populations and to identify potential low penetrance mutations, we reduced the uncertainties associated with array screening and genome-wide association studies. Herein, we show that three HAS1 intron3 SNPs (rs11084110, rs11084109 and rs11669079) are significantly more frequent in patients with systemic B-cell malignancies or in members of a four-generation Icelandic kindred affected by a monoclonal gammopathy-prone phenotype [2;3] than in healthy donors, unaffected Icelandic family members or patients with solid tumors. Overall, the study of 1414 subjects,

including 832 patients and 582 healthy controls, suggests that these inherited changes may predispose to the development of systemic B cell malignancies (multiple myeloma, chronic lympho-cytic leukemia or Waldenstrom macroglobulinemia), but do not predispose to sporadic monoclonal gammopathy of undetermined significance (MGUS) or breast cancer.

Hyaluronan synthase 1 products, encoded by the *HAS1* gene, appear central to the events giving rise to B cell malignancies and to disease progression [1]. HAS1 is aberrantly spliced in malignant cells from multiple myeloma (MM) and Waldenstrom macroglob-ulinemia (WM), but not in their counterparts from healthy donors [4]. HA produced by HAS1 splice variants is likely to contribute to mitotic abnormalities and to malignant spread/migration [1;4;5], suggesting that aberrant splicing may be an important contributor to systemic B cell malignancies. The presence of the aberrant HAS1Vb intronic splice variant correlated with poor survival in MM patients [4]. In transfectants, a HAS1 variant is oncogenic *in vivo* and *in vitro* [6], possibly resulting from induction of chromosomal instability by aberrant intracellular HA and promotion of malignant spread by extracellular HA [1]. Inherited single nucleotide polymorphisms (SNPs) and mutational hotspots in HAS1 exon3 through intron3 influence HAS1 pre-mRNA splicing [7;8]. A major strength of this study is that we have analyzed the *HAS1* polymorphisms in five different disease cohorts and two geographically independent populations (western Canadians and the Icelandic kindred) with their appropriate healthy donor control groups. This is the first report that risk for B-cell malignancies and an inherited monoclonal gammopathy-prone phenotype is directly correlated with intronic *HAS1* SNPs, likely by promoting aberrant HAS1 splicing.

Methods

Study Subjects

Patients with MM, WM or sporadic MGUS were seen at the Cross Cancer Institute and the University of Alberta hospital (Edmonton, AB), and diagnosed according to recommended guidelines [9;10] CLL cells were obtained from the Manitoba CLL Tumor Bank at the Manitoba Institute of Cell Biology. This study was approved by Ethics Review Boards from the University of Alberta, the University of Manitoba, the University of Iceland and Alberta Health Services. Subjects provided written informed consent. Approval for the familial studies was from the Icelandic National Bioethics Committee, license number 8-107-S1, Data Protection Authority: 20096080676. We sequenced DNA from 1,414 individuals (Table 1): this includes a total of 582 healthy control subjects. Controls for B-cell malignancies were 212 anonymous age-matched donors. For breast cancer, 295 anonymous blood samples from patients and 353 matched healthy controls were from the Alberta Research Tumor Bank. For all groups, peripheral blood was taken at the time of diagnosis or at follow-up. We genotyped PB from 34 members from four generations of a monoclonal gammopathy-prone Icelandic family [2;3]. Family members were of both genders; "controls" were the unaffected family members. Affected family members were those with MGUS, MM, WM or a hyper-Ig phenotype. Both the Icelandic kindred and the patients from western Canada are predominantly of Caucasian descent.

Genotyping and Analysis

Peripheral blood mononuclear cells were isolated and genomic DNA was purified from 5×10^6 PBMCs using QIAamp DNA Blood mini kit (QIAGEN). For two Icelandic samples, DNA was isolated from paraffin-embedded tissue, and amplified with whole genome amplification (WGA). Primers were designed based on the consensus human *HAS1* NCBI gene coding sequence (NCBI Reference Sequence: NC_000019.10) (Table S1 in File S1). A *HAS1* gene segment from exon3 to intron3 inclusive was amplified in a 50 µl PCR reaction mix (Table S2 in File S1).

Quality Control

To ensure the genotyping results were accurate, we randomly re-sequenced selected DNA samples. For high fidelity *Taq* DNA polymerase, an enzyme lot was used with an error rate confirmed by us to be 3.0×10^{-4} error/bp. DNA sequencing profiles were analyzed with SeqScape V2.1 for base-calling software/alignment (Applied Biosystems (ABI), CA), confirmed manually by visual inspection of the sequencing profile.

Subcloning and Direct Sequencing

PCR-amplified gene segments were sequenced using two methods: 1) by subcloning in an appropriate vector or 2) by direct sequencing of double or single stranded PCR products. For each patient whose PCR products were subcloned, a minimum of 8 subclones were sequenced in both directions. If a given base was present in all subclones, the two alleles were considered to be homozygous. Heterozygosity was defined as having at least 1/8 subclones with the second allele. 40% of samples were sequenced using plasmid subcloning and 60% were sequenced directly using Big-Dye 3.1 (ABI) on the ABI3130xl DNA analysis system. Obtained sequences were compared to the NCBI *HAS1* reference sequence (NC_000019.10).

Statistical Analysis

Hardy-Weinberg equilibrium (HWE) tests were performed for each SNP. We assessed for deviations from HWE using the chi-square test, with 5 degrees of freedom. The SNPs were only considered for further analysis if the allele frequency conformed to HWE expectation. This ensures that any loss of heterozygosity that might be present in malignant cells is excluded from analysis [11]. The difference in genotype and allele frequencies between patients and healthy controls were analyzed by the Fischer exact test: probability values (P values) of <0.05 were considered statistically significant. The *HAS1* alleles designated as "minor" by NCBI are the most frequent in the populations studied, with the exception of the Icelandic kindred, but we followed the accepted NCBI dbSNP database convention for naming.

Unconditional logistic regression analysis was performed to obtain odds ratios (OR) and 95% confidence interval (CI) to independently estimate relative risks for each SNP, using Statistical Analysis Software (SAS institute). The independent cohorts were

Table 1. Characteristics of study participants (N = 1414).

Study Group	No of samples	Age Range	Sample type
MGUS	98	44–87 (n = 67)	PB
MM	181	46–91 (n = 66)	PB
CLL	169	37–82 (n = 66)	Purified malignant B cells
WM	72	50–82 (n = 66)	PB
Controls	212	Above 60	PB
Icelandic kindred	34	4 generations	PB
Breast cancer cases	295	29–80	PB
Breast cancer Controls	353	29–80	

then combined for Forest plot analysis without any weightage. They show the amount of variation between the studies and an estimate of the overall result. Linkage disequilibrium analysis was done using *Haploview* bioinformatic software (MIT/Harvard Broad Institute). Linked SNPs (rs11084110, rs11084109 and rs11669079) show strong LD patterns in all the four case groups and D' values are above 90. In contrast, the exon3 SNPs (rs61736495, rs11084111) are in equilibrium; only rs11084111 was present in the Icelandic kindred.

Results

HAS1 Polymorphisms

HAS1 gene segments from 1414 individuals were sequenced (Table 1). In the dbSNP database, ten *HAS1* SNPs occur in the region sequenced (Figure 1, Table-S3 in File S1); of these only five met the Hardy-Weinberg Equilibrium criterion of p>0.05; these were two SNPs in exon 3 and three SNPs in intron 3.

HAS1 Genotype and Minor Allele Frequencies in an Icelandic Kindred

We analyzed 34 members of an Icelandic family predisposed to monoclonal gammopathies, including IgM gammopathy, CLL, MM and WM [2;3] (Table 2). Twelve family members showed increased production of immunoglobulin *in vitro*, referred to as hyper-responders [3]. The 12 hyper-responders plus two family members diagnosed MGUS, two with WM and one with MM (a total of 17 family members) were termed "affected" family members. Controls were 17 unaffected family members who lacked any evidence of monoclonal gammopathies and did not have a hyper-responder phenotype. In the Icelandic kindred, the frequencies of the linked intron3 SNPs (rs11084110, rs11084109 and rs11669079) for affected members were significantly different from those of unaffected members (genotype frequencies p = 0.007 for the intron3 SNPs). In contrast, the exon3 SNP rs11084111 is not significantly different between affected and unaffected family members, providing an internal control. The minor allele frequency for the linked intron3 SNPs was 0.74 for affected and 0.32 for unaffected family members (Table 2), a highly significant difference (p = 0.0005).

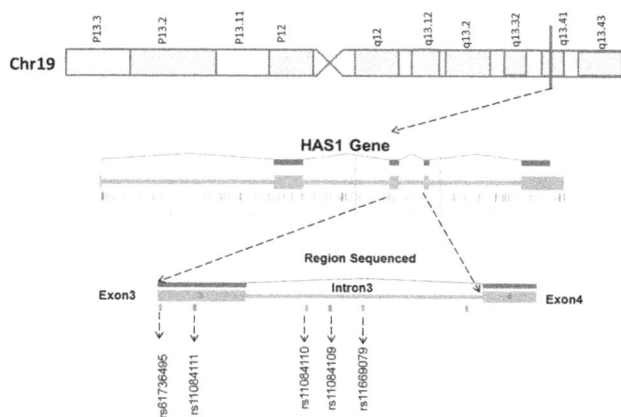

Figure 1. A schematic diagram of HAS1 gene locus in chromosome 19q13. Some parts of Figure 1 were created using Gene Window Software http://genewindow.nci.nih.gov/.

Table 2. Genotype and Allele frequencies of *HAS1* SNPs in Icelandic kindred*.

HAS1 SNP	Status	Genotype frequency				Minor allele frequency		
		Major allele Homozygous	Heterozygous	Minor allele Homozygous	P	Major Allele	Minor Allele	P
rs11084111	Affected	15/17 (88%)	2/17 (12%)	0/17 (0%)	0.36	32 (0.94)	2 (0.06)	0.38
	Unaffected	13/17 (76%)	4/17 (14%)	0/17 (0%)		30 (0.88)	4 (0.12)	
rs11084110	Affected	1/17 (6%)	7/17 (41%)	9/17 (53%)	0.007	9 (0.26)	25 (0.74)	0.0005
	Unaffected	9/17 (53%)	5/17 (29%)	3/17 (18%)		23 (0.68)	11 (0.32)	
rs11084109	Affected	1/17 (6%)	7/17 (41%)	9/17 (53%)	0.007	9 (0.26)	25 (0.74)	0.0005
	Unaffected	9/17 (53%)	5/17 (29%)	3/17 (18%)		23 (0.68)	11 (0.32)	
rs11669079	Affected	1/17 (6%)	7/17 (41%)	9/17 (53%)	0.007	9 (0.26)	25 (0.74)	0.0005
	Unaffected	9/17 (53%)	5/17 (29%)	3/17 18%		23 (0.68)	11 (0.32)	

*P values are calculated using fisher exact test, allele frequencies are shown in parentheses.

Minor Allele Frequencies (MAF) for Study Cohorts

The allele frequencies for patients and their respective control groups were determined (Table 3). For *HAS1* exon3 SNPs the allele distribution between the cancer groups and their controls are not significantly different. In contrast however, the linked *HAS1* intron3 SNPs, the MAF are significantly higher in CLL and WM than they are in the age-matched control group. For all of the intron3 SNPs, the MAF is 0.80 for CLL and 0.81 for WM compared to 0.75 for MM and 0.63 for sporadic MGUS. For MM, sporadic MGUS and the breast cancer group (0.71), the MAFs for the linked *HAS1* intron3 SNPs are not significantly different from their respective control groups. For *HAS1* exon3 SNPs the allele distribution between the cancer groups and their controls are not significantly different.

Association between *HAS1* SNP Genotypes and B-cell Malignancies

Two-tailed unconditional logistic regression was used to determine the effect of *HAS1* SNP genotypes on the presumptive risk of B-cell malignancy (Table 4). No assumptions were made about the effect of the SNPs prior to analysis. Odds ratios (OR) measure the impact of a given *HAS1* SNP on the risk of having a B-cell malignancy (Table 4). Each cancer group was compared to its control group.

As compared to the healthy controls, for the linked *HAS1* intron3 SNPs, the genotypes having the "minor" allele were each associated with an increased risk of B-cell malignancy but not of MGUS, perhaps because only 1–2% of sporadic MGUS transform to MM. For the exon 3 SNPs, there was no association between *HAS1* SNP genotype and B-cell malignancies or MGUS. The intronic *HAS1* SNP rs11084110 was associated with 1.5-fold increase in the risk for MM (OR = 1.53; p = 0.008). The OR was 2.0 for CLL and 2.1 for WM, both of which have a higher familial incidence than does MM. Similar results were observed for the other two intronic SNPs (Table 4). To determine whether or not the linkage between intronic HAS1 SNPs and risk was restricted to B cell malignancies, we also evaluated a cohort of breast cancer patients. There was no difference between breast cancer patients and their matched healthy control group, indicating a lack of association with HAS1 SNPs (Table 5). Comparison of the B-cell cancer group (MM, CLL and WM) with the breast cancer subjects shows that for all the three linked SNPs, the systemic B cell malignancies have a significantly greater association than does breast cancer (p≥0.01). Thus, the solid tumor group and its controls provide a negative control for the patient groups harboring systemic B-cell malignancies. Our findings showed that the linked *HAS1* intron3 SNPs, had a significant association with all B-cell malignancies studied (Table 4), an association that appears restricted to B-cell malignancies.

Pooled Association Analysis

For increased power to demonstrate a relationship between *HAS1* SNPs and the risk of a B-cell malignancy, three case cohorts (MM, CLL and WM) were pooled for analysis (Figure 2). When MM, CLL and WM were evaluated as a single group in comparison with the healthy control group, we found a significant association between the linked *HAS1* intron3 SNPs, and the risk of systemic B-cell malignancy. For the three *HAS1* intronic SNPs (OR = 1.78–1.80; p<0.001), the overall risk was 1.78 (Figure 2, left column of panels) for the group of B cell malignancies. For the Icelandic family members the overall risk was 5.8; no such risk was seen for breast cancer or for the cohort of patients with sporadic MGUS (OR = 0.85 or 0.88, respectively) (Figure 2, right column of panels).

Discussion

Extensive inherited and acquired mutations characterize HAS1 in patients with B-cell malignancies [8]. *HAS1* overexpression has also been reported for some solid tumors, including prostate, ovarian and bladder cancers [1;12–14]. To avoid the uncertainties inherent in genome-wide association studies, we sought susceptibility polymorphisms in a candidate gene, *HAS1*, based on the biology of the gene in cancer patients. By sequencing in 832 patients and 582 healthy controls (a total of 1,414 individuals) a segment of the *HAS1* gene known to influence aberrant HAS1 splicing [7;8], we show that the presence of *HAS1* SNPs is strongly associated with the diagnosis of a systemic B-cell malignancy (range of p = 0.005 to p = 10^{-5}, OR = 1.5 ranging to OR = 2.1, overall risk = 1.78), but not with a solid tumor. For the Icelandic family members the overall risk was 5.8; no such risk was seen for breast cancer or for the cohort of patients with sporadic MGUS that have no known familial predisposition. The observation that HAS1 intronic SNPs do not confer risk to patients with sporadic MGUS likely reflects the fact that only a very small proportion are at risk of transformation to frank malignant disease. It seems likely from the Icelandic familial analysis that if biomarkers were available that preferentially select for only those MGUS that will transform to frank malignancy, a risk association would become detectable. In the Icelandic family kindred, *HAS1* SNPs were more frequent in affected members (those with monoclonal gammopathies or hype-responder phenotype) than in unaffected family members (p = .0005), confirming the association with risk in a four generation family having a shared genetic heritage.

The increased risk associated with minor allele genotypes in *HAS1* intron 3, as first shown here, is supported by our previous work [1;8;15]. In some blood cancer patients, *HAS1* is a hypermutated gene [8] that undergoes aberrant splicing to generate splice variants that correlate with poor survival [4]. *In vitro* mutagenesis of *HAS1* intron3 alters *HAS1* splicing patterns, causing transfectants to acquire the splicing pattern seen in MM patients[7;8]. *In silico* and *in vitro* mutagenesis analyses predict that *HAS1* intron3 plays a central role in clinically relevant splice site selection and consequent aberrant intronic splicing of *HAS1* [7;8]. Intronic SNPs can have a functional impact by affecting gene regulation and splicing mechanisms [16–18], confirming that intronic SNPs have a potentially strong influence on oncogenic events. In MM and WM, *HAS1* genetic variations are distributed in or near splicing elements [8;15] and can direct aberrant splicing of *HAS1* [7;8]. In transfected cells, the properties of aberrant HAS1 variants are dominant over those of the normally expressed HAS1 full length form [6].

The independent Icelandic kindred is a small but relatively homogeneous population with a common ancestry. Affected family members exhibit hyper-Ig synthesis *in vitro* and some have MGUS, WM or MM. The linked *HAS1* intron3 SNP alleles and genotypes of affected members, but not an exon3 SNP, were significantly different from those of unaffected members (genotype frequencies p = 0.007, allele frequencies p = 0.0005).

In the pooled analysis of SNP genotypes for all patient and control groups, the odds ratio for B cell malignancy (OR$_{trend}$) was 1.78 and for affected Icelandic family members, OR was 5.8. These odds ratios, especially when considered in the context of the familial analysis, suggest minimal or no influence of cryptic population stratification. Risk predictions may be directly correlated with the identified SNPs, or may result from unknown

Table 3. Allele frequencies of *HAS1* SNPs in Case cohorts (MGUS, MM, CLL and WM)*.

SNPs	MGUS Cohort			MM Cohort			CLL Cohort			WM Cohort		
	Major Allele	Minor Allele	P	Major Allele	Minor	P	Major Allele	Minor Allele	P	Major Allele	Minor	P
rs61736495												
Case	194 (0.99)	2 (0.01)	0.152	355 (0.98)	7 (0.902)	0.414	329 (0.97)	9 (0.03)	0.88	143 (0.99)	1 (0.01)	0.138
Control	412 (0.97)	12 (0.03)		412 (0.97)	12 (0.03)		412 (0.97)	12 (0.03)		412 (0.97)	12 (0.03)	
rs11084111												
Case	179 (0.91)	17 (0.09)	0.125	329 (0.91)	33 (0.09)	0.04	313(0.93)	25 (0.07)	0.265	132 (0.92)	12 (0.08)	0.204
Control	401 (0.95)	23(0.05)		401 (0.95)	23(0.05)		401 (0.95)	23(0.05)		401 (0.95)	23(0.05)	
rs11084110												
Case	72 (0.37)	126(0.63)	0.44	89(0.25)	273 (0.75)	0.007	68 (0.20)	270 (0.80)	5.0×10^{-5}	28(0.19)	116 (0.81)	5.0×10^{-4}
Control	141 (0.33)	283 (0.67)		141 (0.33)	283 (0.67)		141 (0.33)	283 (0.67)		141 (0.33)	283 (0.67)	
rs11084109												
Case	73 (0.37)	125(0.63)	0.44	90 (0.25)	272(0.75)	0.006	68 (0.20)	270 (0.80)	3.0×10^{-7}	28(0.19)	116 (0.81)	3.7×10^{-4}
Control	143 (0.34)	281 (0.66)		143 (0.34)	281 (0.66)		143 (0.34)	281 (0.66)		143 (0.34)	281 (0.66)	
rs11669079												
Case	72 (0.37)	126(0.63)	0.44	89(0.25)	273 (0.75)	0.007	68 (0.20)	270 (0.80)	5.0×10^{-5}	28(0.19)	116 (0.81)	5.0×10^{-4}
Control	141 (0.33)	283 (0.67)		141 (0.33)	283 (0.67)		141 (0.33)	283 (0.67)		141 (0.33)	283 (0.67)	

*P values are calculated using fisher exact test, allele frequencies are shown in parentheses. Alleles are designated as major or minor based on the NCBI database.

Table 4. HASI SNP genotype associates with risk of B-cell malignancy*.

SNP	Genotype	Controls	MGUS	OR (95% CI) P	MM	OR (95% CI) P	CLL	OR (95% CI) P	WM	OR (95% CI) P
rs61736495	GG	200	96	1.00	174	1.00	160	1.00	71	1.00
HAS1	GA	12	2	0.35 (0.08–1.58) 0.172	7	0.67 (0.25–1.74) 0.4	9	0.93 (0.40–2.25) 0.88	1	0.24 (0.03–1.86) 0.16
	AA	0	0	–	0	–	0	–	0	–
	OR$_{trend}$			0.34 (0.08–1.59) 0.177		0.67 (0.26–1.73) 0.4		0.93 (0.40–2.28) 0.88		0.24 (0.03–1.83) 0.16
rs11084111	CC	189	81	1.00	151	1.00	145	1.00	60	1.00
HAS1	CT	23	17	1.72 (0.90–3.40) 0.116	27	1.46 (0.81–2.66) 0.2	23	1.30 (0.70–2.40) 0.4	12	1.64 (0.77–3.50) 0.19
	TT	0	0	–	3	–	1	–	0	–
	OR$_{trend}$			1.65 (0.86–3.17) 0.129		1.43 (1.00–3.03) 0.05		1.39 (0.70–2.40) 0.26		1.60 (0.76–3.27) 0.21
rs11084110	GG	21	17	1.00	14	1.00	8	1.00	2	1.00
HAS1	GA	99	38	0.47 (0.22–0.99) 0.05	61	0.92 (0.43–1.95) 0.84	52	1.37 (0.60–3.32) 0.47	24	2.54 (0.55–11.6) 0.22
	AA	92	43	0.57 (0.30–1.20) 0.14	106	1.72 (0.83–3.59) 0.14	109	3.11 (1.37–7.35) 0.01	46	5.25 (1.18–23.3) 0.02
	OR$_{trend}$			0.85 (0.60–1.22) 0.39		1.52 (1.14–2.09) **0.008**		2.(1.41–2.76) **1.0×10^{-5}**		2.10 (1.33–3.26) **0.002**
rs11084109	GG	21	18	1.00	14	1.00	8	1.00	2	1.00
HAS1	GA	101	37	0.42 (0.20–0.90) 0.02	62	0.92 (0.43–1.94) 0.82	52	1.37 (0.56–3.25) 0.5	24	2.5 (0.50–11.3) 0.23
	AA	90	43	0.55 (0.30–1.115) 0.11	105	1.75 (0.84–3.64) 0.13	109	3.17 (1.34–7.51) 0.008	46	5.36 (1.20–23.9) 0.02
	OR$_{trend}$			0.85 (0.60–1.22) 0.39		1.53 (1.12–2.10) **0.007**		2 (1.41–2.82) **1.0×10^{-5}**		2.10(1.33–3.30) **0.001**
rs11669079	TT	21	17	1.00	14	1.00	8	1.00	2	1.00
HAS1	TA	99	38	0.47 (0.22–0.99) 0.05	61	0.92 (0.43–1.95) 0.84	52	1.37 (0.60–3.32) 0.47	24	2.54 (0.55–11.6) 0.22
	AA	92	43	0.57 (0.30–1.20) 0.14	106	1.72 (0.83–3.59) 0.14	109	3.11 (1.37–7.35) 0.01	46	5.25 (1.18–23.3) 0.02
	OR$_{trend}$			0.85 (0.60–1.22) 0.39		1.52 (1.14–2.09) **0.008**		2 (1.41–2.76) **1.0×10^{-5}**		2.10 (1.33–3.26) **0.002**

*All comparisons are of case subjects with control subjects. All groups met Hardy Weinberg Equilibrium. Allelic odds ratios and the corresponding 95% confidence intervals were calculated for the association analysis and are shown in the table. CI denotes confidence interval, OR denotes odds ratio. The genome position is based on the National Centre for Biotechnology Information database. For CLL samples, a cohort of 20 patients provided both enriched B cells and buccal cells; both populations gave identical results. No assumptions were made about the effect of the SNPs prior to analysis.

Table 5. *HAS1* SNPs do not associate with breast cancer or ductal carcinoma in situ (DCIS).

SNP	Genotype	Controls	Breast Cancer	OR (95% CI) P	Subset DCIS	OR (95% CI) P	Breast Cancer pooled	OR (95% CI) P
rs61736495	GG	352	237	1.00	55	1.00	292	1.00
HAS1	GA	0	2	–	1	–	3	–
	AA	0	0	–	0	–	0	–
	OR$_{trend}$			–		–		–
rs11084111	CC	339	224	1.00	53	1.00	277	1.00
HAS1	CT	13	15	1.74 (0.81–3.74) 0.15	3	1.47(0.40–5.35) 0.55	18	1.69 (0.81–3.51) 0.15
	TT	0	0	–	0	–	0	–
	OR$_{trend}$			1.72 (0.81–3.65) 0.15		1.47(0.40–5.21) 0.55		1.67 (0.81–3.44) 0.16
rs11084110	GG	26	15	1.00	4	1.00	19	1.00
HAS1	GA	144	104	1.25 (0.63–2.48) 0.52	32	1.44 (0.47–4.42) 0.52	136	1.29 (0.68–2.44) 0.42
	AA	182	120	1.14 (0.58–2.24) 0.69	20	0.71(0.22–2.25) 0.56	140	0.98 (0.52–1.85) 0.96
	OR$_{trend}$			0.99 (0.76–1.28) 0.94		0.69 (0.45–1.05) 0.08		0.88 (0.69–1.12) 0.31
rs11084109	GG	26	15	1.00	4	1.00	19	1.00
HAS1	GA	144	104	1.25 (0.63–2.48) 0.52	32	1.44 (0.47–4.42) 0.52	136	1.29 (0.68–2.44) 0.42
	AA	182	120	1.14 (0.58–2.24) 0.69	20	0.71(0.22–2.25) 0.56	140	0.98 (0.52–1.85) 0.96
	OR$_{trend}$			0.99 (0.76–1.28) 0.94		0.69 (0.45–1.05) 0.08		0.88 (0.69–1.12) 0.31
rs11669079	TT	26	15	1.00	4	1.00	19	1.00
HAS1	TA	144	104	1.25 (0.63–2.48) 0.52	32	1.44 (0.47–4.42) 0.52	136	1.29 (0.68–2.44) 0.42
	AA	182	120	1.14 (0.58–2.24) 0.69	20	0.71(0.22–2.25) 0.56	140	0.98 (0.52–1.85) 0.96
	OR$_{trend}$			0.99 (0.76–1.28) 0.94		0.69 (0.45–1.05) 0.08		0.88 (0.69–1.12) 0.31

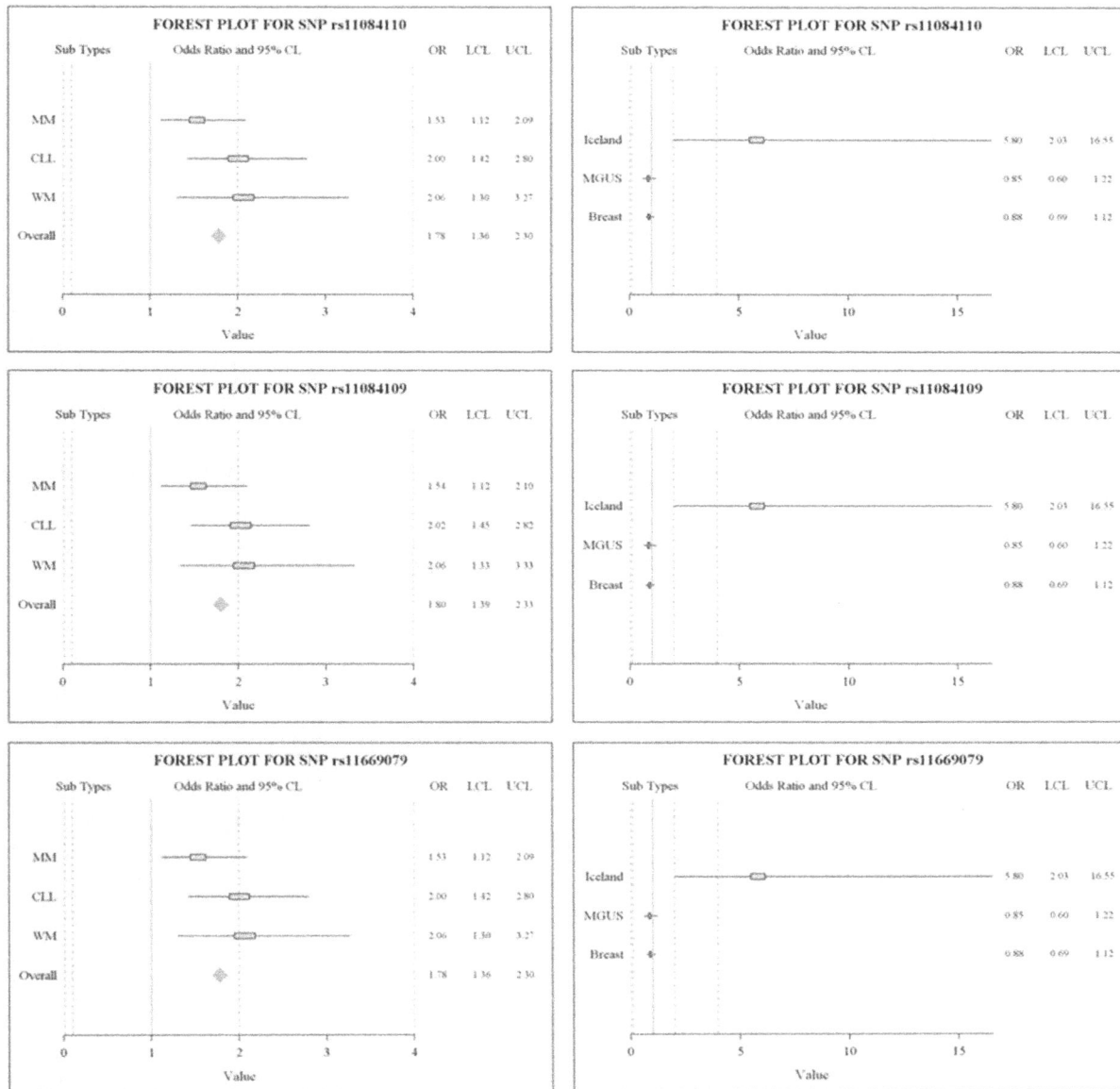

Figure 2. Forest plots of three linked SNPs in B-cell Malignancies, the Icelandic kindred, breast cancer and MGUS. The left column of three panels show the odds ratios of B cell malignancy for the three linked intronic *HAS1* SNPs. The OR denotes the odds of having the minor allele as assessed by genotype. The X-axis corresponds to odds ratio. The horizontal line represents 95% confidence interval. Each box represents the OR point estimate. The diamond represents the odds ratios obtained from pooled analysis with 95% confidence interval. Each group is compared to the appropriate control group. The right column of three panels show odds ratios for the Icelandic kindred, MGUS and breast cancer; each individual group is compared to its own control group as indicated in results. The cumulative risks were not estimated for these last three groups as they are unrelated to each other. These plots show that there were no associations of risk with the three linked SNPs for sporadic MGUS or breast cancer. There was a very strong association of the minor allele with risk for the B cell malignancies (pooled OR = 1.78) and the Icelandic Kindred (OR = 5.8). Note difference in scale values between panels in the two columns.

mutation(s) outside the sequenced region but in linkage disequilibrium with the detected SNPs. The OR for breast cancer patients and MGUS did not differ from unity, suggesting that the increased risk conferred by HAS1 SNPs is selective for systemic B-cell malignancies.

Family members of patients with MGUS or MM have a two-three-fold higher risk of developing MGUS and multiple myeloma [19–22]. CLL and WM include both sporadic and familial forms of the disease [23–26]. Inherited polymorphisms are associated with both CLL and WM [15;25;27–31], and a strongly recurrent

somatic mutation with WM [32]. The odds ratios found here for CLL and WM were considerably more pronounced than those found for MM which appears to have less familial influence. However, this work demonstrates for the first time that an increased frequency of *HAS1* intron3 SNPs is common among all three systemic B-cell malignancies, possibly indicating shared genetic predispositions that culminate in malignant transformation of B-cells.

We employed sequencing for this study because it provides for unequivocal allele calling in each patient, as well as identification of any closely linked rare mutations that might influence risk. An advantage in SNP detection by direct DNA sequencing is the complete information it yields, including haplotype relationships. Recent literature supports our approach [33] and emphasizes the use of sequencing to detect direct associations between disease and casual SNPs [34]. Our analysis was restricted to polymorphisms in *HAS1* exon3 and intron3, a mutation-rich region that is involved in aberrant splicing of *HAS1* exons and introns [7;8]. Our work suggests that the three linked *HAS1* intronic SNPs may predispose to aberrant splicing, or are in linkage disequilibrium with a causative functional variant located outside exon3 and intron3 of HAS1. This study provides strong evidence to support the hypothesis that *HAS1* contributes to a genetic risk of B-cell malignancy.

In conclusion, our findings suggest that genetic variants in *HAS1* are associated with risk of B-cell malignancy in MM, CLL and WM. Because the *HAS1* intron3 SNPs are present at significantly higher frequencies in individuals who have developed a systemic B-cell cancer, these results suggest that intronic *HAS1* SNPs predispose to systemic B-cell cancers and as inherited characteristics may thus act at an early stage of oncogenesis. Although multiple genes are certainly involved, this work supports the idea that *HAS1* intron3 SNPs have a strong impact on molecular events, particularly on aberrant HAS1 pre-mRNA splicing events

that contribute to the malignant phenotype in B-cell cancers. Molecular therapy to target this region of *HAS1* warrants evaluation.

Supporting Information

File S1   Suppporting Tables. Table 1, Primer sequences used for PCR or sequencing reactions. Table S2, Components of PCR mixture. Table S3, HAS1 SNPs observed in this study.

Acknowledgments

We thank all the study participants for their cooperation, Dr. Sunita Ghosh, Biostatistician, Cross Cancer Institute for statistical help and the Manitoba Tumor Bank.

Author Contributions

Conceived and designed the experiments: LMP HK HO AW ARB. Performed the experiments: HK AW EB. Analyzed the data: HK AW EB HO. Contributed reagents/materials/analysis tools: HO HS VH MJM JM JBJ ARB SA. Contributed to the writing of the manuscript: LMP HK HO JM MJM JBJ SA ARB.

References

1. Adamia S, Pilarski PM, Belch AR, Pilarski LM (2013) Aberrant splicing, hyaluronan synthases and intracellular hyaluronan as drivers of oncogenesis and potential drug targets. Curr.Cancer Drug Targets. 13: 347–361.
2. Ogmundsdottir HM, Haraldsdottirm V, Johannesson GM, Olafsdottir G, Bjarnadottir K, et al (2005) Familiality of benign and malignant paraproteinemias. A population-based cancer-registry study of multiple myeloma families. Haematologica 90: 66–71.
3. Ogmundsdottir HM, Johannesson GM, Sveinsdottir S, Einarsdottir S, Hegeman A, et al. (1994) Familial macroglobulinaemia: hyperactive B-cells but normal natural killer function. Scand.J.Immunol. 40:195–200.
4. Adamia S, Reiman T, Crainie M, Mant MJ, Belch A, et al (2005) Intronic splicing of hyaluronan synthase 1 (HAS1): a biologically relevant indicator of poor outcome in multiple myeloma. Blood 105: 4836–4844.
5. Masellis-Smith A, Belch AR, Mant MJ, Turley EA, et al. (1996) Hyaluronan-dependent motility of B cells and leukemic plasma cells in blood, but not of bone marrow plasma cells, in multiple myeloma: alternate use of receptor for hyaluronan-mediated motility (RHAMM) and CD44. Blood 87: 1891–9.
6. Ghosh A, Kuppusamy H, Pilarski LM (2009) Aberrant splice variants of HAS1 (Hyaluronan Synthase 1) multimerize with and modulate normally spliced HAS1 protein: a potential mechanism promoting human cancer. J.Biol.Chem. 284: 18840–18850.
7. Kriangkum J, Warkentin A, Belch AR, Pilarski LM (2013) Alteration of Introns in a Hyaluronan Synthase 1 (HAS1) Minigene Convert Pre-mRNA Splicing to the Aberrant Pattern in Multiple Myeloma (MM): MM Patients Harbor Similar Changes. PLoS.One. 8: e53469.
8. Adamia S, Reichert A, Kuppusamy H, Kriangkum J, Ghosh A, et al. (2008) Inherited and acquired mutations in the hyaluronan synthase-1 (HAS1) gene may contribute to disease progression in multiple myeloma and Waldenstrom's macroglobulinemia. Blood 112: 5111–5121.
9. Smith A, Wisloff F, Samson D (2006) Guidelines on the diagnosis and management of multiple myeloma 2005. Br.J.Haematol. 132: 410–451.
10. Owen RG, Treon SP, Al-Katib A, Fonseca R, Greipp PR, et al. (2003) Clinicopathological definition of Waldenstrom's macroglobulinemia: consensus panel recommendations from the Second International Workshop on Waldenstrom's Macroglobulinemia. Semin.Oncol. 30: 110–115.
11. Wilkins K, LaFramboise T (2011) Losing balance: Hardy-Weinberg disequilibrium as a marker for recurrent loss-of-heterozygosity in cancer. Hum.Mol.Genet. 20: 4831–4839.
12. Yabushita H, Noguchi M, Kishida T, Fusano K, Noguchi Y, et al. (2004) Hyaluronan synthase expression in ovarian cancer. Oncol.Rep. 12: 739–743.
13. Yabushita H, Kishida T, Fusano K, Kanyama K, Zhuo L, et al. (2005) Role of hyaluronan and hyaluronan synthase in endometrial cancer. Oncol.Rep. 13: 1101–1105.
14. Simpson MA, Reiland J, Burger SR, Furcht LT, Spicer AP, et al. (2001) Hyaluronan synthase elevation in metastatic prostate carcinoma cells correlates with hyaluronan surface retention, a prerequisite for rapid adhesion to bone marrow endothelial cells. J.Biol.Chem. 276: 17949–17957.
15. Adamia S, Treon SP, Reiman T, Tournilhac O, McQuarrie, et al. (2005) Single nucleotide polymorphism of hyaluronan synthase 1 gene and aberrant splicing in Waldenstroms macroglobulinemia. Clinical Lymphoma 5: 253–256.
16. Hiratani H, Bowden DW, Ikegami S, Shirasawa S, Shimizu A, et al. (2005) Multiple SNPs in intron 7 of thyrotropin receptor are associated with Graves' disease. J.Clin.Endocrinol.Metab 90: 2898–2903.
17. Berulava T, Horsthemke B (2010) The obesity-associated SNPs in intron 1 of the FTO gene affect primary transcript levels. Eur.J.Hum.Genet. 18: 1054–1056.
18. Zhang Y, Bertolino A, Fazio L, Blasi G, Rampino A, et al. (2007) Polymorphisms in human dopamine D2 receptor gene affect gene expression, splicing, and neuronal activity during working memory. Proc.Natl.Acad.Sci.U.S.A 104: 20552–20557.
19. Landgren O, Kristinsson SY, Goldin LR, Caporaso NE, Blimark C, et al. (2009) Risk of plasma cell and lymphoproliferative disorders among 14621 first-degree relatives of 4458 patients with monoclonal gammopathy of undetermined significance in Sweden. Blood 114: 791–795.
20. Altieri A, Chen B, Bermejo JL, Castro F, Hemminki K (2006) Familial risks and temporal incidence trends of multiple myeloma. Eur.J.Cancer 42: 1661–1670.
21. Kang SH, Kim TY, Kim HY, Yoon JH, Cho HI, et al. (2008) Protective role of CYP1A1*2A in the development of multiple myeloma. Acta Haematol. 119: 60–64.
22. Maggini V, Buda G, Galimberti S, Martino A, Orciuolo E, et al. (2008) Lack of association of NQO1 and GSTP1 polymorphisms with multiple myeloma risk. Leuk.Res. 32: 988–990.
23. Mauro FR, Giammartini E, Gentile M, Sperduti I, Valle V, et al. (2006) Clinical features and outcome of familial chronic lymphocytic leukemia. Haematologica 91: 1117–1120.
24. Speedy HE, Sava G, Houlston RS (2013) Inherited susceptibility to CLL. Adv.Exp.Med.Biol. 792: 293–308.
25. Berndt SI, Skibola CF, Joseph V, Camp NJ, Nieters A, et al. (2013) Genome-wide association study identifies multiple risk loci for chronic lymphocytic leukemia. Nat.Genet. 45: 868–876.
26. Royer RH, Koshiol J, Giambarresi TR, Vasquez LG, Pfeiffer RM, et al. (2010) Differential characteristics of Waldenstrom macroglobulinemia according to patterns of familial aggregation. Blood 115: 4464–4471.
27. Goldin LR, Bjorkholm M, Kristinsson SY, Turesson I, Landgren O (2009) Elevated risk of chronic lymphocytic leukemia and other indolent non-Hodgkin's lymphomas among relatives of patients with chronic lymphocytic leukemia. Haematologica 94: 647–653.
28. Sava GP, Speedy HE, Houlston RS (2014) Candidate gene association studies and risk of chronic lymphocytic leukemia: a systematic review and meta-analysis. Leuk.Lymphoma 55: 160–167.
29. Coombs CC, Rassenti LZ, Falchi L, Slager SL, Strom SS, et al. (2012) Single nucleotide polymorphisms and inherited risk of chronic lymphocytic leukemia among African Americans. Blood 120: 1687–1690.
30. Poulain S, Roumier C, Galiegue-Zouitina S, Daudignon A, Herbaux C, et al. (2013) Genome wide SNP array identified multiple mechanisms of genetic changes in Waldenstrom macroglobulinemia. Am.J.Hematol. 88: 948–954.

31. Liang XS, Caporaso N, McMaster ML, Ng D, Landgren O, et al. (2009) Common genetic variants in candidate genes and risk of familial lymphoid malignancies. Br.J.Haematol. 146:418–423.

32. Treon SP, Xu L, Yang G, Zhou Y, Liu X, et al. (2012) MYD88 L265P somatic mutation in Waldenstrom's macroglobulinemia. N.Engl.J.Med. 367:826–833.

33. McClellan J, King MC (2010) Genetic heterogeneity in human disease. Cell 141: 210–217.

34. Lachance J (2010) Disease-associated alleles in genome-wide association studies are enriched for derived low frequency alleles relative to HapMap and neutral expectations. BMC.Med.Genomics 3: 57.

7

Involvement of Fatty Acid Amide Hydrolase and Fatty Acid Binding Protein 5 in the Uptake of Anandamide by Cell Lines with Different Levels of Fatty Acid Amide Hydrolase Expression: A Pharmacological Study

Emmelie Björklund[1], Anders Blomqvist[1], Joel Hedlin[1], Emma Persson[2], Christopher J. Fowler[1]*

1 Department of Pharmacology and Clinical Neuroscience, Umeå University, Umeå, Sweden, 2 Department of Radiation Sciences, Umeå University, Umeå, Sweden

Abstract

Background: The endocannabinoid ligand anandamide (AEA) is removed from the extracellular space by a process of cellular uptake followed by metabolism. In many cells, such as the RBL-2H3 cell line, inhibition of FAAH activity reduces the observed uptake, indicating that the enzyme regulates uptake by controlling the intra- : extracellular AEA concentration gradient. However, in other FAAH-expressing cells, no such effect is seen. It is not clear, however, whether these differences are methodological in nature or due to properties of the cells themselves. In consequence, we have reinvestigated the role of FAAH in gating the uptake of AEA.

Methodology/Principal Findings: The effects of FAAH inhibition upon AEA uptake were investigated in four cell lines: AT1 rat prostate cancer, RBL-2H3 rat basophilic leukaemia, rat C6 glioma and mouse P19 embryonic carcinoma cells. Semi-quantitative PCR for the cells and for a rat brain lysate confirmed the expression of FAAH. No obvious expression of a transcript with the expected molecular weight of FLAT was seen. FAAH expression differed between cells, but all four could accumulate AEA in a manner inhibitable by the selective FAAH inhibitor URB597. However, there was a difference in the sensitivities seen in the reduction of uptake for a given degree of FAAH inhibition produced by a reversible FAAH inhibitor, with C6 cells being more sensitive than RBL-2H3 cells, despite rather similar expression levels and activities of FAAH. The four cell lines all expressed FABP5, and AEA uptake was reduced in the presence of the FABP5 inhibitor SB-FI-26, suggesting that the different sensitivities to FAAH inhibition for C6 and RBL2H3 cells is not due to differences at the level of FABP-5.

Conclusions/Significance: When assayed using the same methodology, different FAAH-expressing cells display different sensitivities of uptake to FAAH inhibition.

Editor: Patrizia Campolongo, Sapienza University of Rome, Italy

Funding: This work was supported by the Swedish Science Research Council (Grant no. 12158) and the Research Funds of the Medical Faculty. Umeå University is gratefully acknowledged. The funders had no role in study design, data collection and analysis, decision to publish, or preparation of the manuscript.

Competing Interests: The authors have declared that no competing interests exist.

* Email: cf@pharm.umu.se

Introduction

The endogenous cannabinoid ligand anandamide (arachidonoylethanolamide, AEA) is produced "on demand" [1] and removed from the synaptic cleft by a process of cellular uptake followed by metabolism, primarily by the intra-cellular enzyme fatty acid amide hydrolase (FAAH) [2]. The process of the cellular clearance has been widely discussed in the literature (for review, see [3]) and several intracellular AEA transporters such as fatty acid binding protein 5 and 7, heat shock protein 70 and albumin have been proposed [4,5]. An FAAH-like AEA transporter (FLAT) has also been proposed as an intracellular carrier protein [6], although this has been disputed [7].

In 2001, two papers were published linking the uptake of AEA to its FAAH-catalysed breakdown. Day et al. [8] reported that transfection of HeLa cells with FAAH increased the observed rate of AEA uptake, and that inhibition of the enzyme in RBL-2H3

basophilic leukaemia cells reduced the uptake. Deutsch et al. [9] found that uptake was reduced (but not completely blocked) in FAAH-containing C6 glioma and N18 neuroblastoma cells following inhibition of the activity of this enzyme by the admittedly non-specific compounds methylarachidonoylfluorophosphonate and phenylmethylsulfonyl fluoride, whereas these compounds were without effect on the uptake of Hep2 laryngeal carcinoma cells, which lack FAAH. The authors suggested that FAAH gated the uptake of AEA by hydrolysing the intracellularly accumulated compound, and thereby preserving its extra- : intracellular gradient [8,9]. Selective FAAH inhibitors such as URB597 [10] are now available, and a role for FAAH in regulating the uptake of AEA in several cells has been demonstrated using this compound (see e.g. [11,12]) In a recent study, it was reported that AEA applied to the outside of synthetic lipid vesicles could be hydrolysed if FAAH was attached to the inside of the vesicles, and that the rate of hydrolysis was increased if cholesterol was added to the membrane, leading the authors to argue that the endocannabinoid can be internalised and presented to FAAH without the absolute requirement for membrane translocating proteins [13,14].

Although these and other studies clearly argue in favour of a role of FAAH in regulating AEA uptake, other studies have reported the opposite, namely that the presence of FAAH in a cell is not a determinant of the uptake. Thus, almost complete inhibition of FAAH in cortical astrocytes by 25 μM (E)-6-(bromomethylene)tetrahydro-3-(1-naphthalenyl)-2H-pyran-2-one does not affect the uptake of AEA into these cells, and a similar result was seen with 15 μM linoleyl trifluoromethyl ketone [15]. AEA can also be accumulated by synaptosomes from FAAH$^{-/-}$ mice [16–18]. Conversely, AEA uptake into human astrocytoma cells and cultured rat cortical neurones can be completely blocked by AM1172, a compound that is a weak FAAH inhibitor [16] although a subsequent study argued that this compound did not affect the uptake of AEA into RBL-2H3 cells when a short (25 second) incubation time was used [19].

From the above discussion, there are clearly disagreements in the literature concerning the degree to which FAAH contributes to the regulation of cellular AEA uptake. While it is possible that these differences are due to cellular diversity, it is also possible that methodological differences can contribute to the observed differences. One way of distinguishing between these possibilities is to use a standardised method to compare the sensitivity of different FAAH-containing cells to inhibition of the enzyme. This has been undertaken in the present study.

Methods

Compounds

Anandamide [arachidonoyl 5,6,8,9,11,12,14,15-^{3}H] (specific activity 200 Ci/mmol; for the uptake experiments) and anandamide [ethanolamine-1^{3}H] (specific activity 60 Ci/mmol; for the FAAH assay) was obtained from American Radiolabeled Chemicals Inc. (St. Louis, MO, USA). URB597 (3′-carbamoyl-biphenyl-3-yl-cyclohexyl-carbamate) was obtained from the Cayman Chemical Company (Ann Arbor, MI, USA), Compound 33 [20] was provided by Dr. Valentina Onnis, University of Cagliari, Italy. SB-FI-26 was a kind gift from Drs. Dale Deutsch and Iwao Ojima, Stony Brook University, NY, USA.

Cell cultures

All cell types used were grown in 75 cm^2 culturing flasks at 37°C with 5% CO$_2$ in humidified atmospheric pressure. Passage of cells occurred approximately twice a week and medium was changed every other day. Rat basophilic leukaemia RBL-2H3 cells (passage range 13–72), obtained from the American Type Culture Collection (Manassas, VA, USA) were cultured in minimum essential medium with Earle's Salts (MEM), foetal bovine serum (FBS) (15%), penicillin 100 U ml^{-1} + streptomycin 100 μg ml^{-1} (PEST). Rat prostate cancer AT1 cells (passages 34–58) were obtained from Professor Anders Bergh, Department of Medical Biosciences, Umeå University. The cells (sometimes termed R3327 AT1, and originating from the inventor, [21]) were cultured in RPMI 1640 medium, with 10% FBS, 25 nM dexamethasone, 2 mM l-glutamine and PEST. C6 rat glioma cells (passage range 12–38), obtained from the European Collection of Cell Cultures, (Porton Down, UK) were cultured in F-10 Ham supplemented with 10% FBS and PEST. P19 mouse embryonic carcinoma cells (passage 18–33, European Collection of Cell Cultures, Porton Down, UK), were cultured in MEM alpha 22571 with 10% FBS, 1% non-essential amino acids and PEST.

AEA uptake assay

The method of Rakhshan et al. [22] with minor modifications [23] was used. Cells (RBL-2H3, AT1, C6 and P19) were plated at a density of 2×10^5 cells per well in 24-well culture plates and incubated overnight at 37°C in an atmosphere of 5% CO$_2$. One plate of wells containing only medium was also incubated and subsequently used to determine the non-specific retention of [^{3}H]AEA to the plates. After incubation, cells were washed once with Krebs-Ringer Hepes (KRH)-buffer (120 mM NaCl, 4.7 mM KCl, 2.2 mM CaCl$_2$, 10 mM 4-(2-hydroxyethyl)-1-piperazi-neethane-sulfonic acid (HEPES), 0.12 mM KH$_2$PO$_4$, 0.12 mM MgSO$_4$ in milliQ deionised water, pH 7.4) containing 1% bovine serum albumin (BSA) and once with KRH- buffer alone. Cells were preincubated with KRH containing 0.1% fatty acid-free BSA and test compounds or vehicle control (dimethyl sulfoxide for URB597 and SB- FI-26, ethanol for Compound 33; vehicle concentrations are indicated in the figure legends) for 10 minutes at 37°C. [^{3}H-arachidonoyl]AEA (unless otherwise stated; 50 μl, final concentration of 100 nM, in KRH-buffer containing 0.1% fatty acid-free BSA) was added to give a final volume of 400 μl, and the wells were incubated for 4 minutes at 37°C, unless otherwise stated. The plates were put on ice before washing three times with 500 μl of KRH-buffer containing 1% BSA. The buffer was removed, 0.2 M NaOH (500 μl) was added and the plate incubated at 75°C for 15 minutes to solubilise the cells. Aliquots of 300 μl were transferred to scintillation vials and the tritium content was determined by liquid scintillation spectroscopy with quench correction.

FAAH assay

The FAAH assay was carried out essentially as described by Boldrup et al. [24] using lysates from C6 and RBL-2H3 cells. Briefly, 5 μg protein diluted with 10 mM Tris-HCl, 1 mM EDTA pH 7.4, test compound (or vehicle control, final assay concentration 1%) and [^{3}H-ethanolamine]AEA in 10 mM Tris-HCl, 1 mM EDTA, pH 7.4, containing 1% w/v fatty acid-free BSA, final substrate concentration of 0.5 μM were incubated for 10 min at 37°C. Blanks contained buffer instead of membrane preparation. Reactions were stopped by placing the tubes on ice and adding 80 μL activated charcoal mixed in 320 μL of 0.5 M HCl. Samples were mixed and left at room temperature for about 30 min prior to centrifugation at 2500 rpm for 10 min. Aliquots (200 μL) of the supernatants were analysed for tritium content by liquid scintillation spectroscopy with quench correction. Ethical permission for the animal samples was obtained from the local animal research ethical committee (Umeå Ethical Committee for Animal Research, Umeå, Sweden).

For the experiments in intact cells, the assay described above for AEA uptake was used with two changes: a) [^{3}H-ethanolamine]AEA rather than [arachidonoyl 5,6,8,9,11,12,14,15-^{3}H]AEA was used, and b) the reaction was stopped by addition of 120 μL activated charcoal mixed in 480 μL of 0.5 M HCl [25]. Aliquots (600 μL) were pipetted into glass tubes, which were then centrifuged and aliquots (200 μL) of the supernatants were analysed for tritium content by liquid scintillation spectroscopy with quench correction. Blanks were wells alone. An initial experiment using C6 cells indicated that when an initial number (i.e. added to wells and incubated overnight) of 10^5 cells/well were used, the amount of substrate hydrolysed was reasonably linear over time for 30 min, and that at the 10 min time point, the activity was completely blocked by 1 μM URB597. In consequence, this time point and cell density were used in the experiments reported in this paper.

RNA extraction and cDNA synthesis

AT1, C6, RBL-2H3 and P19 cells were plated at a density of 0.7×10^6 cells per well in 6-well plates. After overnight culturing, cells were washed twice in PBS and total RNA was extracted using the miRNeasy Kit (Qiagen, Hilden, Germany, Cat. No. 217004) according to the manufacturer's instructions. Rat prefrontal cortex was lysed using a homogenisator and RNA extracted as described above. The RNA concentration was measured using a NanoDrop ND-1000 instrument (Thermo Scientific, Wilmington, DE, USA). cDNA was synthesized from 2 μg of total RNA using a cDNA synthesis kit with random primers (High capacity cDNA reverse transcription kit; Applied Biosystems, Foster City, CA, USA). Prior to PCR analysis, cDNA from four wells were pooled for each cell line.

Semi-quantitative PCR

For detection of rat and mouse FAAH and FABP5 mRNA, cDNA was amplified in polymerase chain reaction (PCR) using a Taq PCR Core kit (Qiagen, Hilden, Germany, Cat. No. 201223), a Biometra TProfessional Gradient 96 thermocycler (Biometra GmbH, Göttingen, Germany) and the following primers: rat FAAH forward 5'-GTGCTGAGCGAAGTGTGGACC-3', reverse 5'-GGGCCTGGGACAGCTGAGTCT-3', rat FABP5 forward 5'- CGACCGTGTTTTCTTGCACC-3', reverse 5'-TGGCATTGTTCATGACGCAC-3', mouse FAAH forward 5'-GTGGTGCTAACCCCCATGCTGG-3', reverse 5'-TCCACCTCCCGCATGAACCGCAGACA-3', mouse FABP5 forward 5'-GACGGTCTGCACCTTCCAAG-3', reverse 5'-CAGGATGACGAGGAAGCCC-3'. The conditions for PCR were: an initial denaturation step at 94°C for 2 min, followed by 35 cycles with denaturing at 94°C for 40 s, annealing at 60°C for 40 s and elongation at 72°C for 60 s, followed by a final elongation step at 72°C for 3 min. The PCR products were electrophoretically separated on a 1.5% agarose gel, with expected fragment sizes for rat FAAH of 382 bp, rat FABP5 192 bp, mouse FAAH 302 bp, and mouse FABP5 176 bp.

Statistics

Statistical tests (one- or two-way ANOVA for repeated measures with Dunnett's or Šidák's post-hoc multiple tests, as appropriate) were undertaken using GraphPad Prism 5 and 6 for the Macintosh (GraphPad Software Inc., San Diego, CA, USA). The linear regression and Likelyhood ratio analyses of the data with compound 33 were undertaken using the R computer programme [26].

Results

Expression and activity of FAAH in AT1, C6, RBL-2H3 and P19 cells

Semi-quantitative PCR using primers amplifying a PCR product corresponding to the +4 to +385 region of the coding sequence of the rat *faah* gene was performed in order to investigate the expression of FAAH in the three rat cell lines used. As shown in Fig. 1A, the PCR analysis displayed the presence of a band correlating well with the expected fragment size of 382 bp for FAAH mRNA, in all three cell lines and, as a positive control, in rat brain. The expected fragment size of mouse FAAH is 302 bp, and the murine P19 cells expressed a band consistent with this size. In a second experiment (Fig. 1B), the rat cells were run in order to see if a band corresponding to FLAT could be visualised. The top part of the figure shows FAAH expression under conditions of normal exposure. The relative FAAH expression in the samples was AT1<C6<RBL-2H3 cells.

No band at 178 bp (the expected size of FLAT as visualised by this primer pair) was seen for either cells or rat brain; however, a weak band (among other bands) was seen at the appropriate size for the rat brain and AT1 cells when the gels were greatly overexposed (main gel in Fig. 1B). The lack of a band corresponding to FLAT under normal exposures is consistent with a recent study in this Journal using mouse tissues and a different primer pair [7]. FAAH activities were also measured in intact cells as part of the experiments described in section 3.3. After incubation of cells (10^5 per well incubated overnight prior to the experiment) for 10 min with 100 nM added [³H]AEA, C6, RBL-2H3 and AT1 cells the tritium recovered in the aqueous phase per well was 3.3±0.66, 2.1±0.16 and 0.31±0.09 pmol, respectively (means ± s.e.m., n = 3). The corresponding value for P19 cells was 0.70±0.09 pmol. Thus, all four cell lines express FAAH, albeit with different activities.

Inhibition of [³H]AEA uptake in AT1, RBL-2H3, C6 and P19 cells by URB597

In Fig. 1C, the uptake of [³H]AEA in the absence and presence of 1 μM URB597 is shown for the four cell lines and for wells alone. The cells were assayed concomitantly, and a two-way ANOVA matching for URB597 gave significant effects of cell line ($F_{3,16} = 7.96$, P<0.005), URB597 ($F_{1,6} = 256$, P<0.0001) and the interaction term URB597×cell line ($F_{3,16} = 32$, P<0.0001) [the data for the wells alone were not included]. The significant interaction term allows for *post-hoc* comparisons for vehicle and URB597-treated cells. For the vehicle-treated cells, Šidák's multiple comparisons test found significant differences between C6 or RBL2H3 cells and AT1 or P19 cells (P<0.001) but not between C6 and RBL2H3 cells or between AT1 and P19 cells. In contrast, for the URB597 treated cells, there were no significant differences between the cell types. The differences in the URB597-sensitive components of uptake between the cells matches well the observed FAAH activity of the intact cells (see above).

The effect of 1 μM URB597 upon the uptake of AEA into AT1, C6, RBL-2H3 and P19 cells at different incubation times is shown in Fig. 2. For all four cell lines, the rate of uptake was slowed by URB597, as demonstrated by the significant incubation time× treatment interaction term in the two-way repeated ANOVAs (see legend to Fig. 2). Over the period 1–7 min, the rate of uptake for the URB597-treated cells (determined as the slopes of the regression lines for individual experiments) were 30±9, 26±11, 28±5 and 34±4% (means ± s.e.m., n = 3–5) of the corresponding vehicle-treated cells for AT1, C6, RBL-2H3 and P19 cells, respectively.

The effects of reversible FAAH inhibition upon the cellular uptake and hydrolysis of AEA

Compound 33 of [20] is an inhibitor of FAAH without time-dependence, a property which is advantageous when investigating the effects of FAAH inhibition upon uptake in different assays. We used this compound to compare its ability to inhibit AEA hydrolysis in intact AT1, C6 and RBL-2H3 cells with its ability to affect AEA uptake the same cells. A clear relationship was found between the % reduction of AEA hydrolysis and uptake in all three cells, but not the wells (Fig. 3). From the mean data shown in Fig. 3, linear regression analyses were conducted for three different models in all cases with the mean % FAAH inhibition as an explanatory variable for the mean % uptake inhibition: I, where the intercepts and slopes are the same regardless of cell type. II; where the intercepts are different for the cells but the slopes are not; and III, where there is an interaction term between mean %

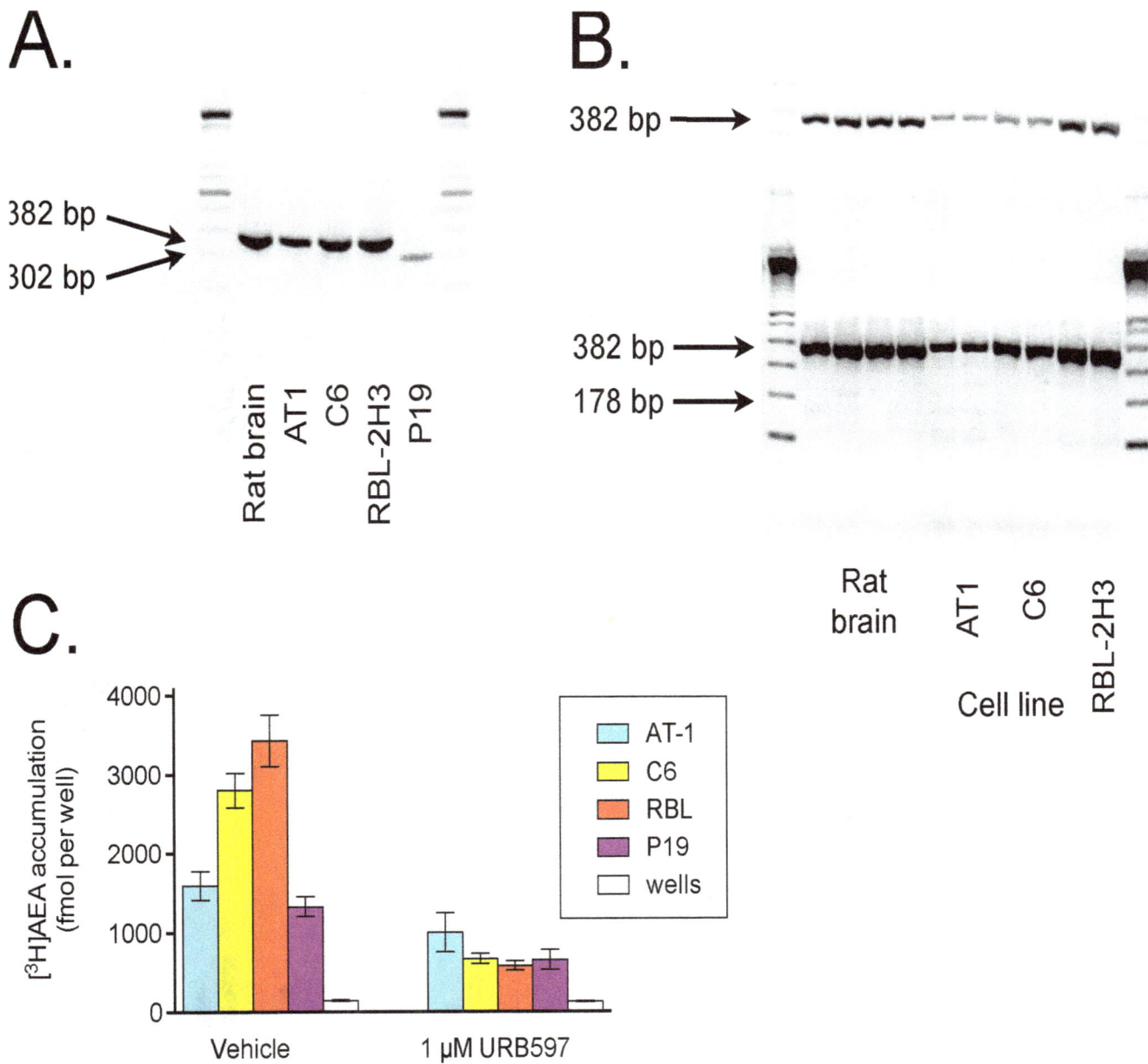

Figure 1. Expression of FAAH and sensitivity of AEA uptake to the FAAH inhibitor URB597 in AT1, C6, RBL-2H3 and P19 cells. In Panels A and B semi-quantitative PCR analysis of the mRNA expression of FAAH are shown for the cells, with rat brain lysates (two different lysates, lanes 2–5, in Panel B) as positive controls. Molecular size markers are also shown. Total RNA was isolated and reverse transcribed into cDNA. Samples were pooled (n = 4) and the PCR analysis was performed using primers designed to recognize rat or mouse FAAH, as appropriate. The PCR products were analyzed by agarose gel electrophoresis and fragment size estimated using a 100 bp marker. The arrows show the expected sizes for FAAH (both Panels) and FLAT (Panel B) with the primer pair used. In Panel B, the main gel shows an overexposure of the gels, with the small panel above showing the band corresponding to FAAH at normal levels of exposure. The photographs have been inverted to show the minor bands. In Panel C, the effect of 1 μM URB597 upon the uptake of [³H]AEA is shown for AT1, C6, RBL2H3 and P19 cells. Cells (or wells alone) were preincubated with URB597 for 10 min 37°C followed by addition of 100 nM [³H]AEA and incubation for further 4 min at 37°C. Shown are means and s.e.m., n = 5. The statistical treatment of the data is presented in Results.

FAAH inhibition and cell type, thus allowing variation of both slopes and intercepts to occur between cell types. Thereafter, the models were compared using a Likelyhood ratio test. According to this test, model II was preferable to model I, and model III was preferred to model II (P<0.005 in both cases, data not shown). In other words, with the proviso that the standard assumptions about normality of data are fulfilled, the sensitivity of uptake to a given degree of FAAH inhibition, is different between the cells. Thus, although RBL-2H3 and C6 cells express similar mRNA levels of FAAH (Fig. 1), the slope for RBL-2H3 cells is flatter than seen for C6 cells. The slope for the AT1 cells, which express much lower mRNA levels of FAAH than the other two rat cell lines (Fig. 1), is approximately mid way between the slopes for the other two cells.

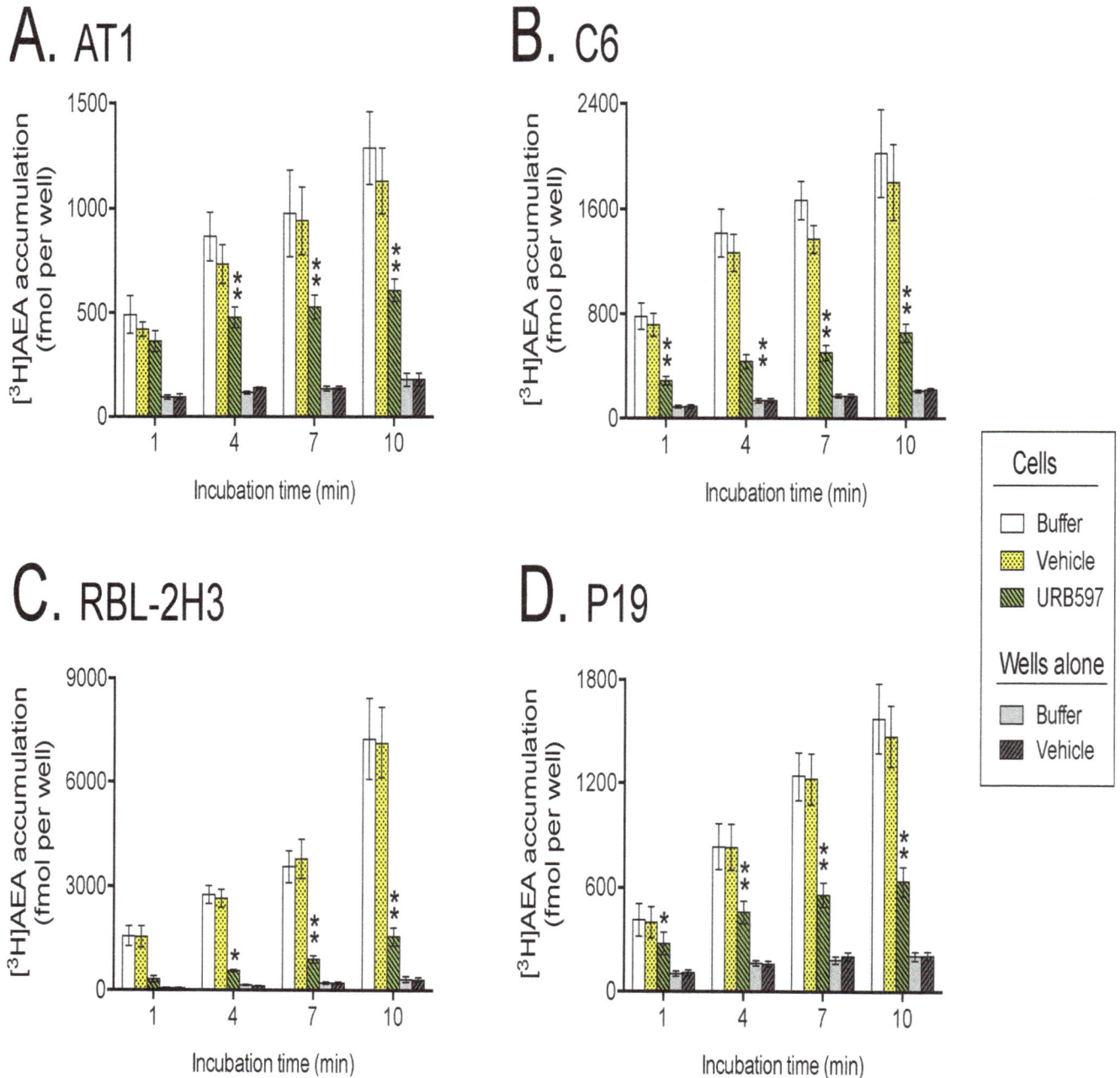

Figure 2. Time-dependent uptake of [³H]AEA in AT1, C6, RBL-2H3 and P19 cells treated with either buffer alone, vehicle, or 1 μM URB597. The cells were preincubated for 10 min with the test compounds and then incubated for 1, 4, 7 or 10 min with [³H]AEA. Values are mean and s.e.m. (when not enclosed by the symbols), n = 4 (AT1, C6), 3 (RBL-2H3), or 5 (P19). The concentration of DMSO for the vehicle was 0.2%. For the cell data with vehicle and 1 μM URB597 as variables, two-way repeated-measure ANOVAs matching both time and treatment indicated significant effects of time (P<0.01 for all cells), treatment (P<0.005 for C6, RBL-2H3 and P19; P<0.05 for AT1) and the interaction term time×treatment (P<0.01 for all cells). *P<0.05, **P<0.01, *post-hoc* comparisons using Šídák's multiple comparison for URB597-treated *vs.* corresponding vehicle-treated cells.

It can be argued that a comparison between AEA labelled in the arachidonoyl part of the molecule (for uptake) *vs.* AEA labelled in the ethanolamine part of the molecule (for FAAH) may be misleading given that the FAAH reaction products will have different subsequent metabolic fates in the cells. Further, the use of different incubation times (4 min for uptake vs. 10 min for hydrolysis) may be a complicating factor, although compound 33 was chosen because of its lack of time-dependency. In conse-

quence, we investigated the effects of compound 33 upon the uptake of [³H]AEA labelled in the ethanolamine part of the molecule by C6 and RBL2H3 cells. Further, we investigated the effects of this compound upon the AEA hydrolytic activity of C6 and RBL2H3 cell lysates (Fig. 4). Compound 33 produced essentially identical levels of FAAH inhibition in the lysates of the two cell types, but the difference in slopes between the cell types seen for the intact cells was retained. Further, the slopes for

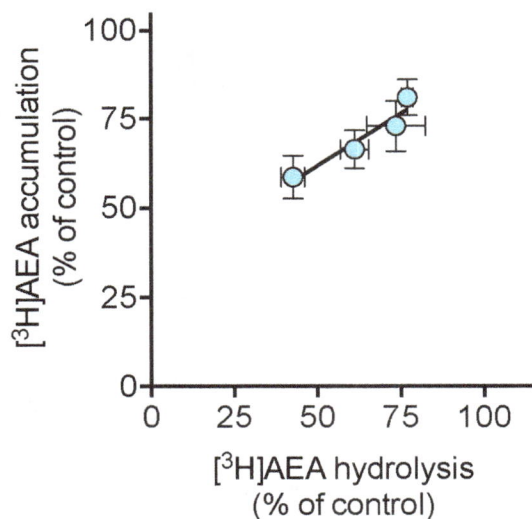

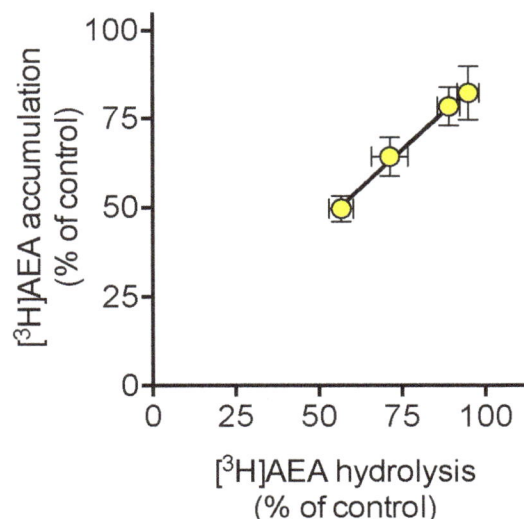

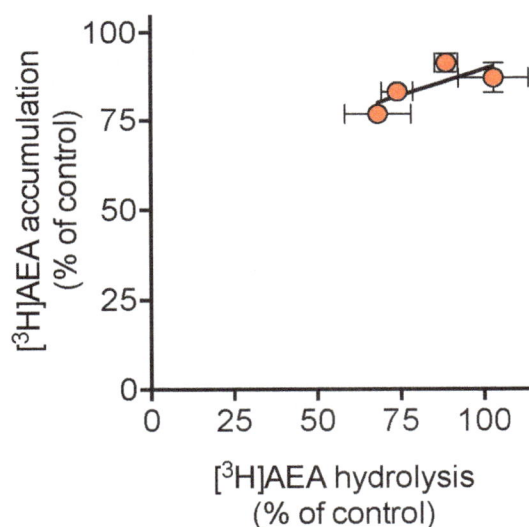

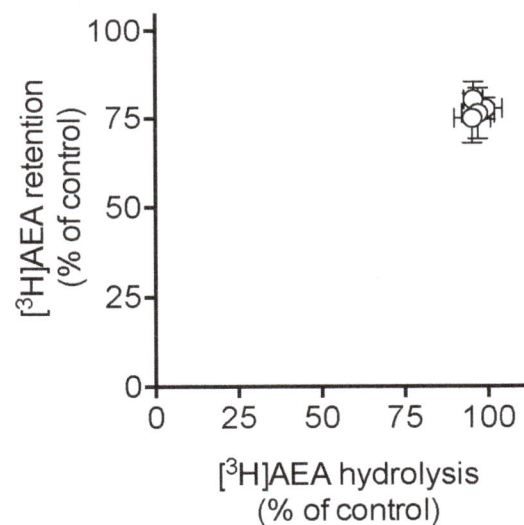

Figure 3. Effect of compound 33 upon AEA uptake and hydrolysis by intact cells. Cells (or wells alone) were pre-incubated with Compound 33, a paracetamol ester with a 2-(4-(2-(trifluoromethyl)pyridin-4-ylamino)phenyl)acetic acid substituent [20], for 10 minutes followed by further incubation with [3H]AEA for an additional 4 (uptake; [3H-arachidonoyl]-AEA) or 10 (hydrolysis, [3H-ethanolamine]-AEA) minutes. The longer time used for the hydrolysis measurements was to allow a sufficient assay: blank ratio. The lack of time-dependency of the inhibition of FAAH by compound 33 [20] permits this difference in incubation times. Shown are means $\pm$ s.e.m., n = 3–4. The concentration of EtOH for the vehicle was 0.2% (cells). The values ($\pm$ s.e.m.) of the slopes determined from the regression lines of the pooled data for each cell were: AT1, 0.58$\pm$0.21; C6, 0.85$\pm$0.18; RBL-2H3, 0.30$\pm$0.12.

the regression lines were the same (for a given cell) for the [3H]AEA labelled in the ethanolamine part as for the [3H]AEA

labelled in the arachidonoyl part of the molecule (see legend to Fig. 4).

A. C6

B. RBL-2H3

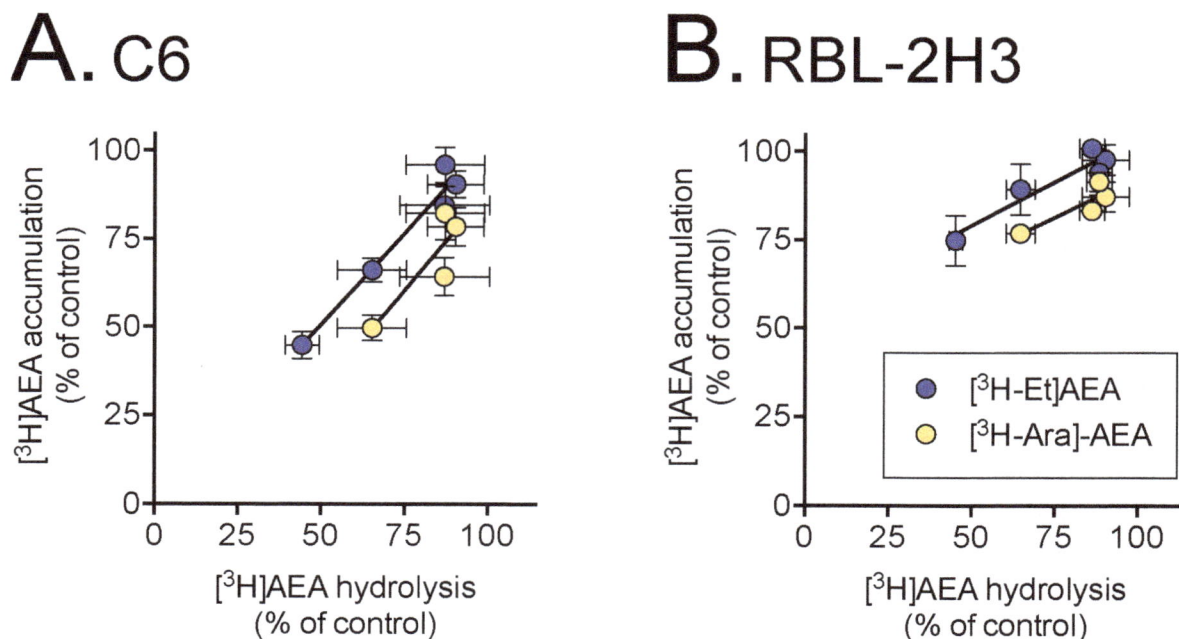

Figure 4. Effect of compound 33 upon AEA uptake using either [³H-ethanolamine]- or [³H-arachidonoyl]- labelled ligand and hydrolysis of [³H-ethanolamine]-AEA by cell lysates. The same conditions as in figure 2 were used. Shown are means ± s.e.m., n = 3–4. The data for [³H-arachidonoyl]- labelled AEA uptake is the same as for Fig. 2, but in this case the x-axes are for cell lysates rather than intact cells. The values (± s.e.m.) of the slopes determined from the regression lines of the pooled data for [³H-ethanolamine]- or [³H-arachidonoyl]- labelled AEA, respectively, were: C6 cells,, 1.03±0.10 and 1.11±0.31; RBL-2H3 cells, 0.49±0.14 and 0.46±0.14. The concentration of EtOH for the vehicle was 0.2% (cells) and 1% (lysates).

Expression of FABP5 by AT1, RBL-2H3, C6 and P19 cells

FABP5 is an important intracellular carrier of AEA [4], raising the possibility that the differential effects seen between C6 and RBL-2H3 cells in Figs. 3 and 4 may reflect differences in expression levels of this protein. In consequence, we investigated the mRNA expression levels and function of FABP5 in the cells, the latter using the FABP5 inhibitor SB-FI-26 [27]. The PCR analysis displayed the presence of a band correlating well with the expected fragment size of 192 bp for rat FABP5 mRNA (rat brain, AT1, C6, RBL-2H3) and 179 bp for mouse FABP5 mRNA (P19 cells). Further, the expression levels were very similar for the different cells (Fig. 5A). The effects of 5, 15 and 50 μM SB-FI-26 upon the uptake of AEA by the cells, and upon the retention of AEA by the wells alone, are shown in Figs. 5B–F (note that the scales on the y-axes are very different for the cells and for the wells). In all cases 50 μM SB-FI-26 reduced the observed uptake, but it even affected the rate of AEA retention by the wells, which complicates interpretation of the data. In the RBL2H3 cells (and wells), the combination of 50 μM SB-FI-26 and 1 μM URB597 produced a greater reduction in uptake than seen with URB597 alone, whereas in the other cells no significant differences were seen at the P<0.05 level.

The effect of 50 μM SB-FI-26 upon the adsorption to the wells is small in absolute terms, and can be further minimised by following the change in uptake/adsorbtion over time. These data are shown with C6 and RBL-2H3 cells and in wells in Fig. 6. Assuming linearity over the 1–7 min incubation times, the rates of uptake (in fmol/min per well) in the absence and presence of 50 μM SB-FI-26, respectively, calculated from the individual experiments were, C6 cells, 382±70 and 260±95; RBL-2H3, 416±58 and 352±54; wells, 23±6 and 15±4. A two-way repeated measures ANOVA of the data for the C6 and RBL-

2H3 cells matching for SB-FI-26 indicated a significant effect of the compound ($F_{1,8}=22$, P<0.005), but not for cell ($F_{1,8}=2.22$, P=0.17) or the interaction term cell×SB-FI-26 ($F_{1,8}=0.57$, P=0.47). Thus, these data do not support the hypothesis that differences in FABP-5 expression or function lie behind the different sensitivities of AEA uptake by C6 and RBL-2H3 cells to reversible inhibition of FAAH.

Discussion

Although the metabolic pathways for AEA are well characterized, the mechanisms responsible for the cellular uptake of AEA still remain to be completely explained (review, see [3]). One point of contention is the degree to which FAAH regulates the uptake of AEA. In the present study, we have investigated this in some detail using cells with different expression levels of the enzyme. Two approaches were taken: in the first, time courses of the reduction of the rate of uptake following irreversible FAAH inhibition were investigated. For all three cell lines, 1 μM URB597 (which completely inhibits hydrolysis in the C6 cells) produced a 70% reduction in the rates of uptake between 1 and 7 min incubations. It is notable that for the C6 cells, a significant effect of URB597 is seen even at the 1 minute incubation time. This would suggest that sufficient AEA has reached FAAH for it to be metabolised by 1 min of incubation; thereby at this time point, the enzyme contributes to the intra- :-extracellular concentration gradient. This is reinforced by our finding that the FABP-5 inhibitor SB-FI-26 also produces a significant reduction in uptake at the 1 min time point, assuming, of course, that FABP5 plays a part in the shuttling of AEA to FAAH in this cell line. More conclusively, it has been shown that in RBL-2H3 and U937 human monocytic leukaemia cells, AEA hydrolysis can be demonstrated at very short

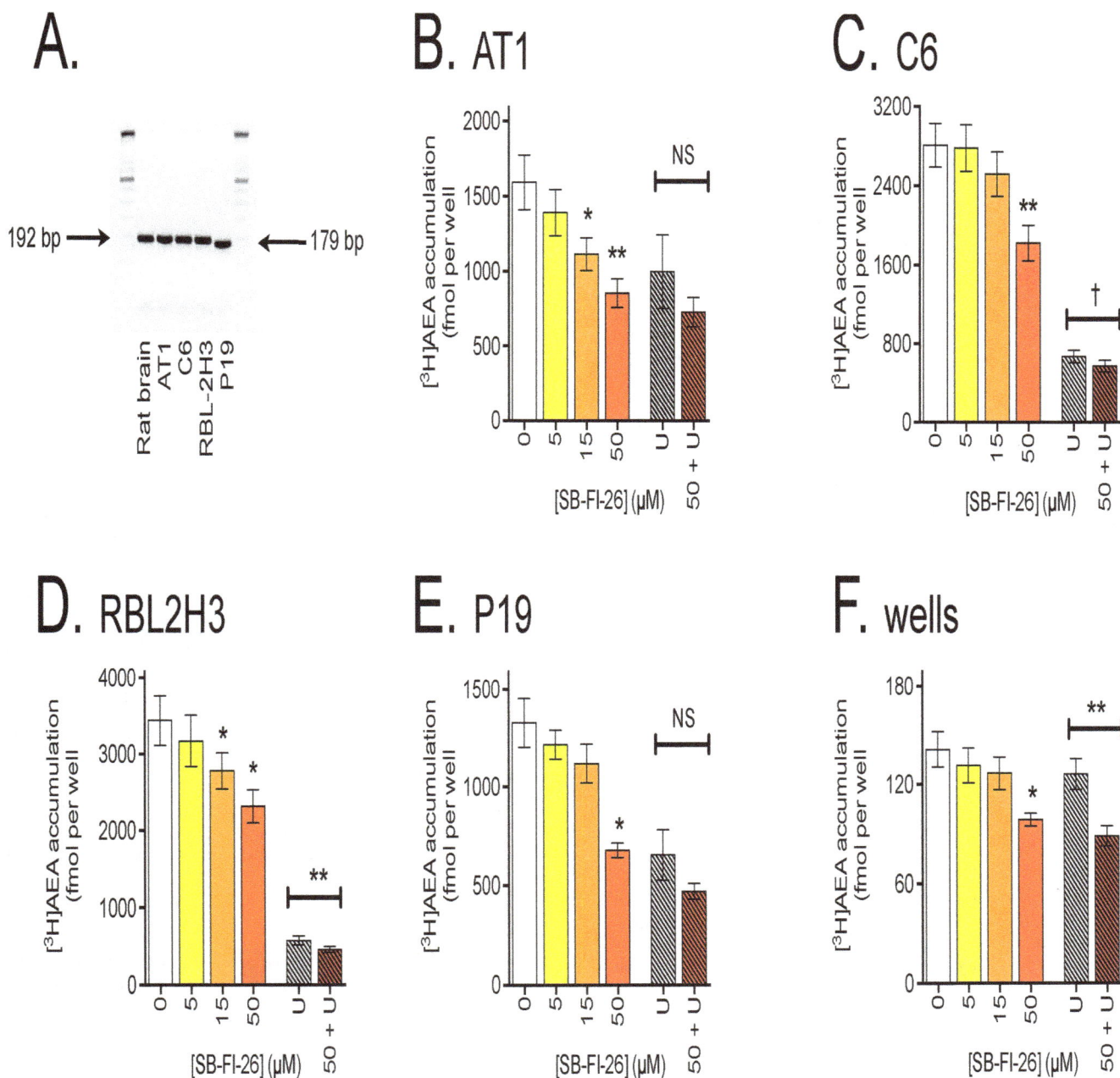

Figure 5. FABP5 expression and function in the cells. In Panel A, semi-quantitative PCR analysis of the mRNA expression of FABP5 is shown for the cells, with a rat brain lysate as positive control. Molecular size markers are also shown. Panels B-E show the effect of SB-FI-26 and 1 µM URB597 ("U") upon the accumulation of [³H]AEA in AT1, C6, RBL2H3, P19 cells and upon the retention of label by wells alone. Note that the scales on the y-axis are different, particularly for the wells, where the rate of accumulation is very low. *$P<0.05$, **$P<0.01$ either Dunnett's multiple comparisons test vs. vehicle control following significant one way repeated measures ANOVA not assuming sphericity (for SB-FI-26 concentration-response data) or paired t-test between 50 µM SB-FI-26+1 µM URB597 vs. URB597 alone (NS, not significant; †, P = 0.054). All values are means ± s.e.m., n = 5. Note that the vehicle control and 1 µM URB597 data are the same as shown in Fig. 1C.

incubation times (25–30 sec) [12,19], and so this explanation seems feasible.

A more surprising finding, however, was the difference in the sensitives of uptake to modest levels of reversible inhibition. The basic finding, that there was a relationship between % inhibition of AEA hydrolysis and uptake is consistent with the study of Kaczocha et al. [19]. These authors compared the % uptake and % hydrolysis using both FAAH inhibitors (three concentra-

tions of CAY10400, two concentrations of URB597) and two concentrations each of uptake inhibitors (OMDM2, AM1172, VDM11 and UCM707), and found a linear relationship for the complete dataset [19]. However, in our study, RBL-2H3 cells were less sensitive than both the C6 cells (which had broadly similar FAAH expression) and the AT1 cells (which have a much lower FAAH expression) to a given level of FAAH inhibition by compound 33. Such a difference indicates that the reported

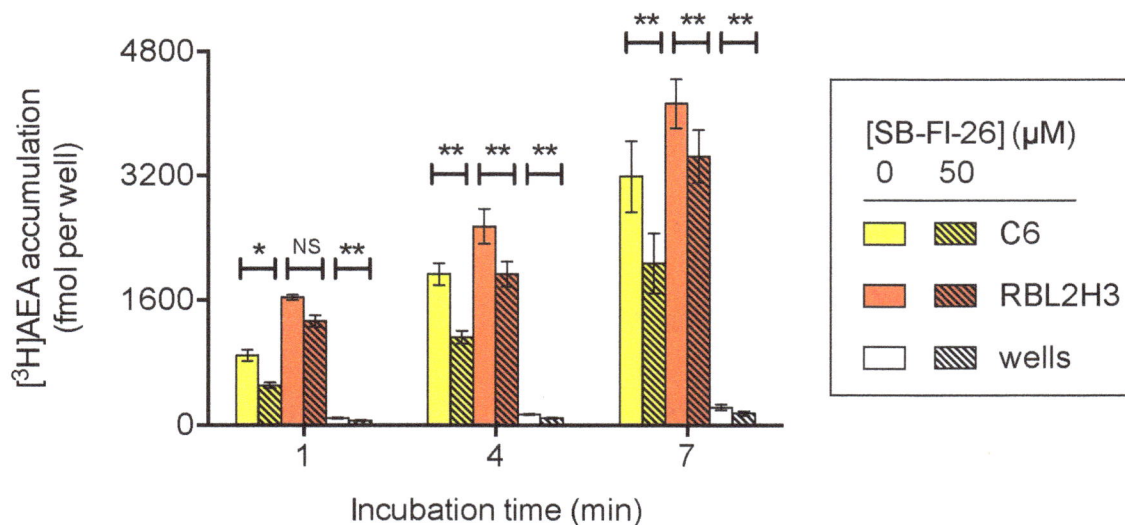

Figure 6. Inhibition of AEA uptake in C6 and RBL-2H3 cells by SB-FI-26 at different incubation times. Shown are means and s.e.m., $n = 5$, for the uptakes measured at each time point. Two-way ANOVA matching for both time and SB-FI-26 were undertaken separately for each cell line and for the wells. **$P < 0.01$, *$P < 0.05$, Šídák's multiple comparison test. Note that for the RBL-2H3 cells, the interaction term time×SB-FI-26 did not reach significance, and so the difference in significance at the different time points should not be over-interpreted. For both cell lines and for the wells, the ANOVA values were significant ($P < 0.005$) for the main effects of time and of SB-FI-26 treatment.

variation in FAAH sensitivities of AEA uptake seen by different authors (see Introduction) need not be ascribed to methodological differences, but instead can reflect the properties of the cells themselves. Given than the maximal inhibition of the rate of uptake seen with 1 μM URB597 between 1 and 7 min is the same in percentage terms for all four cells, the data would suggest that in RBL-2H3 cells, the effect of inhibition of FAAH upon uptake "catches up" following the lag in sensitivity between 0 and 50% inhibition. The difference in sensitivities between the cell lines, in particular between RBL-2H3 and C6 cells, is unlikely to be due to differences in FABP5 involvement, given the similar inhibition profiles with SB-FI-26 in the cells, but this of course does not rule out cell-dependent differences in the involvement of other AEA shuttling pathways. The mechanism(s) by which intracellular AEA is transported to its catabolic and/or sequestration sites is not fully understood, although several molecular targets (in addition to FABP-5) and sequestration sites have been reported, and may be amenable to pharmacological attack [5,28,29]. As argued by

Hillard and Jarrahian [30] cells may accumulate AEA for different reasons depending upon whether this lipid is required for signalling purposes or as a source of arachidonic acid. Although variations in the intracellular fate of AEA presumably explain the subtle differences seen in the present study.

Acknowledgments

The authors are grateful to Drs. Dale Deutsch and Iwao Ojima for their kind gift of SB-FI-26, and Dr. Jenny Häggström for her valuable help and advice concerning the statistical analysis of the data with compound 33.

Author Contributions

Conceived and designed the experiments: EB CJF. Performed the experiments: EB AB JH EP. Analyzed the data: EB AB JH EP CJF. Wrote the paper: EB CJF.

References

1. Muccioli GG (2010) Endocannabinoid biosynthesis and inactivation, from simple to complex. Drug Discov Today 15: 474–483.
2. Deutsch DG, Chin SA (1993) Enzymatic synthesis and degradation of anandamide, a cannabinoid receptor agonist. Biochem Pharmacol 46: 791–796.
3. Fowler CJ (2013) Transport of endocannabinoids across the plasma membrane and within the cell. FEBS J 280: 1895–1904.
4. Kaczocha M, Glaser S, Deutsch D (2009) Identification of intracellular carriers for the endocannabinoid anandamide. Proc Natl Acad Sci USA 106: 6375–6380.
5. Oddi S, Fezza F, Pasquariello N, D'Agostino A, Catanzaro G, et al. (2009) Molecular identification of albumin and Hsp70 as cytosolic anandamide-binding proteins. Chem Biol 16: 624–632.
6. Fu J, Bottegoni G, Sasso O, Bertorelli R, Rocchia W, et al. (2011) A catalytically silent FAAH-1 variant drives anandamide transport in neurons. Nat Neurosci 15: 64–69.
7. Leung K, Elmes MW, Glaser ST, Deutsch DG, Kaczocha M (2013) Role of FAAH-like anandamide transporter in anandamide inactivation. PLoS One 8: e79355.
8. Day T, Rakhshan F, Deutsch D, Barker E (2001) Role of fatty acid amide hydrolase in the transport of the endogenous canabinoid anandamide. Mol Pharmacol 59: 1369–1375.

9. Deutsch D, Glaser S, Howell J, Kunz J, Puffenbarger R, et al. (2001) The cellular uptake of anandamide is coupled to its breakdown by fatty-acid amide hydrolase. J Biol Chem 276: 6967–6973.
10. Kathuria S, Gaetani S, Fegley D, Valiño F, Duranti A, et al. (2003) Modulation of anxiety through blockade of anandamide hydrolysis. Nat Med 9: 76–81.
11. Thors L, Eriksson J, Fowler CJ (2007) Inhibition of the cellular uptake of anandamide by genistein and its analogue daidzein in cells with different levels of fatty acid amide hydrolase-driven uptake. Br J Pharmacol 152: 744–750.
12. Chicca A, Marazzi J, Nicolussi S, Gertsch J (2012) Evidence for bidirectional endocannabinoid transport across cell membranes. J Biol Chem 287: 34660–34682.
13. Kaczocha M, Lin Q, Nelson LD, McKinney MK, Cravatt BF, et al. (2012) Anandamide externally added to lipid vesicles containing-trapped fatty acid amide hydrolase (FAAH) is readily hydrolyzed in a sterol-modulated fashion. ACS Chem Neurosci 3: 364–368.
14. Di Pasquale E, Chahinian H, Sanchez P, Fantini J (2009) The insertion and transport of anandamide in synthetic lipid membranes are both cholesterol-dependent. PLoS ONE 4: e4989.
15. Beltramo M, Stella N, Calignano A, Lin SY, Makriyannis A, et al. (1997) Functional role of high-affinity anandamide transport, as revealed by selective inhibition. Science 277: 1094–1097.

16. Fegley D, Kathuria S, Mercier R, Li C-M, Goutopoulos A, et al. (2004) Anandamide transport is independent of fatty-acid amide hydrolase activity and is blocked by the hydrolysis-resistant inhibitor AM1172. Proc Natl Acad Sci USA 101: 8756–8761.

17. Ligresti A, Morera E, van der Stelt M, Monory K, Lutz B, et al. (2004) Further evidence for the existence of a specific process for the membrane transport of anandamide. Biochem J 380: 265–272.

18. Ortega-Gutiérrez S, Hawkins E, Viso A, López-Rodríguez M, Cravatt B (2004) Comparison of anandamide transport in FAAH wild-type and knockout neurons: evidence for contributions by both FAAH and the CB1 receptor to anandamide uptake. Biochemistry 43: 8184–8190.

19. Kaczocha M, Hermann A, Glaser S, Bojesen I, Deutsch D (2006) Anandamide uptake is consistent with rate-limited diffusion and is regulated by the degree of its hydrolysis by fatty acid amide hydrolase. J Biol Chem 281: 9066–9075.

20. Onnis V, Congiu C, Björklund E, Hempel F, Söderström E, et al. (2010) Synthesis and evaluation of paracetamol esters as novel fatty acid amide hydrolase inhibitors. J Med Chem 53: 2286–2298.

21. Isaacs J, Isaacs W, Feitz F, Scheres J (1986) Establishment and characterization of seven Dunning rat prostatic cancer cell lines and their use in developing methods for predicting metastatic abilities of prostatic cancers. Prostate 9: 261–281.

22. Rakhshan F, Day T, Blakeley R, Barker E (2000) Carrier-mediated uptake of the endogenous cannabinoid anandamide in RBL-2H3 cells. J Pharmacol Exp Ther 292: 960–967.

23. Sandberg A, Fowler CJ (2005) Measurement of saturable and non-saturable components of anandamide uptake into P19 embryonic carcinoma cells in the presence of fatty acid-free bovine serum albumin. Chem Phys Lipids 134: 131–139.

24. Boldrup L, Wilson SJ, Barbier AJ, Fowler CJ (2004) A simple stopped assay for fatty acid amide hydrolase avoiding the use of a chloroform extraction phase. J Biochem Biophys Methods 60: 171–177.

25. Björklund E, Larsson TNL, Jacobsson SOP, Fowler CJ (2014) Ketoconazole inhibits the cellular uptake of anandamide via inhibition of FAAH at pharmacologically relevant concentrations. PLoS ONE 9: e87542.

26. R Core Team (2012). R: A language and environment for statistical computing. R Foundation for Statistical Computing, Vienna, Austria. ISBN 3-900051-07-0, Available: http://www.R-project.org/.

27. Berger WT, Ralph BP, Kaczocha M, Sun J, Balius TE, et al. (2012) Targeting fatty acid binding protein (FABP) anandamide transporters-a novel strategy for development of anti-inflammatory and anti-nociceptive drugs. PLoS One 7: e50968.

28. Oddi S, Fezza F, Pasquariello N, De Simone C, Rapino C, et al. (2008) Evidence for the intracellular accumulation of anandamide in adiposomes. Cell Mol Life Sci 65: 840–850.

29. Kaczocha M, Glaser ST, Chae J, Brown DA, Deutsch DG (2010) Lipid droplets are novel sites of N-acylethanolamine inactivation by fatty acid amide hydrolase-2. J Biol Chem 285: 2796–2806.

30. Hillard C, Jarrahian A (2005) Accumulation of anandamide: evidence for cellular diversity. Neuropharmacology 48: 1072–1078.

8

Decitabine of Reduced Dosage in Chinese Patients with Myelodysplastic Syndrome

Xiao Li[1]*[9], Qiang Song[2][9], Yu Chen[3][9], Chunkang Chang[1], Dong Wu[1], Lingyun Wu[1], Jiying Su[1], Xi Zhang[1], Liyu Zhou[1], Luxi Song[1], Zheng Zhang[1], Feng Xu[1], Ming Hou[2]

1 Department of Hematology, the Sixth People's Hospital affiliated with Shanghai Jiaotong University, Shanghai, China, 2 Department of Hematology, Qilu Hospital affiliated with Shandong University, Jinan, China, 3 Department of Hematology, Ruijin Hospital affiliated with Shanghai Jiaotong University School of Medicine, Shanghai, China

Abstract

Decitabine has been approved for the treatment of all subtypes of myelodysplastic syndrome (MDS). However, the optimal regimen for decitabine treatment is not well established. In this study, an observational, retrospective and multi-center analysis was performed to explore the decitabine schedule for the treatment of MDS. A total of 79 patients received reduced dosage decitabine treatment (15 mg/M^2/day intravenously for five consecutive days every four weeks). Fifty-three out of the 79 patients were defined as intermediate-2/high risk by international prognostic scoring system (IPSS) risk category. 67.1% of MDS patients achieved treatment response including complete response (CR) (n = 23), Partial response (n = 1), marrow CR (mCR) with hematological improvement (HI) (n = 11), mCR without HI (n = 11) and HI alone (n = 7) with a median of 4 courses (range 1–11). The median overall survival (OS) was 18.0 months. The median OS was 22.0, 17.0 and 12.0 months in the patients with CR, those with other response, and those without response, respectively. In addition, this regimen contributed to zero therapy-related death and punctual course delivery, although III or IV grade of cytopenia was frequently observed. In conclusion, the 15 mg/M^2/d×5 day decitabine regimen was effective and safe for Chinese MDS patients with IPSS score of 0.5 or higher.

Editor: Ken Mills, Queen's University Belfast, United Kingdom

Funding: This work was supported by the National High Technology Research and Development Program of China ("863" program, # 2012AA02A505). The funders had no role in study design, data collection and analysis, decision to publish, or preparation of the manuscript.

Competing Interests: The authors have declared that no competing interests exist.

* E-mail: lixiao3326@163.com

9 These authors contributed equally to this work.

Introduction

Myelodysplastic syndrome (MDS) is widely recognized as a clonal hematopoietic stem cell disorder. The hypermethylation of tumor suppressor genes (TSGs) is frequently observed in MDS, which may play a key role in the pathogenesis of MDS [1,2]. Decitabine has been approved for the treatment of MDS of all FAB subtypes and different International Prognostic Scoring System (IPSS) risk groups [3]. The use of decitabine is often limited by its severe toxicity represented by myelosuppression even at relatively low doses [4–6].

Reported number of MDS patients receiving decitabine treatment is still limited at less than 600 cases [7–14]. As a result, ideal regimen is not known [15]. A low-dose 5-day decitabine regimen (20 mg/M^2/d for 5 days every four weeks) is widely used in many oncology centers worldwide and seems to have better efficacy and safety profile in comparison to a high dose 3-day protocol (for a total of 135 mg/M^2 per course) [7,8]. However, treatment-related death is still estimated to occur in 6% of the patients receiving this extended regimen at low dose if the dose and schedule is not adjusted properly [10]. To minimize the risk of myelosuppression and death, treatment must often be postponed at the cost of efficacy [9,11].

In a dosage-exploration trial of small scale [5], reduced decitabine at 15 mg/M^2/d for 10 days (150 mg/M^2 per course) achieved very promising response. Due to severe hematological adverse events, however, the trial was terminated. In a mechanistic study by Yang et al. [6] in patients with hematologic malignancies, decitabine at 15 mg/M^2/d produced comparable degree of hypomethylation of the Alu and LINE1 elements in comparison to 20 mg/M^2/d. This study also showed that low doses at 15 and 20 mg/M^2/d have more efficacious hypomethylation action than at a daily dose of 100 mg/M^2, which seemed to mainly drive a cytotoxic effect. Put together, these findings seem to advocate a daily dose of 15 mg/M^2 but for less duration (than 10 days in a course).

In the current study, we carried out a preliminary assessment of a decitabine regimen at 15 mg/M^2/d for 5 days per course in Chinese MDS patients with IPSS score of 0.5 or higher.

Methods

Patients

This multi-center, retrospective study was approved by the institutional Review Board of all participating centers. All subjects signed written informed consent. Disease subtype was classified based on the French-American-British (FAB) classification [16].

Table 1. Clinical characteristic of MDS patients.

	Values
Regimen	15 mg/M²/d ×5
Tested patients, n	79
Median age, y	60 (28–82)
M:F ratio, n	49:30
De novo MDS, n (%)	74 (93.7)
RAEB plus RAEB-t, n (%)	59 (74.7)
CMML, n (%)	7 (8.9)
IPSS int-1 risk, n (%)	26 (32.9)
IPSS int-2/high risk, n (%)	53 (67.1)
Abnormal chromosome, n (%) according to IPSS	44 (55.7)
Good, n (%)	40 (50.6)
Intermediate, n (%)	19 (24.1)
Poor, n (%)	20 (25.3)
p15^{INK4B} positive, n (%)	40/59 (67.8)

Abbreviations: RAEB, refractory anemia with excess blasts; RAEB-t, refractory anemia with excess blasts in transformation; CMML, chronic myelomonocytic leukemia; IPSS, International Prognostic Scoring System.

The IPSS [17] score was 0.5 or higher. Patients having an Eastern Cooperative Oncology Group performance score of >2, receiving previous hypomethylation therapy, or co-morbid with severe heart-lung diseases were excluded from data analysis.

Ethics Statement

All subjects provided written informed consent between September 2009 and June 2013 from three Chinese hematological institutes. The written informed consent was obtained from patient themselves (blank copy of informed consent in Table S1). The study was approved by the ethics committee of the Sixth People's Hospital affiliated with Shanghai Jiaotong University, Qilu Hospital affiliated with Shandong University and Ruijin Hospital affiliated with Shanghai Jiaotong University School of Medicine.

All patient-relevant research strictly abided by the Declaration of Helsinki.

Treatment

Decitabine was infused intravenously over a one-hour period at a daily dose of 15 mg/M² for five consecutive days every four weeks. Neither dose reduction nor escalation was allowed, but the treatment course was delayed upon grade 4 hematologic toxicities or life-threatening myelosuppression (e.g., bleeding or proven infection). The patients accepted decitabine treatment for at least four courses unless the disease progressed, or the patients experienced intolerable myelosuppression. Prophylactic antimicrobials, hematopoietic growth factors, and other supportive cares were available at the discretion of the physician.

Table 2. Response data (79 patients) by the 2006 IWG Criteria.

Response by IWG 2006 criteria	Patients number (%)
ORR	53 (67.1)
CR	23 (29.1)
PR	1 (1.3)
mCR without HI	11 (13.9)
mCR with HI	11 (13.9)
HI only	7 (8.9)
SD	5 (6.3)
PD	21 (26.6)
Cytogenetic response* n (%)	
CR	17/37 (45.9)
PR	4/37 (10.8)
NR	16/37 (43.2)

*the percentage means the ratio of responder in 37 patients with abnormal karyotypes.
Abbreviations: IWG, International Working Group; ORR, overall response rate; CR, complete response; mCR, marrow CR; PR, partial response; HI, hematologic improvement; SD, stable disease; PD, progressive disease.

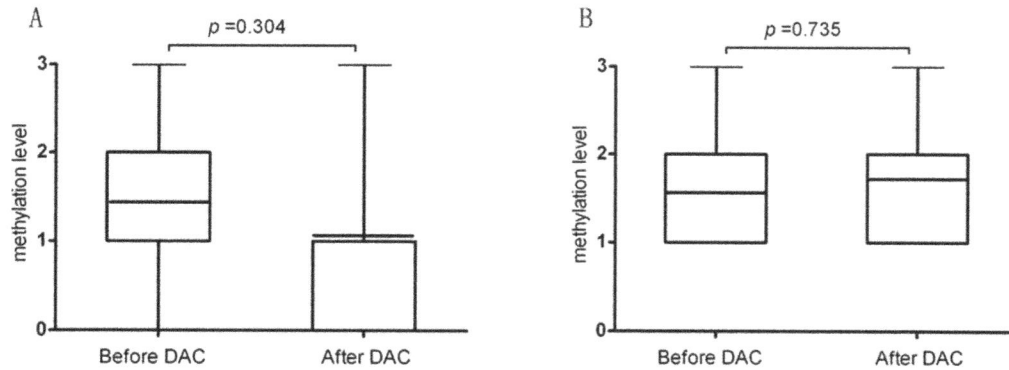

Figure 1. Comparison of P15^Ink4b methylation before and after decitabine regimens. p15 methylation level decreased after decitabine treatment in responders (n = 41) (A); p15 methylation level elevated slightly after decitabine treatment in nonresponders (n = 18) (B).

Response and Hematological Toxicity Evaluation

A routine blood examination was performed twice every week. Bone marrow (BM) was examined with routine aspirate smear and G-banding analysis every 1–2 treatment courses to evaluate responses. The primary endpoint was overall response rate (ORR) using the IWG 2006 criteria [18], and included complete response (CR), partial response (PR), marrow CR (mCR), hematological improvement (HI) and cytogenetic response (including cytogenetic CR (cCR) defined as no detectable cytogenetic abnormality and cPR defined as at least 50% reduction in abnormal metaphases). The secondary endpoints included overall survival (OS), and the rate of acute myeloid leukemia (AML)-free survival at one year from the beginning of treatment [9–11].

Hematological side-effects were assessed using Common Toxicity Criteria version 3.0 [19], including cytopenia, proven infections. Death within 30 days from the beginning of treatment was also calculated.

The p15^INK4B Methylation Status

The methylation status of p15^INK4B was examined in BM mononuclear cells with a methylation-specific PCR (MSP) method, as previously described [20].

Statistical Analysis

The χ^2 test were used to compare categorical variables. Time-to-event was presented using the Kaplan-Meier method and analyzed with a log rank test. All statistical analyses were carried out using the SPSS 16.0 statistical software.

Results

Patient Demographics

A total of seventy-nine patients were treated by decitabine between September 2009 and June 2013 by three Chinese hematological institutes. The median age was 60 years old (range 28–82 years), and the male-to-female ratio was 49:30. The characteristics of these patients were detailed in Table 1. Based on the IPSS risk category, 53 patients had higher-risk MDS (Int-2 and high risk) and the other 26 had lower-risk (Int-1 risk), respectively. Forty-four patients (55.7%) had abnormal karyotypes prior to decitabine treatment, with twenty (25.3%) patients having poor-risk karyotypes based on the IPSS risk category. The median number of decitabine courses was 4 (range 1–11).

Treatment Response

Fifty-three out of the 79 patients (67.1%) responded to the treatment (Table 2): CR in 23 cases (29.1%), PR in one case (1.3%), mCR without HI in 11 cases (13.9%), mCR with HI in 11 cases (13.9%), and HI alone in 7 cases (8.9%). Cytogenetic response was evaluable in 37 patients, and included 17 (45.9%) CR, 4 (10.8%) PR and 16 (43.2%) NR.

Table 3. Hematological adverse effects*.

	Number of patients (%)
Neu III*	13 (16.5)
Neu IV*	43 (54.4)
Neu = 0	6 (7.6)
PLT III	7 (8.9)
PLT VI	46 (58.2)
PLT ≤10×109/L	19 (24.1)
Proven infection	18 (22.8)
Death within 30 days^#	0

*The grading was based on the Common Toxicity Criteria for Adverse Events version 3.0.
^#within 30 days of the start of the initial course of decitabine.

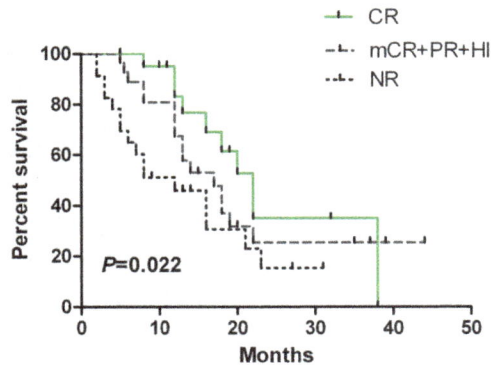

Figure 2. Overall survival according to treatment response type. The overall survival (OS) of the patients who reached CR; or achieved the other response (PR or mCR with/without HI); or got no any response after decitabine treatment; had different OS (22.0 vs. 17.0 vs. 12.0 months, respectively, $P = 0.022$). The patients with CR had longer survival than those without treatment response (22.0 vs. 12.0 months, $P = 0.001$).

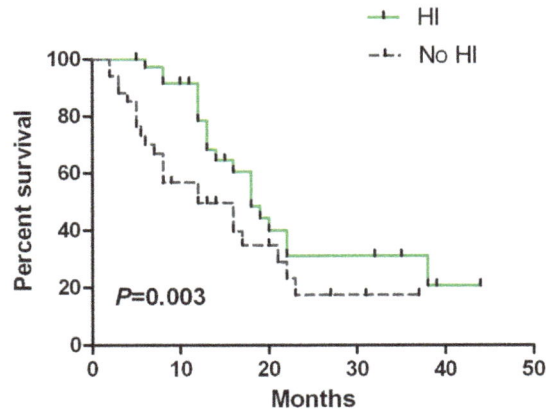

Figure 3. Overall survival according to different patients who achieved HI or did not achieved HI. Patients with HI (CR, PR, mCR with HI or Hi alone) also showed longer OS (18.0 months) than those without HI (mCR alone, failure or PD). (12 months, $P = 0.003$).

Relationship between Treatment Response and p15 Methylation Level

The results (detected by semi-quantitative MSP-PCR) are illustrated from low to high, according to the levels of DNA methylation (M) or unmethylation (U), and were classified as negative (no visible M band, represented by grade 0), weakly positive (M weaker than U, represented by grade 1), positive (M equal to U, represented by grade 2), or strongly positive (M stronger than U, represented by grade 3). Neither ORR nor CR differed between the patients with p15^{INK4B} methylation (ORR 61.7% and CR 23.4%;) vs. without.(ORR 65.6% and CR 28.1%;). Although the P15 methylation level declined for those responders after decitabine treatment, the change did not appear statistically significant. (see Figure 1).

Hematological Toxicity

Major side-effects included cytopenia and cytopenia-related infection (Table 3). Grade III or IV neutropenia (70.9%), and thrombocytopenia (67.1%) were frequently observed. The zero of neutrophil count and thrombocytopenia less than 10×10^9/L occurred in 7.6% and 24.1% of patients, respectively. Non-hematological toxicities were infrequent and reversible. None of the patients died within 30 days of the initiation of decitabine treatment. In addition, although 32 of 79 (40.5%) patients had 58 courses delayed due to grade 4 hematologic toxicities or life-threatening myelosuppression in this study. 63% of the decitabine courses (156/214 courses not including the first 79 courses for the 79 patients) were delivered on schedule, with a median interval between the courses at 28 days (range 28–61 days).

Survival Data

Median OS was 18.0 months (95% CI, 14.7–21.3 months). The rate of OS and AML-free survival at one year was 63.3% and 60.8%, respectively. The median OS was 22.0, 17.0 and 12.0 months in the patients with CR, in those with other types of response (PR or mCR with/without HI), and in those without response to decitabine, respectively ($P = 0.022$). Obvious significance could be observed between the patients with CR and those with NR ($P = 0.001$) (Figure 2). The OS was also longer in the patients with HI (CR, PR, mCR with HI or HI alone) than in

those without HI (mCR alone, failure or PD) (18.0 vs. 12.0 months, $P = 0.003$) (Figure 3).

Comparison of Current Study with Previous Reports

We compared our results with three previously reported data using 5-day regimen (20 mg/M^2/d or 100 mg/M^2/course, Table 4) [9–11]. Our results were similar to the MD. Anderson study [9] on ORR (67.1% vs. 71.0) and CR (29.1% vs. 33.7%). The OS from current study was comparable with data from the other three studies. And our results showed punctual median course interval of 28 days without therapy-related death.

Discussion

The hypermethylation of tumor suppressor genes (TSGs) plays a key role in the pathogenesis of MDS [1,2]. Decitabine reduces DNA methylation, which in turn promotes re-expression of TSGs, and by doing so, inhibits tumor growth [4–6]. Despite of the apparent efficacy, the three-day protocol (135 mg/M^2/course every 6 week) of decitabine lead to high therapy-related death [7,8]. Dose reduction (five-day regimen at 100 mg/M^2/course every four week) reduces therapy-related death to approximately 6%, a level still not satisfying [10]. To minimize life-threatening toxicity, scheduled course often needs to be delayed [9,11]. A pilot dose-finding study indicated that 15 mg/M^2/d is optimal. Similar degree of demethylation was achieved at 15 mg/M^2/d in comparison to 20 mg/M^2/d on Alu and LINE1 elements [4,5]. All together, these information suggested feasibility of the five-day regimen of 15/M^2/d decitabine (75 mg/M^2/course every four weeks).

In this study, fifty-three (67.1%) of the 79 patients achieved treatment response, including 23 patients (29.1%) with CR and 21 patients (21/37, 56.8%) with cytogenetic response. The median OS for the patients receiving decitabine treatment reached 18 months, whereas the median OS in MDS patients receiving the best care in previous report was only 8.5 months [8]. These data suggested that the modified decitabine regimen (15 mg/M^2/d for 5 days) is effective in MDS patients with an IPSS score at 0.5 or higher. Besides, 63% of course delivery could be punctually performed under this regimen (the median course interval was 28 days) without therapy-related death, although III or IV grade of cytopenia was frequently found in over 50% of patients. Our results suggested that this regimen was not only effective, but also

Table 4. Comparison of current study with previous reports.

	Current study	ID-03-0180 MD.Anderson	Daco-020 ADOPT	DIVA study
No. patients	79	95	99	101
Median age, years	60 (28–82)	65 (NM*)	72 (34–87)	65 (23–80)
Eligibility	FAB MDS (IPSS ≥0.5)	FAB MDS (IPSS ≥0.5)	FAB MDS (IPSS ≥0.5)	WHO (IPSS ≥0.5)+CMML
De novo MDS (%)	94	68	89	89
IPSS ≤1.0	32.9%	34.0%	54.0%	52.0%
≥1.5	67.1%	66.0%	46.0%	48.0%
Decitabine regimen	15 mg/M^2/d×5 d	100 mg/M^2/course (3 schedules)	20 mg/M^2/d×5 d	20 mg/M^2/d×5 d
courses, median (range)	4 (1–11)	>7 (1–18)	5 (1–17)	5 (1–18)
Treatment response				
CR	29.1%	33.7%	17.0%	12.9%
PR	1.3%	1.0%	0	1.0%
mCR	27.8%	25.0%	15.0	22.8%
HI	8.9%	13.0%	18.0%	18.8%
ORR	67.1%	71.0%	51.0%	55.4%
Overall survival				
Median	18.0 months	19.0 months	19.4 months	17.7 months
1-year probability	63.3%	56.0%	66.0%	78.6%
1-year % for AML-free survival	60.8%	51.%∞	NM	77.9%
Median Course interval	28 day	35–40 days	28 days	34 days
Death in 30 days (n)	0	0	11#	NM*

11# refer to reference 10. just 6/11 patients death was considered being related to decitabine treatment. NM* means not mentioned; ∞this datum was from a observation at the point of 18 months.

relatively safe. At the same time, it was similar with previous report, that the methylation of p15^{INK4B} in this assay did not predict the decitabine response [4].

A comparison of the current 5-day regimen (75 mg/M^2/course) with previous studies [9–11] showed similar ORR and CR as reported by Kantajian *et al.* [9], and slightly better than that in the Steensma *et al.* [10] and *Lee et al.* [11] studies. A recent study on decitabine treatment containing 66.7% of MDS patients with IPSS Int-1 risk reported only 22.4% ORR and 10.5% CR [21]. ORR and CR in the ADOPT and DIVA trials were relatively low because over 50% of patients in the studies had IPSS low or Int-1 risk.

None of the 79 patients died of decitabine treatment in our study. Also, 63% of the decitabine courses were delivered on schedule (median course interval at 28 days). The data from ADOPT trial [10] and Korea [11], reported a delay of scheduled decitabine treatment (median course interval at 35–40 and 34 days due to severe cytopenia, respectively). The ADOPT trial reported 11 deaths during the initial 30 days of decitabine treatment, with six out of the 11 deaths attributable to decitabine treatment. In

other word, delay in schedule treatment and therapy-related death in the 20 mg/M^2/d regimen may influence the therapeutic effect of decitabine. In comparison to the standard regimen of 20 mg/ M^2/d, a regimen with reduced dosage (15 mg/M^2/d) could achieve similar clinical response but minimize course delay and none-therapy-related death. Although some prognostic factor analysis [22] did not refer to this probably important factor,we considered that the increased adherence to scheduled treatment may contribute to satisfying effects despite of reduced dosage.

Primarily, the reduced decitabine regimen (15 mg/M^2/d for five consecutive day every four weeks) appeared effective and relatively safe in Chinese patients with MDS. But, because of the limitation of an observational and retrospective analysis, some big prospective and double-blind clinical trials are necessary to validate our result.

Author Contributions

Conceived and designed the experiments: XL QS YC. Performed the experiments: CC DW LW JS XZ LZ LS ZZ FX MH. Analyzed the data: XL FX LW. Contributed reagents/materials/analysis tools: XL QS YC MH. Wrote the paper: XL QS YC.

References

1. Baylin SB, Herman JG, Graff JR, Vertino PM, Issa JP (1998) Alterations in DNA methylation: a fundamental aspect of neoplasia. Adv Cancer Res 72: 141–196.
2. Herman JG (1999) Hypermethylation of tumor suppressor genes in cancer. Semin Cancer Biol 9: 359–367.
3. Saba HI. (2007) Decitabine in the treatment of myelodysplastic syndromes. Ther Clin Risk Manag 3: 807–817.

4. Mund C, Hackanson B, Stresemann C, Lübbert M, Lyko F (2005) Characterization of DNA demethylation effects induced by 5-Aza-2'- deoxycytidine in patients with myelodysplastic syndrome. Cancer Res 65: 7086–7090.
5. Issa JP, Garcia-Manero G, Giles FJ, Mannari R, Thomas D, et al. (2004) Phase 1 study of low-dose prolonged exposure schedules of the hypomethylating agent 5-aza-2-deoxycytidine (decitabine) in hematopoietic malignancies. Blood 103: 1635–1640.

6. Yang AS, Doshi KD, Choi SW, Mason JB, Mannari RK, et al. (2006) DNA methylation changes after 5-Aza-2'-Deoxycytidine therapy in patients with leukemia. Cancer Res 66: 5495–5503.

7. Kantarjian H, Issa JP, Rosenfeld CS, Bennett JM, Albitar M, et al. (2006) Decitabine improves patient outcomes in myelodysplastic syndromes: results of a phase III randomized study. Cancer 106: 1794–1803.

8. Lübbert M, Suciu S, Baila L, Rüter BH, Platzbecker U, et al. (2011) Low-dose decitabine versus best supportive care in elderly patients with intermediate- or high-risk myelo- dysplastic syndrome (MDS) ineligible for intensive chemotherapy: final Results of the randomized phase III study of the European Organization for Research and Treatment of Cancer Leukemia Group and the German MDS Study Group. J Clin Oncol 29: 1987–1996.

9. Kantarjian H, Oki Y, Garcia-Manero G, Huang X, O'Brien S, et al. (2007) Results of a randomized study of 3 schedules of low-dose decitabine in higher-risk myelodysplastic syndrome and chronic myelomonocytic leukemia. Blood 109: 52–57.

10. Steensma DP, Baer MR, Slack JL, Buckstein R, Godley LA, et al. (2009) Multicenter study of decitabine administered daily for 5 Days every 4 weeks to adults with myelodysplastic syndromes: the alternative dosing for outpatient treatment (ADOPT) trial. J Clin Oncol 27: 3842–3848.

11. Lee JH, Jang JH, Park J, Park S, Joo YD, et al. (2011) A prospective multicenter observational study of decitabine treatment in Korean patients with myelodysplastic syndrome. Haematologica 96: 1441–1447.

12. Iastrebner M, Jang JH, Nucifora E, Kim K, Sackmann F, et al. (2010) Decitabine in myelodysplastic syndromes and chronic myelomonocytic leukemia: Argentinian/South Korean multi-institutional clinical experience. Leuk Lymphoma 51: 2250–2257.

13. Oki Y, Kondo Y, Yamamoto K, Ogura M, Kasai M, et al. (2012) Phase I/II study of decitabine in patients with myelodysplastic syndrome: A multi-center study in Japan. Cancer Science 103: 1839–1847.

14. Yang H, Zhu HY, Jiang MM, Wang QS, et al. (2013) Clinical observation of decitabine-treating patients with myelodysplastic syndrome and acute myeloid leukemia]. Zhongguo Shi Yan Xue Ye Xue Za Zhi 21: 121–125.

15. Giagounidis AA (2007) Decitabine dosage in myelodysplastic syndromes. Blood 110: 1082–1083.

16. Bennett JM, Catovsky D, Daniel MT, Flandrin G, Galton DA, et al. (1976) Proposals for the classification of the acute leukaemias: French-American-British Cooperative Group. Br J Haematol 33: 451–458.

17. Greenberg P, Cox C, LeBeau MM, Fenaux P, Morel P, et al. (1997) International scoring system for evaluating prognosis in myelodysplastic syndromes. Blood 89: 2079–2088.

18. Tefferi A, Barosi G, Mesa RA, Cervantes F, Deeg HJ, et al. (2006) International Working Group (IWG) consensus criteria for treatment response in myelofibrosis with myeloid metaplasia, for the IWG for Myelofibrosis Research and Treatment (IWG-MRT). Blood 108: 1497–1503.

19. Trotti A, Colevas AD, Setser A, Rusch V, Jaques D, et al. (2003) CTCAE v3.0: development of a comprehensive grading system for the adverse effects of cancer treatment. Semin Radiat Oncol 13: 176–181.

20. Xu F, Li X, Wu L, Zhang Q, Yang R, et al. (2011) Overexpression of the EZH2, RING1 and BMI1 genes is common in myelodysplastic syndromes: relation to adverse epigenetic alteration and poor prognostic scoring. Ann Hematol 90: 643–653.

21. Garcia-Manero G, Jabbour E, Borthakur G, Faderl S, Estrov Z, et al. (2013) Randomized open-label phase II study of decitabine in patients with low- or intermediate-risk myelodysplastic syndromes. J Clin Oncol 31: 2548–2553.

22. Jabbour EI, Garcia-Manero G, Ravandi F, Faderl S, O'Brien S, et al. (2013) Prognostic factors associated with disease progression and overall survival in patients with myelodysplastic syndromes treated with decitabine. CLIN lymphoma myeloma Leuk 13: 131–138.

9

Genomic Inverse PCR for Exploration of Ligated Breakpoints (GIPFEL), a New Method to Detect Translocations in Leukemia

Elisa Fueller[1][9], **Daniel Schaefer**[2][9], **Ute Fischer**[2], **Pina F. I. Krell**[2], **Martin Stanulla**[3], **Arndt Borkhardt**[2]*, **Robert K. Slany**[1]*

1 Department of Genetics, Friedrich Alexander University, Erlangen, Germany, **2** Department of Pediatric Oncology, Hematology and Clinical Immunology, University Children's Hospital, Medical Faculty, Heinrich Heine University, Düsseldorf, Germany, **3** Department of Pediatric Hematology and Oncology, Hannover Medical School, Hannover, Germany

Abstract

Here we present a novel method "Genomic inverse PCR for exploration of ligated breakpoints" (GIPFEL) that allows the sensitive detection of recurrent chromosomal translocations. This technique utilizes limited amounts of DNA as starting material and relies on PCR based quantification of unique DNA sequences that are created by circular ligation of restricted genomic DNA from translocation bearing cells. Because the complete potential breakpoint region is interrogated, a prior knowledge of the individual, specific interchromosomal fusion site is not required. We validated GIPFEL for the five most common gene fusions associated with childhood leukemia (MLL-AF4, MLL-AF9, MLL-ENL, ETV6-RUNX1, and TCF3-PBX1). A workflow of restriction digest, purification, ligation, removal of linear fragments and precipitation enriching for circular DNA was developed. GIPFEL allowed detection of translocation specific signature sequences down to a 10^{-4} dilution which is close to the theoretical limit. In a blinded proof-of-principle study utilizing DNA from cell lines and 144 children with B-precursor-ALL associated translocations this method was 100% specific with no false positive results. Sensitivity was 83%, 65%, and 24% for t(4;11), t(9;11) and t(11;19) respectively. Translocation t(12;21) was correctly detected in 64% and t(1;19) in 39% of the cases. In contrast to other methods, the characteristics of GIPFEL make it particularly attractive for prospective studies.

Editor: Jörn Lausen, Georg Speyer Haus, Germany

Funding: This research was funded by a grant of the German Ministry for Radiation Protection (Bundesministerium für Strahlenschutz, BfS) grant number 3612S70019. The funders had no role in study design, data collection and analysis, decision to publish, or preparation of the manuscript.

Competing Interests: The authors have declared that no competing interests exist.

* Email: arndt.borkhardt@med.uni-duesseldorf.de (AB); robert.slany@fau.de (RKS)

[9] These authors contributed equally to this work.

Introduction

The realization that certain subtypes of leukemia are invariably associated with recurrent genomic abnormalities was a seminal discovery in leukemia research. This was first recognized in conjunction with chronic myeloid leukemia and the paradigmatic Philadelphia chromosome [1]. Nowadays we know that this is a widespread phenomenon. The determination of genotype has become essential for diagnosis, stratification, treatment planning and prognosis of hematological malignancies. Particularly in infant and childhood leukemia almost half of all diagnosed cases are characterized by the persistent appearance of distinctive chromosomal translocations [2].

Because of the importance of these genetic markers for clinical management a series of methods has been devised that allows the detection of the underlying genetic lesion. Cytogenetics and fluorescent in situ hybridization (FISH) are generally applied to demonstrate the presence and overall structure of genomic alterations. However, both approaches require mitotic cells,

cumbersome experimental procedures and experienced operators for success. Alternative methods using archived genetic material have also been developed. Since most translocations create in-frame fusion proteins there are only a limited number of exons within both fusion partners that can be joined productively. This fact has been exploited by PCR based methods that use RNA/cDNA as template [3,4]. In this way the number of primer pairs necessary to interrogate for the presence of a specific translocation is limited and the expected amplification products can be predicted. The drawback is the labile nature of RNA that often precludes successful amplification from stored or aging samples. To avoid this problem DNA based methods have been explored [5,6]. Yet, the actual genomic breakpoints are usually unknown and they are distributed over a large stretch of intronic sequences. This mandates either the use of an unwieldy number of different primer pairs or long range PCR strategies with the disadvantage of non-quantifiable amplicons of unknown length that may well exceed the practicable limits of current PCR.

To avoid these pitfalls, we devised a novel method that can detect chromosomal translocations at the DNA level creating constant, predictable, and quantifiable amplicons. This technique, that we called GIPFEL (genomic inverse PCR for exploration of ligated breakpoints) utilizes the fact that genomic breakpoints are usually confined to defined chromosomal regions. Restriction digest of genomic DNA followed by circularization of resulting fragments will divide even large breakpoint regions into a manageable number of DNA circles. Only cells with translocations will create a "signature" circle that is uniquely characteristic for the nature of the underlying genomic aberration (figure 1). These circles can be quantified by real-time PCR because the sequence of the corresponding ligation joint can be derived from the known genomic sequence and the respective location of the restriction sites within the breakpoint region. Hence corresponding amplicons of suitable size for real-time PCR can be designed. Positive amplification results do not only reveal the presence of a translocation but they also give topical information of the approximate localization of the genomic break. By selecting appropriate restriction enzymes even large breakpoint regions can be covered with relatively few primer/PCR reactions. Here we demonstrate proof-of-principle experiments testing GIPFEL on the five most frequent translocations in childhood leukemia t(4;11), t(9;11), t(11;19), t(12;21), and t(1;19).

Materials and Methods

Circularization of genomic DNA

Genomic DNA from clinical repositories was provided pre-purified. Samples were collected with written informed consent and all institutional and national guidelines for employing human material in research were observed. Patients were enrolled in

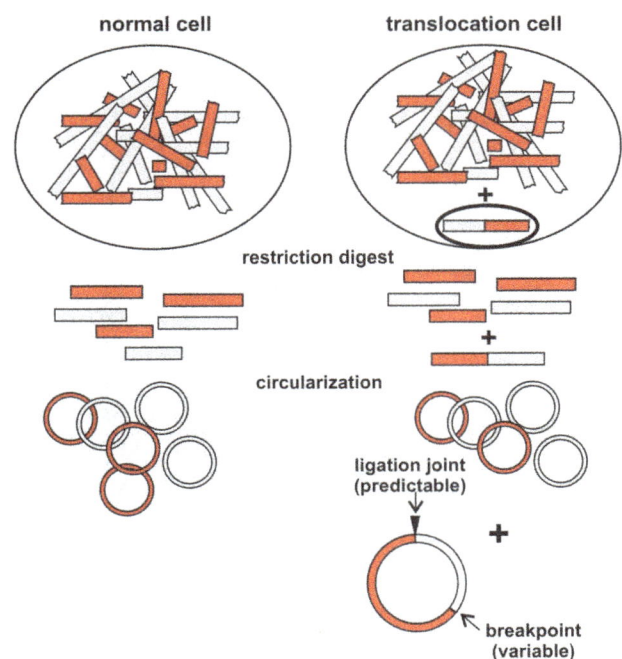

Figure 1. Basic principle of GIPFEL. Upon restriction digest and circularization of genomic DNA only genomic DNA from translocation bearing cells will form circles that join DNA of two different chromosomes. The junction is predetermined by the location of the genomic breakpoint. By probing for all possible ligation junctions with PCR the presence of a translocation can be ascertained.

multicenter trial AIEOP-BFM ALL 2000 on treatment of childhood ALL. Diagnosis, characterization and treatment of ALL were performed as previously described [7,8]. The trial was approved by the institutional review board of Hannover Medical School, Hannover, Germany. Written informed consent for the use of specimen for research was obtained from all study individuals, parents or legal guardians and approved by the institutional review board.

All enzymes used in the procedure were obtained from New England Biolabs (Frankfurt/Main, Germany) and used with the appropriate buffers recommended by the manufacturer. For cell lines and buffy coats DNA was prepared from 1 to 5×10^6 cells with the QIAampDNA Blood Mini Kit exactly according to the instructions of the manufacturer (Qiagen, Hilden, Germany).

If available, e.g. from cell lines, GIPFEL started with 2.5 µg of DNA corresponding to approximately 3.8×10^5 genome equivalents (calculating with 6.6 pg DNA per cell). For detection of translocations in repository DNA, the nucleic acids were either pre-amplified with REPLI-g Ultra Fast Mini Kit according to the manufacturer's (Qiagen) instructions or, when probing for MLL translocations, only 1 µg stored DNA was used directly. The DNA was incubated either with 200 units BamHI-HF (for MLL translocations) or with 200 units of SacI-HF or MfeI-HF for detection of t(12;21) and t(1;19), respectively. Reactions were set up in 100 µl volume using the buffer recommended by the manufacturer and digests were performed for 2 h.

Restriction fragments were isolated by addition of 500 µl buffer PB (Qiagen) to the digestion reaction and a subsequent purification on QIAquick gel extraction columns (Qiagen) according to the instructions of the manufacturer. To improve recovery of longer fragments elution was done with 50 µl of deionized water pre-warmed to 60°C and columns were incubated for 5 minutes at 60°C before final centrifugation.

Religation was performed for 2 h at 24°C in a 100 µl reaction using the total column eluate and 2 µl (800 units) of T4-DNA ligase and the appropriate buffer. After ligation linear DNA fragments were digested by addition of 1 µl (100 units) of exonuclease III and incubation for 30 min at 37°C with a subsequent 5 min heat inactivation at 95°C.

Enriched circular DNA was concentrated by standard alcohol precipitation.

Primer design and semi-nested real time PCR

In silico predictions were done deriving the sequences of all possible ligation junctions that would be created from religation of a genomic fragment carrying a chromosomal breakpoint. Primers spanning ligation sites were designed to generate amplicons suitable for real time PCR (see table 1 and table S1) (https://eu.idtdna.com/analyzer/Applications/OligoAnalyzer/) [9]. To restrict the number of PCRs necessary to include the complete breakpoint region sometimes closely spaced (<1 kb) restriction sites were covered only by a single primer.

All PCR reactions were performed with BrilliantII SYBR green PCR Master Mix from Agilent Technologies (St. Clara, CA, USA) in standard 25 µl reactions using a final primer concentration of 100 nM. For first round PCR 5 µl of circularized DNA corresponding to approximately 1.9×10^5 genome equivalents served as template. Cycle conditions were 10 min initial denaturation, followed by 22 cycles of 15 s 95°C, 30 s 64°C, 30 s 72°C for MLL translocations. Translocation t(12;21) and t(1;19) samples were pre-amplified with 25 cycles.

One µl of primary PCR product was used as input for each secondary PCR. Reactions were monitored on an optical cycler

Table 1. Primers used for GIPFEL.

Name	detection	sequence(5'-3')	GC %	T$_M$ °C	l.	size PCR product
MLL						
MLL-B1r.4	MLL outer pr.	GCTTTCGTGGAGGAGGCTCAC	61.9	69.5	21	
MLL-B1r-n	MLL inner pr.	CTGCTTTTCTTTGGGGCAGGATC	52.2	62.4	23	
MLL-B2f.4	MLL control pr.	TGGGTGAGTTATACACATGATGC	43.4	63.5	23	301
AF4						
AF4-B1f	breakpoints	CTGAAGATGCCTTCTCAGTCAG	50	60.3	22	361
AF4-B2f		TGTGGATTCTTTACTCCCTGTCC	47.8	60.6	23	336
AF4-B3f		GCCACACCATGTGCAGAGACC	61.9	63.7	21	402
AF4-B4f.2		CTTATAGTAGCCCAAGAGGAAAG	43.5	58.9	23	219
AF4-B6f		GTGTGTGTGCTTGTAGTCTTAGC	47.8	60.6	23	426
AF4-B7f		TTGTTCTATTGATTCACCTTCGAC	37.5	63.0	24	257
AF4-B8f		GTATGGCAGGCATTGCATCCAC	54.5	70.5	23	265
AF9						
AF9-B1f.2	breakpoints	TGTTTGTATTTTGCTTGTGTAAAGG	32	62.7	25	199
AF9-B2f.3		GTAATTTAATATAGATTATTGCAGG	24	54.1	25	169
AF9-B3f		ACAGTACAACCATCCAAGTCAGG	47.8	60.6	23	462
AF9-B4f		AGTGGACAAGATAAGAAGGCTCC	47.8	60.6	23	281
AF9-B5f		GTACCTGGCACATAGTTGGTAG	50	60.3	22	429
AF9-B6f.2		CCCACTGGAATGTCACGTTAGG	54.5	67.5	22	183
AF9-B7f		TGTCTTTAAGGAATGGAAAACTGC	37.5	57.6	24	470
AF9-B8f		GAGGAATTACAGCTCTGAGCCC	54.5	62.1	22	287
AF9-B9f		TCGCTAGTGCATAGATTGTTAGG	43.5	58.9	23	318
AF9-B10f		GTTGTACCAGTTACAGTTCAACTG	41.6	59.2	24	317
ENL						
ENL-B6f	breakpoints	GAGCTCCTCTGACTCCCTAGG	61.9	63.4	21	337
ENL-B7f		CTCTGCCTTCTTCTTGGGAACC	54.5	67.1	22	369
ENL-B8f.2		CTCTCTGGACTCCTCTTAATACC	47.8	59	23	243
ENL-B9f		CACTTAGTGCTATGAAGGCGTTG	47.8	60.6	23	324
ENL-B11f		ACTTTGCCGTGGAAGTCAATCC	50	60.3	22	286
ENL-B12f		TGCTGTTTGCTGCTTGTCATCC	50	60.3	22	398
ENL-B13f.2		TCATTGCAGACTCCACCTCTCC	54.5	62.1	22	371
ENL-B14f		CCTAACCACAATATCATTCTGGC	43.4	63.2	23	350
ENL-B15f.7		CTGGGTCTGCAGTGATTGTGG	57.1	61.8	21	94
ENL-B16f.2		GGTGGCATCCCTCCTCGTGG	70	65.5	20	186
ENL-B17f		GTGGAATTCAGGGACAGTTCAG	50	60.3	22	313
ETV6						
ETV6-S1r	ETV6 outer pr.	GATGTGGTTCATGTAAGCCAGGTCTTC	48	68.2	27	
ETV6-S1r-n	ETV6 inner pr.	GGAGGACGCTGGGCAGTGATTATTC	56	69.1	25	
ETV6-S2r	ETV6 outer pr.	AAAGGGACAGTACCTCAAGGCAGAAG	50	67.9	26	
ETV6-S2r-n	ETV6 inner pr.	TGGCAGCACCTTGATGGTCAGCTAG	56	69.1	25	
ETV6-S3r	ETV6 outer pr.	GGGACATTATGCACCTGCTTGGGAG	56	69.1	25	
ETV6-S3r-n	ETV6 inner pr.	TAGGACTGTTCGGGGCCATCTGTC	58	68.5	24	
RUNX1						ETV6-S1/2/3r-n
RUNX1-S1f	breakpoints	CAGAGGCAAGACGGGCTGATAACC	58	68.5	24	512/444/449
RUNX1-S2f		AGGGACTCATGGTGACGGGAGC	64	67.9	22	196/128/133
RUNX1-S3f		GACTCTATATTGGAACCTCGGAAACGC	48	68.2	27	257/189/194
RUNX1-S4f		TTATCTGGTGGGCTGTTAGGAGGCTC	54	69.5	26	267/199/204
RUNX1-S5f		GGTGTGTTTCATAGGGAACTGGTTTTGC	46	68.5	28	169/101/106
RUNX1-S6f		CCCACACCCTAGTTTGCATCGGTTTG	54	69.5	26	131/63/68

Table 1. Cont.

Name	detection	sequence(5′-3′)	GC %	T$_M$ °C	l.	size PCR product
RUNX1-S7f		GAGGTGGAAGTAGTCATTATGGGATAACC	45	69.1	29	670/602/607
RUNX1-S8f		TGGTGACAAGTTGCTTCAGGCTGATG	50	67.9	26	193/125/130
RUNX1-S10f		CCGGGATGACAACAGTTCAAGGAATAC	48	68.2	27	142/74/79
RUNX1-S11f		ACCAGGCACTTGACTCTTAGGATGTTTG	46	68.5	28	229/161/166
RUNX1-S12f		GTGTCATCTCAACCATGGAAAGGGTAC	48	68.2	27	323/255/260
RUNX1-S13f		GGAGGACCTAGTGGGATGCAAGTG	58	68.5	24	159/91/96
RUNX1-S14f		CTGACTGGGCAGCTCCACTATGTC	58	68.5	24	217/149/154
RUNX1-S15f		CCTAGTGAGTTCAGTGTGGTTTTGTCAG	46	68.5	28	174/106/111
RUNX1-S16f		AGTGAGCTGGGGAATCCATTCAAGTG	50	67.9	26	173/105/110
RUNX1-S17f		CGTTTCTAGAAGGAGTGCCGGCAG	58	68.5	24	296/228/233
RUNX1-S18f		GCTACCAGTCAAGTTTCCTTTCGGGC	54	69.5	26	202/134/139
RUNX1-S19f		AGACACAAAAGGTCAGACGCATGACAC	48	68.2	27	314/246/251
RUNX1-S20f		TTGGGGAGAGAAGGATGATGGTCTTG	50	67.9	26	274/206/211
RUNX1-S21f		AGTGGAAAAGGAGGTGGCAAGTACAG	50	67.9	26	152/84/89
RUNX1-S22f		AAGGAAAGAAGCTAGTTGGGGTAGCG	50	67.9	26	272/204/209
RUNX1-S23f		AACAGAGAAGTCGCAATAGTGCAGCAG	48	68.2	27	231/163/168
RUNX1-S24f		TCTCATGTTTTCCAGTTGCTTAGGCGTG	46	68.5	28	230/162/167
RUNX1-S25f		TGTCTTGGGGATCATTCTCGCCTGC	56	69.1	25	185/117/122
RUNX1-S26f		CATCAGGCAGAAAGGAAGAAGGGAAG	50	67.9	26	177/109/114
RUNX1-S27f		TGCAGTCACTTAGAAGCACCCATCTG	50	67.9	26	715/647/652
RUNX1-S28f		CAGAAAATCTTGCAGCAGTCAGCTTGC	48	68.2	27	163/95/100
RUNX1-S29f		TCGGTTAGCTTTCACGGAGGCAGTG	56	69.1	25	135/67/72
RUNX1-S0f	RUNX1 control pr.	CTTGGTTCAGAGTGTATCTCACCCTTG	48	68.2	27	404
RUNX1-S1r	RUNX1 control pr.	GTGAAGCCAGGGACACACACTAAATG	50	67.9	26	404
TCF3						
TCF3-M1r	TCF3 outer pr.	CTGTGCTGGAGCGGGAAGTATGC	61	68.3	23	
TCF3-M1r-n	TCF3 inner pr.	AGCGAGATGAGACCGCAGGAGTG	61	68.3	23	
PBX1						
PBX1-M1f	breakpoints	ACTTAAAACTTGGCCCTAGAGTCCCTC	48	68.2	27	164
PBX1-M2f		GTGAAGCTGAGAAAACTACATGTGTGTCG	45	69.1	29	320
PBX1-M3f		ATGGTGTAAGGATGGGGTGAGTGCTG	54	69.5	26	295
PBX1-M4f		CAAGGATGTAACCTGATGGGGAATAGTG	46	68.5	28	542
PBX1-M5f		TTGGTCTGTGCCTACATGTATGTGCTC	48	68.2	27	217
PBX1-M6f		CCAGGTGTGAGAGGCAGTGTAACATC	54	69.5	26	192
PBX1-M7f		CCATCTGTAAAATTGGGTGGCAGTGTAG	46	68.5	28	228
PBX1-M8f		TCAAGGTAAAGCTCTGAAATCCCACGC	48	68.2	27	239
PBX1-M9f		GATGGTGTCCCAGGAGCAAGCAAC	58	68.5	24	273
PBX1-M10f		GGATTGACACAGACCAAGGGGTCTTG	54	69.5	26	356
PBX1-M11f		AGAGAGGTCAGGAAGGGAAAGGGATG	54	69.5	26	186
PBX1-M12f		CGATCCCACCATTGGTCAACACAGAC	54	69.5	26	247
PBX1-M13f		TAGAATGAGGCAGAGCTTCCAGGATAG	48	68.2	27	224
PBX1-M14f		GAGAGAGACTCAGCTTCAGTAACCTG	50	67.9	26	177
PBX1-M15f		CCCTAGGCTGAACGAAACGAAAACTC	50	67.9	26	727
PBX1-M16f		TCAAAGGCAGGAGTGAGATGTCATCC	50	67.9	26	218
PBX1-M17f		TCTCTGACCTTCTGTCTCTGGGCAC	56	69.1	25	257
PBX1-M18f		CTCTGAGACACGGAACACTAGTTGTG	50	67.9	26	192
PBX1-M19f		TCCCTCTAGTCATATGTCTGTGCTGC	50	67.9	26	183
PBX1-M20f		CAAAGTATGTTGAAGTGTGTTGGCGCC	48	68.2	27	158
PBX1-M21f		GTACATAGGCGTTATCACCTCATTGGAAG	45	69.1	29	279

Table 1. Cont.

Name	detection	sequence(5'-3')	GC %	T$_M$ °C	I.	size PCR product
PBX1-M22f		GACCCCTTCTCTCTTAACTCATAATGGC	46	68.5	28	276
PBX1-M23f		CAGGAACAAGAACAAGAAGGCATGTAGG	46	68.5	28	199
PBX1-M24f		AGCATCATAGGTGACAAGGGGCCATG	54	69.5	26	164
PBX1-M25f		TGCCTGGTGCATGTTAAGCCTCACAG	54	69.5	26	234
PBX1-M26f		TAGAACATGCAGAATGCCCACCGTGG	54	69.5	26	183
PBX1-M27f		TGAGTGTGTTGGTACCGATGTGTGGC	54	69.5	26	147
PBX1-M28f		GTGAATGCCTGTGTGTACACTTAACGTG	46	68.5	28	253
PBX1-M29f		CTGGCGTCATAACAGAAGTAGTCACAG	48	68.2	27	268
PBX1-M30f		TGGCATCTGAAGCACCTGTCCTAATG	50	67.9	26	205
PBX1-M31f		CTGAGCTTGACCTTCCAGTCGTCTTC	54	69.5	26	204
PBX1-M32f		TTGGCATTGTGACCAGGAGATCTATTGC	46	68.5	28	243
PBX1-M33f		GATGCAAGGGAACAATTACTGGACTGTTC	45	69.1	29	346
PBX1-M34f		ACATTCTGAGGAAGATACATGGTTGTTCC	41	67.4	29	177
PBX1-M35f		TGGTGGTAATGGGGTTGGTGGGATAG	54	69.5	26	328
PBX1-M36f		ATACACACATGCACGTAACACCCCAAAG	46	68.5	28	167
PBX1-M0f	PBX1 control pr.	GCCCTGTAACCTGGGAGGTCTATTAG	54	69.5	26	298
PBX1-M1r	PBX1 control pr.	AACCATCTGTGGAGTGCCCGGATTAG	54	69.5	26	298

for 40 to 45 cycles under conditions as in first round PCR reaction. The multiplexing scheme is given in table 2.

To avoid contamination by airborne DNA, all PCR reactions were assembled under clean-room conditions in an UV-sterilized PCR cabinet with separate equipment and rooms for pre- and post-PCR procedures.

Evaluation of results

A sample was scored as PCR-positive if a primer pair specific for a translocation circle yielded a threshold cycle (C$_T$) that was clearly decreased compared to the cohort of all other primer pairs. Positive real time products were run on standard agarose gels for determination of size. In addition DNA was isolated from the gel and sequenced from both sides using the PCR amplification primers.

The higher number of primers necessary to cover the t(12;21) and t(1;19) breakpoint region mandated multiplexing also during the second round of PCR. Therefore positively scoring products obtained with a primer pool were re-tested in a third round PCR using single forward primers.

Results

Validation of the GIPFEL procedure

To generate a genomic DNA preparation enriched in circular ligated DNA a 4-step biochemical procedure was developed (figure 2A). After digestion of genomic DNA and purification of a genome wide population of restriction fragments the nucleic acid was converted to circular form by ligation in a large volume. Remaining linear fragments were removed by digesting with exonuclease III followed by alcohol precipitation to prepare a template for PCR analysis.

PCR was designed in a semi-nested setup (figure 2B) pre-amplifying with an outer anchor primer (three primers for ETV6) binding to sequences of the 5' fusion portion. This primer was paired with pools of downstream primers corresponding to the

predicted 3' fusion sequence. The reaction products of this primary PCR served as input for the next round of PCR. Secondary PCRs were monitored with SYBR green on a real time machine using a 5' inner primer (three primers for ETV6) and either each downstream primer in individual combination (for MLL fusion proteins) or again pools of downstream primers (see Table 1 for primer sequences and Table 2 for multiplexing strategies). Primers amplifying a nearby genomic region unaffected by the translocation were employed alongside as controls. For further evaluation amplified PCR products were sized on agarose gels, isolated and sequenced (figure 2C). A sample was scored positive if the size and the predicted sequence of a PCR product could be unequivocally confirmed (see Table S1 for a list of predicted ligation joint sequences).

To evaluate the efficiency of the overall process we validated the procedure with DNA from three cell lines: MV4;11 carries a t(4;11), REH contains t(12;21) and 697 was used to detect t(1;19). For all lines the exact location of the breakpoint is known obviating the need for multiplexing in the set-up experiments. DNA from cell lines negative for the translocations to be tested (HL60, 697, REH) served as background control. Translocation bearing cells were mixed in various ratios with control cells and the GIPFEL procedure was performed (figure 3). Under these optimal conditions detection of signature circles was possible for all translocations down to a dilution of 1 into 10^{-4}. This dilution is equivalent to a calculated presence of 19 target molecules per PCR reaction (2.5 µg DNA = 3.8×10^5 cells $\times 10^{-4}$ = 38 but because only 50% of the circularization reaction was used as template for PCR, effectively a calculated maximum of 19 template molecules have been present).

To further validate the method on actual patient samples, DNA was obtained from clinical repositories. A collection was assembled encompassing 21 MLL-AF4, 16 MLL-AF9, 18 MLL-ENL, 60 ETV6-RUNX1, and 30 TCF3-PBX1 cases. Five negative control samples were added to each translocation group and the samples were blinded for processing. Because of the limited amount of the

Table 2. Multiplexing strategy for GIPFEL analysis.

	anchor pr.	#1	#2	#3	#4	#5	#6	#7	#8	#9	#10	#11	#12	control
MLLAF4*														
PCR1	MLL-B1r.4+	B1f+B2f+B3f	B4f.2+B6f+B7f	B8f										#4 control MLL-B2f.4
PCR2	MLL-B1r.n +	B1f	B2f	B3f	B4f.2	B6f	B7f							#8 control MLL-B2f.4
MLLAF9*														
PCR1	MLL-B1r.4 +	B1f.2+B2f.3+B3f	B4f+B5f+B6f.2	B7f+B8f+B9f	B10f									#5 control MLL-B2f.4
PCR2	MLL-B1r.n +	B1f.2	B2f.3	B3f	B4f	B5f	B6f.2	B7f	B8f	B9f	B10f			#11 control MLL-B2f.4
MLLENL*														
PCR1	MLL-B1r.4 +	B6f+B7f+B8f.2	B9f+B11+B12f	B13f.2+B14f+15f.7	B16f.2+B17f									#5 control MLL-B2f.4
PCR2	MLL-B1r.n +	B6f	B7f	B8f	B9f	B11f	B12f	B13f.2	B14f	B15f.7	B16f.2	B17f		#12 control MLL-B2f.4
ETV6-RUNX1														
PCR1	ETV6- S1r + S2r + S3r +	S12f + S15f + S17f + S22f + S23f + S26f + S28f	S1f + S4f + S10f + S11f + S14f + S24f + S27f	S2f + S6f + S7f + S8f + S18f + S20f + S29f	S3f + S5f + S13f + S16f + S19f + S21f + S25f									#5 control RUNX1-S0f + S1r (no anchor)
PCR2†	ETV6- S1r-n + S2r-n + S3r-n +	S12f + S15f + S17f + S22f + S23f + S26f + S28f	S1f + S4f + S10f + S11f + S14f + S24f + S27f	S2f + S6f + S7f + S8f + S18f + S20f + S29f	S3f + S5f + S13f + S16f + S19f + S21f + S25f									#5 control RUNX1-S0f + S1r (no anchor)
TCF3-PBX1														
PCR1	TCF3-M1r+	M1f + M6f + M12f + M13f + M26f + M29f + M33f + M36f	M4f + M8f + M9f + M10f + M16f + M21f + M23f	M2f + M11f + M20f + M25f + M28f + M34f + M35f	M3f + M5f + M14f + M18f + M19f + M24f + M32f	M7f + M15f + M17f + M22f + M27f + M30f + M31f								#6 control PBX1-M0f + M1r (no anchor)
PCR2†	TCF3-M1r-n+	M1f + M6f + M12f + M13f + M26f + M29f + M33f + M36f	M4f + M8f + M9f + M10f + M16f + M21f + M23f	M2f + M11f + M20f + M25f + M28f + M34f + M35f	M3f + M5f + M14f + M18f + M19f + M24f + M32f	M7f + M15f + M17f + M22f + M27f + M30f + M31f								#6 control PBX1-M0f + M1r (no anchor)

*for MLL fusion proteins multiplexing was done only in the first round of semi-nested PCR.
†for ETV6-RUNX1 and TCF3-PBX1 multiplexing was done for both rounds of PCR. For samples scoring positive, a third validation round using single primers was added.

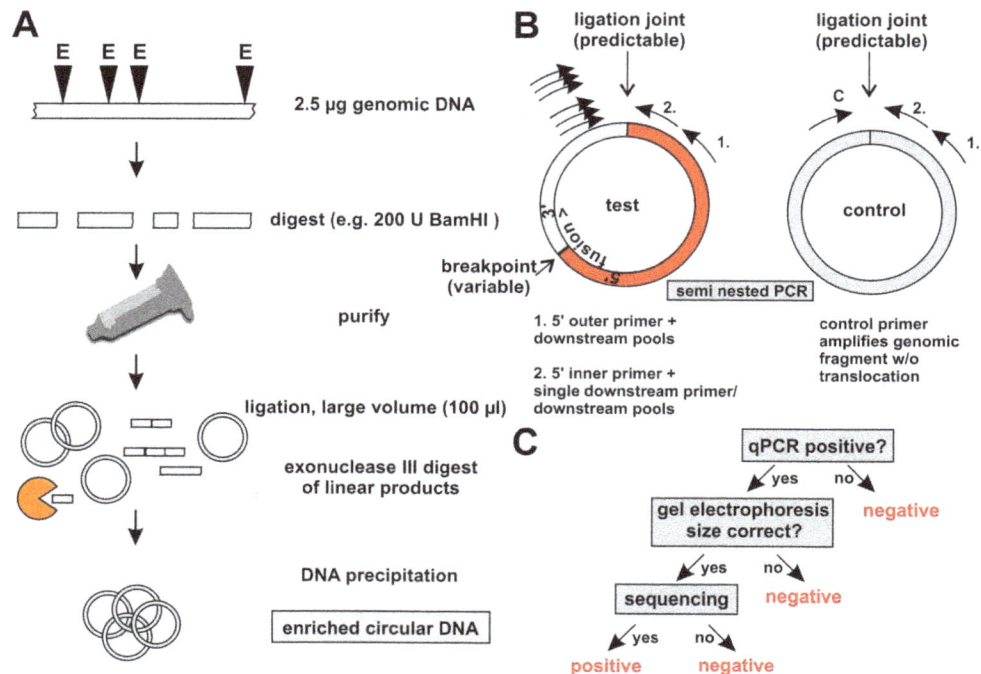

Figure 2. Flow chart of the GIPFEL procedure. A. Biochemical steps for enrichment of circularized DNA. The products of a restriction enzyme (E) digest of genomic material are column purified and ligated in a large volume. Subsequently exonuclease III (presented in yellow) removes remaining linear fragments allowing enrichment for circularized DNA. B. PCR strategy to detect the presence of translocation specific circles. Primer pairs are designed that cover all possible ligation joints of translocation specific ligation products. Semi-nested PCR is performed first with an outer primer corresponding to the 5′ portion of the fusion and pools of downstream primers. The PCR products from these reactions are used as templates for secondary PCRs using a 5′ inner primer and the same downstream primers, yet in different combinations. A control PCR amplifies a ligation joint created from wild-type cells. C. Decision tree for scoring of GIPFEL results.

clinical material the procedure was performed with 1 μg of genomic DNA as input for MLL bearing translocations. For the other translocations the DNA was genome amplified and 2.5 μg were used. Again the three-tiered decision process of real-time PCR, agarose gelelectrophoresis and sequencing was applied to score the results. Representative examples of positive experiments are shown in figure 3D–F. Upon unblinding GIPFEL showed 100% specificity as no false positive results were obtained. As expected, accuracy was lower. For MLL-AF4, MLL-AF9, MLL-ENL, ETV6-RUNX1, and TCF3-PBX1, 83%, 65%, 24%, 64% and 39% of positive samples were correctly called. Sensitivity was comparable to cell line experiments. When tested with selected patient material positive samples still could be successfully called at dilutions between 10^{-3} and 10^{-4}. A summary of patient and cell line data is given in table 3. Because GIPFEL also gives topical information of the breakpoint location depending on the primer pair yielding a positive readout, a breakpoint distribution chart could be assembled (figure 4). As observed previously, chromosomal junction sites were not randomly distributed but clustered in certain areas corresponding to known hotspots of instability giving additional support to the validity of our GIPFEL results [5,10–20].

Discussion

Here we present a proof-of-principle study demonstrating that it is possible to detect the most commonly occurring translocations in childhood leukemia using small amounts of DNA without having to resort to long range PCR or unstable RNA. The GIPFEL method relies on the prior knowledge of the genomic region where breaks occur. As long as this information is available it can be

adapted to any recurrent translocation. At the same time this is also a drawback of the technique. Breaks outside of the pre-defined genomic region will not be detected. Likewise, more complicated genomic rearrangements might elude discovery because they alter the predicted ligation joints. Translocations resulting from more complicated reshuffling of the genome have been described [21]. During our study we serendipitously detected at (11;19) breakpoint where material of chromosome 5 had been interspersed at the junction site of chromosome 11 and 19 (not shown). Events of this type are the most likely explanation for the false negative rate in the present study. In addition the fact that occasionally only one of two closely spaced restriction sites was covered by primer pairs also causes small "blind spots". However, compared to the size of most breakpoint regions it is highly improbable that these tiny regions <1 kb should have a major impact on the sensitivity of the assay.

The biochemical preparation of circular ligated DNA seems to be close to the optimum. Reactions that contained less than 20 calculated template molecules still yielded a positive readout indicating that all previous preparatory steps worked with near perfect efficiency. Therefore the sensitivity of GIPFEL seems to be mainly limited by the amount of total template DNA that can be fed per PCR reaction. This restricts the practical threshold of GIPFEL to about 1 in 10^4 cells which falls in the range of most DNA based methods. We estimate this sensitivity should suffice to discover most clinically meaningful cases.

Another current constraint is the number of PCR reactions that need to be manually assembled to cover a translocation region. However, for this aspect improvements are in sight as new developments like digital droplet PCR should be easily adaptable to GIPFEL allowing the simultaneous screening for multiple

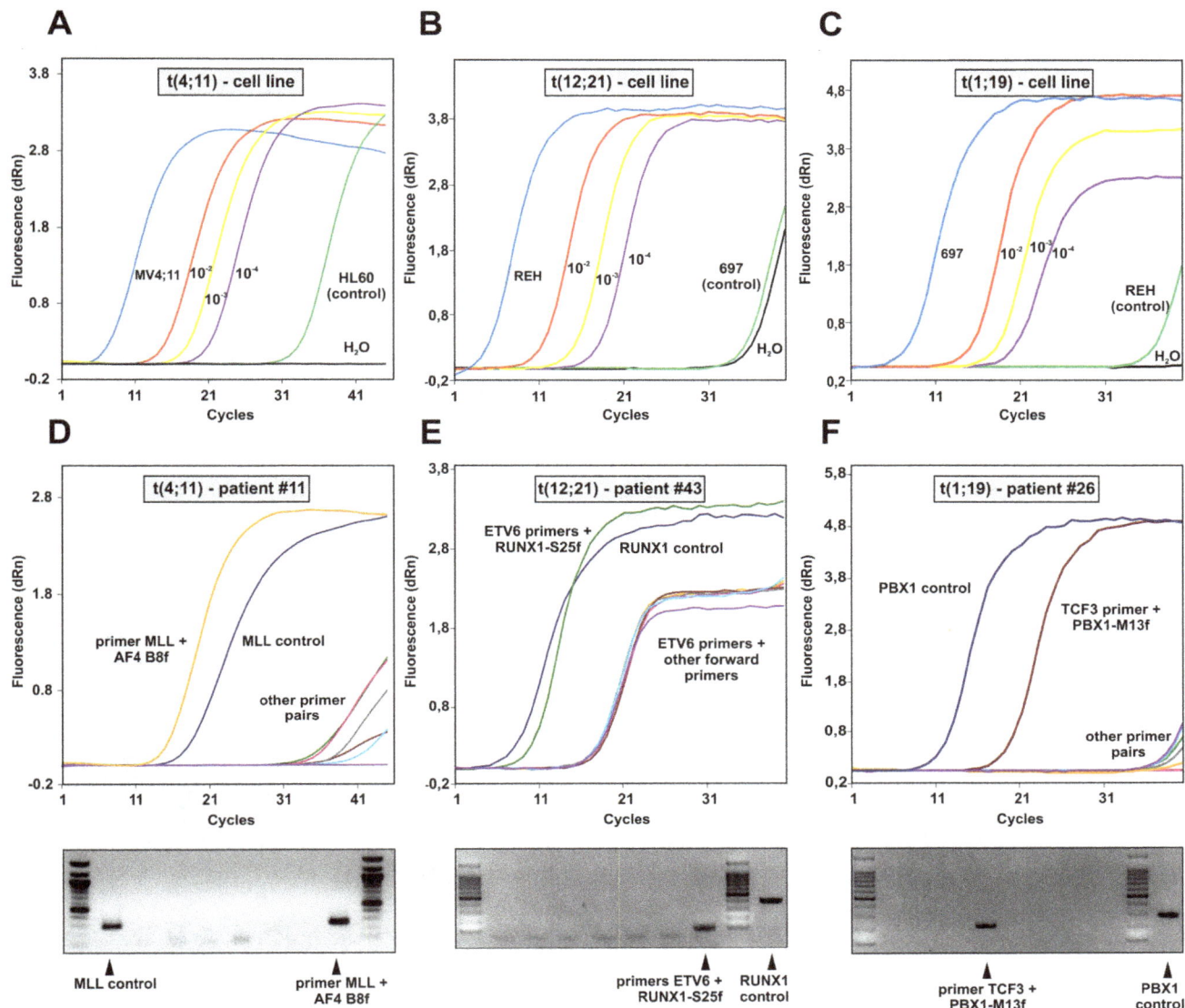

Figure 3. Examples of GIPFEL results. A. Sensitivity test. Circularized genomic DNA was produced from MV4;11 cells a cell line with a known t(4;11) translocation and from HL60 cells as "non-translocation" control as well as from various mixtures "diluting" MV4;11 cells in a population of HL60 as indicated. GIPFEL was performed and real-time amplification curves are shown. B. As in "A" with REH t(12;21) cells and 697 cells instead of HL60 cells. C. As in "A" with 697 t(1;19) and REH cells. D. Example for a GIPFEL result using patient DNA. Upper panel: Amplification chart of a typical GIPFEL experiment with patient DNA. Amplification is achieved with the genomic MLL control primer and a translocation specific primer pair. Lower panel: Agarose gel electrophoresis of the 8 individual secondary PCRs interrogating the (4;11) breakpoint region. E. Results presented as in "D" for a t(12;21) breakpoint. F. Results for a t(1;19) patient sample.

translocations in a high-throughput fashion. Despite the fact that t(11;19) and t(1;19) do not read out optimally in our assay, most cases of the much more frequently occurring t(4;11), t(9;11) and particularly t(12;21) will be recorded. In addition actual population based frequencies of the less easily detectable translocations may be extrapolated from the incidence as detected by GIPFEL corrected by the respective accuracy rate. In addition it is to be expected that NGS data from actual breakpoint regions will beome increasingly available. This information will aid in developing better primers for GIPFEL thus increasing precision of this method.

In summary GIPFEL could become a valuable tool particularly in prospective settings. Patients that have been exposed to topoisomerase inhibitors during the treatment of non-blood related neoplastic diseases are at a higher risk developing 11q23 translocation-positive secondary malignancies. Similarly, persons exposed to ionizing radiation might be screened for the appearance of translocation positive clones. Finally, GIPFEL may be used to solve the ongoing scientific discussion about the actual frequency of pre-leukemic events in healthy newborns, who never develop leukemia in later life. For this purpose birth cohorts might be screened for the presence of interchromosomal fusion sequences in apparently healthy newborns. Previous studies gave highly divergent results ranging from 1:100 ETV6-RUNX1 positive cases [22] to less than 1 in 1417 cord blood samples [23,24]. In all these cases GIPFEL may detect the appearance of translocation positive clones allowing for follow up and maybe early treatment.

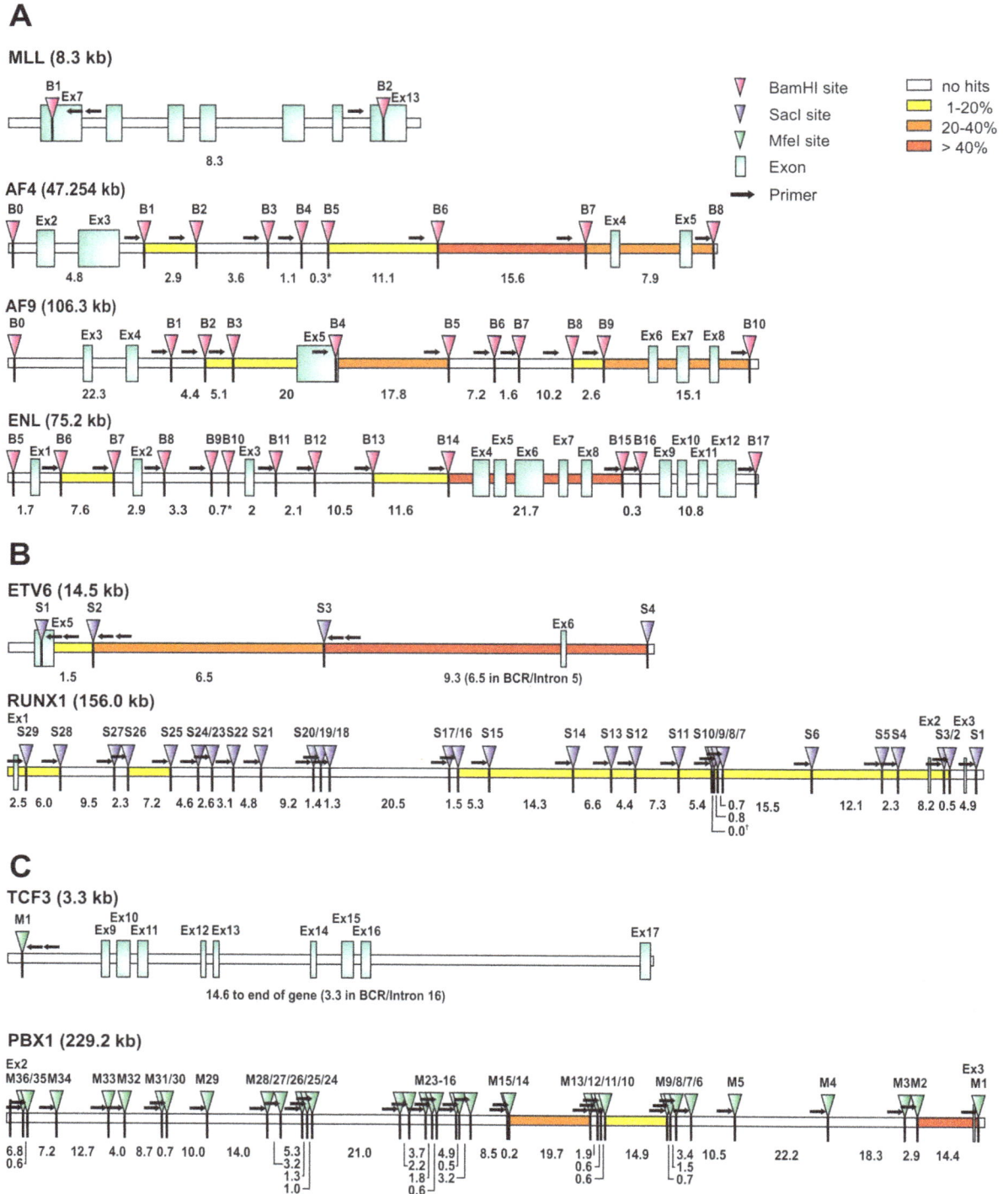

Figure 4. Breakpoint distribution, restriction site and primer locations for individual translocations. A. Schematic depiction of the 11q23 breakpoint region covered by GIPFEL. Consecutively numbered BamHI sites (B), primer locations (arrows) and exons (squares) involved are depicted. Numbers denote the size in kb between restriction sites. * Note: For restriction fragments <1 kb no primers were designed. B. Schematic depiction of the t(12;21) breakpoint regions covered by GIPFEL. SacI sites (S), primer locations and exons involved are depicted as described in A. Numbers denote the size in kb between restriction sites. † Note: Restriction sites S9 and S10 were 4 bp apart. No primer was designed for site S9. C. Schematic depiction of the t(1;19) breakpoint covered by GIPFEL. Presentation as in A and B. Digest was carried out with MfeI (M). The heatmap indicates the frequency of the breakpoints detected in the respective region.

Table 3. GIPFEL results summary.

MLLAF4 (n = 23) Breakpoint region:	# patient samples + cell lines
B0–B1	0
B1–B2	2
B2–B4	0
B5–B6	1
B6–B7	9*+1
B7–B8	7*+1
not detected	3
MLLAF9 (n = 17) Breakpoint region:	
B0–B2	0
B2–B3	1
B3–B4	1
B4–B5	4*
B5–B8	0
B8–B9	1
B9–B10	5*+1
not detected	5
MLLENL (n = 17) Breakpoint region:	
B5–B6	0
B6–B7	1
B7–B13	0
B13–B14	1
B14–B15	2
B15–B17	0
not detected	13
ETV6RUNX1 (n = 61)	
Breakpoint region RUNX1:	
S1–S2	0
S2–S3	2
S3–S4	1
S4–S5	3
S5–S6	3
S6–S7	2
S7–S8	0
S8–S9	2
S10–S11	4
S11–S12	3
S12–S13	1
S13–S14	2+1
S14–S15	5
S15–S16	1
S16–S25	0
S25–S26	2
S26–S28	0
S28–S29	6
S29–S30	1
not detected	22
Breakpoint Region ETV6:	
S1–S2	6*
S2–S3	11*+1
S3–S4	22

Table 3. Cont.

MLLAF4 (n = 23) Breakpoint region:	# patient samples + cell lines
not detected	22
TCF3PBX1 (n = 31)	
Breakpoint region:	
M1–M2	5+1
M2–M9	0
M9–M10	2
M10–M13	0
M13–M14	4
M14–M37	0
not detected	19

* = two different breakpoints were detected in a patient sample.

Acknowledgments

The authors wish to thank Sabine Hornhardt for valuable support and advice.

Author Contributions

Conceived and designed the experiments: AB RKS. Performed the experiments: EF DS UF PF. Analyzed the data: EF DS UF PF MS AB RKS. Contributed reagents/materials/analysis tools: MS. Contributed to the writing of the manuscript: EF DS UF PF MS AB RKS.

References

1. Rowley JD (2013) Genetics. A story of swapped ends. Science 340: 1412–1413.
2. Pui CH, Carroll WL, Meshinchi S, Arceci RJ (2011) Biology, risk stratification, and therapy of pediatric acute leukemias: an update. J Clin Oncol 29: 551–565.
3. Akao Y, Isobe M (2000) Molecular analysis of the rearranged genome and chimeric mRNAs caused by the t(6;11)(q27;q23) chromosome translocation involving MLL in an infant acute monocytic leukemia. Genes Chromosomes Cancer 27: 412–417.
4. Cimino G, Rapanotti MC, Biondi A, Elia L, Lo Coco F, et al. (1997) Infant acute leukemias show the same biased distribution of ALL1 gene breaks as topoisomerase II related secondary acute leukemias. Cancer Res 57: 2879–2883.
5. Langer T, Metzler M, Reinhardt D, Viehmann S, Borkhardt A, et al. (2003) Analysis of t(9;11) chromosomal breakpoint sequences in childhood acute leukemia: almost identical MLL breakpoints in therapy-related AML after treatment without etoposides. Genes Chromosomes Cancer 36: 393–401.
6. Megonigal MD, Rappaport EF, Jones DH, Kim CS, Nowell PC, et al. (1997) Panhandle PCR strategy to amplify MLL genomic breakpoints in treatment-related leukemias. Proc Natl Acad Sci U S A 94: 11583–11588.
7. Conter V, Bartram CR, Valsecchi MG, Schrauder A, Panzer-Grumayer R, et al. (2010) Molecular response to treatment redefines all prognostic factors in children and adolescents with B-cell precursor acute lymphoblastic leukemia: results in 3184 patients of the AIEOP-BFM ALL 2000 study. Blood 115: 3206–3214.
8. Schrappe M, Valsecchi MG, Bartram CR, Schrauder A, Panzer-Grumayer R, et al. (2011) Late MRD response determines relapse risk overall and in subsets of childhood T-cell ALL: results of the AIEOP-BFM-ALL 2000 study. Blood 118: 2077–2084.
9. Kibbe WA (2007) OligoCalc: an online oligonucleotide properties calculator. Nucleic Acids Res 35: W43–46.
10. Felix CA, Kim CS, Megonigal MD, Slater DJ, Jones DH, et al. (1997) Panhandle polymerase chain reaction amplifies MLL genomic translocation breakpoint involving unknown partner gene. Blood 90: 4679–4686.
11. Kobayashi H, Espinosa R 3rd, Thirman MJ, Gill HJ, Fernald AA, et al. (1993) Heterogeneity of breakpoints of 11q23 rearrangements in hematologic malignancies identified with fluorescence in situ hybridization. Blood 82: 547–551.
12. Meyer C, Schneider B, Reichel M, Angermueller S, Strehl S, et al. (2005) Diagnostic tool for the identification of MLL rearrangements including unknown partner genes. Proc Natl Acad Sci U S A 102: 449–454.
13. Rodic N, Zampella JG, Cornish TC, Wheelan SJ, Burns KH (2013) Translocation junctions in TCF3-PBX1 acute lymphoblastic leukemia/lymphoma cluster near transposable elements. Mob DNA 4: 22.
14. Stanulla M, Wang J, Chervinsky DS, Thandla S, Aplan PD (1997) DNA cleavage within the MLL breakpoint cluster region is a specific event which occurs as part of higher-order chromatin fragmentation during the initial stages of apoptosis. Mol Cell Biol 17: 4070–4079.
15. Thandla SP, Ploski JE, Raza-Egilmez SZ, Chhalliyil PP, Block AW, et al. (1999) ETV6-AML1 translocation breakpoints cluster near a purine/pyrimidine repeat region in the ETV6 gene. Blood 93: 293–299.
16. van der Burg M, Beverloo HB, Langerak AW, Wijsman J, van Drunen E, et al. (1999) Rapid and sensitive detection of all types of MLL gene translocations with a single FISH probe set. Leukemia 13: 2107–2113.
17. von Goessel H, Jacobs U, Semper S, Krumbholz M, Langer T, et al. (2009) Cluster analysis of genomic ETV6-RUNX1 (TEL-AML1) fusion sites in childhood acute lymphoblastic leukemia. Leuk Res 33: 1082–1088.
18. Wiemels JL, Hofmann J, Kang M, Selzer R, Green R, et al. (2008) Chromosome 12p deletions in TEL-AML1 childhood acute lymphoblastic leukemia are associated with retrotransposon elements and occur postnatally. Cancer Res 68: 9935–9944.
19. Wiemels JL, Leonard BC, Wang Y, Segal MR, Hunger SP, et al. (2002) Site-specific translocation and evidence of postnatal origin of the t(1;19) E2A-PBX1 fusion in childhood acute lymphoblastic leukemia. Proc Natl Acad Sci U S A 99: 15101–15106.
20. Emerenciano M, Meyer C, Mansur MB, Marschalek R, Pombo-de-Oliveira MS (2013) The distribution of MLL breakpoints correlates with outcome in infant acute leukaemia. Br J Haematol 161: 224–236.
21. Ghosh S, Bartenhagen C, Okpanyi V, Gombert M, Binder V, et al. (2013) Recurrent involvement of ring-type zinc finger genes in complex molecular rearrangements in childhood acute myelogeneous leukemia with translocation t(10;11)(p12;q23). Leukemia 27: 1745–1748.
22. Mori H, Colman SM, Xiao Z, Ford AM, Healy LE, et al. (2002) Chromosome translocations and covert leukemic clones are generated during normal fetal development. Proc Natl Acad Sci U S A 99: 8242–8247.
23. Lausten-Thomsen U, Hjalgrim H, Marquart H, Lutterodt M, Petersen BL, et al. (2008) ETV6-RUNX1 transcript is not frequent in early human haematopoiesis. Eur J Haematol 81: 161–162.
24. Lausten-Thomsen U, Madsen HO, Vestergaard TR, Hjalgrim H, Nersting J, et al. (2011) Prevalence of t(12;21)[ETV6-RUNX1]-positive cells in healthy neonates. Blood 117: 186–189.

10

Increased *P16* DNA Methylation in Mouse Thymic Lymphoma Induced by Irradiation

Wengang Song[1], Yongzhe Liu[2], Ying Liu[3], Cong Zhang[4], Bao Yuan[5], Lianbo Zhang[6]*, Shilong Sun[4]

1 Beihua University, Jinlin, China, 2 Department of Toxicology, School of Public Health, Tianjin Medical University, Tianjin, China, 3 Department of Toxicology, School of Public Health, Jilin University, Changchun, China, 4 Ministry of Health, Key Laboratory of Radiobiology, Jilin University, Changchun, China, National Laboratory of Medical Molecular Biology, Tsinghua University, Beijing, PR China, 5 College of Animal Sciences, Jilin University, Changchun, China, 6 Department of Plastic and Reconstructive Surgery, China-Japan Union Hospital of Jilin University, Changchun, China

Abstract

DNA methylation is an important part of epigenetics. In this study, we examined the methylation state of two CpG islands in the promoter of the *p16* gene in radiation-induced thymic lymphoma samples. The mRNA and protein levels of P16 were significantly reduced in radiation-induced thymic lymphoma tissue samples. Twenty-three CpG sites of the CpG islands in the *p16* promoter region were detected, and the methylation percentages of -71, -63, -239, -29, -38, -40, -23, 46 CpG sites were significantly higher in radiation-induced thymic lymphoma tissue samples than those in matched non-irradiated thymus tissue samples. This study provides new evidence for the methylation state of *p16* in the radiation-induced thymic lymphoma samples, which suggests that the methylation of these CpG sites in the *p16* promoter may reduce its expression in the thymic lymphoma after irradiation.

Editor: Dajun Deng, Peking University Cancer Hospital and Institute, China

Funding: This paper is supported by a grant from the National Science Foundation of China (No. 81372068) and the Science and Technology research projects of the Education Department of Jilin province. The funders had no role in study design, data collection and analysis, decision to publish, or preparation of the manuscript.

Competing Interests: The authors have declared that no competing interests exist.

* E-mail: doctorzhanglianbo@163.com

Introduction

Radiation, as a definite factor in carcinogenesis, has been widely investigated and studied, but the epigenetic regulation mechanisms of many radiation sensitive genes have not been clearly explored. The tumor suppressor gene *p16* (also known as CDKN2, INK4a, p14ARF, p19Arf, p16INK4, p16INK4a, and CDKN2A), located on chromosome 9p21, is the most commonly altered gene in human malignancies [1]. The *p16* gene encoding 148 amino acid protein contains 4 ankyrin repeats, and is a cell cycle regulator through inhibiting the G_1-S phase transition [2]. The *p16* (INK4a) protein acts as a cyclin-dependent kinase inhibitor (CDKI) that impedes the mitosis at G_1-S transition by inactivation of specific cyclin-protein kinase complexes including cyclin D1, CDK4, and CDK6. *p16* functions as an important tumor suppressor. The loss of *p16* activity through homologous deletion, point mutation, negative regulation of MicroRNAs (miRNAs) or methylation-induced promoter silencing, is a common step in tumor development and progression, which has been widely observed in cancer cell lines and many malignant tumors [3], including acute lymphoblastic leukemia, melanoma, pancreatic cancer, esophagus cancer, lung cancer, bladder cancer, and cervical cancer [4–7].

Cytosine methylation is a common form of epigenetic mechanism. CpG sites are the DNA regions where a cytosine nucleotide occurs next to a guanine nucleotide in the linear sequence of bases along its length. Cytosines in CpG dinucleotides can be methylated by DNA methyltransferases to form 5-methylcytosine. The regions in the genome with a higher concentration of CpG sites are named as CpG islands [8]. Many genes have CpG islands in their promoter regions from the upstream of the transcription start site to within the first exon [9]. DNA methylation in the promoter regions is associated with the down-regulation of some genes [10–12]. Many transcription factor binding sites have CpG dinucleotides, and methylation of these sites alters their binding to cognate transcription factors [11–13]. Methylation of CpG islands around transcription start sites (TSS) represses gene expression epigenetically and plays crucial roles in cell differentiation, development and pathogenesis [14]. However, the mechanistic insights for the role of DNA methylation in carcinogenesis are still unknown. Attempts to analyze the aberrant methylation and its extension patterns within CpG islands in carcinogenesis, especially in the radiation-induced carcinogenesis, have not been successfully achieved. Aberrant methylation of CpG islands is the main reason for *p16* inactivation in multiple human cancers. Aberrant *p16* methylation is an early event in carcinogenesis and has been shown to significantly increase the risk of malignant transformation of epithelial dysplasia in the stomach, oral cavity and other organs in many studies [15–17]. Although *p16* methylation is one of the well-studied epigenetic events [18–20], most of studies employed in vitro cell culture system. The methylation is not often detectable in tissue samples, especially in the radiation-induced carcinogenesis. In the present study, we studied the relationship between the natural methylation signatures of *p16* CpG islands in the *p16* gene promoter region (from 400 nucleotides upstream to 200 nucleotides downstream of the TSS) and thymic lymphomas.

Materials and Methods

Subjects and irradiation

Male wild-type BALB/c mice, 5–6 weeks of age, were purchased from Jilin university (Changchun, China). All mice were housed in a pathogen-free facility for all experiments. All efforts were made to minimize the number of animals used as well as their suffering. This study was carried out in strict accordance with the recommendations in the Guide for the Care and Use of Laboratory Animals of the National Institutes of Health. The protocol was approved by the Committee on the Ethics of Animal Experiments of the Jilin university (Permit Number: 2011034). All surgery was performed under sodium pentobarbital anesthesia, and all efforts were made to minimize suffering. A fraction of the mice (about 100) were left as controls. Other mice (about 100) were subjected to whole body irradiation split into four weekly sub-lethal doses of 1.75 Gy (Dose rate: 0.58 Gy/min) using a 4-MV linear accelerator (Clinac 4/100, Varian, Palo Alto, CA). Thymic lymphomas were observed to develop at regular intervals of up to 6 months and we find that in our experimental conditions, a global incidence of 43.51% was observed after 6 month (Figure 1A). Thymic lymphoma in mice has been extensively studied as a model of radiation induced carcinogenesis since it was first described by Kaplan et al. in 1953 [21]. Immunological markers and morphologic criteria of thymic lymphoma induced by irradiation have also been commonly described in many studies [22,23]. In our study, histopathology of thymic lymphoma showed that Thymus inherent structure was replaced by diffuse proliferative lymphoma cells compared with the normal thymus in our study (Figure 1B).

mRNA expression profile analysis by Illumina Bead Array and quantitative RT-PCR analysis

Total RNA was extracted from the thymic lymphoma tissue samples or thymus tissue samples using the TRIzol method according to the manufacturer's protocol. Labeling was achieved by use of the incorporation of biotin-16-UTP (Perkin Elmer Life and Analytical Sciences, Boston, MA) present at a ratio of 1:1 with unlabeled UTP. Labeled, amplified material (700 ng per array) was hybridized to a pilot version of the Illumina Sentrix Mouse-6 Expression BeadChip according to the Manufacturer's instructions (Illumina, Inc., San Diego, CA). Amersham fluorolink streptavidin-Cy3 (GE Healthcare Bio-Sciences, Little Chalfont, UK) following the BeadChip manual. Arrays were scanned with an Illumina Bead array Reader confocal scanner according to the Manufacturer's instructions. Array data processing and analysis were performed using Illumina Bead Studio software. More information can be obtained from the Web: http://www.illumina.com/.Total RNA was reverse transcribed to cDNA using Superscript II reverse transcriptase (Invitrogen) and oligonucleotide primers. Quantitative real-time PCR (RT-PCR) analysis of gene expression was performed in a 25 µl reaction volume containing cDNA, SYBR Premix Ex Taq (Takara Bio Inc., Shiga, Japan), TaqMan Universal PCR Master Mixture and primers for each gene.The primers for the *p16* gene were as follows: 5'-GCAGATTCGAACTGCGAG-3' (forward) and 5'-CAC-GATGTCTTGATGTCCC-3' (reverse); The β-actin was used as a reference gene and its PCR primers included: 5'-ATATCGCTGCGCTGGTCGTC-3' (forward) and 5'- AG-GAGTCCTTCTGACCCATTC -3' (reverse).The relative quantitative method was used for the quantitative analysis and fold change (FC) was used to present data.

Western blotting

Thymic lymphoma tissue samples induced by irradiation were harvested and lysed after 6 month; proteins were separated on a SDS/polyacrylamide gel and transferred into a PVDF membrane (Bio-Rad, Hercules, CA). After blocking, the membranes were incubated with the primary antibody, anti-P16 polyclonal antibody (Santa Cruz Biotechnology, Santa Cruz, CA). The membranes were extensively washed and incubated with a horseradish peroxidase conjugated secondary antibody (Bio-Rad). The antigen antibody complexes were visualized by West-Q-Chemiluminescent Sub Kit Plus (BIOTANG, Waltham, MA).

Isolation and bisulfite treatmentof thymus DNA

DNA was extracted from BALB/c mouse thymus using the Gentra Puregene kit (Qiagen GmbH, Hilden, Germany) according to the manufacturer's protocol. Determination of Percent Methylated Cytosine Genomic DNA (300 ng) was treated with sodium bisulfate using the EZ-96 DNA Methylation Kit D5004 (Zymo Research, Orange, CA) according to the manufacturer's protocol. The final bisulfite-treated DNA was eluted in 40 ml M-Elution Buffer. Primers for amplifying the upstream *p16* CpG island using bisulfite-treated DNA were designed using Methyl Primer Express v1.0 (Applied Biosystems, Foster City, CA) and Vector NTI Advance 10 (Invitrogen, Carlsbad, CA). Amplification was performed with 1 µl bisulfite-treated DNA, 1 µM of each primer (primer : 5'-GTTAAAGGGTGATTAGGTATGG-3' and :5'-ACCCCAACTTCCAACAATAC- 3', 250 µM each of dATP, dCTP, dGTP, and TTP, 50 µM KCl, 4 µM MgCl2, 0.625 U AmpliTaq Gold (Applied Biosystems), and 10 µM Tris-HCl (pH 8.3) in 50 µl. Amplification consisted of 5 min at 95°C, 40

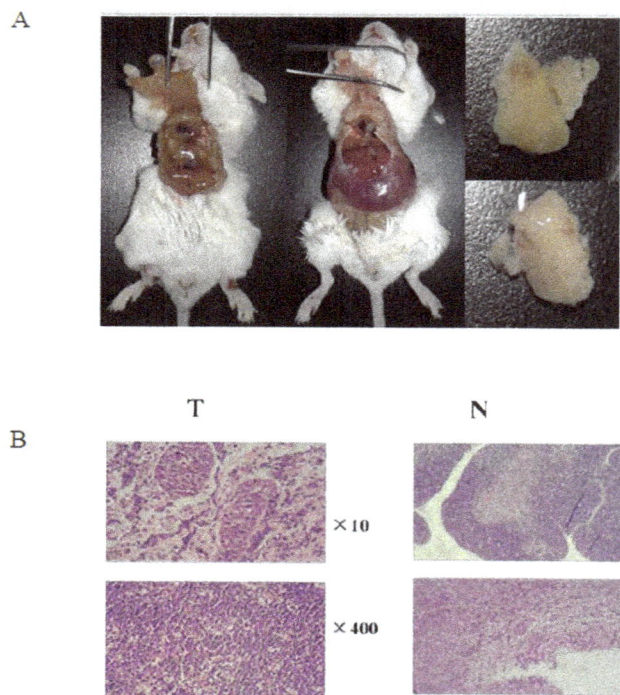

Figure 1. A. Gross image of a thymic lymphoma in a dissected mouse. B. Histological section of a thymic lymphoma stained with Hematoxylin and Eosin (H&E). N: normal control non-irradiated thymus tissue samples. T: radiation induced thymic lymphoma tissue samples.

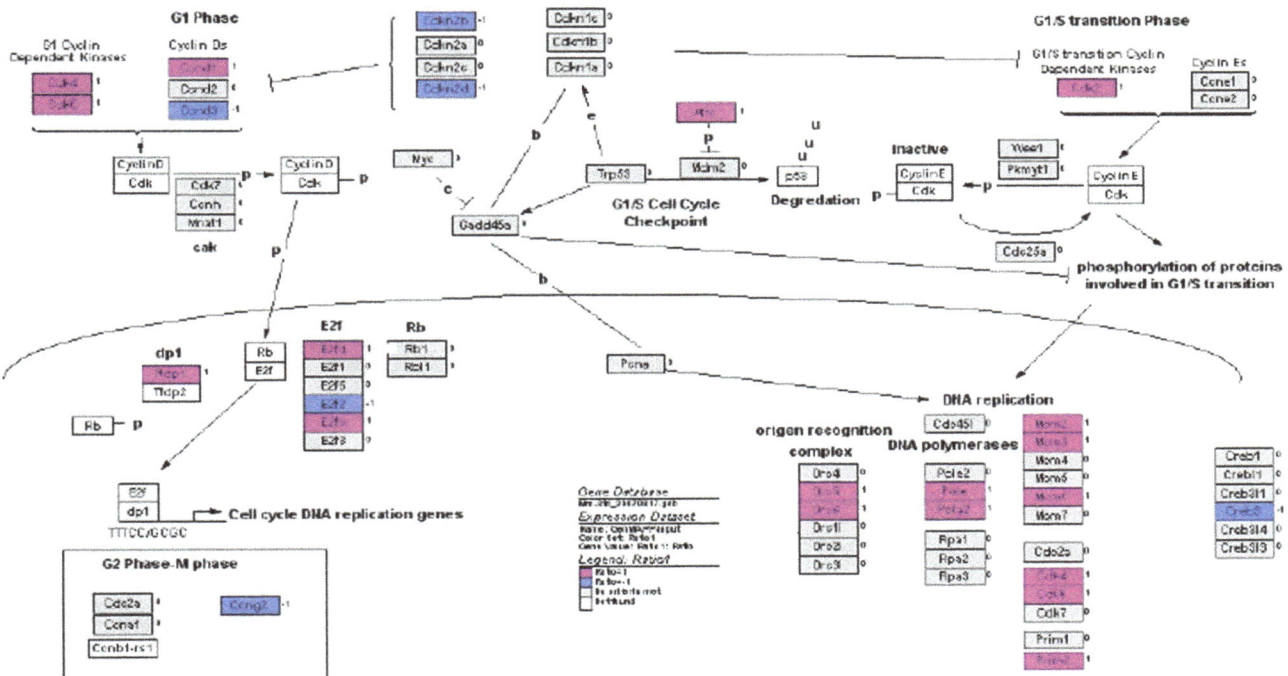

Figure 2. Analysis of mRNA expression profile by the Illumina Sentrix Mouse-6 Expression BeadChip in G1/S cell cycle. Blue: expression down-regulated; Pink: expression up-regulated.

cycles of 15 sat 95°C, 15 s at 52°C, and 30 s at 72°C, followed by a final elongation step at 72°C for 7 min.

Cloning of PCR Fragments and Sequencing

Amplified DNA fragments, 474 bp in size, were cloned using the TA Cloning Kit into the pCRII plasmid (Invitrogen).The

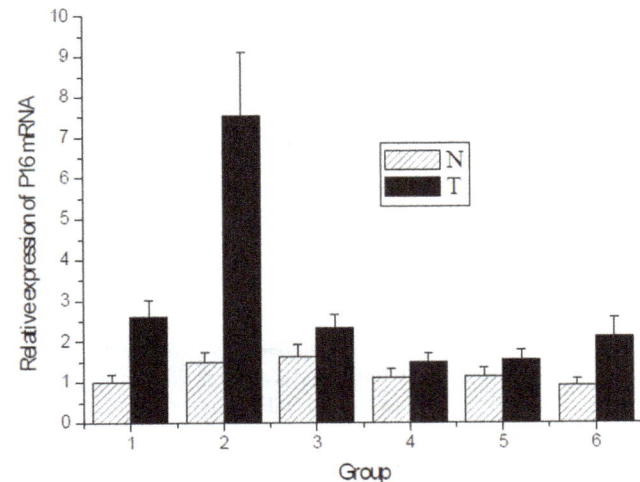

Figure 3. Quantitative RT-PCR analysis of *P*16 mRNA expression in thymic lymphoma tissue samples radiation induced irradiation and normal control non-irradiated thymus tissue samples. N: normal control non-irradiated thymus tissue samples. T: radiation induced thymic lymphoma tissue samples. (T vs N, $P<0.05$).

amplicons were cloned into the PCR-blunt vector, transformed into E. coli, and sequenced using an ABI 3730 Analyzer. At least 6clones were then randomly selected and sequenced for each sample. To demonstrate the initiation and extension of de novo methylation of *p16* CpG islands, the methylation status of each clone was analyzed as a independent variable. There are23 tested CpG sites in the promoter region of *p16* gene.

Sequence Analysis

The amplified region of *p16* was analyzed for predicted transcription factor-binding sites using Transcription Element Search System (TESS; Schug and Overton, 1977).

Statistical analysis

All the statistical tests were performed using the SPSS for Windows 11.0 software package (SPSS, Chicago, IL,USA), including descriptive statistics, t- test, the Chi-square test and one-way analysis of variance (ANOVA). The significant level was set at a P-value of <0.05.

Result

p16 is down-regulated in radiation-induced thymic lymphoma tissues

The mRNA expression of tumor suppressor gene *p16* in radiation-induced thymic lymphoma tissues and normal non-irradiated thymus tissue samples was examined by qRT-PCR analysis, while the mRNA expression profiles in two groups were analyzed by microarray. Of 45000 mouse genes in the microarray, we found 2876 genes showed significantly different expression between radiation-induced thymic lymphoma samples and normal non-irradiated thymus samples. The expression patterns of *p16* are

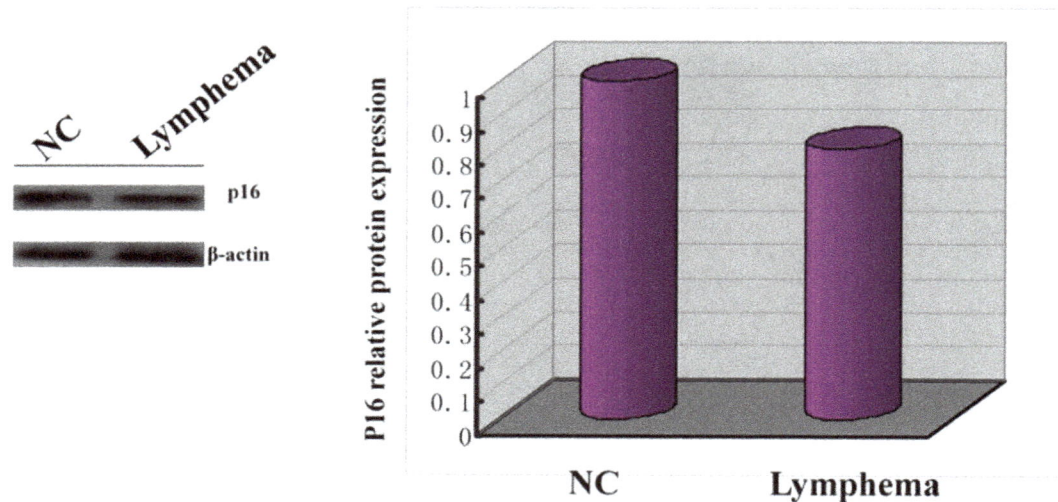

Figure 4. Reduced of *P*16 protein expression in thymic lymphoma induced by irradiation.

shown in the G_1-S pathway (Figure 2), and the important results of microarray were given in Table 1 in detail. We detected the mRNA expression of *p16* in 6 tissue samples from both groups (Figure 3). Moreover, *p16* mRNA expression level was significantly lower in the radiation-induced thymic lymphoma tissue samples compared with matched normal non-irradiated thymus tissue samples. P16 protein expression in both groups was examined by western blot, we found that P16 protein expression level was significantly lower in the radiation-induced thymic lymphoma tissues than that in matched normal non-irradiated thymus tissues (Figure 4).

The methylation pattern in the promoter of the *p16* gene

We also examined the methylation state of CpG islands in the *p16* promoter. Two CpG islands were found from 400 nucleotides upstream to 200 nucleotides downstream of the *p16* TSS (Figure 5A). The CpG islands were located from nucleotides −355 to78 (relative to the A of the ATG translation start site). We identified 23 CpG dinucleotides located at nucleotides of −355, −342, −331, −320, −309, −268, −239, −174, −162, −71, −63, −55, −40, −38, −29, −23, 9, 32, 35, 46, 57, 61 and 78 in the *p16* gene promoter. To test the methylation state of a CpG island in the *p16* promoter, DNA samples from both groups were treated with bisulfite to convert unmethylated cytosines to uracil and leave methylated cytosines unmodified. The region containing two CpG islands was amplified by PCR, cloned into T vector, and sequenced. The methylation pattern of CpG islands in the *p16* promoter was shown in Figure 5B. By using the Chi-square test, we found that the methylation percentages of −71, −63, −239, −29, −38, −40, −23, 46 CpG sites were significantly higher in radiation-induced thymic lymphoma tissue samples compared with matched control non-irradiated thymus tissue samples (P<0.05, P<0.01, Figure 5). The highest methylation was at the −29 CpG site.

Discussion

Ionizing-radiation-induced leukemogenesis and lymphomagenesis is a complex process involving both genetic and epigenetic changes [24]. Ionizing radiation induces genomic instability, which is mainly characterized as cell necrosis, chromosomal aberration, increased apoptosis, micronucleus formation, changes in gene expression, and abnormal DNA methylation [25,26]. Currently, the genetic changes have been clarified by several studies, whereas the studies on epigenetic changes have recently been carried out due to the limitations in detection technology. DNA methylation is an important part of epigenetics. Extensive genomic hypomethylation, hypomethylation of CpG islands in the promoter region of oncogenes, and hypermethylation of CpG

Table 1. Data of mRNA expression with significant difference in G_1/S cell cycle by the Illumina Sentrix Mouse-6 Expression Bead Chip.

Gene	N.AVG_Signal	T.AVG_Signal	Differnt Score	Differnt Ratio
Cdk4	2480.164	6887.145	63.27042	2.776891
Cdk6	47.29345	220.5876	39.11695	4.664231
Cdkn2b	304.7015	75.08892	−38.45883	0.2464344
Cdkn2d	2720.639	709.1175	−55.01941	0.2606437
Cdk2	3130.801	5331.355	29.05482	1.702872
Atm	300.9656	626.6469	22.72435	2.082121
E2f2	7689.074	3044.281	−36.05586	0.395923
E2f4	1116.279	1935.731	24.09156	1.734093
E2f6	1321.134	2664.024	27.10226	2.016467
Ccnd1	881.3447	2146.841	56.64333	2.43587
Ccnd3	10626.85	4594.292	−29.83043	0.4323286
Tfdp1	4279.905	7409.138	25.3472	1.731146
Pola2	1227.237	2374.903	36.0864	1.935163
Pole	176.3562	360.9415	21.78839	2.046663
Orc5l	1144.603	1950.801	26.35427	1.704348
Orc6l	3755.128	8224.204	35.02106	2.190126
Mcm2	3782.601	6463.503	26.67579	1.708746
Mcm3	1091.692	1804.522	22.5774	1.65296
Mcm6	1852.818	3947.626	24.63652	2.130607

N: normal control non-irradiated thymus tissue samples. T: radiation induced thymic lymphoma tissue samples.

(A) , (B) and (C)

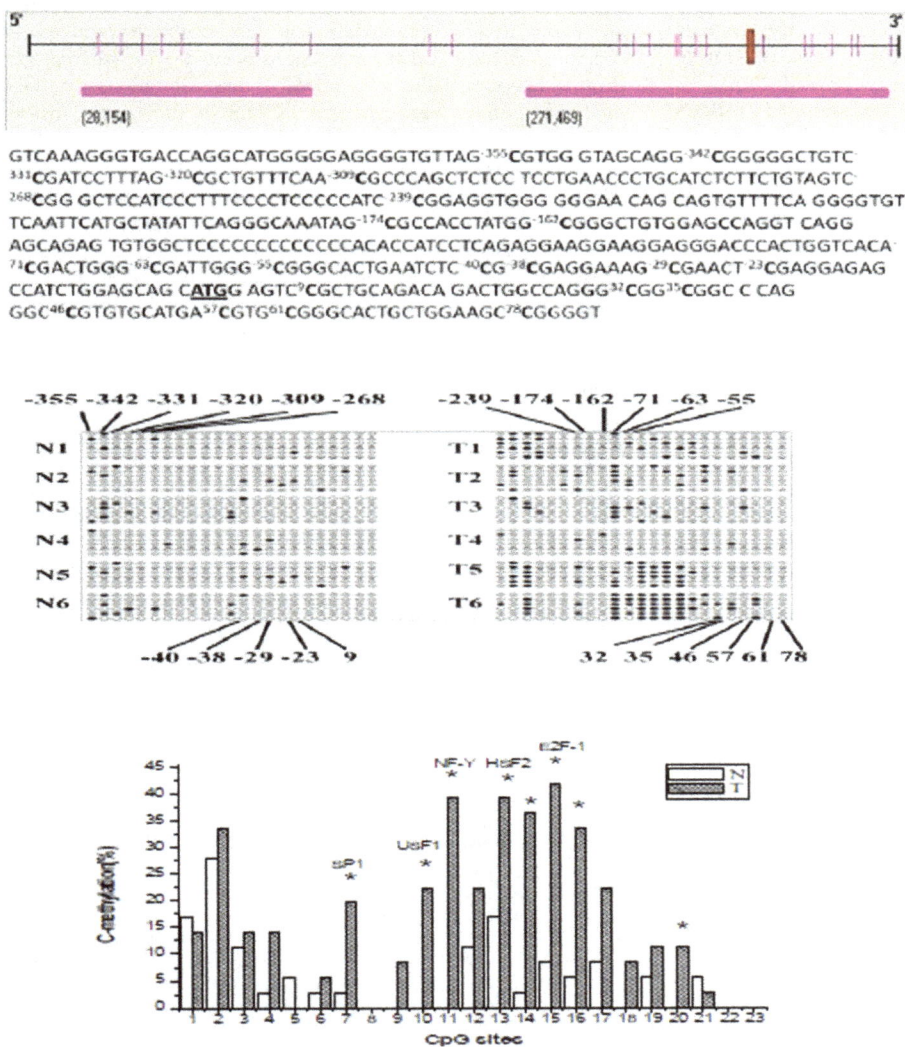

Figure 5. The P16 promoter region and Methylation at the 23 CpG sites. (A) Schematic of the P16 gene promoter region (from 400 nucleotides upstream to 200 nucleotides downstream of the transcription start site) is presented in the upper diagram. The two CpG islands are boxed. The CpG dinucleotides are indicated as |. The major transcription start site is located at −355 upstream to 78 downstream of the ATG translation start site. The 16 CpG sites analyzed for cytosine methylation (bold) with their position relative to the A (chr4: NC_000070, 12509) of the ATG translation start site (underlined) are indicated. (B) Analysis of cloned amplified bisulfite-treated DNA from 6 pairs of radiation induced carcinogenesis tissue samples and normal control non-irradiated thymus tissues. Solid circles are methylated CpG sites. The location of these sites is shown relative to their location in the amplified P16 region. (C) Percent methylation of 16 CpG dinucleotides in the p16 promoter region. CpG sites in Sp1, USF-1, NF-Y, HSF2 and E2F-1 binding sites are indicated. *$p < 0.05$. The numbers 1 to 23 represented 23 methylation sites sequentially (−355 to 78). N: normal control non-irradiated thymus tissue samples. T: radiation induced thymic lymphoma tissue samples.

islands in the promoter region of the tumor suppressor genes are frequent in hematological malignancies caused by radiotherapy, or in other tumors. It has been suggested that the change in DNA methylation status plays an important role in the process of tumor occurrence and development [27].

The fate of cells is tightly controlled by a series of cytokines, of which CDK4 is the key enzyme controlling the process of G₁ phase. CDK4 activity is regulated by P16 protein encoded by *p16* gene. P16 protein prevents cell S phase entry by specifically inhibiting CDK4 and inducing cell cycle arrest, thus *p16* acts as a tumor suppressor gene. Once P16 is inactivated, cell growth is accelerated and proliferation becomes abnormal, eventually leading to tumorigenesis [28]. Methylation of CpG islands in the

promoter region of tumor suppressor genes is one of the important factors for the inactivation of tumor suppressor genes. It is involved in the occurrence and development of a variety of tumors [29]. Previous studies revealed that *p16* gene hypermethylation plays an important role in the development of a variety of tumors [30–32]. The changes in *p16* gene methylation status in radiation-induced tumorigenesis have not widely been investigated, although the changes in *p16* gene methylation status may be important in the process of ionizing-radiation-induced tumorigenesis. In contrast, Kovalchuk et al. showed that methylation in the promoter of *p16* was increased significantly in the normal liver tissues of mice exposed acute and chronic low dose irradiation [33]. Our study tended to find the changes of every single CpG point in the promoter of *p16* in the process of ionizing-radiation-induced tumorigenesis. When the methylation rate is increased, the affinity of the gene-transcription-factor binding sites for the cognate transcription factor is reduced, thus the gene transcription is inhibited and the protein expression level is decreased [34].

Our study showed that 6 months after irradiation, *p16* mRNA and protein levels in the mouse thymocytes were significantly inhibited compared with control group. P16 protein expression levels in thymic lymphoma cells were downregulated. Twenty-three CpG sites of the CpG islands in the promoter region of *p16* gene were identified. DNA methylation at -71, -63, -239, -29, -38, -40, -23 and 46 CpG sites in thymic lymphoma cells was significantly increased after irradiation, but there was no significant change at other sites. DNA sequence analysis using TESS software showed that the -239, -40, -71, -63 and -38 CpG sites corresponded to the binding sites for transcription factors SP1, HSF2, USF1, NF-Y and E2F- 1, respectively. Increased methylation at the -239, -40, -71, -63 and -38 sites in the *p16* promoter region may inhibit the binding of corresponding transcription factors to the transcription factor binding sites of the promoter region, and then down regulate *p16* gene and protein expression. Thus, the inhibitory effect of P16 protein on the cell cycle is reduced and cell proliferation is uncontrolled, and thus eventually leads to tumorigenesis. The *p16* promoter region CpG islands hypermethylation of mouse liver tissue could be induced by low dose whole body irradiation [33]. At the same time, in many studies of radiation, hypermethylation of promoter region and hypomethylationof global DNA could be induced by irradiation in many cell lines including normal cell lines [35–37]. These studies provided important information on alterations in DNA methylation as one of the determinants of radiation effects, which may be associated with altered gene expression, especially *p16* gene. Since alterations in DNA methylation have also emerged as one of the most consistent molecular alterations in cancer, these data also suggest the possibility that radiation-induced carcinogenic risk might be affected by complicated DNA methylation. Combined with the results, we concluded that the *p16* promoter region CpG islands hypermethylation is one of the important epigenetic changes in tumorigenesis of mouse thymus caused by radiation. However, further studies are needed to analyse and detect the initiation factors under the influence of above five CpG sites, and to explore the effects of CpG island hypermethylation in the *p16* gene promoter region on ionizing-radiation-induced tumorigenesis.

Acknowledgments

The authors thank members of the Laboratory of National Laboratory of Medical Molecular Biology, Institute of Basic Medical Sciences, Chinese Academy of Medical Sciences for discussions and Q Xu for help and discussions.

Author Contributions

Conceived and designed the experiments: LZ. Performed the experiments: WS Ying Liu BY CZ. Analyzed the data: SS Yongzhe Liu. Contributed reagents/materials/analysis tools: LZ SS. Wrote the paper: SS.

References

1. Hirama T, Koeffler HP (1995): Role of the cyclin-dependent kinase inhibitors in the development of cancer. Blood 86(3):841–854.
2. Serrano M, Hannon G, Beach D (1993) A new regulatory motif in cell-cyclecontrol causing specific inhibition of cyclin D/CDK4. Nature 366: 704–707.
3. Silva SD, Nonogaki S, Soares FA, Kowalski LP (2012) p16 (INK4a) has clinicopathological and prognostic impact on oropharynx and larynx squamous cell carcinoma. Braz J Med Biol Res 45(12):1327–33.
4. Smith EM, Rubenstein LM, Hoffman H, Haugen TH, Turek LP (2010) Human papillomavirus, p16 and p53 expression associated with survival of head and neck cancer. Infect Agent Cancer 5: 4.
5. Rother J, Jones D (2009) Molecular markers of tumor progression in melanoma. Curr Genomics 10: 231–239.
6. Salam I, Hussain S, Mir MM, Dar NA, Abdullah S, et al. (2009) Aberrant promoter methylation and reduced expression of p16 gene in esophageal squamous cell carcinoma from Kashmir valley: a high-risk area. Mol Cell Biochem 332: 51–58.
7. Attaleb M, El hamadani W, Khyatti M, Benbacer L, Benchekroun N, et al. (2009) Status of p16 (INK4a) and E-cadherin gene promoter methylation in Moroccan patients with cervical carcinoma. Oncol Res 18: 185–192.
8. Francisco Antequera, Adrian Bird (1993) Number of CpG islands and genes in human and mouse. PNAS 90(24):11995–9.
9. Gardiner-Garden M, Frommer M (1987) CpG islands in vertebrate genomes. J Mol Biol 196(2):261–82.
10. Jaenisch R, Bird A (2003) Epigenetic regulation of gene expression: how the genome integrates intrinsic and environmental signals. Nat Genet Suppl:245–54.
11. Douet V, Heller MB, Le Saux O (2007) DNA methylation and Sp1 binding determine the tissue-specific transcriptional activity of the mouse Abcc6 promoter. Biophys Res Commun 354(1):66–71.
12. Michelotti GA, Brinkley DM, Morris DP, Smith MP, Louie RJ, et al. (2007) Epigenetic regulation of human alpha1d-adrenergic receptor gene expression: a role for DNA methylation in Sp1-dependent regulation. FASEB 21(9):1979–93.
13. Alikhani-Koopaei R, Fouladkou F, Frey FJ, Frey BM (2004) Epigenetic regulation of 11 beta-hydroxysteroid dehydrogenase type 2 expression. J Clin Invest 114(8):1146–57.
14. Lu ZM, Zhou J, Wang X, Guan Z, Bai H, et al. (2012) Nucleosomes correlate with in vivo progression pattern of de novo methylation of p16 CpG islands in human gastric carcinogenesis. PLoS One 7(4):e35928.
15. Bai H, Gu LK, Zhou J, Deng DJ (2003) p16 hypermethylation during gastric carcinogenesis of Wistar rats by N-methyl-N9-nitro-N-nitrosoguanidine. Mutation Research-Genetic Toxicology and Environmental Mutagenesis 535: 73–78.
16. Sun Y, Deng DJ, You WC, Bai H, Zhang L, et al. (2004) Methylation of p16 CpG islands associated with malignant transformation of gastric dysplasia in a population-based study. Clinical Cancer Research 10: 5087–5093.
17. Cao J, Zhou J, Gao Y, Gu LK, Meng HX, et al. (2009) Methylation of p16 CpG Island Associated with Malignant Progression of Oral Epithelial Dysplasia: A Prospective Cohort Study. Clinical Cancer Research 15: 5178–5183.
18. Deng DJ, Li QA, Wang XH (2010) Methylation and demethylation of Ink4 locus in cancer development. Chinese Journal of Cancer Research 22: 245–252.
19. Li Q, Wang X, Lu Z, Zhang B, Guan Z, et al. (2010) Polycomb CBX7 Directly Controls Trimethylation of Histone H3 at Lysine 9 at the p16 Locus. PLoS ONE 5: e13732.
20. Hinshelwood RA, Melki JR, Huschtscha LI, Paul C, Song JZ, et al. (2009) Aberrant de novo methylation of the p16INK4A CpG island is initiated post gene silencing in association with chromatin remodelling and mimics nucleosome positioning. Hum Mol Genet 18: 3098–3109.
21. Kaplan HS, Brown MB, Paull J (1953) Influence of post irradiation thymectomy and of thymic implants on lymphoid tumor incidence in C57BL mice. Cancer Res 13(9):677–80.
22. Pattengale PK, Frith CH (1983) Immunomorphologic classification of spontaneous lymphoid cell neoplasms occurring in female BALB/c mice. J Nat Cancer Inst 70:169–179.
23. Pattengale P, Leder A, Kuo A, Stewart T, Leder P (1986) Lymphohematopoietic and other malignant neoplasms occurring spontaneously in transgenic mice carrying and expressing MTV/myc fusion genes. Curr Topics Microbiol Immunol 132:9–16.
24. Koturbash I, Pogribny I, Kovalchuk O (2005) Stable loss of global DNA methylation in the radiation-target tissue—A possible mechanism contributing to radiation carcinogenesis? Biochem Biophys Res Commun 337(2): 526–33.
25. Mosesso P, Palitti F, Pepe G, Piñero J, Bellacima R, et al. (2010) Relationship between chromatin structure, DNA damage and repair following X-irradiation of human lymphocytes. Muta Res 701(1): 86–91
26. Kaup S, Grandjean V, Mukherjee R, Kapoor A, Keyes E, et al. (2006) Grandjean V, Mukherjee R, et al. Radiation-induced genomic instability is associated with DNA methylation changes in cultured human keratinocytes. Mutat Res 597(1–2): 87–97.
27. Voso MT, D'Alò F, Greco M, Fabiani E, Criscuolo M, et al. (2010) Epigenetic changes in therapy-related MDS/AML. Chem Biol Interact 184 (1–2):46–9.
28. Feng Z, Chen J, Wei H, Gao P, Shi J, et al. (2011) The risk factor of gallbladder cancer: Hyperplasia of mucous epithelium caused by gallstones associates withp16/CyclinD1/CDK4 pathway. Exp Mol Pathol 91(2): 569–77.
29. Das PM, Singal R (2004) DNA Methylation and Cancer. J Clin Oncol 22(22): 4632–42.

30. Shim YH, Yoon GS, Choi HJ, Chung YH, Yu E (2003) p16 Hypermethylation in the early stage of hepatitis B virus- associated hepatocarcinogenesis. Cancer lett 190(2): 213–9.
31. Vidaurreta M, Maestro ML, Sanz-Casla MT, Maestro C, Rafael S, et al. (2008) Inactivation of p16 by CpG hypermethylation in renal cell carcinoma. Urol Oncol 2008, 26(3): 239–45.
32. Sharma G, Mirza S, Prasad CP, Srivastava A, Gupta SD, et al. (2007) Promoter hypermethylation of p16INK4A, p14ARF, CyclinD2 and Slit2 in serum and tumor DNA from breast cancer patients. Life Sci 80(20): 1873–81.
33. Kovalchuk O, Burke P, Besplug J, Slovack M, Filkowski J, et al. (2004) Methylation changes in muscle and liver tissues of male and female mice exposed to acute and chronic low-dose X-ray-irradiation. Mutat Res 14;548(1–2):75–84.
34. Nielsen DA, Yuferov V, Hamon S, Jackson C, Ho A, et al. (2009) Increased OPRM1 DNA methylation in lymphocytes of methadone-maintained former heroin addicts. Neuropsychopharmacology 34(4):867–73.
35. Kumar A, Rai PS, Upadhya R, Vishwanatha, Prasada KS, et al. (2011) γ-radiation induces cellular sensitivity and aberrant methylation in human tumor cell lines. Int J RadiatBiol 87(11):1086–96.
36. Goetz W, Morgan MN, Baulch JE (2011) The effect of radiation quality on genomic DNA methylation profiles in irradiated human cell lines. RadiatRes 175(5):575–87.
37. Krakowczyk L, Blamek S, Strzelczyk JK, Plachetka A, Maciejewski A, et al. (2010) Effects of X-ray irradiation on methylation levels of p16, MGMT and APC genes in sporadic colorectal carcinoma and corresponding normal colonic mucosa. Med SciMonit 16(10):469–74

11

Rapid Detection of *DNMT3A* R882 Mutations in Hematologic Malignancies using a Novel Bead-Based Suspension Assay with BNA(NC) Probes

Velizar Shivarov[1]*[9], Milena Ivanova[2][9], Elissaveta Naumova[2]

1 Laboratory of Hematopathology and Immunology, National Hematology Hospital, Sofia, Bulgaria, **2** Department of Clinical Immunology, Alexandrovska University Hospital, Medical University, Sofia, Bulgaria

Abstract

Mutations in the human DNA methyl transferase 3A (*DNMT3A*) gene are recurrently identified in several hematologic malignancies such as Philadelphia chromosome-negative myeloproliferative neoplasms (MPN), myelodysplastic syndromes (MDS), MPN/MDS overlap syndromes and acute myeloid leukemia (AML). They have been shown to confer worse prognosis in some of these entities. Notably, about 2/3 of these mutations are missense mutations in codon R882 of the gene. We aimed at the development and validation of a novel easily applicable in routine practice method for quantitative detection of the *DNMT3A* p.R882C/H/R/S mutations bead-based suspension assay. Initial testing on plasmid constructs showed excellent performance of BNA(NC)-modified probes with an optimal hybridization temperature of 66°C. The method appeared to be quantitative and showed sensitivity of 2.5% for different mutant alleles, making it significantly superior to direct sequencing. The assay was further validated on plasmid standards at different ratios between wild type and mutant alleles and on clinical samples from 120 patients with known or suspected myeloid malignancies. This is the first report on the quantitative detection of *DNMT3A* R882 mutations using bead-based suspension assay with BNA(NC)-modified probes. Our data showed that it could be successfully implemented in the diagnostic work-up for patients with myeloid malignancies, as it is rapid, easy and reliable in terms of specificity and sensitivity.

Editor: Ken Mills, Queen's University Belfast, United Kingdom

Funding: This work was supported financially by Project ID_09_157 (Contract 5/16.12.2009) from the National Science Fund, Bulgaria. The funders had no role in study design, data collection and analysis, decision to publish, or preparation of the manuscript.

Competing Interests: The authors have declared that no competing interests exist.

* E-mail: vshivarov@abv.bg

[9] These authors contributed equally to this work.

Introduction

Somatic mutations in the DNA methyltransferase 3A (DNMT3A) gene have been reported as recurrently associated with myeloid malignancies. The frequency of mutations varies between different entities. In adult acute myeloid leukemia (AML) *DNMT3A* mutations are found in 14–34% of cases from different series [1], 5–15% of MDS cases [2], 10% of chronic myelomonocytic leukemia (CMML) patients [3], 5.7% of primary myelofibrosis (PMF) patients [4], 12% of cases with systemic mastocytosis [5] and about 18% of T cell acute lymphoblastic leukemia (T-ALL) cases [6]. Approximately 2/3 of the *DNMT3A* are missense mutations at codon R882 [7]. Most of the current literature supports the notion that the presence of *DNMT3A* mutations is an adverse prognosis biomarker at least in adult AML and may be an important parameter of the integral molecular genetics profiling in these patients [8,9,10]. These lines of evidence necessitate the development of methods for reliable detection of *DNMT3A* mutations that are easily applicable and affordable for routine use together with the testing for other mutations. The most frequently reported techniques used for *DNMT3A* mutations include direct sequencing, high-resolution melting analysis and next generation sequencing. Sanger sequencing is particularly well-established technique [7,11] for the identification of previously unreported mutations but its relatively low sensitivity (~10–20% mutant allele burden) may be problematic for detection of low frequency somatic mutations. High resolution melting (HRM) technique has also been adapted for detection of *DNMT3A* mutations and is also good for screening for unknown mutations in a single tube format with a sensitivity of about 4% [12,13]. However, it requires well-established standards and eventually verification of the result through direct sequencing. Targeted amplicon resequencing on next generation sequencing (NGS) platforms has also been used for *DNMT3A* mutations [14,15]. The obvious advantages of NGS as the digital allele burden output, theoretically very high sensitivity, the possibility for identification of novel mutations are currently limited by the costly equipment and the necessity for a strong bioinformatic support. Simple approaches such as restriction fragment length polymorphism (RFLP) based assay have also been developed [16], whose relatively low sensitivity could be overcome by coupling with quantitative PCR (qPCR)[17]. Another less frequently used technique for verification of *DNMT3A* mutations confirmation

Table 1. Primary sequence of the tested oligonucleotides and the predicted melting temperatures (Tm).

Modification	Probe designation/Codon change	Sequence	Tm
LNA	WT (CGC)	5'-CGCCAAGCGGCTCAT-3'	68°C
	R882C (CGC->TGC)	5'-CGCCAAGCAGCTCAT-3'	66°C
	R882H (CGC->CAC)	5'-CGCCAAGTGGCTCAT-3'	66°C
	R882P (CGC->CCC)	5'-CGCCAAGGGGCTCAT-3'	67°C
	R882S (CGC->AGC)	5'-CGCCAAGCTGCTCAT-3'	66°C
BNA(NC)	WT (CGC)	5'-CGCCA+AGCG+GCTCATGTT-3'	70°C
	R882C (CGC->TGC)	5'-CGCC+A+AGCAG+CTC+ATGTT-3'	70°C
	R882H (CGC->CAC)	5'-CGCC+A+AGTG+GCTC+ATGTT-3'	70°C
	R882P (CGC->CCC)	5'-CGCCA+AGGGG+CTCATGTT-3'	70°C
	R882S (CGC->AGC)	5'-CGCC+A+AGCTG+CTC+ATGTT-3'	70°C

The character "+N" denotes the position of any BNA(NC) modified nucleotide. The positions of LNA modification are proprietary property of Exiqon, Denmark and are, therefore, not disclosed.

was denaturing high-performance liquid chromatography (DHPLC) [18].

In our view a particularly suitable for routine diagnostics could be the detection of somatic mutations in hematologic malignancies using a microsphere-based suspension array. It allows single tube quantitative detection of mutations in one or several amplicons in a mid-throughput format, making it a rapid and affordable method. Here we report the development and validation of a sensitive multiplexed bead-based suspension assay for quantitative detection of *DNMT3A* R882 mutations. The method appeared to be applicable to clinical samples from patients with myeloid malignancies.

Materials and Methods

Ethics statement

The study was conducted in accordance with the principles of the Declaration of Helsinki. Written informed consent was obtained from all patients. Blood and bone marrow sampling as well as molecular testing were part of the routine diagnostic procedures approved by the Institutional Review Board (IRB) at Alexandrovska University Hospital, Sofia, Bulgaria.

Patients

A total of 120 peripheral blood or bone marrow samples of consecutive patients with known or suspected myeloid malignancies were collected between January 2010 and June 2013. Patients were classified according to the WHO criteria as follows: Acute myeloid leukemia (AML) (n = 21), Chronic myeloid leukemia (CML) (n = 1), Myelodysplastic syndrome (MDS) (n = 6), Myeloproliferative neoplasm (MPN) (n = 81), Overlap MPN/MDS (n = 5), and others with suspected but unproven MPN (n = 6).

DNA extraction

All samples were collected using sodium citrate-containing blood sampling tubes (BD Biosciences) and stored at room temperature for no more than 4 hours before processing. Genomic DNA was extracted from whole blood using a iPrep (Invitrogen) automated system. Genomic DNA samples were stored at −20°C before further analyses.

DNMT3A exon 23 sequencing

Exon 23 of the human *DNMT3A* gene was amplified from genomic DNA as reported before [5] using the following primers: DNMT3A (forward): 5'-TCCTGCTGTGTGGTTAGACG and DNMT3A (reverse): 5'-ACAGAAAACCCCTCTGAAAAG. Amplification in 25 µl reactions included the following: 100 ng genomic DNA; 1.5 U Taq polymerase (Invitrogen); 3 mM $MgCl_2$; 0.2 mM dNTP mixture; and 10 pmol of each primer. The amplification conditions were as follows: 95°C for 5 min; 35 cycles of 95°C for 30 sec, 58°C for 40 sec, 72°C for 2 min and final extension at 72°C for 10 min. PCR products were purified using Exo-SAP (Applied Biosystems, USA) and sequenced bidirectionally with the same set of primers. The sequencing reaction was performed in a final volume of 10 µL using 2 µL of the purified PCR product, 3.2 pmol of one the primers and 2 µL of Big Dye terminator cycle-sequencing kit v3.1 (Applied Biosystems, USA). The sequencing program was 25 cycles of denaturation at 96°C for 10 s, annealing at 50°C for 5 s and extension at 60°C for 4 min. The sequence detection was conducted using the ABI Prism 3100 Genetic Analyzer (Applied Biosystems, USA). Sequences alignment and analysis were performed using Sequencher v. 5.0. (GeneCodes, USA).

Bead-based assay

The bead-based assay was performed as described before [19,20,21]. Briefly, the exon 23 *DNMT3A* fragment was amplified from either genomic or plasmid DNA samples using a 5'-botinylated forward primer. The same primers and PCR conditions as described above for the sequencing analysis were applied. Genotyping was performed by direct hybridization with 5 LNA- or BNA(NC)-modified oligonucleotide probes, specific for the wild type or the mutant alleles. LNA-modified oligonucleotides were designed and synthesized by Exiqon, Denmark, and the BNA(NC)-modified oligonucleotides were designed by us and synthesized by BioSynthesis, USA. The sequences and the melting temperatures (Tm) of all oligonucleotides are shown in Table 1. All probes were synthesized with 5'-amino group and 20 bases as a spacer sequence for the purpose of covalent binding to the carboxylated microspheres (Luminex, USA). The coupling of the amine modified probe to the carboxylated surface of the beads was performed using a standard carbodiimine-coupling procedure [22]. Mixtures of 5 sets of coupled microspheres were prepared by

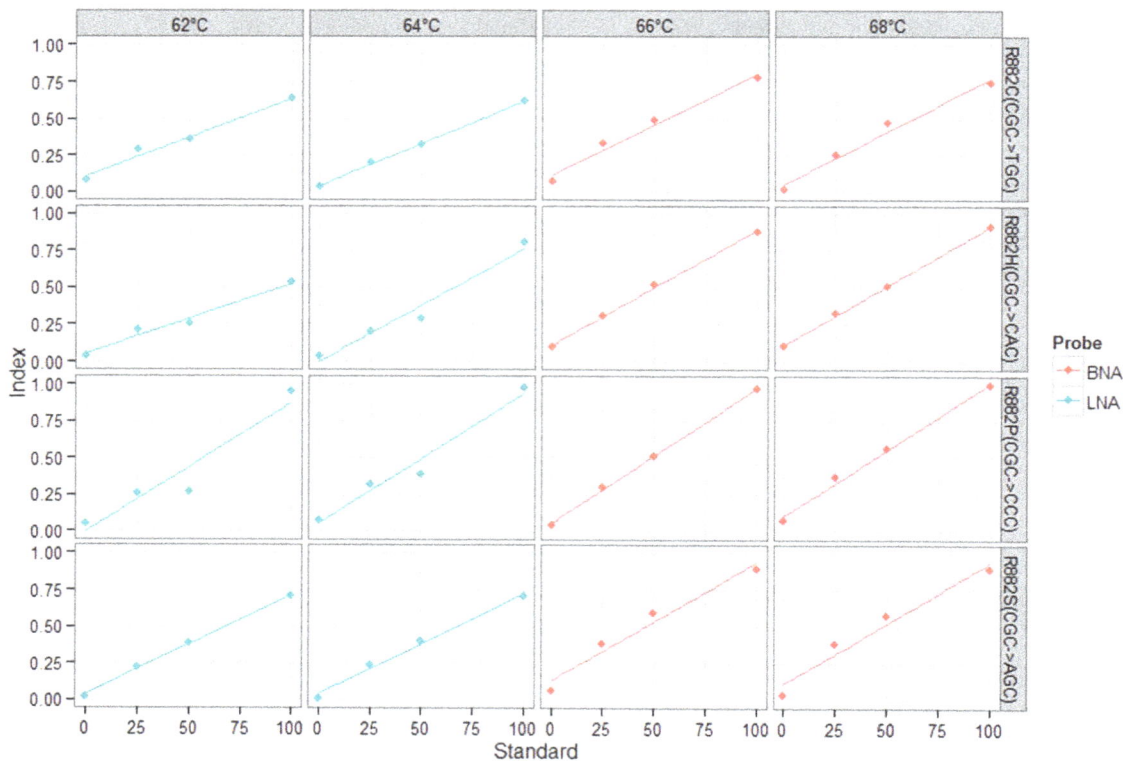

Figure 1. Fitted linear standard curves from the test assays for determination of the best performing probe set and the optimal hybridization temperature.

combining equal volumes of each set of the microspheres. Approximately, 160 beads of each type/µl were used for the analysis of one sample. Five µl of PCR product; 20 µl Hybridization buffer (Wakunaga Pharmaceuticals, Japan); 3 µl Bead mixture and 2 µl of streptavidin-phycoerythrine (SAPE) (Wakunaga Pharmaceuticals, Japan) were combined per well of a 96-well Thermowell plate and hybridization was performed at 62°C, 64°C, 66°C or 68°C for 30 min in a thermocycler (Applied Biosystems, USA). After incubation, 75 µl Washing buffer (Wakunaga Pharmaceuticals, Japan) were added to each well. The supernatants were removed after plate centrifugation at 4000 rpm for 2 min. Finally, the microspheres were resuspended in 75 µl Washing buffer (Wakunaga Pharmaceuticals, Japan) and acquired on a LabScan^{200} flow platform (Luminex, USA). A minimum of 100 events per bead region of interest was collected. For each set of reactions a background control of a sample containing only the respective sets of microspheres was included. The background median fluorescence intesity (MFI) values were subtracted from the MFI values for each sample. The resulting values were used for the calculation of the relative fluorescence indices for each mutant allele according to the following equation: Index (mutant allele$_i$) = MFI (mutant allele$_i$)/[MFI (mutant allele$_1$) + … +MFI (mutant allele$_4$) + MFI (wild type allele)].

Determination of the cut-off index values of the assay

Sensitivity and specificity of the assay for each mutant as well as the optimal threshold values for mutant allele indices were determined using Receiver Operating Characteristic (ROC) analysis [23]. All indices for positive and negative samples for each mutant from five independent runs of the assay were used for the analysis. The optimal cut-off point was determined by the

Fisher's test implemented through the R language-based web tool Cutoff Finder (http://molpath.charite.de/cutoff/) [24]. Analysis of the sensitivity in terms of percent mutant allele burden was performed by plotting the range of indices for each mutant at concentration 1%, 2.5% and 5% and 12.5% versus the already determined optimal cut-off value.

Results

Determination of the optimal probes set and hybridization conditions

The development of any hybridization-based assay for detection of single nucleotide changes (e.g. SNPs, point mutations) is particularly challenging because of the need to design highly specific probes that are able to discriminate between the different alleles with high accuracy. The task becomes even more complicated when more than two alleles are to be discriminated in a multiplex fashion. The design of the probes is also influenced by the overall nucleotide content of the fragment of interest and in some instances even single nucleotide changes can lead to a high variability in the melting temperatures. So, the primary goal of the optimal probe set design is to select probes with high and uniform Tm. Traditionally, this could be achieved through variation of probe length, which is a time and labor-consuming process. To overcome this limitation a number of chemically modified bases have been used to design oligonucleotide probes. For the purpose of developing a bead-based assay for detection of *DNMT3A* R882 mutations we tested the performance of two sets of oligonucleotide probes with synthetically modified nucleotides. The first set comprised of 1st generation bridged nucleic acids (BNA), known also as locked nucleic acids (LNA)-oligonucleotides, *i.e.* they

Table 2. Parameters of the fitted linear models shown in Fig. 1.

Modification	LNA							
Temperature	62°C				64°C			
Mutant	R882C	R882H	R882P	R882S	R882C	R882H	R882P	R882S
Intercept	0.1041	0.0526	−0.0033	0.0322	0.0393	−0.0017	0.0535	0.0373
Slope	0.0053	0.0047	0.0088	0.0068	0.0058	0.0076	0.0088	0.0069
R²	0.9812	0.9717	0.9179	0.9972	0.9984	0.966	0.967	0.9922

Modification	BNA(NC)							
Temperature	66°C				68°C			
Mutant	R882C	R882H	R882P	R882S	R882C	R882H	R882P	R882S
Intercept	0.1139	0.1074	0.0525	0.1277	0.0508	0.1105	0.1045	0.1086
Slope	0.0069	0.0078	0.0092	0.0081	0.0072	0.008	0.009	0.0082
R²	0.9779	0.9976	0.999	0.9648	0.9793	0.9996	0.9932	0.964

contain one or more 2′-O,4′-C-methylene-β-D-ribofuranosyl monomer(s) [25]. These probes were designed and synthesized by the LNA patent holder Exiqon, Denmark. The second set of in-house designed probes included third generation BNA oligonucleotides, known also as 3rd generation bridged nucleic acids (BNA(NC)), i.e. they contain more than one 2′-O,4′-aminoethylene-β-D-ribofuranosyl monomers [26]. The design of the BNA(NC) oligonucleotides was performed following the published recommendations (http://www.biosyn.com/faq/BNA-general-design-guidelines.aspx) and they were synthesized by BioSynthesis Inc., USA.

As shown in Table 1 the BNA(NC) probes had uniform Tm of 70°C, whereas the LNA probes had slightly lower Tm values varying between 66°C and 68°C. Based on our previous experience with Luminex-based hybridization assays[21] we expected the optimal performance of each set of probes to be around 2°C–4°C below the expected Tm. Indeed, to determine the optimal hybridization conditions for each set of probes we used dilutions of 100%, 50%, 20%, and 0% of each mutant plasmid in the wild-type plasmid. For the LNA probes set we tested 62°C and 64°C hybridization temperatures and for the BNA(NC) probes we tested 66°C and 68°C hybridization temperatures. Mutant allele indices for each sample were calculated and linear regression model was fitted for each mutant at every hybridization temperature (Fig. 1). The parameters for every linear model fit are presented at Table 2. The BNA(NC) probes set performed better than the LNA probes and the former was selected for further testing. The 66°C and 68°C hybridization temperature levels tested for the BNA(NC) probes were actually identical in terms of the parameters of the fitted linear models (Table 2). We selected the 66°C for all subsequent runs of the assay as at this level the raw MFI values were higher than those at the 68°C level.

Determination of the index threshold value and assay sensitivity

To determine the mutant allele index threshold values we used Receiver Operating Characteristic (ROC) analysis. ROC curves were based on the analysis of the index values from plasmid samples with wild type only (true negative samples) and wild type and mutant alleles samples (true positive samples) as described above. ROC curves for all mutants are shown at Fig. 2. The determined areas under the curve (AUC) were indicative for an excellent performance of the assay with all values being over 0.9 as follows: p.R882C (0.94), p.R882H (0.98), p. R882P (0.94), and p. R882S (0.97). The corresponding specificity and sensitivity at the selected cut-off index values are shown in Fig. 2. In order to determine the corresponding sensitivity of the assay for each mutant in terms of mutant allele burden we assayed plasmid standards with 1%, 2.5%, 5%, and 12.5% of each mutant plasmid on wild type background. The sensitivity was defined as the lowest mutant allele burden whose range of index values was above the determined respective threshold. As shown in Fig. 3 the determined sensitivity was 2.5% for all *DNMT3A* mutants.

Concordance of the bead-based assay with direct sequencing using genomic DNA

We further tested the performance of our bead-based assay on a set of genomic DNA samples from 120 patients with known or suspected myeloid malignancies. We identified a total of two R882 missense mutations (one p.R882C and one p.R882Q) (Fig. 4). Both cases were AML. The results from the bead-based assay for all cases were compared with direct sequencing of exon 23 of *DNMT3A*. The sequencing data confirmed the presence of the two

Index (R882C) as positive marker for Presence (R882C)

Index (R882H) as positive marker for Presence (R882H)

Index (R882P) as positive marker for Presence (R882P)

Index (R882S) as positive marker for Presence (R882S)

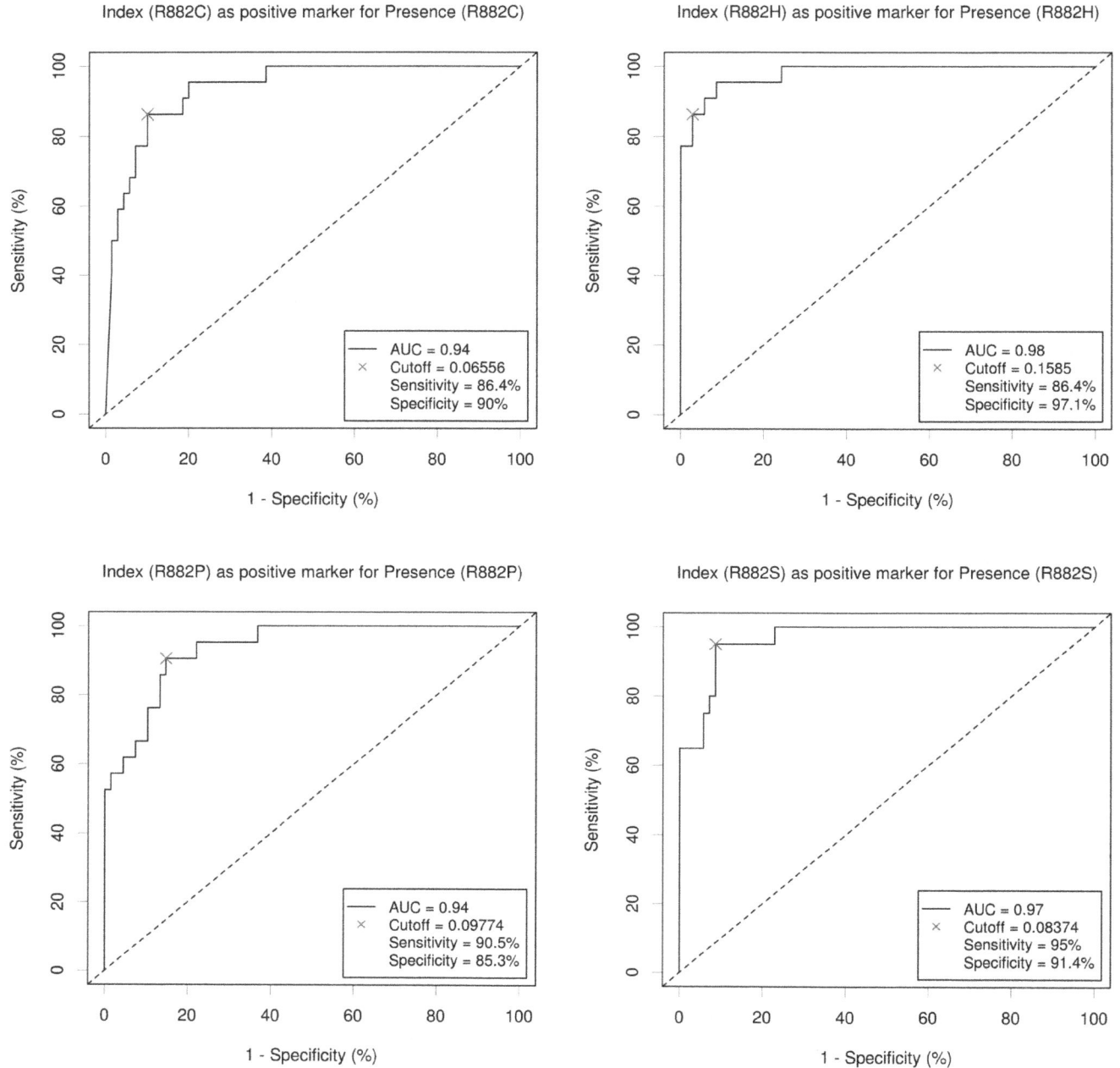

Figure 2. ROC curves for the determination of the overall performance of the assay and the optimal cut-off value for each mutant's index.

R882 mutations but also identified another unreported heterozygous synonymous mutation p.Q886Q (c.2658G>A). This patient was also diagnosed with AML. All other cases were negative for R882 mutations on both the microsphere-based assay and direct sequencing. This straightforward comparison validated the applicability of our assay for the detection of R882 mutations in clinical settings.

Discussion

Recent advances in genomic profiling technologies showed that genes encoding enzymes involved in epigenetic regulation are frequently affected by the mutational process in myeloid malignancies [27]. *DNMT3A* is a key gene for the epigenetic regulation of human cells as the encoded enzyme is known to be a major player in the de novo DNA methylation at CpG sites [28]. *DNMT3A* mutational status has recently been included in several studies on the prognostic power of integrated molecular profiling in AML [9,10,29]. Most of the studies used targeted sequencing of exon 23 of the gene spanning the mutational hotspot, codon R882. From a clinical standpoint the restriction of molecular testing for *DNMT3A* mutations only to the mutational hotspot, codon R882, is justified by three lines of evidence: i) approximately 2/3 of all reported *DNMT3A* mutations are affecting codon R882 (with

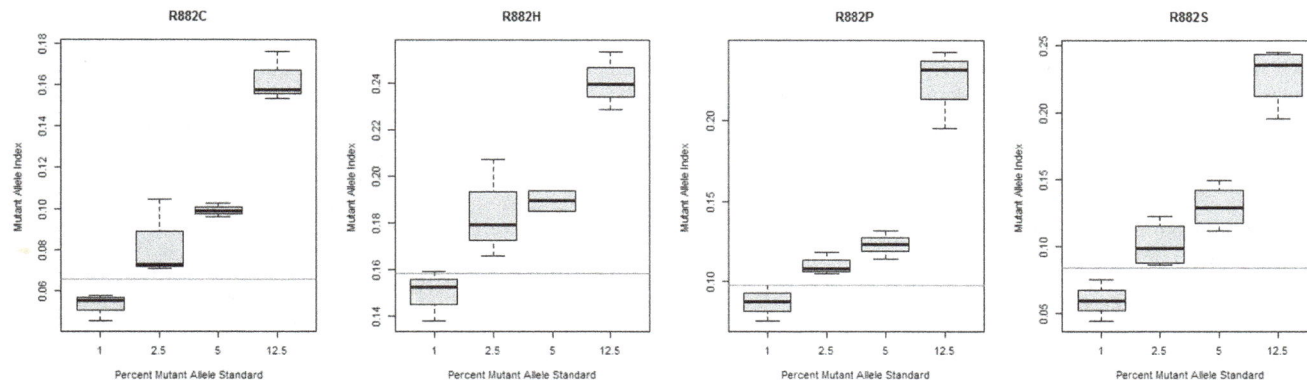

Figure 3. Determination of the sensitivity of the assay as expressed in percent mutant allele. The horizontal lines denote the threshold level for each mutant's index.

p.R882H and p.R882C being the most frequent ones); ii) R882 missense mutations perturb the normal molecular function of the enzyme; and iii) R882 mutations may differ in their prognostic effect from non-R882 mutations [18].

It was shown recently that the most frequent *DNMT3A* mutation, R882H, disrupted the dimerization interface of the enzyme. This leads to a several fold drop down in its activity as a processive CpG methylase [30]. However, *DNMT3A* R882 mutations are not just hypomorphic and they seem to exert also dominant negative effect as the expression of the analogous mouse *DNMT3A* R878H mutations in embryonic stem (ES) cells containing endogenous DNMT3A or DNMT3B caused hypomethylation [31]. Xu et al. [32] just showed that the transplantation of hematopoietic stem cells (HSCs) transduced retrovirally with R882H mutant and transplanted to immunodeficient mice caused CMML disease with characteristic hypomethylation patterns. A number of retrospective clinical studies assessed the prognostic power of *DNMT3A* in AML. Only a few of them, however, compared R882 mutations with non-R882 mutations, but the conclusions regarding their prognostic power are not consistent. For instance, Gaidzik et al. [7] showed that R882-mutated cases may be prognostic for unfavorable OS vs. non-R882-mutated cases. Other studies, however, did not find such a

difference between different types of DNMT3A mutations [33]. Taken together, the clinical and experimental evidence suggest the relevance of *DNMT3A* mutations detection in the work-up for AML (and eventually other related myeloid malignancies).

To address the rapidly growing need for testing the *DNMT3A* R882 in clinical settings we adapted the bead-based flow platform developed by the Luminex Corporation, USA. This system utilizes barcoding of various analytes recognizing molecules (antibodies, ligands, oligonucleotides) through coupling with fluorescently labeled microbeads [34]. In the cases of direct hybridization based method the amplified DNA fragment is either directly labeled with Cy3/PE or with biotin with subsequent streptavidin-phycoerythrine (SAPE) labeling. A number of recent reports demonstrated the applicability of this technique for detection and/or quantitation of somatic mutations associated with malignant diseases such as *KRAS* and *BRAF* [35,36], *NPM1, JAK2, MPL, IDH1/2* [19,20,21,37,38,39] and for detection of chromosomal translocations [40,41] and even for CpG methylation profiling [42]. The greatest advantage of this method is the opportunity for multiplexing in a single tube the detection of up to 100 analytes. A nice demonstration of that advantage for detection of cancer-associated mutations has recently been provided by Bando et al. [43] who performed multiplex single tube testing for 36 mutations

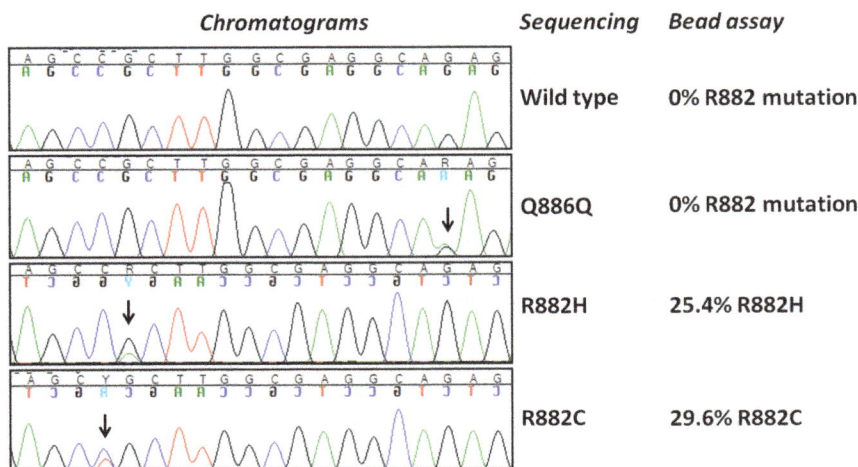

Figure 4. Comparison of the bead-based assay to direct sequencing in selected genomic DNA samples. The vertical arrows show the positions of the identified mutations.

in *KRAS*, *NRAS*, *BRAF* and *PIK3CA*. Unfortunately, they did not provide any data on the analytical sensitivity of the assay. The greatest challenge in the development of such assays is the design of probes that could specifically discriminate between sequences differing in just one nucleotide base. In the last decade a working strategy to overcome this limitation appeared to be the use of synthetic nucleotides that can increase the specificity and the Tm of the oligonucleotide probes they are incorporated in. The LNA-containing oligonucleotides have been reported to be successfully coupled with Luminex beads for SNP or somatic mutations detection. Here, to the best of our knowledge we reported for the first time the use of BNA(NC)-containing oligonucleotides coupled with micro-beads and resolved on the Luminex platform. Our in-house designed BNA(NC) probe set appeared to be superior to an LNA probe set intended for the same purpose. The BNA(NC) incorporation allowed for more uniform Tm of the probes in the set resulting in better sensitivity and specificity as demonstrated by the very high linearity between the mutant allele standards and the obtained mutant allele indices (Fig. 1 and Table 2). This BNA(NC)-modified probes superiority in comparison to the LNA-modified ones might not be considered surprising as this has already been shown for RNA silencing application [44].

We further used a state-of-the art technique to determine the index cut-off value for presence of any of the specific mutant alleles. Notably, all the cut-off values translated in 2.5% mutant allele burden sensitivity, which is of clinical relevance, as this value would mean 5% heterozygous mutant carrier cells in the sample. In principle enhancement of the sensitivity of the assay is possible through use of mutant-enrichment PCR protocols (COLD-PCR) or signal amplification techniques (e.g. use of PE-labeled anti-biotin antibodies). This would, however, increase the work load associated with the assay. We also validated our multiplex assay on clinical samples from patients with known or suspected myeloid malignancies. We were able to identify two R882 mutations, both in AML patients. This result was concordant with the direct sequencing read-out which also confirmed the presence of these mutations. Expectedly, sequencing appeared to be superior in detecting other mutations beyond the R882 codon. We identified a synonymous p.Q886Q mutation (c.2658G>A), which is obviously of no clinical relevance.

In conclusion, here we demonstrated the applicability of BNA(NC) probes coupled with fluorescently labeled beads for quantitative detection of DNMT3A R882 mutations. This method is rapid (taking up to 5 hours from DNA extraction to data acquisition) and allows processing of samples in a mid-throughput format (in 96 or 384 well plates). The demonstrated sensitivity of 2.5% for each mutant allele is well suited for the clinical practice. The greatest advantage of this assay is the opportunity for further multiplexing of the assay for simultaneous detection of many clinically relevant mutations. Therefore, it may become a valuable tool in the era of integrated integrated mutational profiling of myeloid malignancies especially for laboratories not having access to NGS platforms.

Author Contributions

Conceived and designed the experiments: VS MI. Performed the experiments: VS MI. Analyzed the data: VS MI EN. Contributed reagents/materials/analysis tools: VS MI EN. Contributed to the writing of the manuscript: VS MI.

References

1. Shivarov V, Gueorguieva R, Stoimenov A, Tiu R (2013) DNMT3A mutation is a poor prognosis biomarker in AML: results of a meta-analysis of 4500 AML patients. Leuk Res 37: 1445–1450.
2. Itzykson R, Kosmider O, Fenaux P (2013) Somatic mutations and epigenetic abnormalities in myelodysplastic syndromes. Best Pract Res Clin Haematol 26: 355–364.
3. Jankowska AM, Makishima H, Tiu RV, Szpurka H, Huang Y, et al. (2011) Mutational spectrum analysis of chronic myelomonocytic leukemia includes genes associated with epigenetic regulation: UTX, EZH2, and DNMT3A. Blood 118: 3932–3941.
4. Vannucchi AM, Lasho TL, Guglielmelli P, Biamonte F, Pardanani A, et al. (2013) Mutations and prognosis in primary myelofibrosis. Leukemia 27: 1861–1869.
5. Traina F, Visconte V, Jankowska AM, Makishima H, O'Keefe CL, et al. (2012) Single nucleotide polymorphism array lesions, TET2, DNMT3A, ASXL1 and CBL mutations are present in systemic mastocytosis. PLoS One 7: e43090.
6. Grossmann V, Haferlach C, Weissmann S, Roller A, Schindela S, et al. (2013) The molecular profile of adult T-cell acute lymphoblastic leukemia: mutations in RUNX1 and DNMT3A are associated with poor prognosis in T-ALL. Genes Chromosome Canc 52: 410–422.
7. Gaidzik VI, Schlenk RF, Paschka P, Stölzle A, Späth D, et al. (2013) Clinical impact of DNMT3A mutations in younger adult patients with acute myeloid leukemia: results of the AML Study Group (AMLSG). Blood 121: 4769–4777.
8. Patel JP, Gonen M, Figueroa ME, Fernandez H, Sun Z, et al. (2012) Prognostic relevance of integrated genetic profiling in acute myeloid leukemia. N Engl J Med 366: 1079–1089.
9. Kihara R, Nagata Y, Kiyoi H, Kato T, Yamamoto E, et al. (2014) Comprehensive analysis of genetic alterations and their prognostic impacts in adult acute myeloid leukemia patients. Leukemia "In press".
10. Hou HA, Lin CC, Chou WC, Liu CY, Chen CY, et al. (2014) Integration of cytogenetic and molecular alterations in risk stratification of 318 patients with de novo non-M3 acute myeloid leukemia. Leukemia 28: 50–58.
11. Marcucci G, Metzeler KH, Schwind S, Becker H, Maharry K, et al. (2012) Age-related prognostic impact of different types of DNMT3A mutations in adults with primary cytogenetically normal acute myeloid leukemia. J Clin Oncol 30: 742–750.
12. Singh RR, Bains A, Patel KP, Rahimi H, Barkoh BA, et al. (2012) Detection of high-frequency and novel DNMT3A mutations in acute myeloid leukemia by high-resolution melting curve analysis. J Mol Diagn 14: 336–345.
13. Lin J, Yao DM, Qian J, Chen Q, Qian W, et al. (2011) Recurrent DNMT3A R882 mutations in Chinese patients with acute myeloid leukemia and myelodysplastic syndrome. PLoS One 6: e26906.
14. Luthra R, Patel KP, Reddy NG, Haghshenas V, Routbort MJ, et al. (2013) Next generation sequencing based multi-gene mutational screen foracute myeloid leukemia using miseq: applicability for diagnostics anddisease monitoring. Haematologica "In press".
15. Grossmann V, Roller A, Klein HU, Weissmann S, Kern W, et al. (2013) Robustness of amplicon deep sequencing underlines its utility in clinical applications. J Mol Diagn 15: 473–484.
16. Brewin JN, Horne GA, Bisling KE, Stewart HJ, Chevassut TJ (2013) Rapid detection of DNMT3A R882 codon mutations allows early identification of poor risk patients with acute myeloid leukemia. Leuk Lymphoma 54: 1336–1339.
17. Bisling KE, Brewin JN, McGovern AP, Horne GA, Rider T, et al. (2014) DNMT3A mutations at R882 hotspot are only found in major clones of acute myeloid leukemia. Leuk Lymphoma 55: 711–714.
18. Ribeiro AF, Pratcorona M, Erpelinck-Verschueren C, Rockova V, Sanders M, et al. (2012) Mutant DNMT3A: a marker of poor prognosis in acute myeloid leukemia. Blood 119: 5824–5831.
19. Ivanova MI, Shivarov VS, Hadjiev EA, Naumova EJ (2011) Novel multiplex bead-based assay with LNA-modified probes for detection of MPL exon 10 mutations. Leuk Res 35: 1120–1123.
20. Shivarov V, Ivanova M, Hadjiev E, Naumova E (2011) Rapid quantification of JAK2 V617F allele burden using a bead-based liquid assay with locked nucleic acid-modified oligonucleotide probes. Leuk Lymphoma 52: 2023–2026.
21. Shivarov V, Ivanova M, Hadjiev E, Naumova E (2013) Novel multiplex bead-based assay for detection of IDH1 and IDH2 mutations in myeloid malignancies. PLoS One 8: e76944.
22. Ivanova M, Ruiqing J, Matsushita M, Ogawa T, Kawai S, et al. (2008) MBL2 single nucleotide polymorphism diversity among four ethnic groups as revealed by a bead-based liquid array profiling. Hum Immunol 69: 877–884.
23. Fawcett T (2006) An introduction to ROC analysis. Pattern Recogn Lett 27: 861–874.
24. Budczies J, Klauschen F, Sinn BV, Gyorffy B, Schmitt WD, et al. (2012) Cutoff Finder: a comprehensive and straightforward Web application enabling rapid biomarker cutoff optimization. PLoS One 7: e51862.
25. Koshkin AA, Nielsen P, Meldgaard M, Rajwanshi VK, Singh SK, et al. (1998) LNA (locked nucleic acid): An RNA mimic forming exceedingly stable LNA: LNA duplexes. J Am Chem Soc 120: 13252–13253.

26. Rahman SM, Seki S, Obika S, Yoshikawa H, Miyashita K, et al. (2008) Design, synthesis, and properties of 2′,4′-BNA(NC): a bridged nucleic acid analogue. J Am Chem Soc 130: 4886–4896.

27. Murati A, Brecqueville M, Devillier R, Mozziconacci MJ, Gelsi-Boyer V, et al. (2012) Myeloid malignancies: mutations, models and management. BMC Cancer 12: 304.

28. Okano M, Bell DW, Haber DA, Li E (1999) DNA methyltransferases Dnmt3a and Dnmt3b are essential for de novo methylation and mammalian development. Cell 99: 247–257.

29. Patel JP, Gönen M, Figueroa ME, Fernandez H, Sun Z, et al. (2012) Prognostic relevance of integrated genetic profiling in acute myeloid leukemia. N Eng J Med 366: 1079–1089.

30. Holz-Schietinger C, Matje DM, Reich NO (2012) Mutations in DNA methyltransferase (DNMT3A) observed in acute myeloid leukemia patients disrupt processive methylation. J Biol Chem 287: 30941–30951.

31. Kim SJ, Zhao H, Hardikar S, Singh AK, Goodell MA, et al. (2013) A DNMT3A mutation common in AML exhibits dominant-negative effects in murine ES cells. Blood 122: 4086–4089.

32. Xu J, Wang YY, Dai YJ, Zhang W, Zhang WN, et al. (2014) DNMT3A Arg882 mutation drives chronic myelomonocytic leukemia through disturbing gene expression/DNA methylation in hematopoietic cells. Proc Natl Acad Sci U S A "In press".

33. Ley TJ, Ding L, Walter MJ, McLellan MD, Lamprecht T, et al. (2010) DNMT3A mutations in acute myeloid leukemia. N Eng J Med 363: 2424–2433.

34. Dunbar SA (2006) Applications of Luminex xMAP technology for rapid, high-throughput multiplexed nucleic acid detection. Clin Chim Acta 363: 71–82.

35. Laosinchai-Wolf W, Ye F, Tran V, Yang Z, White R, et al. (2011) Sensitive multiplex detection of KRAS codons 12 and 13 mutations in paraffin-embedded tissue specimens. J Clin Pathol 64: 30–36.

36. Wu S, Zhu Z, He J, Luo X, Xu J, et al. (2010) A novel mutant-enriched liquidchip technology for the qualitative detection of somatic mutations in KRAS gene from both serum and tissue samples. Clin Chem Lab Med 48: 1103–1106.

37. Hafez M, Ye F, Jackson K, Yang Z, Karp JE, et al. (2010) Performance and clinical evaluation of a sensitive multiplex assay for the rapid detection of common NPM1 mutations. J Mol Diagn 12: 629–635.

38. Shivarov V, Ivanova M, Yaneva S, Petkova N, Hadjiev E, et al. (2013) Quantitative bead-based assay for detection of JAK2 exon 12 mutations. Leuk Lymphoma 54: 1343–1344.

39. Paradis FW, Simard R, Gaudet D (2010) Quantitative assay for the detection of the V617F variant in the Janus kinase 2 (JAK2) gene using the Luminex xMAP technology. BMC Med Genet 11: 54.

40. Wallace J, Zhou Y, Usmani GN, Reardon M, Newburger P, et al. (2003) BARCODE-ALL: accelerated and cost-effective genetic risk stratification in acute leukemia using spectrally addressable liquid bead microarrays. Leukemia 17: 1411–1413.

41. Shackelford RE, Jackson KD, Hafez MJ, Gocke CD (2013) Liquid bead array technology in the detection of common translocations in acute and chronic leukemias. Methods Mol Biol 999: 93–103.

42. Wertheim GB, Smith C, Figueroa ME, Kalos M, Bagg A, et al. (2014) Microsphere-based multiplex analysis of DNA methylation in acute myeloid leukemia. J Mol Diagn 16: 207–215.

43. Bando H, Yoshino T, Shinozaki E, Nishina T, Yamazaki K, et al. (2013) Simultaneous identification of 36 mutations in KRAS codons 61 and 146, BRAF, NRAS, and PIK3CA in a single reaction by multiplex assay kit. BMC Cancer 13: 405.

44. Yamamoto T, Yasuhara H, Wada F, Harada-Shiba M, Imanishi T, et al. (2012) Superior Silencing by 2′,4′-BNA(NC)-Based Short Antisense Oligonucleotides Compared to 2′,4′-BNA/LNA-Based Apolipoprotein B Antisense Inhibitors. J Nucleic Acids 2012: 707323.

12

ATO/ATRA/Anthracycline-Chemotherapy Sequential Consolidation Achieves Long-Term Efficacy in Primary Acute Promyelocytic Leukemia

Zi-Jie Long[1⑨], Yuan Hu[1⑨], Xu-Dong Li[1], Yi He[1], Ruo-Zhi Xiao[1], Zhi-Gang Fang[1], Dong-Ning Wang[1], Jia-Jun Liu[1], Jin-Song Yan[3], Ren-Wei Huang[1*], Dong-Jun Lin[1*], Quentin Liu[1,2*]

1 Department of Hematology, Third Affiliated Hospital, Sun Yat-sen University, Sun Yat-sen Institute of Hematology, Sun Yat-sen University, Guangzhou, China, 2 Institute of Cancer Stem Cell, Dalian Medical University, Dalian, China, 3 Department of Hematology, Second Affiliated Hospital, Dalian Medical University, Dalian, China

Abstract

The combination of all-trans retinoic acid (ATRA) and arsenic trioxide (As_2O_3, ATO) has been effective in obtaining high clinical complete remission (CR) rates in acute promyelocytic leukemia (APL), but the long-term efficacy and safety among newly diagnosed APL patients are unclear. In this retrospective study, total 45 newly diagnosed APL patients received ATRA/chemotherapy combination regimen to induce remission. Among them, 43 patients (95.6%) achieved complete remission (CR) after induction therapy, followed by ATO/ATRA/anthracycline-based chemotherapy sequential consolidation treatment with a median follow-up of 55 months. In these patients, the estimated overall survival (OS) and the relapse-free survival (RFS) were 94.4%±3.9% and 94.6%±3.7%, respectively. The toxicity profile was mild and reversible. No secondary carcinoma was observed. These results demonstrated the high efficacy and minimal toxicity of ATO/ATRA/anthracycline-based chemotherapy sequential consolidation treatment for newly diagnosed APL in long-term follow-up, suggesting a potential frontline therapy for APL.

Editor: Francesco Bertolini, European Institute of Oncology, Italy

Funding: The authors have no support or funding to report.

Competing Interests: The authors have declared that no competing interests exist.

* Email: liuq9@mail.sysu.edu.cn (QL); lindj@mail.sysu.edu.cn (DJL); huangrw56@163.com (RWH)

⑨ These authors contributed equally to this work.

Introduction

Acute promyelocytic leukemia (APL), characterized by the t (15, 17) chromosomal translocation and leukemogenic PML-RARα fusion protein, is accumulated of abnormal promyelocytes in the bone marrow and causes severe bleeding tendency [1]. The treatment of APL with chemotherapy achieved complete remission (CR) in two-thirds of newly diagnosed patients, however, the 5-year disease-free survival (DFS) was still very poor [1–3]. The induction of all-trans retinoic acid (ATRA) in the treatment and optimization of the anthracycline-based regimens resulted in terminal differentiation of APL cells with a 90–95% CR and the 5-year DFS up to 74% [1,4,5], although approximately 5–30% of patients developed disease recurrence [6].

As one of the most potential drugs in APL, arsenic trioxide (As_2O_3, ATO) targets PML/RARα and exerts dose-dependent dual effects on APL cells, with low concentrations inducing differentiation and high concentrations triggering apoptosis [7]. Since 1990s, the use of ATO has improved the clinical benefit of refractory or relapsed as well as newly diagnosed APL [8–11]. ATO injection for APL patients who developed disease recurrence or failed to respond to standard treatment was later approved by the US FDA. Moreover, molecular remission is obtainable in patients from 72% to 91% after CR by ATO alone [12,13]. Strong synergistic anti-leukemic effects of ATO in combination with ATRA were found in both APL cell lines and APL animal models, with induction catabolism of the PML-RARα fusion protein [14–17]. Importantly, previous clinical trials showed that the combination of ATO and ATRA yielded a longer survival rate compared to either ATRA or ATO monotherapy [18–23]. Moreover, ATO consolidation therapy spared anthracycline exposure [24], and improved both event-free survival (EFS) and overall survival (OS) in newly diagnosed APL [25]. Yet, a standard ATO/ATRA consolidation regimen for newly diagnosed APL remains to be further validated.

In this retrospective study, ATRA/chemotherapy combination regimen was applied to induce remission for newly diagnosed APL patients. A regimen consisting of ATO, ATRA and anthracycline-based chemotherapy was used sequentially as consolidation therapy for the patients who obtained CR. The long-term efficacy and safety of ATO/ATRA/anthracycline-based chemotherapy consolidation regimen were evaluated.

Methods

Patients

This retrospective study consisted of 45 patients with newly diagnosed APL in the Third Affiliated Hospital, Sun Yat-sen University, from March 1, 2000 to August 31, 2012. The median age was 29 years (10–62 years). Pertinent patient clinical reports of this study were obtained with patients' written consent and the approval of the Ethical Board of The Third Affiliated Hospital,

Sun Yat-sen University ([2013]2-69). Parental written consent was obtained for underage participants.

APL diagnosis was established according to clinical presentations, morphological criteria of the French-American-British classification, cytogenetic assay for t (15; 17) (q22; q21) and RT-PCR analysis for PML-RARα transcripts. The exclusion criteria for this retrospective study included: dysfunction of liver or kidney; any heart diseases or cardiac functional insufficiency; patients who died before initiation of the therapy. Standard induction therapy was administered for the 45 newly diagnosed APL patients (Figure 1). Two patients died during induction treatment. The remaining 43 patients received consolidation therapy. The clinical features of patients were described in Table 1.

Remission Induction Therapy

Induction therapy for these newly diagnosed patients with APL was a combination of ATRA and daunorubicin plus cytarabine. Once the diagnosis was suspected on the basis of clinical features and the peripheral blood smear, ATRA was administered orally at 40 mg/m^2/day (divided into two equal doses) until CR was achieved. Patients with WBC counts $\geq 10 \times 10^9$/L additionally received hydroxycarbamide orally until the WBC count was down to less than 10×10^9/L. ATRA was continued for 3 to 15 days to ameliorate the coagulopathy before initiating chemotherapy (daunorubicin 40 mg/m^2/day for 3 days, cytarabine 100 mg/q12 h for 7 days).

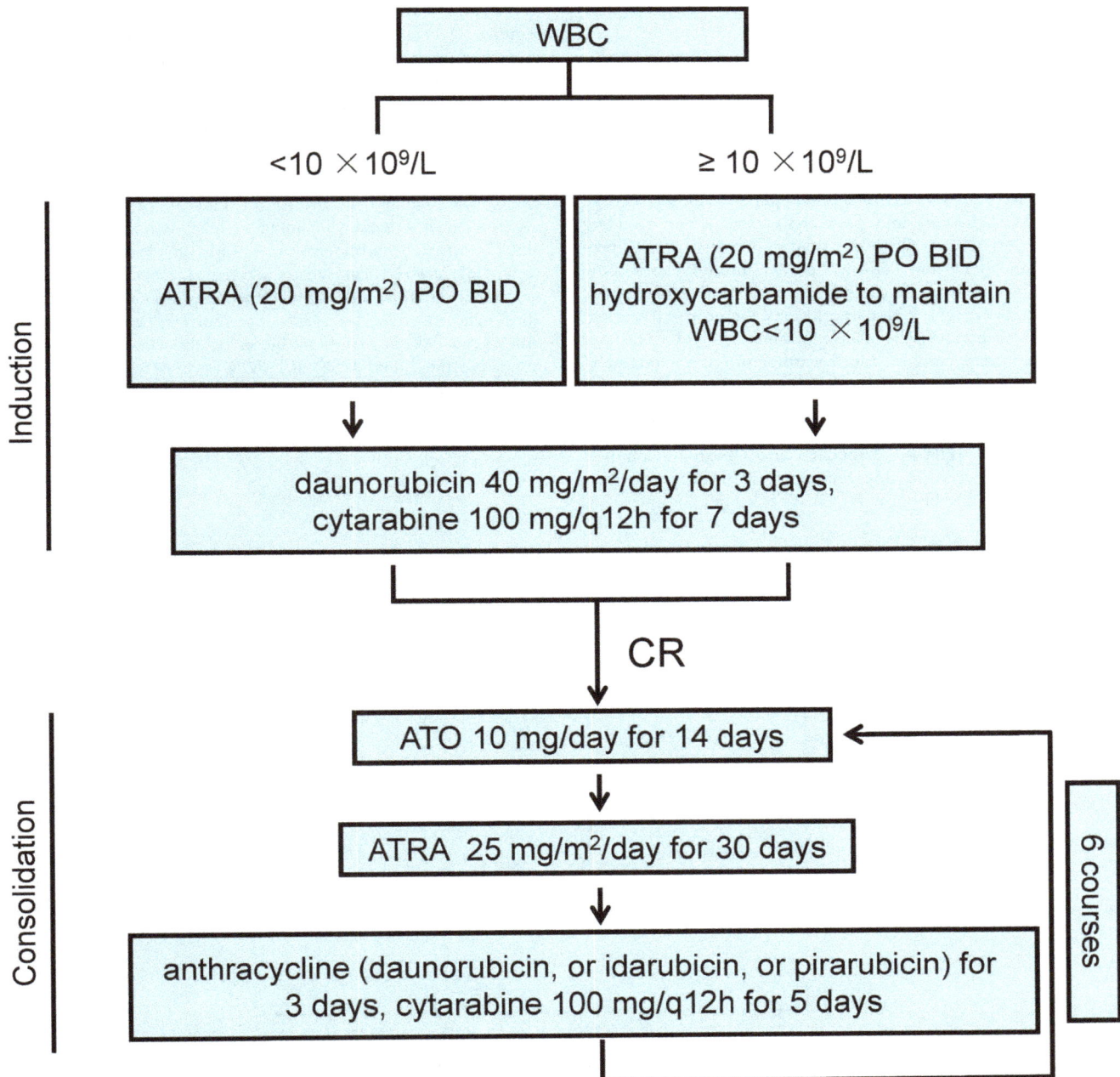

Figure 1. A chart review of patients treated with standard of induction and consolidation therapy.

Table 1. Clinical data of the patients.

	N = 45
Gender, male/female	20/25
Median age, years	29 (10–62)
WBC, ×109/L	
Median	2.3 (0.2–47.5)
<10	1.9 (0.2–7.8, 84.4%)
≥10	37.9 (13.2–47.5, 15.6%)
Median Hb, g/L	81.0 (38.0–120.0)
Median platelet, ×109/L	23.0 (5.0–120.0)
Clinical CR	95.6%
Median days to clinical CR	30 (20–60)
Median months to molecular CR	6 (2–12)

Supportive Care

During induction of remission, examinations including whole peripheral blood cell counts, renal and hepatic function tests were performed. Coagulation and fibrinolysis parameters including fibrinogen, D-dimmers, fibrin degradation product (FDP), prothrombin time (PT), and activated partial thromboplastin time (APTT) were monitored to identify the requirement of platelet, fresh plasma, or cryoprecipitate transfusions. Supportive treatment was based on maintaining platelet counts $>30 \times 10^9/L$ until coagulopathy disappearance. Electrocardiogram and sonography were used for monitoring the cardiac function for patients. APL differentiation syndrome (APLDS) was treated with prednisone or dexamethasone until clear resolution of symptoms. Drug toxicities were documented using the National Cancer Institute-Common Toxicity Criteria, version 3.0. Symptomatic therapy was performed for the side effects of ATO, ATRA and anthracycline.

Patients with chronic hepatitis B were treated with lamivudine or telbivudine for prevention of virus activation.

Consolidation Therapy

Patients were monitored to confirm that the bone marrow morphology and recovery of peripheral blood cell counts. Consolidation therapy included 6 courses was initiated once CR was achieved, and each course included three consecutive regimens: (1) ATO, 10 mg/day for 14 days intravenously; (2) ATRA, 25 mg/m^2/day for 30 days orally; (3) anthracycline-based regimens: daunorubicin (40 mg/m^2/day), or idarubicin (8 mg/m^2/day), or pirarubicin (25 mg/m^2/day) for 3 days plus cytarabine 100 mg/q12 h for 5 days. The three regimens of consolidation therapy were administered sequentially every month in the first year after achieving CR. In the second year, each regimen of consolidation therapy was administered sequentially every two months. Six courses were given totally.

All patients received intrathecal therapy (methotrexate 15 mg, cytarabine 50 mg, dexamethasone 8 mg) when CR was achieved. Prophylaxis was performed 4–6 times altogether.

Response Definition

CR was defined according to clinical presentations and morphological criteria, including cellular bone marrow blasts and abnormal promyelocytes ≤5% with an absolute neutrophil count $\geq 1.0 \times 10^9/L$ and platelet count $\geq 100 \times 10^9/L$. Clinical recurrence was defined as the presence of ≥5% blasts, or abnormal promyelocytes in the bone marrow, or the appearance of leukemic cells in peripheral blood, or abnormal promyelocytes in cerebrospinal fluid (CSF). RT-PCR for the PML-RARα fusion transcript was performed on the bone marrow follow-up every 2 months for monitoring molecular remission. After molecular remission, the examination was still performed every 3 months for monitoring relapse.

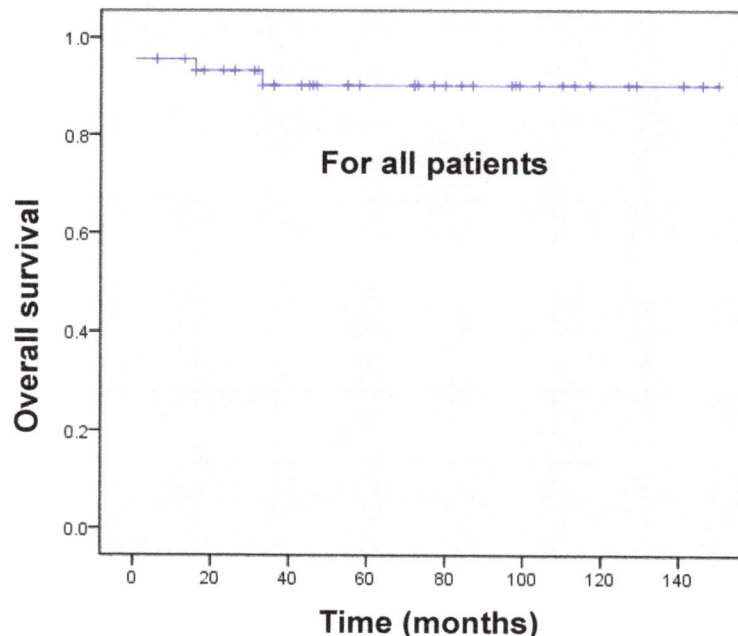

Figure 2. Survival analysis. The OS for all 45 patients.

A

B

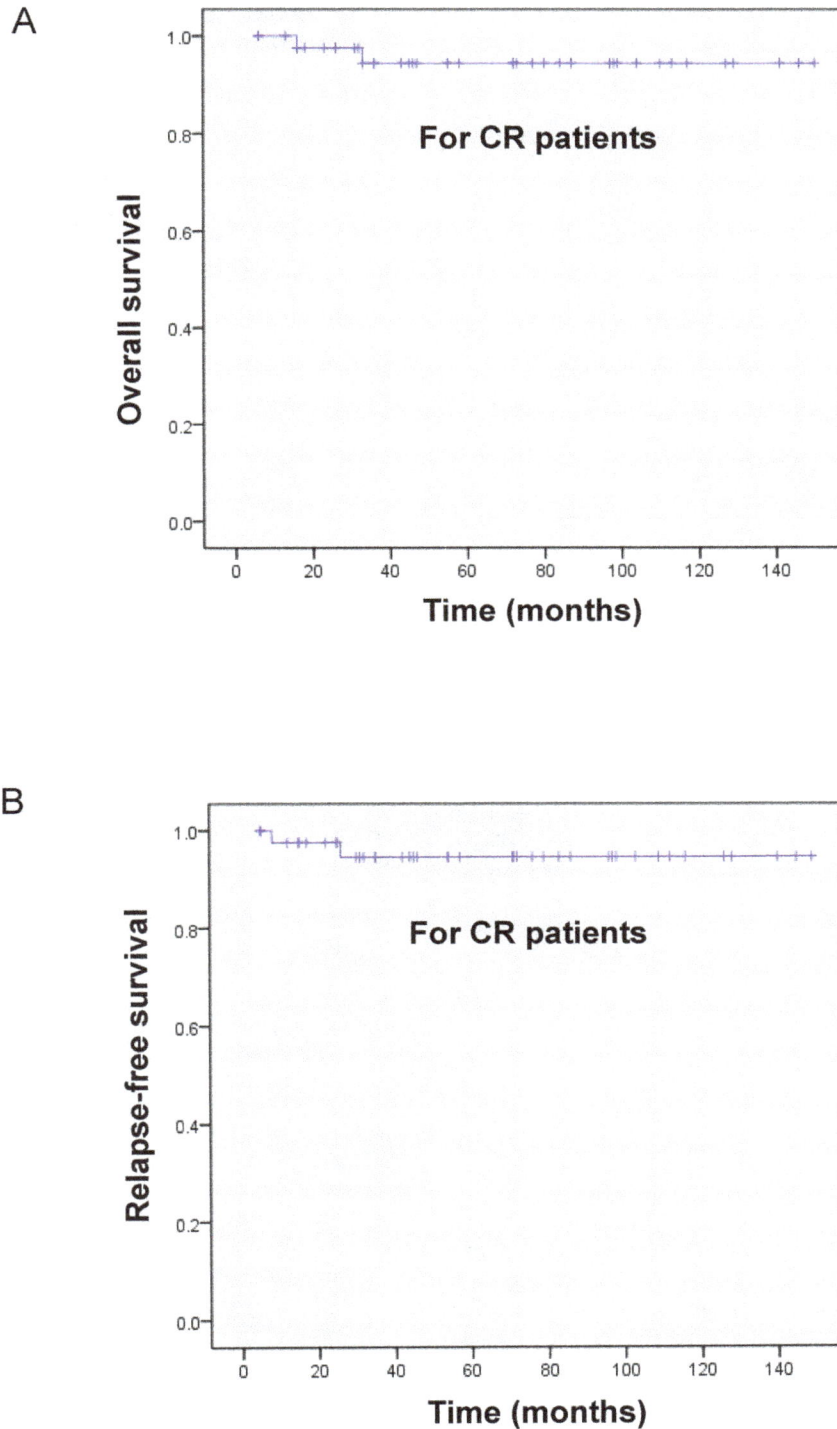

Figure 3. Survival analysis. The OS (A) and RFS (B) for the 43 patients who obtained CR.

Statistical Analysis

OS was defined as the time from the initiation of induction therapy to death. RFS was defined as the time from CR to relapse. Survival analysis was performed using Kaplan-Meier estimate methods. Statistical analysis was performed using SPSS16.0 for windows software.

Results

Outcomes

As seen in Table 1, among total 45 patients, 43 (95.6%) achieved CR in remission introduction therapy. The median time to achieve CR was 30 days (range: 20–60 days). Two patients suffered from early death within 15 days during the induction

Table 2. Toxicity profile.

	N = 43
Hepatotoxicity	7 (16.3%)
Grade I	6 (14.0%)
Grade II	1 (2.3%)
Grade III	0 (0%)
Grade IV	0 (0%)
Skin reaction	19 (44.2%)
Headache	13 (30.2%)
Neutropenia	8 (18.6%)
Gastrointestinal reaction	6 (14.0%)
Cardiac arrhythmia	1 (2.3%)
APLDS	2 (4.7%)
Fever	4 (9.3%)

therapy due to intracranial hemorrhage (1 case), or acute tumor lysis syndrome (1 case). For the 43 patients who entered CR, all received ATO/ATRA/anthracycline-based chemotherapy for consolidation therapy. The median follow-up was 55 months (range: 6–150 months), and the median months to molecular CR was 6 months (range: 2–12 months). Till the end of this study, 41 patients remained in good clinical and molecular remission. Two patients relapsed: one presented with central nervous system (CNS) leukemia in the 27th month and the other developed full bone marrow relapse in the 10th month. Both patients died 6 months after relapse. No patient developed a secondary myelodysplastic syndrome or carcinoma.

As shown in Figure 2 and Figure 3, the estimated 3-year OS rates for all 45 patients and for those who achieved CR (n = 43) were 90.2% ± 4.7% (Figure 2) and 94.4% ± 3.9% (Figure 3A), respectively. The RFS rates for CR patients were 94.6 ± 3.7% (Figure 3B).

Toxicity Profile

The main side effect of ATRA is the APLDS whereas that of ATO is liver dysfunction. Both ATRA- and ATO- based treatments were tolerated well in the present study. As shown in Table 2, APLDS was diagnosed in 2 patients (4.7%). Other side effects of ATRA, such as skin reactions (19 patients, 44.2%), headache (13 patients, 30.2%), gastrointestinal tract reactions (6 patients, 14.0%) and fever (4 patients, 9.3%), were mild and overcame by administration of symptomatic medication. During consolidation, 6 of 41 patients developed tolerable and reversible grade I liver dysfunction and 1 patients developed grade II liver dysfunction, whereas no grade III–IV liver toxicity was observed. Hepatic function returned to normal in all of these patients after supportive therapy. No one needed termination of ATO therapy because of severe liver damage. Therapy-related neutropenia were observed in 8 patients (18.6%). One 62-year-old patient presented with chronic cardiac insufficiency in the 18th month after CR, which might be due to the accumulation of anthracycline for the elderly. In addition, all the 8 hepatitis B patients did not show any virus reactivation during consolidation.

Discussion

ATRA in combination with anthracycline-based chemotherapy is considered as the standard for the induction and consolidation

therapy of newly diagnosed APL. However, cumulative incidence of relapse still occurs in one third of the patients who have obtained CR. ATO induced catabolism of the PML-RARα fusion protein, demonstrating an effective targeted therapy in APL. In 1990s, the possibility of using a triad of chemotherapy, ATRA, and ATO for newly diagnosed patients in APL was discussed at a meeting in Shanghai. Then studies in the mouse model showed that this combination could dramatically prolong the survival or even eradicate disease. These results encouraged physicians to conduct new therapeutic approaches based on ATO/ATRA/anthracycline-based chemotherapy combination for the treatment of newly diagnosed APL patients.

Indeed, since the introduction of ATRA/ATO-based combination treatment for newly diagnosed APL and recurrence, the CR rate and the 5-year DFS have been greatly improved [18–23,26]. In this study, the ATRA/chemotherapy combination regimen was administered to induce remission, and the ATO plus ATRA and anthracycline-based chemotherapy consolidation regimen was used to maintain long-term efficacy for newly diagnosed APL patients. In 45 *de novo* patients, CR was achieved in 43 patients (95.6%), whereas the median time to achieved CR was 30 days. The estimated 3-year OS rate for all patients was 90.2% ± 4.7%. For patients who achieved CR (n = 43), the OS and RFS rates were 94.4% ± 3.9% and 94.6% ± 3.7%, respectively. Our data were consistent with recent studies [23], which reported a long-term outcome in the ATRA/ATO-based regimen.

The therapeutic benefit of ATO as a single agent for the treatment of APL has been reported previously [27,28], thus using ATO as the post-remission therapy for the APL patients in CR was reasonable. Importantly, ATO consolidation produced a good survival rate no matter which method was used in CR induction and eliminated the need for maintenance therapy [29–31]. However, the relatively high incidence of ATO-induced hepatotoxicity during remission induction remains unclear and worthy of note, though the side effects of ATO were considered to be moderate. Reversible grade III–IV hepatotoxicity was seen in a small proportion of patients [27]. Overtreatment in the majority of patients was potentially associated with a risk of treatment-related death during early disease remission as well as longer-term risks of secondary carcinoma or anthracycline-related cardiomyopathy. Thus in the present study, ATRA-based induction regimen was applied and ATO was not added to the remission regimen. Either the daily or the total dosage of ATO for consolidation was minimal (10 mg/day for 14 days each course), which APL patients could benefit from ATO by consolidation without overtreatment during each course. In fact, during the consolidation, no grade III–IV hepatotoxicity was documented in our patients. Only 7 patients developed tolerable and reversible grade I–II liver dysfunction, and their hepatic function returned to normal after consolidation therapy. Other side effects were minimal during post-remission treatment. Another major concern associated with long-term exposure to ATO is secondary tumors, and we found no cases in the present study developed secondary tumors. Besides, our analysis showed that incorporation of ATRA drastically achieved long-term efficacy. Importantly, patients in our study showed a very low incidence of APLDS (4.7%). While the dosage of ATO was relatively small, APL patients could benefit from the consolidation with ATO and ATRA, thus usage of ATO/ATRA combination as the post-remission therapy for the APL patients in CR contributed to high efficacy and low side effects.

The therapeutic benefit of ATRA/ATO use in relapsed APL has been described previously [32–35]. However, in a randomized study of 10 cases, the ATRA/ATO combination regimen failed to induce synergistic effect [36]. In our study, the beneficial effects

Table 3. Review of clinical studies of APL in different groups.

Clinical Studies	No. of patients	Age (median)	Sanz Risk (low/int/high)	Induction Therapy	CR	Consolidation Therapy	Maintenance Therapy	Survival Outcome
Long ZJ, et al. present study	45 (20/25)	29 (10–62)	low/int 38; high 7	ATRA+DNR+Ara-C	95.6%	ATO+ATRA+IDA+Ara-C, 6 courses		3-year OS 90.2%, RFS 94.6%
Zhang YM, et al. 2013 [37]	33 (18/15)	65 (60–79)	6/22/5	ATO	87.9%	ATO, 4 years		10-year OS 69.3%, DFS 64.8%, CSS 84.8%
Lo-Coco F, et al. 2013 [38]	A: 77 (40/37); B: 79 (36/43)	A: 44.6 (19.1–70.2); B: 46.6 (18.7–70.2)	A: low/int 33/44; B: low/int 27/52	A: ATRA+ATO; B: ATRA+IDA	A: 100%; B: 95%	A: ATO+ATRA, 28 weeks; B: ATRA+IDA/MTZ, 3 cycles	B: MTX, 6-MP, ATRA, 2 years	A: 2-year OS 99%, DFS 97%; B: 2-year OS 91%, DFS 90%
Iland HJ, et al. 2012 (APML4) [39]	124 (62/62)	44 (3–78)	32/67/24	ATRA+IDA+ATO	95%	ATO+ATRA, 2 cycles	ATRA, MTX, 6-MP, 8 cycles	2-year RFS 97.5%, FFS 88.1%, OS 93.2%
Avvisati G, et al. 2011 (AIDA 0493) [40]	828 (438/390)	37.2 (1.4–74.7)	157/432/231	ATRA+IDA	94.3%	IDA+Ara-C, MTZ+VP-16, IDA+Ara-C+6-TG, 3 courses	6-MP, MTX, ATRA, 2 years	12-year EFS 68.9%, OS 76.5%, DFS 70.8%
Sanz MA, et al. 2010 (LPA2005) [41]	402 (209/193)	42 (3–83)	84/200/118	ATRA+IDA	99%/95%/83%	IDA, ATRA, MTZ, Ara-C, 3 courses	6-MP, MTX, ATRA, 2 years	4-year DFS 90% (93%/92%/82%), OS 88% (96%/91%/79%)
Powell BL, et al. 2010 (C9710) [25]	A: 244 (123/121); B: 237 (124/113)	15–60 year 207/197; >60 year 37/40	A: 69/120/55; B: 67/112/58	A: ATRA+Ara-C+DNR; B: ATRA+Ara-C+DNR	A: 90%; B: 90%	A: ATO, 2 cycles+(ATRA+DNR), 2 cycles; B: (ATRA+DNR), 2 cycles	ATRA±6-MP/MTX, 1 year	3-year EFS 80%/63%, OS 86%/81%, DFS 90%/70%
Hu J, et al. 2009 [23]	85 (47/38)	>55 year 14; ≤55 year 71	low/int 66; high 19	ATRA+ATO	94.1%	DNR+Ara-C, Ara-C pulse, HHT+Ara-C, 3 cycles	ATRA, ATO, MTX/6-MP, 5 cycles	5-year OS 91.7%, RFS 94.8%.
Lengfelder E, et al. 2009 142 (AMLCG) [42]	142 (59/83)	40 (16–60)	33/72/37	ATRA+TAD (6-TG, Ara-C, DNR)+HAM (Ara-C, MTZ)	low/int 95.2%; high 83.8%	TAD, 1 cycle	Ara-C, DNR, 6-TG, CTX, 3 years	6-year EFS 78.3%/67.3%, OS 84.4%/73.0%, RFS 82.1%/80.0%
Asou N et al. 2007 (APL97) [31]	283 (158/125)	48 (15–70)	low/int 232; high 51	ATRA±IDA/Ara-C	94%	MTZ+Ara-C, DNR+VP-16+Ara-C, IDA+Ara-C, 3 courses	BHAC, DNR, 6-MP, MTZ, VP-16, VDS, ACR, 6 courses	6-year DFS 68.5%, OS 83.9%

Abbreviations: low/int/high: low/intermediate/high; OS: overall survival; DFS: disease-free survival; CSS: cause-specific survival; FFS: failure-free survival; Ara-C: cytarabine; BHAC: behenoyl Ara-C; DNR: daunorubicin; IDA: idarubicin; MTX: methotrexate; 6-MP: mercaptopurine; MTZ: mitoxantrone; VP-16: etoposide; VDS: vindesin; ACR: aclarubicin; 6-TG: 6-thioguanine; HHT: homoharringtonine; CTX: cyclophosphamide.

were observed in the newly diagnosed APL, in contrast to that report. The reason might be that majority of the relapsed patients lost sensitivity to ATRA due to previous exposure, making it difficult to expect a full efficacy of the synergism between ATRA and ATO in those patients. In addition, parts of recent studies about different risks of patients were summarized in Table 3 [23,25,31,37–42] to make a comparison and we found that there was no strong evidence about the recommended strategy for different risk groups. However, the addition of ATO was proved to improve the long-term survival of patients with different risks, which gave support to our present study.

Mechanically, ATRA and ATO targets PML/RARα and exerts dose-dependent differentiation and apoptosis. Microarray, proteomics, and bioinformatics revealed that synergistic effect in combination therapy was due to transcriptional remodeling induced by ATRA-induced differentiation and ATO-related proteome level change. Importantly, enhanced degradation of PML-RARα might be considered for the efficacy of combination therapy in patients: ATO targeted PML, while ATRA aimed to RARα. Besides RA signaling and ubiquitin-proteasome pathway,

some self-renewal and differentiation related molecules were newly revealed to be involved in the ATO/ATRA synergistic effect, such as c-myc, Bmi-1 [14,43]. Thus, further studies should attempt to identify the network by which ATO/ATRA regulates in APL cells.

In summary, we reported that the ATO/ATRA-based regimen incorporating chemotherapy for consolidation therapy for newly diagnosed APL yielded an encouraging long-term survival rate with alleviated side effects, thus reinforcing its potential use as frontline therapy for APL.

Acknowledgments

We thank members of Department of Hematology, Third Affiliated Hospital, Sun Yat-sen University for their critical comments.

Author Contributions

Conceived and designed the experiments: QL RWH DJL. Performed the experiments: XDL YH RZX ZGF DNW JJL. Analyzed the data: ZJL YH XDL. Contributed reagents/materials/analysis tools: QL DJL RWH. Wrote the paper: ZJL YH JSY.

References

1. Wang ZY, Chen Z (2008) Acute promyelocytic leukemia: From highly fatal to highly curable. Blood 111: 2505–2515.
2. Cunningham I, Gee TS, Reich LM, Kempin SJ, Naval AN, et al. (1989) Acute promyelocytic leukemia: treatment results during a decade at Memorial Hospital. Blood 73: 1116–1122.
3. Sanz MA, Jarque I, Martin G, Lorenzo I, Martínez J, et al. (1988) Acute promyelocytic leukemia: therapy results and prognostic factors. Cancer 61: 7–13.
4. Huang ME, Ye YC, Chen SR, Chai JR, Lu JX, et al. (1988) Use of all-trans retinoic acid in the treatment of acute promyelocytic leukemia. Blood 72: 567–572.
5. Tallman MS, Andersen JW, Schiffer CA, Appelbaum FR, Feusner JH, et al. (2002) All-trans retinoic acid in acute promyelocytic leukemia: Longterm outcome and prognostic factor analysis from the North American Intergroup protocol. Blood 100: 4298–4302.
6. Tallman MS (2007) Treatment of relapsed or refractory acute promyelocytic leukemia. Best Pract Res Clin Haematol 20: 57–65.
7. Chen GQ, Shi XG, Tang W, Xiong SM, Zhu J, et al. (1997) Use of arsenic trioxide (As₂O₃) in the treatment of acute promyelocytic leukemia (APL): As2O3 exerts dosedependent dual effects on APL cells. Blood 89: 3345–3353.
8. Shen ZX, Chen GQ, Ni JH, Li XS, Xiong SM, et al. (1997) Use of arsenic trioxide (As₂O₃) in the treatment of acute promyelocytic leukemia (APL): II. Clinical efficacy and pharmacokinetics in relapsed patients. Blood 89: 3354–3360.
9. Sun HD, Ma L, Hu XC, Zhang TD (1992) Ai-Lin I treated 32 cases of acute promyelocytic leukemia. Chin J Integrat Chin West Med 12: 170–171.
10. Zhang P, Wang SY, Hu LH (1996) Arsenic trioxide treated 72 cases of acute promyelocytic leukemia. Chin J Hematol 17: 58–62.
11. Niu C, Yan H, Yu T, Sun HP, Liu JX, et al. (1999) Studies on treatment of acute promyelocytic leukemia with arsenic trioxide: remission induction, follow-up, and molecular monitoring in 11 newly diagnosed and 47 relapsed acute promyelocytic leukemia patients. Blood 94: 3315–3324.
12. Shigeno K, Naito K, Sahara N, Kobayashi M, Nakamura S, et al. (2005) Arsenic trioxide therapy in relapsed or refractory Japanese patients with acute promyelocytic leukemia: updated outcomes of the phase II study and postremission therapies. Int J Hematol 82: 224–229.
13. Soignet SL, Frankel SR, Douer D, Tallman MS, Kantarjian H, et al. (2001) United States multicenter study of arsenic trioxide in relapsed acute promyelocytic leukemia. J Clin Oncol 19: 3852–3860.
14. Zheng PZ, Wang KK, Zhang QY, Huang QH, Du YZ, et al. (2005) Systems analysis of transcriptome and proteome in retinoic acid/arsenic trioxide-induced cell differentiation/apoptosis of promyelocytic leukemia. Proc Natl Acad Sci USA 102: 7653–7658.
15. Gianni M, Koken MH, Chelbi-Alix MK, Benoit G, Lanotte M, et al. (1998) Combined arsenic and retinoic acid treatment enhances differentiation and apoptosis in arsenic-resistant NB4 cells. Blood 91: 4300–4310.
16. Jing Y, Wang L, Xia L, Chen GQ, Chen Z, et al. (2001) Combined effect of all-trans retinoic acid and arsenic trioxide in acute promyelocytic leukemia cells in vitro and in vivo. Blood 97: 264–269.
17. Lallemand-Breitenbach V, Guillemin MC, Janin A, Daniel MT, Degos L, et al. (1999) Retinoic acid and arsenic synergize to eradicate leukemic cells in a mouse model of acute promyelocytic leukemia. J Exp Med 189: 1043–1052.
18. Shen ZX, Shi ZZ, Fang J, Gu BW, Li JM, et al. (2004) All-trans retinoic acid/As₂O₃ combination yields a high quality remission and survival in newly

diagnosed acute promyelocytic leukemia. Proc Natl Acad Sci USA 101: 5328–5335.
19. Aribi A, Kantarjian HM, Estey EH, Koller CA, Thomas DA, et al. (2007) Combination therapy with arsenic trioxide, all-trans retinoic acid, and gemtuzumab ozogamicin in recurrent acute promyelocytic leukemia. Cancer 109: 1355–1359.
20. Estey E, Garcia-Manero G, Ferrajoli A, Faderl S, Verstovsek S, et al. (2006) Use of all-trans retinoic acid plus arsenic trioxide as an alternative to chemotherapy in untreated acute promyelocytic leukemia. Blood 107: 3469–3473.
21. Wang G, Li W, Cui J, Gao S, Yao C, et al. (2004) An efficient therapeutic approach to patients with acute promyelocytic leukemia using a combination of arsenic trioxide with low-dose all-trans retinoic acid. Hematol Oncol 22: 63–71.
22. Li X, Sun WJ, Li ZJ, Zhao YZ, Li YT, et al. (2007) A survival study and prognostic factors analysis on acute promyelocytic leukemia at a single center. Leuk Res 31: 765–771.
23. Hu J, Liu YF, Wu CF, Xu F, Shen ZX, et al. (2009) Long-term efficacy and safety of all-trans retinoic acid/arsenic trioxide-based therapy in newly diagnosed acute promyelocytic leukemia. Proc Natl Acad Sci U S A 106 (9): 3342–3347.
24. Gore SD, Gojo I, Sekeres MA, Morris L, Devetten M, et al. (2010) Single cycle of arsenic trioxide-based consolidation chemotherapy spares anthracycline exposure in the primary management of acute promyelocytic leukemia. J Clin Oncol 28(6): 1047–1053.
25. Powell BL, Moser B, Stock W, Gallagher RE, Willman CL, et al. (2010) Arsenic trioxide improves event-free and overall survival for adults with acute promyelocytic leukemia: North American Leukemia Intergroup Study C9710. Blood 116(19): 3751–3757.
26. Quezada G, Kopp L, Estey E, Wells RJ (2008) All-trans-retinoic acid and arsenic trioxide as initial therapy for acute promyelocytic leukemia. Pediatr Blood Cancer 51: 133–135.
27. Mathews V, George B, Lakshmi KM, Viswabandya A, Bajel A, et al. (2006) Single-agent arsenic trioxide in the treatment of newly diagnosed acute promyelocytic leukemia: Durable remissions with minimal toxicity. Blood 107: 2627–2632.
28. Ghavamzadeh A, Alimoghaddam K, Ghaffari SH, Rostami S, Jahani M, et al. (2006) Treatment of acute promyelocytic leukemia with arsenic trioxide without ATRA and/or chemotherapy. Ann Oncol 17: 131–134.
29. Dai CW, Zhang GS, Shen JK, Zheng WL, Pei MF, et al. (2009) Use of all-trans retinoic acid in combination with arsenic trioxide for remission induction in patients with newly diagnosed acute promyelocytic leukemia and for consolidation/maintenance in CR patients. Acta Haematol 121 (1): 1–8.
30. Coutre SE, Othus M, Powell B, Willman CL, Stock W, et al. (2014) Arsenic trioxide during consolidation for patients with previously untreated low/intermediate risk acute promyelocytic leukaemia may eliminate the need for maintenance therapy. Br J Haematol doi: 10.1111/bjh.12775.
31. Asou N, Kishimoto Y, Kiyoi H, Okada M, Kawai Y, et al. (2007) A randomized study with or without intensified maintenance chemotherapy in patients with acute promyelocytic leukemia who have become negative for PML-RARalpha transcript after consolidation therapy: the Japan Adult Leukemia Study Group (JALSG) APL97 study. Blood 110(1):59–66.
32. Au WY, Chim CS, Lie AK, Liang R, Kwong YL (2002) Combined arsenic trioxide and all-trans retinoic acid treatment for acute promyelocytic leukaemia recurring from previous relapses successfully treated using arsenic trioxide. Br J Haematol 117: 130–132.

33. Grigg A, Kimber R, Szer J (2003) Prolonged molecular remission after arsenic trioxide and all-trans retinoic acid for acute promyelocytic leukemia relapsed after allogeneic stem cell transplantation. Leukemia 17: 1916–1917.

34. Galimberti S, Papineschi F, Carmignani A, Testi R, Fazzi R, et al. (1999) Arsenic and all-trans retinoic acid as induction therapy before autograft in a case of relapsed resistant secondary acute promyelocytic leukemia. Bone Marrow Transplant 24: 345–348.

35. Rock N, Mattiello V, Judas C, Huezo-Diaz P, Bourquin JP, et al. (2014) Treatment of an acute promyelocytic leukemia relapse using arsenic trioxide and all-trans-retinoic in a 6-year-old child. Pediatr Hematol Oncol 31(2):143–148.

36. Raffoux E, Rousselot P, Poupon J, Daniel MT, Cassinat B, et al. (2003) Combined treatment with arsenic trioxide and all-trans-retinoic acid in patients with relapsed acute promyelocytic leukemia. J Clin Oncol 21: 2326–2334.

37. Zhang Y, Zhang Z, Li J, Li L, Han X, et al. (2013) Long-term efficacy and safety of arsenic trioxide for first-line treatment of elderly patients with newly diagnosed acute promyelocytic leukemia. Cancer 119(1):115–125.

38. Lo-Coco F, Avvisati G, Vignetti M, Thiede C, Orlando SM, et al. (2013) Retinoic acid and arsenic trioxide for acute promyelocytic leukemia. N Engl J Med 369(2):111–121.

39. Iland HJ, Bradstock K, Supple SG, Catalano A, Collins M, et al. (2012) All - trans-retinoic acid, idarubicin, and IV arsenic trioxide as initial therapy in acute promyelocytic leukemia (APML4). Blood 120(8):1570–1580.

40. Avvisati G, Lo-Coco F, Paoloni FP, Petti MC, Diverio D, et al. (2011) AIDA 0493 protocol for newly diagnosed acute promyelocytic leukemia: very long-term results and role of maintenance. Blood 117(18):4716–4725.

41. Sanz MA, Montesinos P, Rayón C, Holowiecka A, de la Serna J, et al. (2010) Risk-adapted treatment of acute promyelocytic leukemia based on all-trans retinoic acid and anthracycline with addition of cytarabine in consolidation therapy for high-risk patients: futher improvements in treatment outcome. Blood 115(25): 5137–5146.

42. Lengfelder E, Haferlach C, Saussele S, Haferlach T, Schultheis B, et al. (2009) High dose ara-C in the treatment of newly diagnosed acute promyelocytic leukemia: long-term results of the German AMLCG. Leukemia 23(12):2248–2258.

43. Dos Santos GA, Kats L, Pandolfi PP (2013) Synergy against PML-RARa: targeting transcription, proteolysis, differentiation, and self-renewal in acute promyelocytic leukemia. J Exp Med 210(13):2793–2802.

13

Clinicopathologic Characterization of Diffuse-Large-B-Cell Lymphoma with an Associated Serum Monoclonal IgM Component

M. Christina Cox[1]*[◆], Arianna Di Napoli[2◆], Stefania Scarpino[2], Gerardo Salerno[3], Caterina Tatarelli[1], Caterina Talerico[2], Mariangela Lombardi[2], Bruno Monarca[1], Sergio Amadori[4], Luigi Ruco[2]

1 Hematology Unit, Sant'Andrea Hospital, Department of Clinical and Molecular Medicine La Sapienza University, Rome, Italy, 2 Pathology Unit, Department of Clinical and Molecular Medicine, Sant'Andrea Hospital, La Sapienza University, Rome, Italy, 3 Clinical Pathology Unit, Department of Clinical and Molecular Medicine Sant'Andrea Hospital, La Sapienza University, Rome, Italy, 4 Hematology Department, Tor Vergata University, Rome, Italy

Abstract

Recently, diffuse-large-B-cell lymphoma (DLBCL) associated with serum IgM monoclonal component (MC) has been shown to be a very poor prognostic subset although, detailed pathological and molecular data are still lacking. In the present study, the clinicopathological features and survival of IgM-secreting DLBCL were analyzed and compared to non-secreting cases in a series of 151 conventional DLBCL treated with R-CHOP. IgM MC was detected in 19 (12.5%) out of 151 patients at disease onset. In 17 of these cases secretion was likely due to the neoplastic clone, as suggested by the expression of heavy chain IgM protein in the cytoplasm of tumor cells. In IgM-secreting cases immunoblastic features (p<.0001), non-GCB-type (p = .002) stage III-IV(p = .003), ≥2 extra nodal sites (p<.0001), bone-marrow (p = .002), central-nervous-system (CNS) involvement at disease onset or relapse (p<.0001), IPI-score 3–5 (p = .009) and failure to achieve complete remission (p = .005), were significantly more frequent. FISH analyses for BCL2, BCL6 and MYC gene rearrangements detected only two cases harboring BCL2 gene translocation and in one case a concomitant BCL6 gene translocation was also observed. None of the IgM-secreting DLBCL was found to have L265P mutation of MYD88 gene. Thirty-six month event-free (11.8% vs 66.4% p<.0001), progression-free (23.5% vs 75.7%, p<.0001) and overall (47.1% vs 74.8%, p<.0001) survivals were significantly worse in the IgM-secreting group. In multivariate analysis IgM-secreting (p = .005, expB = 0.339, CI = 0.160-0.716) and IPI-score 3–5 (p = .010, expB = 0.274, CI = 0.102–0.737) were the only significant factors for progression-free-survival. Notably, four relapsed patients, who were treated with salvage immmunochemotherapy combined with bortezomib or lenalidomide, achieved lasting remission. Our data suggests that IgM-secreting cases are a distinct subset of DLBCL, originating from activated-B-cells with terminally differentiated features, prevalent extra nodal dissemination and at high risk of CNS involvement.

Editor: Kristy L. Richards, University of North Carolina at Chapel Hill, United States of America

Funding: Fondi di ricerca di Ateneo. The funders had no role in study design, data collection and analysis, decision to publish, or preparation of the manuscript.

Competing Interests: The authors have declared that no competing interests exist.

* E-mail: chrisscox@gmail.com

◆ These authors contributed equally to this work.

Introduction

Diffuse-Large-B-cell Lymphoma (DLBCL) is a biologically heterogeneous entity [1],that is still homogeneously treated with Rituximab-Cyclophosphamide-Adriamycin-Vincristine-Prednisone (R-CHOP) immunochemotherapy [2]. Since the combination of rituximab and CHOP became the gold standard for DLBCL treatment, the International-Prognostic-Index score (IPI-score) has proved to be less powerful [3]. Moreover, the IPI variables [4] do not provide insight into DLBCL biology. A pivotal step in unveiling DLBCL biology and clinical heterogeneity was achieved in 2000 when Alizadeh et al. identified by gene-expression-profiling (GEP) two main groups of DLBCL with substantially different outcomes: Activated-B-cell type (ABC-type) and Germinal-Center-B-cell type (GCB-type) [5]. Since then considerable efforts have been made in order to translate the complexity of GEP-derived information into fewer data readily

achievable by routine tests. However, this attempt is still in progress [6], and the choice of shifting towards an upfront intensified treatment remains largely based on the IPI-score or on IPI-derived scores [7,8]. Notwithstanding, new biomarkers and scores are needed to identify very poor-risk DLBCL sub-groups [9–12]. During the course of 2011 we noticed that three newly diagnosed DLBCL patients who shared poor presenting features and early relapse after R-CHOP, had a serum IgM monoclonal component (MC) at disease onset. In the literature only few occasional studies describing IgM-secreting DLBCL associated to haemolytic anemia or other paraproteinemia related events were reported [13–15]. In order to find out whether our observation was just an incidental finding, we started to search for similar cases in our database. In 2011 Maurer et al. [16], showed that in DLBCL increased serum free light chain (FLC) represented an independent adverse prognostic factor and in 2013 Jardin et al. [17] found that an abnormal IgMκ/IgMλ ratio was associated with survival in patients with DLBCL. In this study we have further increased and characterized a series of DLBCL with an associated IgM MC [18], reporting detailed analysis of their clinical, histological and molecular features.

Methods

Patients

This is a retrospective study evaluating the incidence of IgM-secreting DLBCL and comparing this subset with a non-secreting control group for clinicopathological features and survival. The study was approved by our Institutional Review Board (procedure code: RS 44/2013, Sant'Andrea Hospital Ethics Committee) and was conducted in accordance with the regulations of health information protection policies. Patients were asked to sign a written consent at disease onset in order to collect their data on an electronic database and to allow further pathological characterization of biological material harvested for diagnostic purposes. Clinical data, including HCV and HBV markers screening, were prospectively collected and obtained from corresponding medical records. A hundred and fifty-one patients (68F/83M, median age 62 years) diagnosed with conventional *de novo* DLBCL [19] between 2005 and February 2013 at Sant'Andrea Hospital of Rome were enrolled in the study. All 151 patients were analyzed for serum protein electrophoresis at disease onset, and those who had a likely monoclonal band in the serum were further investigated by serum immunofixation (methods are fully described in File S1). From the 151 patients a set of 107 consecutive non-secreting DLBCL were selected as control cases for survival analysis. All these cases had a follow up time ≥24 months, unless a DLBCL–related event (i.e. primary refractoriness, relapse or death) had occurred earlier. Immunodeficiency-associated lymphomas, patients who had been previously treated with radiotherapy or chemotherapy for low-grade lymphoma and patients with stage I non-bulky were excluded from the study.

High risk patients younger than 61 years were treated with R-CHOP every 14 days [20], all other patients with R-CHOP every 21 days [2]. Patients with central nervous system (CNS) involvement were treated with R-CHOP every 21 days plus high dose methotrexate at day +8. Patients with IPI score 4–5 or involvement of bone marrow, testis, and craniofacial sites or with involvement of ≥2 extra nodal sites, received intrathecal prophylaxis with 4–6 injections of 12 mg methotrexate.

HCV and HBV test

Before chemotherapy all patients were tested for hepatitis B surface antigen and its antibody (HBsAg, HBsAb), antibodies to the core antigen (HBcAb, total and IgM), and for hepatitis C virus (HCV) antibodies. Commercially available enzyme immunoassays were used for HBV and HCV determinations (Architect, Abbott Diagnostics, Italy). All cases were tested for hepatitis B virus deoxyribonucleic acid polymerase chain reaction (Amplicor Roche, Italy- lower limit of detection <200 cp/ml). Only cases that were positive for HCV antibodies were further investigated for HCV–RNA (Amplicor Roche, Italy). Either active, inactive or occult HBV carriers [21] were classified as HBV-positive. Cases were considered HCV-positive if HCV antibodies were positive (Table 1).

Morphological and Immunohistochemical analyses

Classification and subtyping of all tumors followed the definitions of the 2008 WHO classification of DLBCL [19]. Immunostainings for CD3, CD5, CD20, CD79a, CD10, MUM1, BCL2, BCL6, kappa and lambda light chains and heavy chain IgM (all purchased by DAKO, Denmark) were performed using Dako automated immunostainer (DAKO, Denmark). Immunohistochemistry with anti-MYC (clone Y69, Ventana-Roche, Italy) was conducted using BenchMark Ultra automated immunostainer (Ventana Medical Systems, Tucson, AZ, USA). The Hans algorithm [22] was used in order to classify cases as GCB-type or non GCB-type. Immunostaining results for BCL2 and MYC were recorded as the percentage of positive cells in increments of 10% regardless of the intensity of the staining. Cases were considered as negative if <5% of tumor cells were positive. Immunohistochemical and morphological analyses were independently evaluated by two experienced hematopathologists (LR, ADN). Disagreements were resolved by joint review on a multi-head microscope.

FISH and molecular analyses

Since the aim of this study was to define the clinicopathologic features of the IgM-secreting subset, the analyses of recurring chromosomal translocations, MYD88 gene mutation, the BCL2/MYC immunhistochemical score, and the presence of EBV-infection were carried out only in the IgM-secreting subset and in a small control group of non-secreting DLBCL cases (Table S1 in File S1). FISH analyses in tissue paraffin sections were carried out with the following probes: MYC dual color break-apart, BCL6 dual color break-apart; IGH/BCL2 dual color fusion (Vysis, Abbott Molecular Inc. US), and BCL2 dual color break-apart (Kreatech Diagnostics, The Netherlands). The cut-off values for the interphase FISH analyses were established following the criteria of Ventura [23]. In situ hybridization for EBV-encoded RNA (EBER) was performed on paraffin sections using Epstein - Barr virus (EBER) PNA Probe/Fluorescein, and FITC/HRP (DAKO, Denmark)

Allele-specific polymerase chain reaction (AS-PCR) was performed using two reverse primers designed to recognize the mutant and the wild-type allele of MYD88 L265P as previously described [24]. The mutant-specific reverse primer was 5′-CCT TGT ACT TGA TGG GGA aCG-3′ and the wild-type-specific reverse primer was 5′-GCC TTG TAC TTG ATG GGG AAC A-3′. The common forward primer was 5′-AAT GTG TGC CAG GGG TAC TTA G-3′. PCR reaction was performed using AmpliTaq Gold PCR Master Mix (Applied Biosystems, Forster City, CA, USA) in a final volume of 25 mL with 50 nM of each primer and 100 ng of DNA. Thermal cycling conditions were as follow: 2 min. at 94°C, followed by 40 cycles of 94°C for 30 s, 57° for 30 s. and a final extension at 68°C for 5 min. The amplified PCR products (159 bp) were separated on 2% agarose gel. One case of Waldenström macroglobulinemia was used as MYD88 L265P mutation positive control (Detailed methodologies are fully described in File S1).

Statistics

Categorical data were compared using Fisher's exact test and two-sided p-value, whereas for ordinal data, non-parametric tests were used. The definitions of complete response (CR), event free survival (EFS), progression free survival (PFS) and overall survival (OS) were the standard [25]. The actuarial survival analysis was carried out according to the method described by Kaplan and Meier and the curves compared by the log-rank test [26]. The multivariate analyses for survival were carried out by using the stepwise proportional hazards model [27]. Statistical analyses were done with IBM SPSS Statistics 19 (SPSS Inc. Chicago, IL, USA).

Table 1. Comparison of clinicopathological features in DLBCL subgroups.

Features (cases investigated)	IgM-secreting	Non-secreting	P-value[1]	IgM+/non secreting	P-value[2]
	n = 17	n = 134		n = 34	
ALC ≤0.840. 10⁹/L³ (n = 143)	47%(7/15)	24%(31/128)	.118	23%(7/30)	.265
BULKY>7.5 cm (n = 151)	23%(4/17)	36%(48/134)	.248	41%(14/34)	.320
HBV+ (n = 148)	25%(4/16)	13.6%(18/132)	.261	18%(18/34)	.707
HCV+ (n = 141)	19%(3/16)	13%(16/125)	.368	9%(3/34)	.370
Anemia <12 g/dL (n = 139)	71%(12/17)	42%(51/122)	.036	39%(13/33)	.072
Sex female (n = 151)	70%(13/17)	41%(134)	.008	47%(16/34)	.072
COO⁴: non-GCB-type (n = 41)	100%(17/17)	54.4%(49/90)	.001	85%(29/34)³	.357
COO: GCB-type (n = 66)	0%(0/17)	45.5%(41/90)	.001	12%(4/34)	.357
Immunoblastic-Morphology (n = 151)	76%(13/17)	3%(4/134)	<.0001	9%(n = 3/34)	<.0001
Bone Marrow+ (n = 149)	71% (12/17)	28%(37/132)	.002	23.5% (8/34)	.002
CNS⁵ (n = 124)	41%(7/17)	4%(4/107)	<.0001	9%(3/34)	.010
Age >60 (n = 151)	82%(14/17)	54%(75/134)	.040	62%(21/34)	.203
LDH abnormal (n = 148)	56%(9/16)	52%(69/132)	.797	48%(16/33)	.762
Extra nodal sites ≥2 (n = 151)	82%(14/17)	34%(46/134)	<.0001	32% (11/34)	.001
Stage 3–4 (n = 150)	100%(17/17)	68%(91/134)	.003	73%(24/33)	.020
ECOG-PS⁶≥2 (n = 151)	59%(10/17)	33%(44/134)	.057	32%(11/34)	.130
IPI 3–5⁷ (n = 149)	88%(15/17)	55%(73/133)	.009	47%(16/34)	.006
Complete Remission (n = 151)	47%(8/17)	80.5%(108/134)	.005	79%(27/34)	.027

p-value[1]: comparison of clinical features in IgM-secreting and non-secreting DLBCL subgroups.
p-value[2] comparison of clinical features in IgM-secreting and IgM+/non-secreting DLBCL subgroups.
ALC³: absolute lymphocyte count.
COO⁴:: cell of origin based on the Hans algorithm.
CNS⁵ central nervous system involvement at diagnosis or relapse.
ECOG-PS⁶≥2: performance status following the ECOG nomenclature.
IPI 3–5⁷: International prognostic index score 3–5.

Results

IgM serum levels at diagnosis and during follow-up

In 19 out of 151 (12.6%) DLBCL a serum monoclonal IgM component was detected. The serum level of monoclonal IgM at diagnosis varied from 2.5 g/dL to 0.22 g/dL (median value 0.42 g/dL). Eleven out of 19 (58%) patients were monitored by serum immunofixation and FLC k/λ ratio during the course of treatment and follow-up. After 1-3 cycles of R-CHOP the monoclonal IgM component disappeared and the FLC k/λ ratio returned to the normal range in all of these patients. Three out of four patients (75%) at tumor recurrence were negative for serum monoclonal IgM and had a normal FLC k/λ ratio. In the remaining case the reappearance of a monoclonal IgM and of FLC k/λ abnormal ratio preceded relapse. Four patients who are in continuous complete remission are persistently negative for both. Two patients with an IgM MC not related to the neoplastic clone (Table 2) showed no disappearance of the IgM MC during and after treatment.

Pathological Features

One-hundred and seven out of 151 (71%) DLBCL were suitable to be classified for the cell-of-origin (COO) using the Hans algorithm [22]. Of these, 66 out of 107 cases (61.6%) were classified as non-GCB-type and 41 out of 107 (38.3%) as GCB-type. The same cases were also analyzed for the expression of cytoplasmic IgM chains, except for five cases (4.7%) in which one of the two assessments was not achievable (Figure 1). Fifty-one out of 107 DLBCL (47.6%) showed IgM expression in the cytoplasm of tumor cells (IgM+ cases); of these, 47 cases (92%) were classified as non-GCB-type and four cases (7.8%) as GCB-type. Within the IgM+ group 17/51 (33.3%) DLBCL had an associated serum IgM monoclonal component. Immunostaining of paraffin tissue sections allowed to detect in the tumor cells the same type of heavy chain IgM, and of light chain κ (n = 15) or λ(n = 2) found in patient's serum. These findings suggest that the serum monoclonal IgM component was related to the DLBCL clone. These 17 cases are from here on referred as IgM-secreting DLBCL (Table 1). The remaining 34/51 cases (66.6%) are referred as IgM+/non-secreting DLBCL. Two additional patients had a monoclonal IgM component in the serum although, tumors stained negative for cytoplasmic IgM (Table 2). All 17 IgM-secreting cases were CD10 negative and MUM1 positive and were classified as non-GCB-type. Moreover, based on the morphology 13 out of the 17 (76%) cases were classified as immunoblastic DLBCL (Figure S1 in File S1) compared to only 4 out of 134 (3%) cases in the control group (p<.0001) and 3 out of 34 (9%) in the IgM+/non-secreting subset (p<.0001) (Table 1). Nine patients out of 134 (6.8%) in the non IgM-secreting group and one out of 17 (5.8%) in the IgM-secreting group had composite lymphoma at diagnosis with the simultaneous presence of DLBCL and a low-grade B-cell lymphoma.

Molecular analyses

Molecular analyses were performed in the IgM-secreting DLBCL and in a control group of non-secreting DLBCL (Table

Table 2. Clinicopathological features of 19 DLBCL with a serum monoclonal IgM protein.

Cases	Extra nodal sites	Morphology	COO[2]	IgM-I[3]	EBER	LMP1	HIV	MYC-I[4]	BCL2-I[5]	MYC-f[6]	BCL2-f[7]	BCL6-f[8]	MYD88[9]	FUP-[10]	Status
1	CNS[1], Liver	Immunoblastic	Non-GCB	+	neg	neg	neg	90%	70%	NE[11]	NE	NE	WT[16]	5	Died in progression
2	Marrow, Liver, Lung, CNS	Immunoblastic	Non-GCB	+	neg	neg	neg	50%	40%	NE	NT[12]	NE	WT	5	Died in progression
3	Bone, Marrow, PB, CNS	Immunoblastic	Non-GCB	+	neg	neg	neg	90%	80%	NT	T[13]	T	WT	19	Died in progression
4	Lung, Marrow, CNS	Immunoblastic	Non-GCB	+	neg	neg	neg	70%	neg	NE	NE	NE	WT	1	Early death
5	Bone, CNS, Marrow	Immunoblastic	Non-GCB	+	NE	NE	neg	NE	NE	NT	NT	NT	NE	14	Died in progression
6	Kidney, Gut, Adrenal gland, CNS	Immunoblastic	Non-GCB	+	neg	neg	neg	20%	20%	NT	T	NT	WT	4	Died in progression
7	Intestine, mesenter	DLBCL	Non-GCB	+	neg	neg	neg	40%	>90%	NT	NT	NT	WT	60	CCR1[14]
8	Bone, Marrow, PB, bones	Immunoblastic	Non-GCB	+	neg	neg	neg	40%	50%	NT	NT	NT	WT	18	CCR1
9	Marrow, PB	Immunoblastic	Non-GCB	+	neg	neg	neg	60%	70%	NT	NT	NT	WT	38	CCR1
10	Lung, Marrow	Immunoblastic	Non-GCB	+	neg	neg	neg	10%	60%	NT	NT	NT	WT	29	CCR2[15]
11	Pharynx	Immunoblastic	Non-GCB	+	neg	neg	neg	30%	>90%	NT	NT	NT	WT	41	CCR2
12	Marrow, PB	Immunoblastic	Non-GCB	+	neg	neg	neg	20%	neg	NT	NE	NE	WT	60	CCR2
13	Pharynx, Marrow	Immunoblastic	Non-GCB	+	neg	neg	neg	40%	50–60%	NT	NT	NT	WT	22	CCR2
14	None	T-cell rich	Non-GCB	+	neg	neg	neg	10–20%	80%	NT	NT	NT	WT	35	Died in progression
15	None	Immunoblastic	Non-GCB	+	neg	neg	neg	40%	>90%	NT	NT	NT	WT	1	Early death
16	Kidney, intestine, peritoneum, bone	DLBCL	Non-GCB	+	NE	NE	neg	NE	60%	NE	NE	NE	NE	2	Died refractory
17	Marrow, pharynx, CNS	DLBCL	Non-GCB	+	neg	neg	neg	60–70%	>90%	NT	NT	NT	WT	5	On treatment
18	Marrow, Uterus	Centroblastic	GCB	-	neg	neg	neg	4%	>90%	NT	NT	NE	WT	16	Died in progression
19	Bone	DLBCL	Non-GCB	-	neg	neg	neg	20–30%	60%	NE	NE	NT	WT	7	On treatment

CNS[1]: Central nervous system involvement at diagnosis or during relapse progression.
COO[2]: Cell of Origin defined by the Hans algorithm.
IgM-I[3]: heavy chain IgM expression assessed by immunohistochemistry.
MYC-I[4]: MYC protein expression by immunohistochemistry.
BCL2-I[5]: BCL2 protein expression by immunohistochemistry.
MYC-f[6]: MYC gene translocation by FISH analysis.
BCL2-f[7]: BCL2 gene translocation by FISH analysis, carried out by both IGH/BCL2 and BCL2 break apart probes.
BCL6-f[8]: BCL6 gene translocation by FISH analysis.
MYD88[9]: MYD88 gene analyzed for L265P mutation.
FUP[10]: Follow-up.
NE[11]: Not evaluable.
NT[12]: Not translocated.
T[13]: Translocated.
CCR1[14],1st Continuous complete remission.
CCR2[15], 2nd Continuous complete remission.
WT[16]: wild type.

	IgM-secreting DLBC	Non-secreting DLBC	IgM IHC	COO	Survival Analysis
Protein Electrophoresis	17	134	107	107	124
Survival Analysis	17	107	107	107	
COO	17	90	102		
IgM IHC	17	90			

Figure 1. The cross table diagram shows in the colored rectangles the type of analysis that was carried out or the subgroup of DLBCL (non-secreting and IgM-secreting). The white rectangles show the number of cases that match the crossing of horizontal and vertical rows.

S1 in File S1). A total of 35 cases were studied for EBV-status, 45 cases for common chromosomal translocations and 30 cases for L265P somatic mutation of MYD88 gene respectively. The results of these analyses did not differ from data reported in the literature [28–30]. In the 19 DLBCL patients with a serum IgM MC (Table 2), EBER and LMP1 were evaluable in 17 cases (89.5%) and all of them were negative. None of the 16 evaluable IgM-secreting DLBCL showed MYD88 L265P mutation (Figure S2 File S1). In cases with serum IgM MC FISH analyses were feasible for MYC and BCL2 translocations in 14/19 (74%), and for BCL6 gene rearrangements in 13/19 (68.4%) cases respectively. Two IgM-secreting cases harbored BCL2 translocation; one of these had concomitant translocation of BCL6 gene (Table 2). None of the IgM-secreting cases investigated was found to be rearranged for MYC. Overall, the incidence of chromosomal translocations, and of MYD88 L265P mutation (Figure S2 in File S1) were lower in the IgM-secreting group compared to the control group although the differences were not statistically significant.

Clinical features and outcome

All the DLBCL (n = 151) were analyzed for clinical characteristics and prognostic scores (Table 1). One-hundred and twenty-four patients out of 151 (82%) with a follow-up ≥24 months or a DLBCL–related event (i.e. primary refractoriness, relapse or death) were considered suitable for survival analysis (Figure 2a). One-hundred and seven patients out of the 124 cases included in the survival analysis (Figure 1) were tested for COO and IgM expression. All the 17 IgM-secreting cases were of the non-GCB-type (100%) in contrast to only 50/90 (55%) in the non-secreting tumors (p = .002). The following clinicopathological features were significantly more frequent in the IgM-secreting group compared to the non-secreting group and also compared to the IgM+/non-secreting subset: immunoblastic morphology, advanced stage of disease, IPI score 3–5, extra nodal involvement ≥2, bone marrow and central nervous system (CNS) involvement, failure to achieve complete remission after R-CHOP. Anemia, female sex and age> 60 years were significantly more frequent in the IgM-secreting compared to the non-secreting group (Table 1). Sixteen out of 17 IgM-secreting DLBCL (94%) were *de-novo* DLBCL without a

previous history of low-grade lymphoma. One patient was diagnosed with nodal marginal zone lymphoma ten years earlier, but she did not receive any treatment before transformation into DLBCL. One patient had autoimmune hemolytic anemia related to the monoclonal IgM antibody; another with massive kidney infiltration by DLBCL presented a nephrotic syndrome with intact monoclonal IgM in the urine. In the remaining 15 cases no other paraproteinemia-related signs were observed.

Fifteen out of 17 (88.2%) IgM-secreting patients had a DLBCL-related event compared to 36 out of 107 (33.6%) control cases (p< .0001). Nine out of 17 (53%) IgM-secreting patients and 27 out of 107 (25%) control cases died (p<.0001). In the IgM-secreting group, seven patients died with primary refractory or relapsed lymphoma. Two patients died within one month from the start of treatment for toxicity: one patient was in very poor conditions with diffuse meningeal and brain involvement, while the other died of ischemic stroke during treatment. Worthy of note, seven out of 17 IgM-secreting patients (41%) had CNS localization at disease onset (2/17 cases) or during progression/relapse (5/17 cases) (Table 2). One of these patients achieved partial remission on third line treatment with low dose bendamustine and lenalidomide but died in progression after eight months. Eight out of 17 IgM-secreting patients (47%) are alive. Two patients who relapsed within eight months from diagnosis are progression free at +33 and +21 months respectively after second line salvage treatment with bortezomib-rituximab-DHAP [31] followed by high dose therapy (HDT) and peripheral blood stem cell (PBSC) rescue. One patient is progression free at +36 months after second line salvage treatment with rituximab-bendamustine and lenalidomide maintenance [32].One patient who relapsed ten months after diagnosis is in 2nd complete remission at +12 months after rituximab-DHAP and lenalidomide maintenance. One patient, who achieved less than partial remission after four cycles of R-CHOP, is presently in 1st CR after two cycles of RMAD [33] at +15 months. One patient had CNS progression after two cycles of R-CHOP and is responding to high-dose methotrexate. Only two patients are progression free after first line R-CHOP at +60 and +38 months respectively. Of the two patients who had a monoclonal IgM component in the serum but were negative for heavy chain IgM

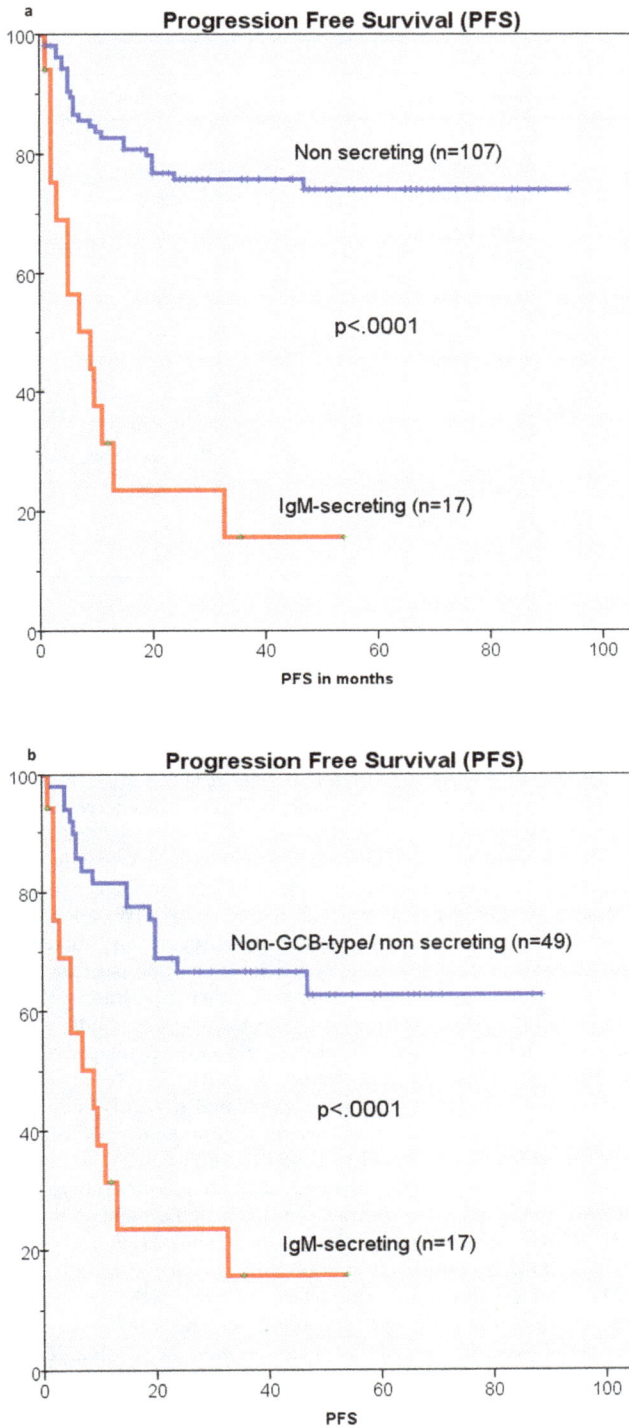

Figure 2. Kaplan-Meier estimates of progression free survival (PFS) in IgM-secreting and in non-secreting DLBCL patients. a) PFS of IgM-secreting and non-secreting DLBCL patients; b) PFS of IgM-secreting and non-GCB-type DLBCL patients.

expression by IHC (Table 2), one died with resistant relapse 16 months after diagnosis, while the other is in complete remission seven months after diagnosis (Table 2).

Survival analysis

The estimated 36-month PFS (23.5% vs 75.7%, p<.0001) (Figure 2a) and OS (47.1% Vs 74.8%, p<.0001) were significantly worse for the IgM-secreting compared to the non-secreting group (Table 3). The differences in survival remained significant even when the IgM-secreting group was compared to the non–GCB-type (Figure 2b). In multivariate analysis (Table 4), IgM-secreting (p = .005, expB = 0.339, CI = 0.160–0.716) and IPI-score 3–5 (p = .010, expB = 0.274, CI = 0.102–0.737) were the only significant factors for PFS; while IPI-score 3–5 was the only significant factor for OS (p = .001, expB = 0.186, CI = 0.071–0.484). A subset of 107/124 (86%) patients who were investigated by IHC for heavy chain IgM expression in tumor samples, were analyzed for the relevance of this factor. The expression of IgM was a significant prognostic factor in univariate analysis (Figure 3a) for PFS (p = .009) and OS (p = .024). However, when patients were subdivided into three sub-groups: 1) IgM-negative (n = 56); 2) IgM+/non-secreting (n = 34) and 3) IgM-secreting (n = 17) survival analysis showed a significant difference only between the IgM-secreting group versus the other two groups (Figure 3b and Figure S3 in File S1).

Discussion

The identification of poor-prognostic subgroups correlated to defined biological tumor characteristics is the aim of modern oncological research. In the case of DLBCL this issue is presently a matter of intense development and debate. Several prognostic factors and scores have been proposed to better stratify patients who would benefit from more intensive treatment than R-CHOP [5,10,11]. We had previously reported on a subset of conventional DLBCL associated with a serum monoclonal IgM component characterized by advanced disease and poor prognosis after R-CHOP [18]. In this study we described its clinical, pathological and, molecular features more in depth.

DLBCL with serum IgM MC represented a sizable subset of our series. The majority of these cases were defined as IgM-secreting DLBCL since same type of heavy chain IgM and κ or λ light chains were detected in tumor cells. Most patients had advanced disease, involvement of several extra nodal sites including bone marrow and high IPI-score. Worthy of note, the incidence of CNS involvement at diagnosis or during relapse/progression was surprisingly high. Most of these poor prognostic features remained significantly more frequent in the IgM-secreting subset even when compared to the IgM+/non-secreting subset. Monitoring patients by immunofixation and FLC κ/λ ratio during and after therapy was of little value for predicting relapse. All IgM-secreting cases were classified as non-GCB-type and the great majority showed Immunoblastic morphology.

L265P mutation of MYD88 gene has been reported within 6.5% and 17% of unselected DLBCL [28–30]. More recently, this mutation has been shown to be very common in DLBCL originating in extra nodal sites [30]. Since L265P mutation of MYD88 gene was prevalent in IgM-secreting Waldenström macroglobulinemia [24], and it was reported in up to 29% of DLBCL with an ABC-type [34], we expected to find this mutation in the IgM-secreting DLBCL subset. Surprisingly, none of IgM-secreting DLBCL showed L265P mutation of MYD88 gene. This result suggests that other molecular pathways may be involved in IgM-secreting DLBCL [35].

Recurring chromosomal translocations have been reported in DLBCL [36–40]. In our series of IgM-secreting DLBCL these were not a distinct feature. None of the tumors showed MYC rearrangement and only two cases harbored BCL2 translocation.

Table 3. Survival analyses comparison for main predictors.

Predictors	36-month rate	P-value
Progression free survival		
Non-GCB[1] (yes vs no)	54.5% vs 85%	<.0001
IgM-secreting (yes vs no)	23.5% vs 75.7%	<.0001
Immunoblastic Morphology (yes vs no)	23.5% vs 75.7%	<.0001
Anemia HB<12 g/dL (yes vs no)	52.7% vs 80.7%	.001
IPI[2] (0–2 vs 3–5)	52.8% vs 90.4%	<.0001
ALC[3] ≤0.840. 10^9/L (yes vs no)	51.6% vs 75.3%	.003
Bone marrow involvement (yes vs no)	46.3% vs 79%	.001
Overall survival		
IgM-secreting (yes vs no)	47.1% vs 74.8%	<.0001
Immunoblastic Morphology (yes vs no)	47.1% vs 74.8%	<.0001
IPI (0–2 vs 3–5)	56.9% vs 90.4%	<.0001
ALC ≤0.840. 10^9/L (yes vs no)	61.3% vs 76.5%	.022
Bone marrow involvement (yes vs no)	58.5% vs 76.5%	.024

Non-GCB[1] = Non Germinal Center type, evaluated on the basis of the Hans' algorithm.
IPI[2] = international prognostic index scores 0–2 and 3–5.
ALC[3] = absolute lymphocyte count.

In 2011 Maurer et al [16], showed that increased serum FLC, present in 32% of DLBCL was an independent adverse prognostic factor. More recently, after the introduction of a new sensitive method for immunoglobulin heavy chain detection, a prospective study showed elevated IgMκ or IgMλ or an abnormal IgMκ/IgMλ ratio to occur in 9.3% and 19.1% of DLBCL respectively [17]. Similarly to us, they found a lower PFS and OS in patients with IgM serological abnormalities. Although the two methods are not perfectly comparable, patients with a serum monoclonal IgM detected by immunofixation, as we did in our study, should reasonably have an abnormal IgMκ/IgMλ ratio and possibly also an elevated IgMκ or IgMλ immunoglobulin. The lower sensitivity of our method and the fact that we carried out serum immunofixation only in those patients who had an abnormal protein electrophoresis could explain why the proportion of IgM-secreting DLBCL in our series was somewhat lower compared to that with an abnormal IgMκ/IgMλ ratio described by Jardin et al. [17]. Conversely, Jardin et al. using a very sensitive detection method (Binding Site's Hevylite assay, San Diego, CA, USA) could have possibly found cases with an abnormal IgMκ/IgMλ ratio or an elevated IgMκ or IgMλ without a real clinical significance.

The expression of the heavy chain IgM gene was shown in the Wright signature to be one of the most discriminating genes between GCB and ABC DLBCL subtypes [41–42]. It has been also reported that IgM isotype expression in tumor tissues is a more powerful prognostic marker than the Hans algorithm [43]. In our series the expression of heavy chain IgM in tumor cells was found in less than half of the patients. IgM+ cases were mostly classified as non-GCB-type and a third of the cases belonging to this group were also IgM-secreting. Survival analyses of IgM+/non-secreting subset was similar to that of IgM-negative patients. Although we could not analyze all the series by IHC for heavy chain IgM, our data suggests that the poor prognosis attributed to IgM+ cases could be at least in part related to those patients who are IgM-secreting. Notably, monitoring patients by immunofixation and FLC κ/λ ratio during and after therapy was of little value for predicting tumor relapse. Indeed, even in overt relapse, three out of four patients were found negative for serum IgM monoclonal component. It can be speculated that this finding is the result of a clonal evolution of lymphoma cells during progression leading to loss of secretion capability.

Recently, it has been identified a plasmablastic subtype of DLBCL thought to derive from terminally differentiated B-cells [44]. This subset is frequently associated with HIV and EBV infection and is considered a very poor prognostic group. The IgM-secreting subset we characterized, was HIV and EBV negative [45–46] and did not show the morphological and immunophenotypic findings of plasmablastic lymphoma. Conversely, the majority of IgM-secreting cases showed immunoblastic

Table 4. Multivariate analyses for the response and survival.

Progression free survival	Exp(B) (95%CI)	P-value
IPI (3–5)[1]	0.274(0.102–0.737)	.010
IgM-secreting	0.339(0.160–0.716)	.005
Overall survival		
IPI (3-5)	0.186 (0.071–0.484)	0.001

IPI[1] (3–5): International prognostic score index value 3–5.

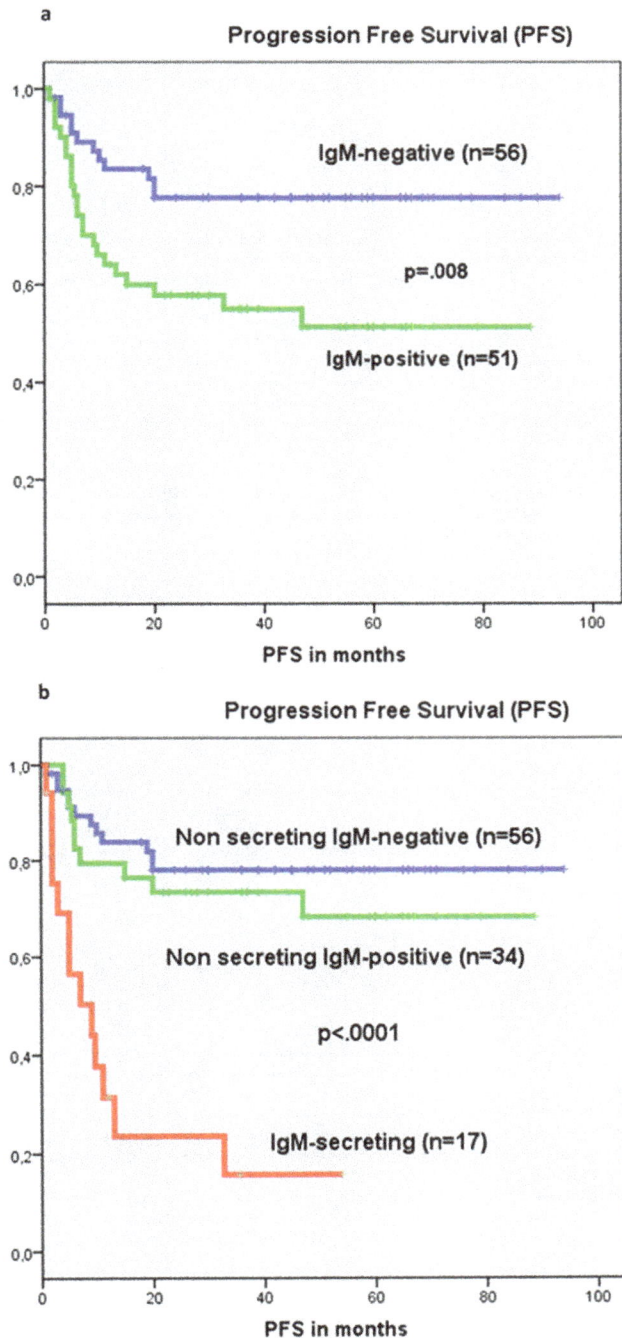

Figure 3. a) Kaplan-Meier estimates of progression free survival (PFS) in patients who are positive for heavy chain IgM (IgM+) by Immunohistochemistry (IHC) and in patients who are negative for heavy chain IgM (IgM-negative) by IHC. b) Kaplan-Meier estimates of PFS in patients negative for heavy chain IgM expression by IHC (IgM-negative), in patients positive for heavy chain IgM expression by IHC but non-secreting (IgM+/non-secreting) and in patients positive for heavy chain IgM expression by IHC and IgM-secreting (IgM-secreting).

features. This finding is in accordance with the notion that secreting capability is acquired by B-cells during end-stage differentiation and that terminally differentiated high grade lymphoma has a poor prognosis [44,47–48].

In our series of IgM-secreting DLBCL, we found a strikingly high incidence of CNS involvement. This finding is in keeping with previous studies showing that primary lymphoma of the central nervous system expresses an IgM isotype [49–51], and with the detection of FLC in the cerebrospinal fluid of patients with CNS lymphoma [52]. If our observation will be validated by further studies, an intensified CNS prophylaxis should be recommended in patients with IgM-secreting DLBCL.

Outcome after R-CHOP was disappointing in IgM-secreting patients with most relapses occurring within one year from diagnosis. Interestingly, four patients who relapsed without CNS involvement achieved lasting complete remission when treated with immunochemotherapy combined with biological drugs such as bortezomib or lenalidomide [31–32].This fact might suggest that these combinations could be more effective and less toxic than high-intensity treatments in this very poor risk group.

Finally, we speculate that IgM-secretion in DLBCL has since been underrated because it is easily missed by clinicians given the rarity of associated clinical signs, its low entity at diagnosis and rapid disappearance during treatment.

The main limitations of our study pertain to its retrospective nature. IgM expression analysis and COO subtyping were not assessable in all the cases because of the lack of suitable material. Moreover, we classified tumors basing on the Hans' algorithm, which is less sensitive and specific than GEP analysis [5]. We also regret that during follow-up serum immunofixation and FLC k/λ ratio were done only in roughly half of the patients.

In DLBCL patients the identification of reliable prognostic markers that may guide in selecting a more specific treatment is of considerable importance [53]. Widely used and inexpensive routine analysis could easily detect serum monoclonal IgM component. Further confirmation by immunohistochemistry or by other molecular detection assays of IgM expression by tumor cells [43,54] would allow to identify IgM-secreting DLBCL. We believe that IgM-secreting capability represents a very robust prognostic marker, since it is related to a defined biological characteristic of DLBCL derived from terminally differentiated B-lymphocytes.

Acknowledgments

We are deeply in debt with Professor Vincenzo Ambrogi for scientific advice in editing this paper and with Claudia Cippitelli for technical support.

Author Contributions

Conceived and designed the experiments: MCC ADN LR. Analyzed the data: MCC C. Tatarelli SS SA. Wrote the paper: MCC ADN LR BM GS SA. Contributed to morphological, FISH, immunohistochemistry and serological analyses: ADN SS C. Talerico GS LR ML.

References

1. Campo E, Swerdlow SH, Harris NL, Pileri S, Stein H, et al. (2011) The 2008 WHO classification of lymphoid neoplasms and beyond: evolving concepts and practical applications. Blood 117: 5019–32.
2. Fu K, Weisenburger DD, Choi WW, Perry KD, Smith LM, et al. (2008) Addition of rituximab to standard chemotherapy improves the survival of both the germinal center B-cell-like and non-germinal center B-cell-like subtypes of diffuse large B-cell lymphoma. J Clin Oncol 2628: 4587–94.
3. Sehn LH, DJ, Chanabhai M, Fitzgerald C, Gill K, Klasa R, et al. (2005) Introduction of combined CHOP plus rituximab therapy dramatically improved outcome of diffuse large B-cell lymphoma in British Columbia. J ClinOncol 23: 5027–5033.
4. Project, TIN-HsLPF (1993) A predictive model for aggressive non-Hodgkin's lymphoma The International Non-Hodgkin's Lymphoma Prognostic Factors Project. N Engl J Med 329: 987–994.
5. Alizadeh AA, Davis EM, Ma RE, Lossos C, Rosenwald A, et al. (2000) Distinct types of diffuse large B-cell lymphoma identified by gene expression profiling. Nature 3; 403: 503–511.
6. Visco C, LY, Xu Monette ZY, Miranda RN, Green TM, Li Y, et al. (2012) Comprehensive gene expression profiling and immunohistochemical studies support application of immunophenotypic algorithm for molecular subtype classification in diffuse large B-cell lymphoma: a report from the International DLBCL Rituximab-CHOP Consortium Program Study. Leukemia 269: 2103–2113.
7. Advani RH, Habermann CH, Morrison TM, Weller VA, Fisher EA, et al. (2010) Comparison of conventional prognostic indices in patients older than 60 years with diffuse large B-cell lymphoma treated with R-CHOP in the US Intergroup Study ECOG 4494, CALGB 9793: consideration of age greater than 70 years in an elderly prognostic index E-IPI. Br J Haematol 1512: 143–151.
8. Cox MC, Nofroni I, Ruco L, Amodeo R, Ferrari A, et al. (2008) Low absolute lymphocyte count is a poor prognostic factor in diffuse-large-B-cell-lymphoma. Leuk Lymphoma 499:1745–51.
9. Barrans S, Crouch S, Smith A, Turner K, Owen R, et al. (2010) Rearrangement of MYC is associated with poor prognosis in patients with diffuse large B-cell lymphoma treated in the era of rituximab J Clin Oncol 2820: 3360–65.
10. Green TM, Young KH, Visco C, Xu-Monette ZY, Orazi A, et al. (2012) Immunohistochemical Double-Hit Score Is a Strong Predictor of Outcome in Patients With Diffuse Large B-Cell Lymphoma Treated With Rituximab Plus Cyclophosphamide, Doxorubicin, Vincristine, and Prednisone. J Clin Oncol 3028: 3460–7
11. Johnson NA, Slack GW, Savage KJ, Connors JM, Ben-Neriah S, et al. (2012) Concurrent expression of MYC and BCL2 in diffuse large B-cell lymphoma treated with rituximab plus cyclophosphamide, doxorubicin, vincristine, and prednisone. J Clin Oncol 3028: 3452–59.
12. Horn H, Becher ZM, Barth C, Bernd TF, Feller HW, et al. (2013) MYC status in concert with BCL2 and BCL6 expression predicts outcome in diffuse large B-cell lymphoma. Blood 121: 2253–63.
13. Noguchi M, Yamazaki S, Suda K, Sato N, Oshimi K, et al. (2003) Multifocal motor neuropathy caused by a B-cell lymphoma producing a monoclonal IgM autoantibody against peripheral nerve myelin glycolipids GM1 and GD2b. Br J Haematol 1234: 600–605.
14. Lin P, Hao S, Handy BC, Bueso-Ramos CE, Medeiros J, et al. (2005) Lymphoid neoplasms associated with IgM paraprotein: a study of 382 patients Am J Clin Pathol 1232: 200–205.
15. Eskazan AE, Akmurad H, Ongoren S, Ozer O, Ferhanoglu B (2011). Primary gastrointestinal diffuse large B cell lymphoma presenting with cold agglutinin disease. Case Rep Gastroenterol 52: 262–266.
16. Maurer MJ, Micallef INM, Cerhan JR, Katzmann JA, Link BK, et al. (2011) Elevated serum free light chains are associated with event-free and overall survival in two independent cohorts of patients with diffuse large B-cell lymphoma. J Clin Oncol 2912: 1620–1626.
17. Jardin F, Molina TJ, Copie Bergman C, Brièr J, Petrella T, et al. (2013) Immunoglobulin heavy chain/light chain pair measurement is associated with survival in diffuse large B-cell lymphoma. *Leuk Lymphoma* 54:1898–907.
18. Cox MC, Di Napoli A, Scarpino S, Cavalieri E, Naso V, et al. (2012) Diffuse-Large-B-Cell Lymphoma Patients With Secreting IgM Monoclonal Component is A Very Poor Prognostic Subset. Blood 120: 2659
19. Swerdlow SH, Campo E, Harris NL, Jaffe ES, Pileri S, et al. (2008) WHO classification of Tumors of Haematopoietic and lymphoid Tissues. IARC press, Lyon.
20. Pfreundschuh M, Trümper L, Kloess M, Schmits R, Feller AC, et al. (2004). Two-weekly or 3-weekly CHOP chemotherapy with or without etoposide for the treatment of young patients with good-prognosis (normal LDH) aggressive lymphomas: results of the NHL-B1 trial of the DSHNHL. Blood 104: 626–33.
21. Marzano A, Angelucci E, Andreone P, Brunetto M, Bruno R, et al. (2007) Italian Association for the Study of the Liver. Prophylaxis and treatment of hepatitis B in mmunocompromised patients. Dig Liver Dis 39: 397–408.
22. Hans CP, Weisenburger DD, Greiner TC, Gascoyne RD, Delabie J, et al. (2004). Confirmation of the molecular classification of diffuse large B-cell lymphoma by immunohistochemistry using a tissue microarray. Blood 103(1):275–82.
23. Ventura RA, Martin-Subero JI, Jones M, McParland J, Gesk S, et al. (2006) FISH analysis for the detection of lymphoma-associated chromosomal abnormalities in routine paraffin-embedded tissue. J Mol Diagn 82:141–51.
24. Xu L, Hunter ZR, Yang G, Zhou Y, Cao Y, et al. (2013) Monoclonal gammopathy, and other B-cell lymphoproliferativeMYD88 L265P in Waldenström macroglobulinemia, immunoglobulin M disorders using conventional and quantitative allele-specific polymerase chain reaction. Blood 121: 2051–58.
25. Cheson BD, Pfistner B, Juweid ME, Gascoyne RD, Specht L, et al. (2007) Revised response criteria for malignant lymphoma. J Clin Oncol 255: 579–86.
26. Kaplan EL (1958) Meier P Non-parametric estimation from incomplete observations J Am Stat Assoc 53: 457–81.
27. Cox D (1972) Regression models and life tables. J R Stat Assoc 34: 187–220.
28. Choi JW, Kim Y, Lee JH, Kim YS (2013) MYD88 expression and L265P mutation in diffuse large B-cell lymphoma. Hum Pathol 44: 1375–81.
29. Lohr JG, Stojanov P, Lawrence MS, Auclair D, Chapuy B, et al. (2012) Discovery and prioritization of somatic mutations in diffuse large B-cell lymphoma DLBCL by whole-exome sequencing. Proc Natl Acad Sci U S A 10910: 3879–84.
30. Kraan W, Horlings HM, van Keimpema M, Schilder-Tol EJ, Oud ME, et al. (2013) High prevalence of oncogenic MYD88 and CD79B mutations in diffuse large B-cell lymphomas presenting at immune-privileged sites. Blood Cancer J doi: 10.1038/bcj.2013.28.
31. Zinzani PL, PC, Merla E, Ballerini F, Fabbri A, Guarini A, et al. (2012) Bortezomib as salvage treatment for heavily pretreated relapsed lymphoma patients: a multicentre retrospective study. Hematological Oncology, in press.
32. Rigacci L, Vitolo U, Cox MC, Devizzi L, Fabbri A, et al. (2012) Lenalidomide Is Effective in Heavily Pretreated Non Hodgkin Lymphoma NHL: Analysis of a Retrospective Data Collection. Blood 120: 3694.
33. Vitolo U, Angelucci E, Rossi G, Liberati AM, Cabras MG, et al. (2009) Dose-dense and high-dose chemotherapy plus rituximab with autologous stem cell transplantation for primary treatment of diffuse large B-cell lymphoma with a poor prognosis: a phase II multicenter study. Haematologica 949: 1250–1258.
34. Ngo VN, Young RM, Schmitz R, Jhavar S, Xiao W, et al. (2011) Oncogenically active MYD88 mutations in human lymphoma. Nature 470:115–9.
35. Randen U, Trøen G, Tierens A, Steen C, Warsame A, et al. (2014) Primary cold agglutinin-associated lymphoproliferative disease: a B-cell lymphoma of the bone marrow distinct from lymphoplasmacytic lymphoma. Haematologica 99: 497–504.
36. Kramer MH, Hermans J, Wijburg E, Philippo K, Geelen E, et al. (1998) Clinical relevance of BCL2, BCL6, and MYC rearrangements in diffuse large B-cell lymphoma. Blood 92: 3152–3162.
37. Copie-Bergman C, Gaulard P, Leroy K, Briere J, Baia M, et al. (2009) Immuno-fluorescence in situ hybridization index predicts survival in patients with diffuse large B-cell lymphoma treated with R-CHOP: a GELA Study. J Clin Oncol 27: 5573–5579.
38. Barrans SL, Evans PA, O'Connor SJ, Kendall SJ, Owen RG, et al. (2003) The t(14;18) is associated with germinal center-derived diffuse large B-cell lymphoma and is a strong predictor of outcome. Clin Cancer Res 9: 2133–2139.
39. Akyurek N, Uner A, Benekli M, Barista I (2012) Prognostic significance of MYC, BCL2, and BCL6 rearrangements in patients with diffuse large B-cell lymphoma treated with cyclophosphamide, doxorubicin, vincristine, and prednisone plus rituximab. Cancer 118: 4173–83.
40. Pedersen MO, Gang AO, Poulsen TS, Knudsen H, Lauritzen AF, et al. (2014) MYC translocation partner gene determines survival of patients with large B-cell lymphoma with MYC- or double-hit MYC/BCL2 translocations. Eur J Haematol 92: 42–8.
41. Lenz G, Siebert R, Roschke AV, Sanger W, Wright GW, et al. (2007) Aberrant immunoglobulin class switch recombination and switch translocations in activated B cell-like diffuse large B cell lymphoma. J Exp Med 2043: 633–643.
42. Wright G, Tan B, Rosenwald A, Hurt EH, Wiestner A, et al. (2003) A gene expression-based method to diagnose clinically distinct subgroups of diffuse large B cell lymphoma. Proc Natl Acad Sci USA 100: 9991–9996.
43. Ruminy P, Couronné L, Parmentier F, Rainville V, Mareschal S, et al. (2011) The isotype of the BCR as a surrogate for the GCB and ABC molecular subtypes in diffuse large B-cell lymphoma Leukemia 254: 681–688.
44. Montes-Moreno S, Rodriguez Pinilla MA, Maestre SM, Sanchez Verde L, Roncador G, et al. (2010) Aggressive large B-cell lymphoma with plasma cell differentiation: immunohistochemical characterization of plasmablastic lympho-ma and diffuse large B-cell lymphoma with partial plasmablastic phenotype. Haematologica 958: 1342–1349.
45. Hoeller S, Tzankov A, Pileri SA, Went P, Dirnhofer S, et al. (2010) Epstein-Barr virus-positive diffuse large B-cell lymphoma in elderly patients is rare in Western populations. Hum Pathol 41:352–357.
46. Ahn JS, Yang DH, Duk Choi Y, Jung SH, Yhim HY, et al. (2013) Clinical outcome of elderly patients with Epstein-Barr virus positive diffuse large B-cell lymphoma treated with a combination of rituximab and CHOP chemotherapy. Am J Hematol 88:774–9.
47. Lennert K, Feller A (1992) Histopathology of Non-Hodgkin's Lymphomas. New York: Springer Verlag.

48. Ott G, Ziepert M, Klapper W, Horn H, Szczepanowski M, et al. (2010) Immunoblastic morphology but not the immunohistochemical GCB/non-GCB classifier predicts outcome in diffuse large B-cell lymphoma in the RICOVER-60 trial of the DSHNHL. Blood 116: 4916–25.

49. Kohyama S, NH, Shima K, Shimazaki H (2001) Primary central nervous system lymphoma with paraproteinemia. Surg Neurol 565: 325–328.

50. Montesinos-Rongen M, Courts SR, Stenzel CW, Bechtel D, Niedobitek G, et al. (2005) Absence of immunoglobulin class switch in primary lymphomas of the central nervous system. Am J Pathol 1666:1773–9.

51. Ria R, Occhiogrosso G, Ciappetta P, Ribatti D, Vacca A, et al. (2009) Monoclonal gammopathy as a marker of primary cerebral lymphoma. Eur J Clin Invest 397: 627–629.

52. Schroers R, Baraniskin A, Heute C, Kuhnhenn J, Alekseyev A, et al. (2010) Detection of free immunoglobulin light chains in cerebrospinal fluids of patients with central nervous system lymphomas. Eur J Haematol 853:236–242.

53. Martelli M, Ferreri A, Agostinelli C, Di Rocco A, Pfreundschuh M, et al. (2013) Diffuse large B-cell lymphoma. Crit Rev Oncol Hematol 87:146–71.

54. Koens L, Willemze R, Jansen PM (2010) IgM expression on paraffin sections distinguishes primary cutaneous large B-cell lymphoma, leg type from primary cutaneous follicle center lymphoma. Am J Surg Pathol 347: 1043–1048.

14

Identification of Novel Genomic Aberrations in AML-M5 in a Level of Array CGH

Rui Zhang[1,2], Ji-Yun Lee[2,3], Xianfu Wang[2], Weihong Xu[2], Xiaoxia Hu[2], Xianglan Lu[2], Yimeng Niu[1], Rurong Tang[1], Shibo Li[2], Yan Li[1]*

1 Department of Hematology, The First Affiliated Hospital of China Medical University, Shenyang, Liaoning, P.R. China, **2** Department of Pediatrics, University of Oklahoma Health Sciences Center, Oklahoma City, Oklahoma, United States of America, **3** Department of Pathology, College of Medicine, Korea University, Seoul, South Korea

Abstract

To assess the possible existence of unbalanced chromosomal abnormalities and delineate the characterization of copy number alterations (CNAs) of acute myeloid leukemia-M5 (AML-M5), R-banding karyotype, oligonucelotide array CGH and FISH were performed in 24 patients with AML-M5. A total of 117 CNAs with size ranging from 0.004 to 146.263 Mb was recognized in 12 of 24 cases, involving all chromosomes other than chromosome 1, 4, X and Y. Cryptic CNAs with size less than 5 Mb accounted for 59.8% of all the CNAs. 12 recurrent chromosomal alterations were mapped. Seven out of them were described in the previous AML studies and five were new candidate AML-M5 associated CNAs, including gains of 3q26.2-qter and 13q31.3 as well as losses of 2q24.2, 8p12 and 14q32. Amplication of 3q26.2-qter was the sole large recurrent chromosomal anomaly and the pathogenic mechanism in AML-M5 was possibly different from the classical recurrent 3q21q26 abnormality in AML. As a tumor suppressor gene, *FOXN3*, was singled out from the small recurrent CNA of 14q32, however, it is proved that deletion of *FOXN3* is a common marker of myeloid leukemia rather than a specific marker for AML-M5 subtype. Moreover, the concurrent amplication of *MLL* and deletion of *CDKN2A* were noted and it might be associated with AML-M5. The number of CNA did not show a significant association with clinico-biological parameters and CR number of the 22 patients received chemotherapy. This study provided the evidence that array CGH served as a complementary platform for routine cytogenetic analysis to identify those cryptic alterations in the patients with AML-M5. As a subtype of AML, AML-M5 carries both common recurrent CNAs and unique CNAs, which may harbor novel oncogenes or tumor suppressor genes. Clarifying the role of these genes will contribute to the understanding of leukemogenic network of AML-M5.

Editor: Javier S. Castresana, University of Navarra, Spain

Funding: This work was supported by the "Science and Technology Project of Shenyang" grant (grant number: F12-277-1-21) (URL: www.systplan.gov.cn) and the National Natural Science Foundation of China (NSFC)(grant number: 81170519). The supplementary FISH and PCR tests in this study were supported by these funders. The funders had no role in study design, data collection and analysis, decision to publish, or preparation of manuscript.

Competing Interests: The authors have declared that no competing interests exist.

* E-mail: liyan2@medmail.com.cn

Introduction

Acute monocytic leukemia, also named acute myeloid leukemia-M5 (AML-M5), is one of the most common subtypes of AML defined by the French-American-British (FAB), which is comprised by more than 80% of monoblasts (AML-M5a) or 30–80% monoblasts with (pro)monocytic differentiation (AML-M5b). Responses to chemotherapy and prognosis in AML-M5 patients are varied. The recently proposed World Health Organization (WHO) classification attempts to associate the prognostic variance with cytogenetic abnormalities [1–2]. However, rather than t(8;21) in AML-M2, t(15;17) in AML-M3 and inv(16)/t(16;16) in AML-M4eo, specific subtype-associated translocation is lacking in AML-M5. It has been described that a part of AML-M5 patients carry 11q23 (MLL gene) rearrangement with a wide spectrum of recurrent translocation partner chromosomes [3–4]. In this sense, it is reasonable to assume that unbalanced chromosomal abnormalities might play a major role in the leukemogenesis of AML-M5. Especially those cryptic alterations, which are invisible for traditional banding analysis, are not rare in AML with normal karyotype [5–6].

It is necessary to evaluate the chromosomal changes in a whole genomic level. However, banding analysis, currently as the first choice to evaluate the genomic abnormalities of AML, is frequently to get inconclusive results due to chromosome condensation, imperfect banding, and the presence of few metaphases. FISH is a more sensitive technique, but is limited by the genomic coverage properties. Array CGH provides some distinct advantages including the potential for comprehensive genomic profiling and the ability to delimit the boundaries of specific genomic aberrations. Recently, it is considered as a powerful method to analyze genomic imbalances in hematopoietic malignancies, especially to determine cryptic and recurrent anomalies not observed by routine techniques [7–11].

The primary aim of present study is to assess, by means of array CGH assay, the possible existence of unbalanced chromosomal abnormalities, and delineate the copy number alterations (CNAs) in 24 cases of adult AML-M5 patients. Besides this, recurrent CNAs harboring cancer genes are also analyzed. The novel candidate oncogenes and tumor suppressor genes aberrations which might be implicated in the leukemogenesis of AML-M5 were revealed in this study.

Results

Normal karyotype was in the majority of AML-M5 cases

Karyotypes were available for 16 AML-M5 cases (Table S1 in File S1). 11 of them (10 newly diagnosed cases and 1 relapsed case) had normal karyotypes and 5 cases carried 2 or 3 chromosomal abnormalities. t(9;11)(p22;q23) as the recurrent chromosomal change was presented in 3 cases.

Array CGH delineated the genomic imbalances of AML-M5

A total of 117 CNAs with size ranging from 0.004 to 146.263 Mb were recognized in 12 of 24 cases, involving all chromosomes other than chromosome 1, 4, X and Y (Figure 1 and Table S1 in File S1). The cryptic chromosomal aberrations less than 5 Mb took up 59.8% of all CNAs (Figure 1). It was worth noting that in the 10 newly diagnosed cases with normal karyotype, microduplications spanning 11q23.3 carrying MLL and 5q35.3 carrying AGXT2L2 and COL23A1 were detected in case #8 and case #16, respectively. 12 recurrent CNAs were mapped in Figure 1 and listed in Table 1. Notably, in contrast to the most common recurrent CNAs reported by 8 representative genomic studies of MDS and AML using oligonucleotide array CGH or SNP array [5,12–18] (Table 2), novel CNAs including gains of 3q26.2-qter and 13q31.3 as well as losses of 2q24.2, 8p12 and 14q32 were proposed in the present study. Except that gain of 3q26.2-qter is a large chromosomal abnormality, all the other recurrent CNAs were cryptic and harbored interesting genes.

Translocation and inversion rather than partial duplication of 3q26.2 were identified by FISH

By array CGH, 3q26.2-qter was identified as a recurrent chromosomal anomaly. To investigate whether the gain of 3q26.2-qter, was closely associated with AML-M5 or other subtypes of AML, FISH with EVI (3q26.2) break-apart probe was hybridized in bone marrow cells of 69 cases of de novo AMLs (Table S2 in File S1). Normal two fusion signals were observed in 67 cases and abnormal FISH signal pattern with two fusion signals plus an extra red signal (TEL'EVI1) was shown in another two cases. One of the cases (ID: 37) was AML-M5, containing 89% of abnormal cells in the interphase. t(3;21) in the metaphase were proven by subsequent FISH with ETV6/AML1 probe (Figure S1A–F in File S1). The other one (ID: 65) was AML-M6, which carried 93% of abnormal cells produced by inv(3)(p25;q26) (Figure S1G–I in File S1). No partial duplication of 3q involving EVI gene was observed.

Candidate oncogenes and tumor suppressor genes were inferred by array CGH

Oncogenes and tumor suppressor genes that have been reported to be implicated in carcinogenesis or leukemogenesis were further singled out from the cryptic recurrent CNAs (Table 3). Micro-deletion of 0.209 Mb and large terminal deletion of 51.233 Mb encompassing FOXN3 gene at 14q were observed in two cases (case #13 and #24) (Figure 2). We subsequently investigated the expression levels of the FOXN3 in a cohort of acute leukemia samples including 78 AMLs and 19 ALLs (Table S3 in File S1). In comparison with healthy controls (HCs) (1.80±0.27), significantly lower expression of FOXN3 was found in the AML group (0.90±0.12) ($p < 0.05$) (Figure S2 in File S1). No significant difference was observed between AML-M5 and non-AML-M5 (Figure S3 in File S1). A low tendency toward expression of FOXN3 was detected in the ALL group (1.16±0.65), but the expression was not significantly different from the controls nor the AML groups ($p > 0.05$) (Figure S2 in File S1). Gain of 11q23.3 containing MLL gene was observed in 3 cases with size ranging from 0.004 Mb to 23.133 Mb. Cryptic chromosomal losses of 9p21.3 or a large deletion of 9p involving CDKN2A and MTAP were observed in 3 cases. Strikingly, gains of 11q23.3 and losses of 9p21.3 coexisted in two cases. To confirm the concurrent deletion of 9p21.3 and amplification of 11q23.3 inferred by array CGH, FISH analysis using MLL and CDKN2A probes was performed on case #18 (Figure 3). Consistent with array CGH, amplication of MLL with three or four fusion signals was shown in 69.5% of the 200 nuclei. Homogenous and heterogenous deletion of CDKN2A, indicated by loss of double or single red signal, was observed in 71.5% and 19% of 200 examined nuclei respectively. Totally, MLL amplication and CDKN2A deletion concurred in 68.5% of 200 nuclei.

Correlation of CNAs number and clinico-biological parameters

To investigate the prognostic value of the number of array CGH aberrations, 22 cases of newly diagnosed AML-M5 were grouped based on the numbers of CNA. As the median of CNAs per case was four, cases with four or less CNAs were grouped apart from cases with five or more. The numbers of CNA in the two groups were correlated with clinico-biological parameters which suggest a poor prognosis. These parameters included age>60 years old, white blood cell (WBC) count $>10 \times 10^9$/L, hemoglobin concentration <80 g/L, platelet count $<50 \times 10^9$/L, higher percent of blast cells in bone marrow (comparing to the average blast ratio in bone marrow) and responses to treatment, such as number of CR. By statistic analysis, no significant difference was observed between the two groups (table 4).

Discussion

In the last few years, the classification of AML has developed from a single morphological level to a MICM basis. As one of the diagnostic methods, genetic abnormality examination plays an important role in further sub-classification of AML and gives more clues to therapy selection and prognosis [1–2]. The cohort of patients of our study is in a special subgroup of AML, AML-M5, which is characterized by variable therapy responses and low incidence of recurrent chromosomal abnormalities at the level of conventional cytogenetic method. The present study refined the genomic aberrations of AML-M5 by an integration of chromosome, FISH and array CGH procedure. The majority of the genomic alterations are cryptic and invisible to G-banding analysis, indicating that high-resolution array CGH approach is necessary to provide more precise description of chromosomal aberrations in AML-M5. Particularly, in the patients with normal karyotype, array CGH has been able to unveil the small CNAs. However, similar with the previous studies, the recurrence of the small CNAs is very low [19–20]. Normal genomes are observed in nearly half of the AML-M5s, inferring that additional studies, such as gene sequencing or epigenetic analysis, might be necessary to investigate the underlying mechanism of AML-M5.

Array CGH improves the detectable rate of chromosomal abnormalities, which make it easier to map the recurrent chromosomal aberrations of AML-M5. As a subtype of AML, it seems that AML-M5 carries both the common recurrent CNAs which have been reported in the previous AML studies and novel recurrent CNAs which are noted as candidate AML-M5 associated CNAs. However, whether these novel recurrent CNAs are specially associated with AML-M5 are needed to be clarified. Gain of 3q26.2-qter is the sole large recurrent chromosomal

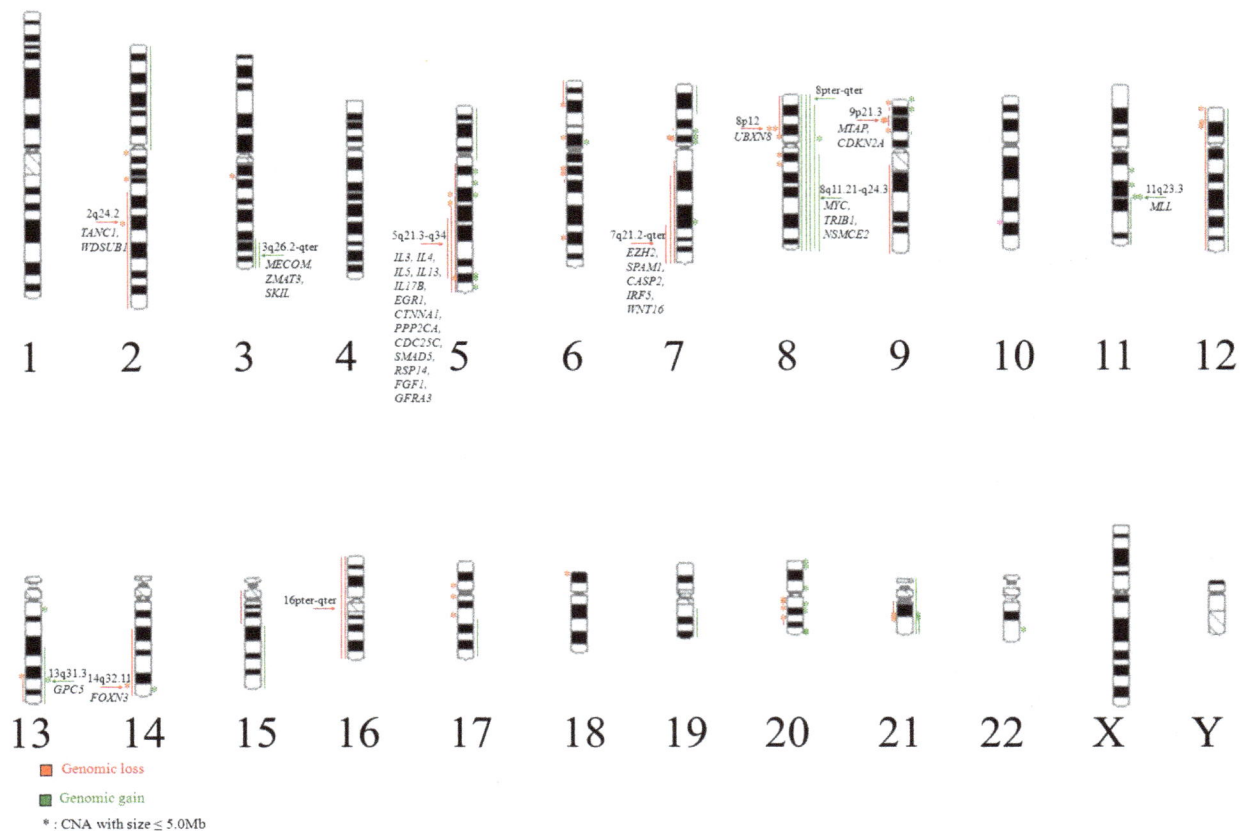

Figure 1. Distribution of CNAs recognized by array CGH in 24 patients with AML-M5. A total of 117 CNAs with 51 genomic gains (43.1%) and 66 genomic losses (56.9%) was observed. 70 CNAs (59.8%) were cryptic with size less than 5 Mb and invisible to karyotype. The arrows indicated recurrent CNAs and harbored interesting genes.

Table 1. The recurrent chromosomal abnormalities of 24 cases of AML-M5.

Chromosome Region	Genomic coordinates (NCBI Build 36.3)	Size(Mb)		Number of cases (case #)	Interesting genes
		Gain	Loss		
2q24.2*	159,772,558→159,847,666		0.075	2 (#11, #13)	TANC1, WDSUB1
3q26.2-qter*	170,262,958→199,381,714	29.119		2 (#12, #18)	MECOM, ZMAT3, SKIL, SOX2, EVI1
5q21.3-q34	104,803,921→163,613,351		58.809	3 (#7, #11, #19)	IL3, IL4, IL5, IL13, IL17B, EGR1,CTNNA1, PPP2CA, CDC25C, SMAD5, RSP14, FGF1, GFRA3
7q21.2-qter	92,258,287→158,816,03		66.558	3 (#7, #11, #12)	EZH2, SPAM1, CASP2, IRF5, WNT16
8p12*	30,721,389→30,765,786		0.044	3 (#11, #13, #18)	UBXN8
8q11.21-q24.3	50,233,257→142,198,258	91.965		2 (#11and #24)	MYC,TRIB1, NSMCE2
8pter-qter	71,702→146,264,232	146.257		3 (#14, #17, #19)	N/A
9p21.3	21,819,027→21,986,390		0.167	3 (#7, #13, #18)	MTAP, CDKN2A
11q23.3	117,844,729→117,849,872	0.004		3 (#7, #8, #18)	MLL
13q31.3*	90,024,777→91,278,708	1.254		2 (#11, #17)	GPC5
14q32.11*	89,027,534→89,236,808		0.209	2 (#13 and #24)	FOXN3
16pter-qter	18,227→88,715,037		88.802	2 (#7 and #19).	N/A

N/A: not applicable;
*recurrent CNA first rep°rted by this study.

Table 2. Recurrent CNAs reported by previous studies of MDS/AML and this study.

Genomic aberrations	Common recurrent CNAs of MDS/AML[*]	Recurrent CNAs of AML-M5 in this study
Gain	8q24.13-q24.21(MYC), 11q23.3(MLL), 12p13.32(CCND2), 21q22.2(ERG, TMPRSS2)	3q26.2-qter, 8q11.21-q24.3, 8pter-qter, 11q23.3, 13q31.3
Loss	5q, 7q, 9p21.3(CDKN2A), 12p13.31-p13.2(ETV6), 16q22.1(CBFB), 17p13(TP53), 17q11.2(NF1), 18p11.2(PTPN2), 21q22.12(RUNX1)	2q24.2, 5q21.3-q34, 7q21.2-qter, 8p12, 9p21.3, 14q32.11, 16pter-qter

*: data based on eight representative genomic studies of MDS and AML using oligonucleotide array CGH or SNP array.

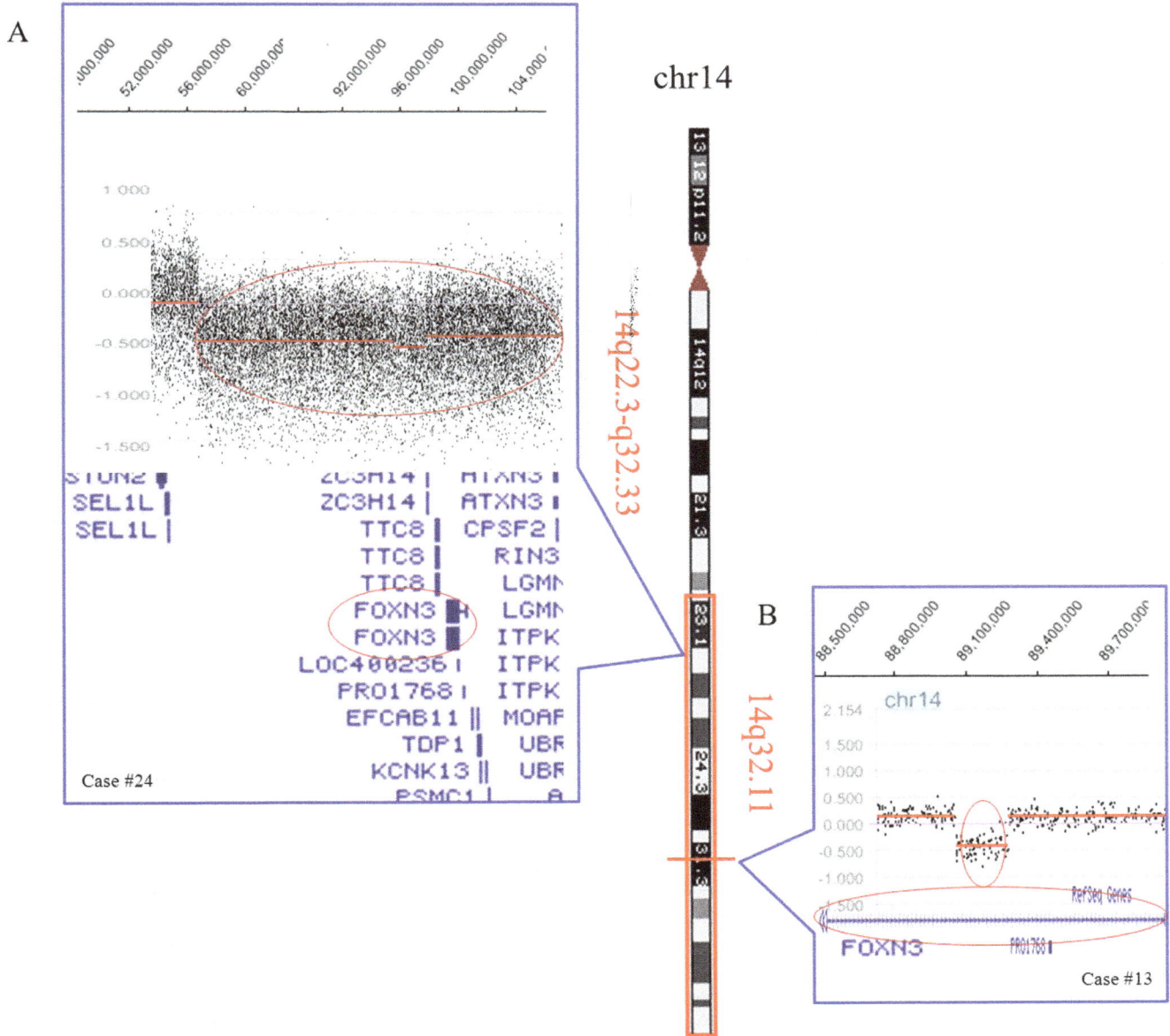

Figure 2. FOXN3 gene (14q31.3-q32.11) deletions in two patients with AML-M5. (A) Array CGH showed a lower signal ratio spanning 14q22.3-q32.33 (55,109,046–106,342,076 bp). FOXN3 gene was one of the genes located at the deleted region. (B) The microdeletion of 14q32.11 (89,027,534–89,236,808 bp) involving FOXN3 gene was inferred by array CGH.

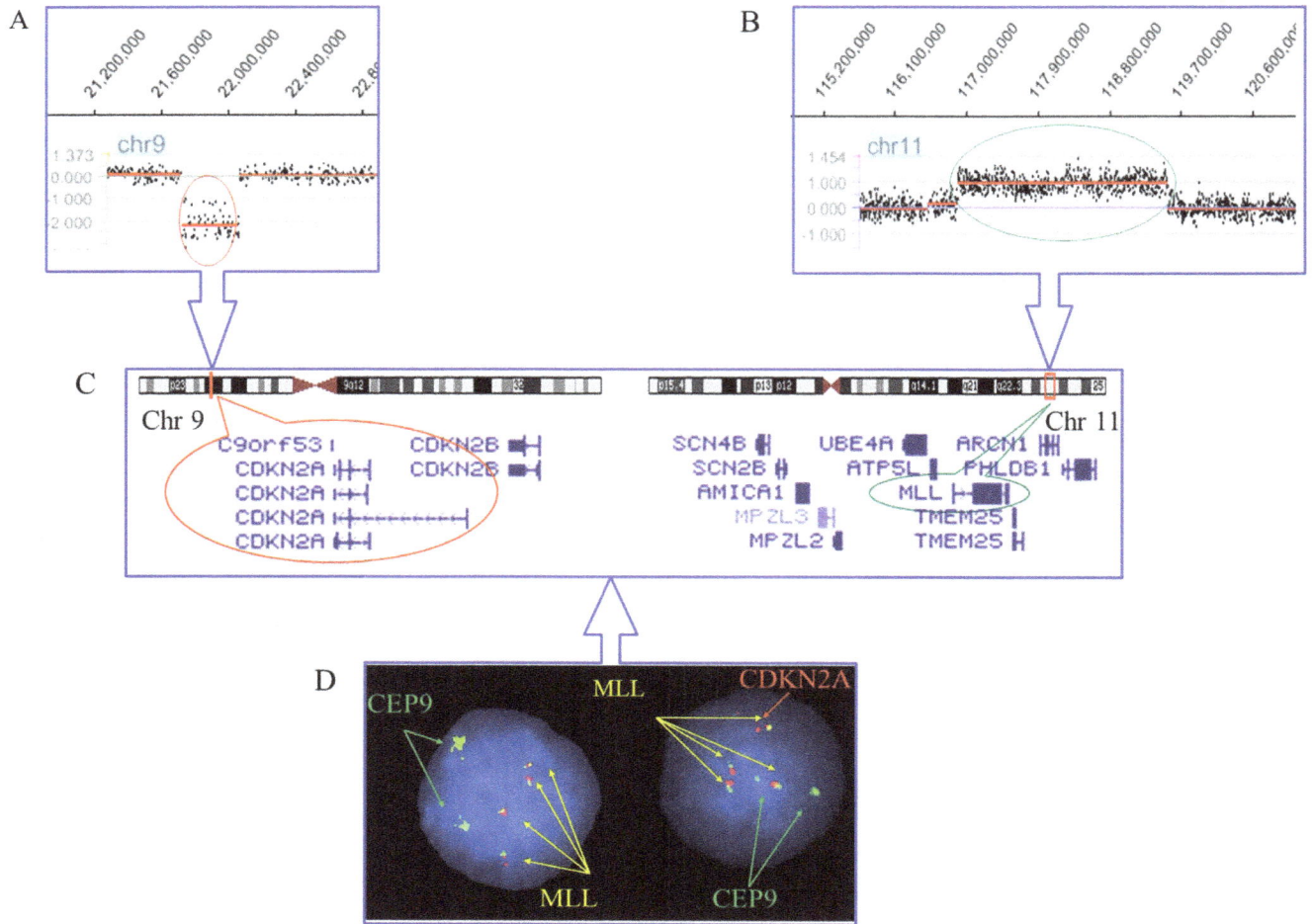

Figure 3. Gain of 11q23.3 and loss of 9p21.3 coexisting in case #18. (A) Lower signal of 21,755,226–22,097,452 on chromosome 9 was recognized by array CGH analysis. (B) A gain in the region of 116,893,506–119,524,806 was observed on chromosome 11 by array CGH. (C) UCSC genome browser (hg18) indicated the RefSeq genes involved *CDKN2A/B* genes and *MLL* gene. (D) FISH analysis showed the concurrent *CDKN2A* gene deletion and *MLL* gene amplification in interphase nuclei. The left nucleus showed the homogenous deletion of *CDKN2A* and the right nucleus demonstrated the heterogenous deletion of *CDKN2A*.

change in the present study. There is an overlap between 3q26.2-qter in case 12 and 3q21.1-qter in case 18. It is known that 3q21q26 anomaly is the most common karyotype in acute myeloid patients with 3q abnormalities [21–22]. *RPN1* gene at the breakpoint of 3q21.3 juxtaposing to *EVI1* gene at the breakpoint of 3q26.2 is the key mechanism of this type of AML. However, the significance of 3q26.2-qter amplification is not well known in AML

although it is considered as a recurrent chromosomal abnormality in several solid tumors [23–25]. This study inferred a possible recurrent amplification of 3q26.2-qter, which is associated with *EVI* gene by array CGH. However, neither its recurrence in AML nor its specific association with AML-M5 was confirmed by FISH. There's limitation on the confirmatory FISH analysis since it only focus on *EVI* gene. Recent study by Hussenet and his colleagues

Table 3. Candidate AML-M5 associated genes inferred by array CGH.

Genomic aberrations	Gene symbol	Gene name	Chromosome location	Function
Gain	MLL	mixed-lineage leukemia	11q23.3	Regulation of hematopoiesis
Loss	CDKN2A	Cyclin-dependent kinase inhibitor 2A	9p21.3	Cell cycle regulation, tumor suppressor
	MTAP	Methylthioadenosine phosphorylase	9p21.3	Deficient in many cancers because this gene and the tumor suppressor CDKN2A gene are co-deleted.
	FOXN3	Forkhead box N3	14q31.3-q32.11	Cell cycle regulation

Table 4. Comparative clinico-biological parameters and number of CR by number of CNAs.

Number of CNA	Total number	Age>60(ys)	WBC>10×10⁹/L	Hb<80 g/L	PLT<50× 10⁹/L	Blast%>0.72 in bone marrow	Number of CR
≤4 CNAs	17	2	12	6	9	11	8
>5 CNAs	5	2	5	2	2	3	1
p value	–	0.2089	0.2899	1.0000	1.0000	1.0000	0.3602

reported that *SOX2* is an oncogene activated by recurrent 3q26.3 amplifications in human lung squamous cell carcinomas [26]. Therefore, amplication of 3q26.2-qter might serve as a novel recurrent 3q abnormalities and it possibly has a different leukemogenic mechanism from the classical 3q21q26 anomaly in AML.

By the advantages of array CGH, the candidate genes in the cryptic recurrent CNAs have been singled out. It is the first time that *FOXN3* deletion is observed in leukemia. The *FOXN3* acts as a transcriptional repressor and has been implicated in DNA damage-inducible cell cycle arrests in saccharomyces cerevisiae [27]. However, the physiological functions of *FOXN3* in mamals are not known. Reduced expression of *FOXN3* has been reported in several cancers, such as renal cell carcinoma and oral squamous cell carcinoma [28–29]. Scott *et al.* found that *FOXN3* recruited SKIP, which played a role in cell growth and differentiation through the TGF-β pathway and repressed genes important for tumorigenesis [30]. The deletion of *FOXN3* gene is recurrent in this study, suggesting that *FOXN3* possibly serves as a novel TSG and contributes to the leukemogenesis. However, subsequent expression study suggested that reduced expression of *FOXN3* was not only presented in AML-M5 but also other subtypes of AML, indicating that the *FOXN3* encodes a myeloid marker rather than a specific leukemogenic protein of AML-M5. The *MLL* gene is reported to be highly associated with AML with complex karyotypes [31]. In this study, it suggests that the amplication of *MLL* frequently co-exists with the deletion of *CDKN2A*. *CDKN2A* encode cyclin-dependent kinase inhibitor, which have emerged as an important effecter in aging as well as a potent tumor suppressor. The main genetic alterations involving *CDKN2A* are deletions by bi- or monoallele or hypermethylation of 5′ GpG island in its promotor [32–34]. In AML, hypermethylation of *CDKN2A* has been reported, but deletion of *CDKN2A* is rare [35–37]. It is intriguing to reveal the coexistence of *MLL* amplication and *CDKN2A* deletions in AML-M5 and the cooperation of these genes rearrangements in leukemogenesis of AML-M5 needs to be further clarified.

Due to the limitation of case number, no statistical difference was shown between the number of CNAs and clinico-biological parameters in our analysis. More cases are necessary to evaluate the clinical significance of the number of CNAs.

In summary, we genetically defined AML-M5 by karyotype, FISH and array CGH. Array CGH is necessary to complement the traditional cytogenetic analysis in revealing the cryptic genomic alterations in AML-M5. As a subtype of AML, AML-M5 carries both common recurrent CNAs coexisting in AML and novel CNAs in AML-M5. The recurrent CNAs harbor oncogenes or tumor suppressor genes. Further studies are needed to understand the role of these genes in the leukemogenic network of AML.

Methods

Patients and clinical data

This research project was approved by both the Ethical Committee of the First Affiliated Hospital of China Medical University and the Institutional Review Board (IRB) at the University of Oklahoma Health Sciences Center (OUHSC) (IRB #13100). Before data collection a written informed consent from was obtained from each participant. Bone marrow samples were collected from 24 adults with AML-M5 (n = 22 at diagnosis, n = 2 at relapse) who referred to the First Affiliated Hospital of China Medical University between May 2009 and December 2010. The patients aged <14 years old were excluded in this study. The diagnosis was made according to the French-American-British (FAB) Cooperative Group criteria [38]. The ratio of males and females is 15:9 and the median age of patients was 47 years old (range, 15 to 72 years). The average value of blast count in bone marrow was 0.72 (range, 0.40 to 0.98). The clinical information of the patients is summarized in Table S4 in File S1.

Therapy

Twenty two patients were newly diagnosed and received a single course of daunorubicin plus cytarabine (DA) or idarubicin plus cytarabine (IA) regimen for induction treatment. For the patients who failed to achieve complete remission (CR) or relapsed from CR, salvage therapy was used, including low-dose cytarabine, aclarubicin and granulocyte colony-stimulating factor (G-CSF) (CAG) or fludarabine, cytarabine and G-CSF (FLAG) regimen. Intermediated dose cytarabine (IDAra-C) ± antharcycline, mitoxantrone plus cytarabine (MA) and DA were chosen as postremission therapy for patients achieved CR and it lasted for 6–8 courses. No further therapy was applied to patients remaining in remission after postremission therapy. The details of each regimen were listed in Table S5 in File S1.

Criteria of response and definition of relapse

For response assessment, bone marrow aspiration was performed between days 21 and 28 after induction therapy. CR was defined as a bone marrow with normal hematopoiesis, blasts in bone marrow less than 5%, granulocyte count ≥1.0×10⁹/L, platelet count ≥100×10⁹/L, no myeloid blasts in the peripheral blood and no extramedullary disease. Patients who did not fulfill the above criteria were defined as unremission. Relapse was defined as the reappearance of more than 5% blasts in bone marrow aspirates or extramedullary leukemia in patients with a previously documented CR.

Ficoll gradient separation and cryopreservation

Bone marrow mononuclear cells (MNCs) were isolated by Ficoll-paque gradient centrifugation (TAKARA Biotechnology, Dalian, China), aliquoted into fetal calf serum (FCS) with 10%

DMSO, and cryopreserved in the liquid phase of a liquid nitrogen tank.

Preparation of Sample DNA and RNA

Liquid nitrogen-cryopreserved (liquid phase) bone marrow mononuclear cells were washed and recovered by centrifugation. Following that, DNA was extracted with phenol-chloroform, and precipitated with ammonium acetate, ethanol and glycogen. RNA was prepared from approximately 2×10^5 to 2×10^6 blasts with Trizol (TAKARA Biotechnology, Dalian, China), and resuspended in 50 μl DEPC-treated water. Complementary DNA was made from ~20 ng of RNA using the SuperScript III first strand synthesis kit and oligo-dT priming [Promega Corporation, an affiliate of Promega (Beijing) Biotech, China].

Cytogenetics

Short-term cultures of unstimulated bone marrow samples were prepared and fixed according to our standard laboratory protocols. Karyotype analysis was performed by R banding technique. Chromosome study could not been performed on six bone marrow samples due to the limitation of cell number. The cytogenetic abnormalities were described according to the International System for Human Cytogenetic Nomenclature.

Array CGH

Array CGH analysis was performed on all DNA samples obtained from 24 patients with AML-M5 following the manufacturer's protocol with minor modifications, (Roche NimbleGen System Inc., Madison, WI). The array consisted of approximately 720,000–mer oligonucleotide probes that spanned both coding and noncoding sequences with average genome coverage of approximately 2 kilobases. A commercially available pooled normal control DNA was used (Promega Corporation, Madison, WI) for reference. The patients and the reference DNA were labeled with either Cyanine 3 (Cy-3) or Cyanine 5 (Cy-5) by random priming (Trilink Biotechnologies, San Diego, CA) and then hybridized to the chip via incubating in the MAUI hybridization system (BioMicro Systems, Salt Lake City, UT). After 40-hours hybridization at 42°C, the slides were washed and scanned using a GenePix 4000B (Molecular Devices, Sunnyvale, CA). NimbleScan version 2.4 and the SignalMap version 1.9 were applied for data analysis (NimbleGen System Inc, Madison, WI). The genomic locations were retrieved from National Center for Biotechnology Information (NCBI) build 36 (hg 18). Frequently affected regions recently detected as copy number polymorphisms were excluded from data analysis according to the Chromosome Number Variation (CNV) database in our lab and genomic variants in human genome (Build 36: Mar. 2006). The genomic data of array CGH are available in NCBI Gene Expression Omnibus (GEO) under accession number GSE53429.

Fluorescence In Situ Hybridization (FISH)

Confirmatory FISH analysis was performed using different probes. (1) vysis LSI MLL dual color break apart rearrangement probe and vysis LSI CDKN2A (9p21)/CEP9 probe (Abbott Molecular Inc., Des Plaines, IL) on case #18. (2) EVI t(3;3) inv(3) Break, Dual-Color Probe (Kreatech Diagnostics, Amsterdam, TN) on 69 de novo AML patients' bone marrow cells. The FAB subtypes and karyotypes of the patients were showed in Table S2 in File S1. (3) Vysis LSI ETV6(TEL)/RUNX1(AML1) ES Dual Color Translocation Probe (Abbott Molecular Inc., Des Plaines, IL) on the case with ID 37 in Table S2 in File S1.

Expression of FOXN3 determined by Quantitative real-time PCR (qRT-PCR)

qRT-PCR was performed to determine the expression of FOXN3 on bone marrow MNCs of 97 patients with acute leukemia and 16 normal controls who had normal myelograms (Table S3 in File S1). Complementary DNAs were made from ~20 ng of RNA using the Superscript I II first strand synthesis kit (Invitrogen) and oligo-dT priming. Primers and TaqMan-based probes were purchased from Applied Bio-systems (Applied Biosystems, Beijing, China) and listed in Table S6 in File S1. Duplicate amplification reactions were done with an ABI 7500 Real time PCR System (Applied Biosystems, Foster City, CA, USA) and the data were analyzed by the ABI 7500 system SDS software (1.4 Version).

Statistical analysis

The Fisher's exact test was employed to assess the association of CNAs numbers per case with clinico-biological parameters. The correlation of the expression levels of FOXN3 and the subtypes of acute leukemia was analyzed by the student's t-test. All statistical analyses were performed using GraphPad Prism5 and p-value ≤0.05 was considered as statistically significant.

Supporting Information

File S1   Figure S1, 3q anomaly identified by karyotype and FISH in two of the 69 de novo AMLs. (A)–(F) showed t(3;21) in case with ID 37 and (G)–(I) showed inv(3) in case with ID 65. Arrows indicated the der(3)t(3;21) (A) and der(21)t(3;21) (B) observed by R-banding. FISH with EVI(3q26) probe showed two fusion signals plus an extra red signal (TEL'EVI1) in interphase (C) and translocation of chromosome 3 with a variant breakpoint of EVI gene in metaphase (D). Hybridization with TEL/AML1 probe demonstrated an extra red signal in interphase (E) and translocation of chromosome 21 in metaphase (F). (G) Arrow indicated the derivative inv(3) showed by R-banding. FISH with EVI(3q26) probe showed two fusion signals plus an extra red signal (TEL'EVI1) in interphase (H) and inv(3) with a variant breakpoint of EVI gene in metaphase (I). Figure S2, The comparisons of FOXN3 Levels in health control, ALL and AML. The significantly reduced FOXN3 level was observed between AML and health controls. *: p<0.05. The FOXN3 level was lower in ALL than health control whereas no significantly difference was observed. Figure S3, The comparisons of FOXN3 Levels in health control, M5 and non-M5. No significantly difference was observed on the FOXN3 levels between AML-M5 and non-AML-M5 (p>0.05). Table S1, The results of karyotype and array CGH in 24 AML-M5. Table S2, FAB subtypes, karyotypes and FISH with EVI (3q26) probe analysis on 69 de novo AML patients. Table S3, Clinical information and FOXN3 expression levels of 97 acute leukemia samples and 16 normal controls. Table S4, The clinical characterizations of 24 cases of AML-M5. Table S5, Drug dose and duration of chemotherapy. Table S6, Primers in qRT-PCR for FOXN3.

Author Contributions

Conceived and designed the experiments: RZ SBL YL. Performed the experiments: RZ XFW WHX XXH XLL YMN RRT. Analyzed the data: RZ JYL XFW WHX. Contributed reagents/materials/analysis tools: SBL YL. Wrote the paper: RZ.

References

1. Vardiman JW, Harris NL, Brunning RD (2002) The World Health Organization (WHO) classification of the myeloid neoplasms. Blood 100: 2292–2302. PubMed: 12239137.

2. Vardiman JW (2010) The World Health Organization (WHO) classification of tumors of the hematopoietic and lymphoid tissues: an overview with emphasis on the myeloid neoplasms. Chem Biol Interact 184: 16–20. doi:10.1016/j.cbi.2009.10.009. PubMed: 19857474.

3. Huret JL (2003) 11q23 rearrangements in leukaemia. Atlas Genet Cytogenet Oncol Haematol. Available: http://AtlasGeneticsOncology.org/Anomalies/11q23ID1030.html. doi: 10.4267/2042/38020

4. Huret JL (2005) MLL (myeloid/lymphoid or mixed lineage leukemia). Atlas Genet Cytogenet Oncol Haematol. Available: http://AtlasGeneticsOncology.org/Genes/MLL.html. doi: 10.4267/2042/38290

5. Tyybäkinoja A, Elonen E, Piippo K, Porkka K, Knuutila S (2007) Oligonucleotide array-CGH reveals cryptic gene copy number alterations in karyotypically normal acute myeloid leukemia. Leukemia 21: 571–574. PubMed: 17268525.

6. Gross M, Mkrtchyan H, Glaser M, Fricke HJ, Höffken K, et al. (2009) Delineation of yet unknown cryptic subtelomere aberrations in 50% of acute myeloid leukemia with normal GTG-banding karyotype. Int J Oncol 34: 417–423. PubMed: 19148476.

7. Yasar D, Karadogan I, Alanoglu G, Akkaya B, Luleci G, et al. (2010) Array comparative genomic hybridization analysis of adult acute leukemia patients. Cancer Genet Cytogenet 197: 122–129. PubMed: 20193845.

8. Kearney L, Horsley SW (2005) Molecular cytogenetics in haematological malignancy: current technology and future prospects. Chromosoma 114: 286–294. PubMed: 16003502.

9. Usvasalo A, Elonen E, Saarinen-Pihkala UM, Räty R, Harila-Saari A, et al. (2010) Prognostic classification of patients with acute lymphoblastic leukemia by using gene copy number profiles identified from array-based comparative genomic hybridization data. Leuk Res 34: 1476–1482. PubMed: 20303590.

10. Armengol G, Canellas A, Alvarez Y, Bastida P, Toledo JS, et al. (2010) Genetic changes including gene copy number alterations and their relation to prognosis in childhood acute myeloid leukemia. Leuk Lymphoma 51: 114–124. doi:10.3109/10428190903350397. PubMed: 20001230.

11. Matteucci C, Barba G, Varasano E, Vitale A, Mancini M, et al. (2010) GIMEMA Acute Leukaemia Working Party, Italy. Rescue of genomic information in adult acute lymphoblastic leukaemia (ALL) with normal/failed cytogenetics: a GIMEMA centralized biological study. Br J Haematol 149: 70–78. doi: 10.1111/j.1365-2141.2009.08056.x. PubMed: 20067559.

12. Suela J, Alvarez S, Cifuentes F, Largo C, Ferreira BI, et al. (2007) DNA profiling analysis of 100 consecutive de novo acute myeloid leukemia cases reveals patterns of genomic instability that affect all cytogenetic risk groups. Leukemia 21: 1224–1231. PubMed: 17377590.

13. Bajaj R, Xu F, Xiang B, Wilcox K, Diadamo AJ, et al. (2011) Evidence-based genomic diagnosis characterized chromosomal and cryptic imbalances in 30 elderly patients with myelodysplastic syndrome and acute myeloid leukemia. Mol Cytogenet 4: 3–12. doi: 10.1186/1755-8166-4-3. PubMed: 21251322.

14. Slovak ML, Smith DD, Bedell V, Hsu YH, O'Donnell M, et al. (2010) Assessing karyotype precision by microarray-based comparative genomic hybridization in the myelodysplastic/myeloin proliferative disorders. Mol Cytogenet 3: 23–36. doi: 10.1186/1755-8166-3-23. PubMed: 21078186.

15. Starczynowski DT, Vercauteren S, Telenius A, Sung S, Tohyama K, et al. (2008) High-resolution whole genome tiling path array CGH analysis of CD34+ cells from patients with low-risk myelodysplastic syndromes reveals cryptic copy number alterations and predicts overall and leukemia-free survival. Blood 112: 3412–3424. doi: 10.1182/blood-2007-11-122028. PubMed: 18663149.

16. Akagi T, Ogawa S, Dugas M, Kawamata N, Yamamoto G, et al. (2009) Frequent genomic abnormalities in acute myeloid leukemia/myelodysplastic syndrome with normal karyotype. Haematologica 94: 213–223. doi: 10.3324/haematol.13024. PubMed: 19144660.

17. Walter MJ, Payton JE, Ries RE, Shannon WD, Deshmukh H, et al. (2009) Acquired copy number alterations in adult acute myeloid leukemia genomes. Proc Natl Acad Sci U S A 106: 12950–12955. doi:10.1073/pnas.0903091106. PubMed: 19651600.

18. Radtke I, Mullighan CG, Ishii M, Su X, Cheng J, et al. (2009) Genomic analysis reveals few genetic alterations in pediatric acute myeloid leukemia. Proc Natl Acad Sci U S A 106: 12944–12949. doi: 10.1073/pnas.0903142106. PubMed: 19651601.

19. Itzhar N, Dessen P, Toujani S, Auger N, Preudhomme C, et al. (2011) Chromosomal minimal critical regions in therapy-related leukemia appear different from those of de novo leukemia by high-resolution aCGH. PLoS One 6: e16623. doi:10.1371/journal.pone.0016623. PubMed: 21339820.

20. Suela J, Alvarez S, Cigudosa JC (2007) DNA profiling by arrayCGH in acute myeloid leukemia and myelodysplastic syndromes. Cytogenet Genome Res 118: 304–309. PubMed: 18000384.

21. Lu Y, Chen ZM, Xu WL, Mu QT, Jin J (2010) Clinical analysis of 24 cases of acute myeloid leukemia with 3q abnormalities. Zhejiang Da Xue Xue Bao Yi Xue Ban 39: 241–245. PubMed: 20544984.

22. De Braekeleer E, Douet-Guilbert N, Le Bris MJ, Ianotto JC, Berthou C, et al. (2013) Double Inv(3)(q21q26), a rare but recurrent chromosomal abnormality in myeloid hemopathies. Anticancer Res 33: 639–642. PubMed: 23393360.

23. Noutomi Y, Oga A, Uchida K, Okafuji M, Ita M, et al. (2006) Comparative genomic hybridization reveals genetic progression of oral squamous cell carcinoma from dysplasia via two different tumourigenic pathways. J Pathol 210: 67–74. PubMed: 16767698.

24. Huang KF, Lee WY, Huang SC, Lin YS, Kang CY, et al. (2007) Chromosomal gain of 3q and loss of 11q often associated with nodal metastasis in early stage cervical squamous cell carcinoma. J Formos Med Assoc 106: 894–902. PubMed: 18063510.

25. Ueno T, Tangoku A, Yoshino S, Abe T, Toshimitsu H, et al. (2002) Gain of 5p15 detected by comparative genomic hybridization as an independent marker of poor prognosis in patients with esophageal squamous cell carcinoma. Clin Cancer Res 8: 526–533. PubMed: 11839673.

26. Hussenet T, Dali S, Exinger J, Monga B, Jost B, et al. (2010) SOX2 is an oncogene activated by recurrent 3q26.3 amplifications in human lung squamous cell carcinomas. PloS One 5: e8960. doi: 10.1371/journal.pone.0008960. PubMed: 20126410.

27. Pati D, Keller C, Groudine M, Plon SE (1997) Reconstitution of a MEC1-independent checkpoint in yeast by expression of a novel human fork head cDNA. Mol Cell Biol 17: 3037–3046. PubMed: 9154802.

28. Struckmann K, Schraml P, Simon R, Elmenhorst K, Mirlacher M, et al. (2004) Impaired expression of the cell cycle regulator BTG2 is common in clear cell renal cell carcinoma. Cancer Res 64: 1632–1638. PubMed: 14996721.

29. Chang JT, Wang HM, Chang KW, Chen WH, Wen MC, et al. (2005) Identification of differentially expressed genes in oral squamous cell carcinoma (OSCC): overexpression of NPM, CDK1 and NDRG1 and underexpression of CHES1. Int J Cancer 114: 942–949. PubMed: 15645429.

30. Scott KL, Plon SE (2005) CHES1/FOXN3 interacts with Ski-interacting protein and acts as a transcriptional repressor. Gene 359: 119–126. PubMed: 16102918.

31. Mrózek K (2008) Cytogenetic, molecular genetic, and clinical characteristics of acute myeloid leukemia with a complex karyotype. Semin Oncol 35: 365–377. doi: 10.1053/j.seminoncol.2008.04.007. PubMed: 18692687.

32. Kim M, Yim SH, Cho NS, Kang SH, Ko DH, et al. (2009) Homozygous deletion of CDKN2A (p16, p14) and CDKN2B (p15) genes is a poor prognostic factor in adult but not in childhood B-lineage acute lymphoblastic leukemia: a comparative deletion and hypermethylation study. Cancer Genet Cytogenet 195: 59–65. doi: 10.1016/j.cancergencyto.2009.06.013. PubMed: 19837270.

33. Schiffman JD, Wang Y, McPherson LA, Welch K, Zhang N, et al. (2009) Molecular inversion probes reveal patterns of 9p21 deletion and copy number aberrations in childhood leukemia. Cancer Genet Cytogenet 193: 9–18. doi: 10.1016/j.cancergencyto.2009.03.005. PubMed: 19602459.

34. Chim CS, Tam CY, Liang R, Kwong YL (2001) Methylation of p15 and p16 genes in adult acute leukemia: lack of prognostic significance. Cancer 91: 2222–2229. PubMed: 11413509.

35. Toyota M, Kopecky KJ, Toyota MO, Jair KW, Willman CL, et al. (2001) Methylation profiling in acute myeloid leukemia. Blood 97: 2823–2829. PubMed: 11313277.

36. Usvasalo A, Ninomiya S, Räty R, Hollmén J, Saarinen-Pihkala UM, et al. (2010) Focal 9p instability in hematologic neoplasias revealed by comparative genomic hybridization and single-nucleotide polymorphism microarray analyses. Genes Chromosomes Cancer 49: 309–318. doi:10.1002/gcc.20741. PubMed: 20013897.

37. Krug U, Ganser A, Koeffler HP (2002) Tumor suppressor genes in normal and malignant hematopoiesis. Oncogene 21: 3475–3495. PubMed: 12032783.

38. Bennett JM, Catovsky D, Daniel MT, Flandrin G, Galton DA, et al. (1976) Proposals for the classification of the acute leukaemias. French-American-British (FAB) co-operative group. Br J Haematol 33: 451–458. PubMed: 188440.

15

S100A8 Contributes to Drug Resistance by Promoting Autophagy in Leukemia Cells

Minghua Yang[1]*, Pei Zeng[1], Rui Kang[3], Yan Yu[1], Liangchun Yang[1], Daolin Tang[2,3], Lizhi Cao[1]*

1 Department of Pediatrics, Xiangya Hospital, Central South University, Changsha Hunan, China, **2** Department of Infectious Diseases, Xiangya Hospital, Central South University, Changsha, Hunan, China, **3** Department of Surgery, University of Pittsburgh Cancer Institute, Pittsburgh, Pennsylvania, United States of America

Abstract

Autophagy is a double-edged sword in tumorigenesis and plays an important role in the resistance of cancer cells to chemotherapy. S100A8 is a member of the S100 calcium-binding protein family and plays an important role in the drug resistance of leukemia cells, with the mechanisms largely unknown. Here we report that S100A8 contributes to drug resistance in leukemia by promoting autophagy. S100A8 level was elevated in drug resistance leukemia cell lines relative to the nondrug resistant cell lines. Adriamycin and vincristine increased S100A8 in human leukemia cells, accompanied with upregulation of autophagy. RNA interference-mediated knockdown of S100A8 restored the chemosensitivity of leukemia cells, while overexpression of S100A8 enhanced drug resistance and increased autophagy. S100A8 physically interacted with the autophagy regulator BECN1 and was required for the formation of the BECN1-PI3KC3 complex. In addition, interaction between S100A8 and BECN1 relied upon the autophagic complex ULK1-mAtg13. Furthermore, we discovered that exogenous S100A8 induced autophagy, and RAGE was involved in exogenous S100A8-regulated autophagy. Our data demonstrated that S100A8 is involved in the development of chemoresistance in leukemia cells by regulating autophagy, and suggest that S100A8 may be a novel target for improving leukemia therapy.

Editor: Spencer B. Gibson, University of Manitoba, Canada

Funding: This work was supported by The National Natural Sciences Foundation of China (81100359 to MY, 30973234 and 31171328 to LC) and a grant from the National Institutes of Health (R01CA160417 to DT). The funders had no role in study design, data collection and analysis, decision to publish, or preparation of the manuscript.

Competing Interests: The authors have declared that no competing interests exist.

* E-mail: yamahua123@163.com (MY); caolizhi318@163.com (LC)

Introduction

Autophagy is a catabolic process involving the degradation of intracellular aggregated or misfolded proteins, and damaged organelles through lysosomal machinery in response to stress or starvation [1,2]. Deregulation of autophagy is implicated in several human diseases including cancers. Depending on the type of tumor and stage of disease, autophagy induces both tumor cell survival and death during the initiation, progression, maturation and maintenance of cancer [3].

It has been well documented that autophagy plays an important role in the resistance of cancer cells to chemotherapy [4]. Consequently, pharmacological inhibition of autophagy enhances chemotherapeutic drug-induced cytotoxicity and apoptosis in leukemia cells [4–6]. We recently found that damage associated molecular pattern molecules (DAMPs) such as high mobility group box 1 (HMGB1) contribute to chemotherapy resistance though upregulating autophagy in leukemia [7]. S100A8 (also designated MRP8 or calgranulin A) is a member of DAMPs, differentially expressed in a wide variety of cell types and abundant in myeloid cells [8,9]. S100A8 is involved in the progression of various cancers, including leukemia, and induces cell death by functional linkage with Bcl-2 family members [10–14]. We previously found that the expression level of S100A8 correlates with poor clinical outcomes in childhood acute myeloblastic leukemia (AML). Accordingly, knockdown of S100A8 by siRNA-treated myeloid leukemia cells showed sensitization to arsenic trioxide, accompa-

nied with the attenuation of autophagy and disassociation of the BECN1-Bcl-2 complex [14]. The data suggest that S100A8 contributes to chemoresistance *via* regulating the autophagy in leukemia.

In this study, we found that S100A8 enhances drug resistance by upregulating autophagy through promoting the formation of BECN1-PI3KC3 [PI3KC3, phosphatidylinositol 3-kinase class 3] complex, providing a novel potential target for the treatment of leukemia.

Materials and Methods

Antibodies and reagents

The antibodies against S100A8 and p62 were obtained from Santa Cruz Biotechnology (Sana Cruz, CA, USA). The antibodies to Actin, BECN1, PI3KC3, C-PARP, ULK1, Bcl-2 and P-ULK1 were from Cell Signaling Technology (Boston, MA, USA). The antibodies to LC3 and TLR-4 were purchased from Abcam (Cambridge, MA, USA). Anti-Atg7 antibody was from Novus (Denver-Littleton, CO, USA). Vincristine (VCR), adriamycin (ADM), rotenone (Rot), thenoyltrifluoroacetone (TTFA), antimycin A (AA), E64D, anti-RAGE antibody and pepstatin were from Sigma (Milpitas, CA, USA). Full-length human S100A8 cDNA (pLPCX-S100A8) was a gift from Dr. RW Stam (Erasmus Medical Center/Sophia Children's Hospital, Netherlands). FITC-Annexin V Apoptosis Detection kit and the Nuclear and Cytoplasmic Protein Extraction kit were purchased form Beyotime Institute of

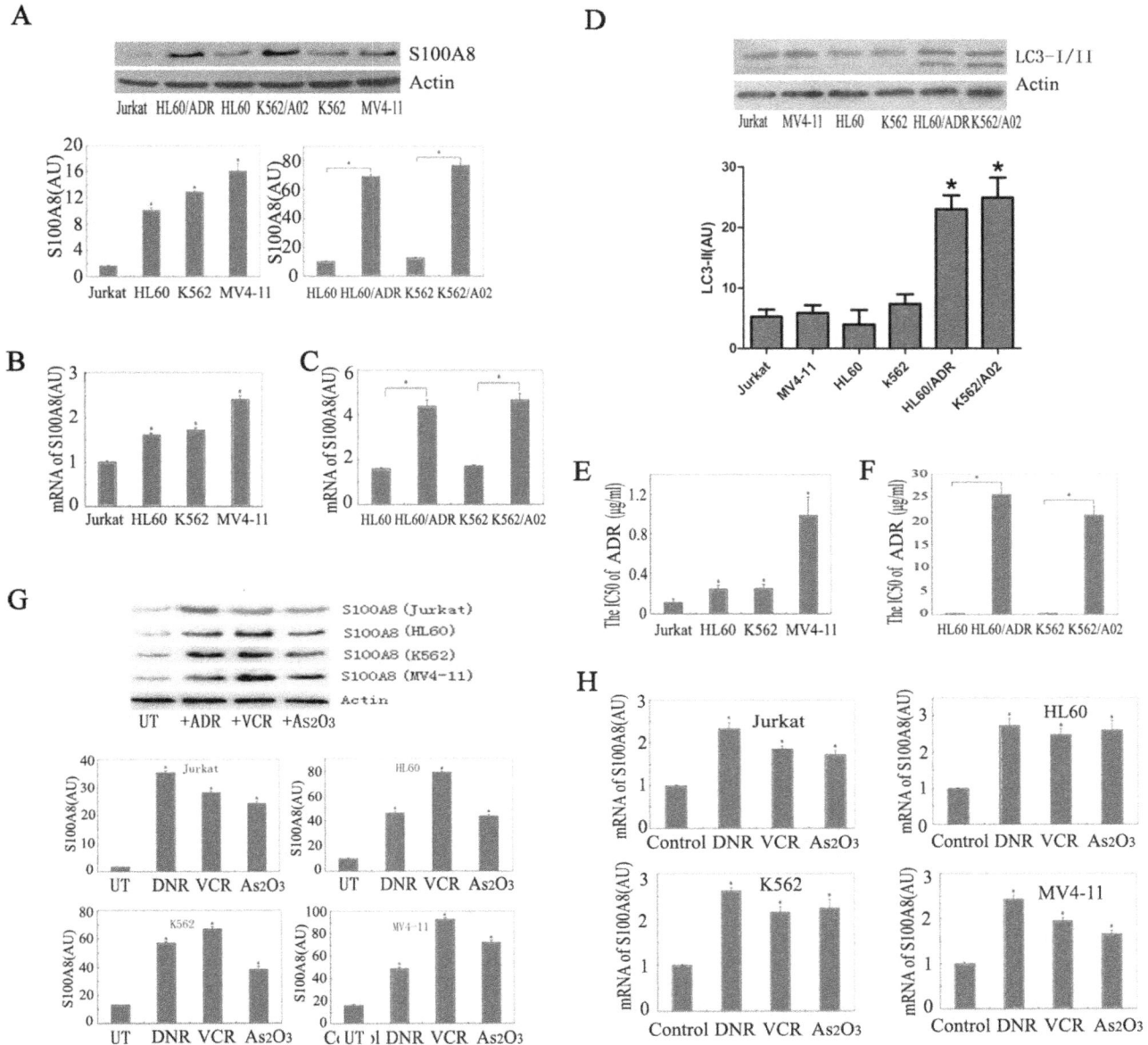

Figure 1. S100A8 was elevated in drug resistance leukemia cells and chemotherapy agents induced S100A8 expression in leukemia cells. (A) Protein level of S100A8 was analyzed by Western blotting in Jurkat, HL-60, K562 and MV4-11 cells (n = 3, *$P<0.05$). (B and C) S100A8 mRNA level in leukemia cells was analyzed by real time RT-PCR (n = 3, *$P<0.05$ versus Jurkat cells in **B** and *$P<0.05$ versus HL-60 or K562 in **C**, Jurkat group set as 1). (**D**) Basal LC3-I/II level was analyzed by Western blotting in leukemia cells (n = 3, *$P<0.05$ *versus* Jurkat cells). (**E and F**) IC50 levels of adriamycin (ADR) in Jurkat, K562, HL-60, MV4-11, K562/A02, and HL-60/ADR cells (n = 3, *$P<0.05$ versus Jurkat cells in **E**, *$P<0.05$ versus HL-60 or K562 in **F**). (**G**) Jurkat, HL-60, K562 and MV4-11 cells were treated with ADR (1 µg/ml), VCR (1 µg/ml) or As2O3 (5 µM) for 24 hours and S100A8 protein level was analyzed by Western blotting (n = 3, *P<0.05 vs. UT, untreated group). AU, arbitrary unit. (**H**) Jurkat, HL-60, K562 and MV4-11 cells were treated with ADR (1 µg/ml), vincristine (VCR, 1 µg/ml) or arsenic trioxide (As2O3, 5 µM) for 24 hours and S100A8 mRNA level was analyzed by real time RT-PCR (n = 3, *P<0.05 versus control group, control group set as 1).

Biotechnology (Beijing, China). S100A8 protein was obtained from Novus Biologicals. Contaminating LPS was removed by Triton X-114 extraction. LPS content was always below 0.5 ng/mg protein, which did not cause an effect in our assays.

Cell culture

The human leukemia cell lines, K562 (chronic myeloid leukemia cells), HL-60 (acute myeloid leukemia cells), MV-4-11 (biphenotypic B myelomonocytic leukemia cells), Jurkat (T-cell acute lymphoblastic leukemia cells), and K562/A02 (multidrug resistance K562) were from the American Type Culture Collection; HL-60/ADR (multidrug resistance HL-60) was from the Institute of Hematology & Blood Diseases Hospital of Chinese Academy of Medical Sciences & Peking Union Medical College. Cells were cultured in RPMI-1640 medium supplemented with 10% heat-inactivated FBS and 2 mM glutamine in a humidified incubator with 5% CO2 and 95% air.

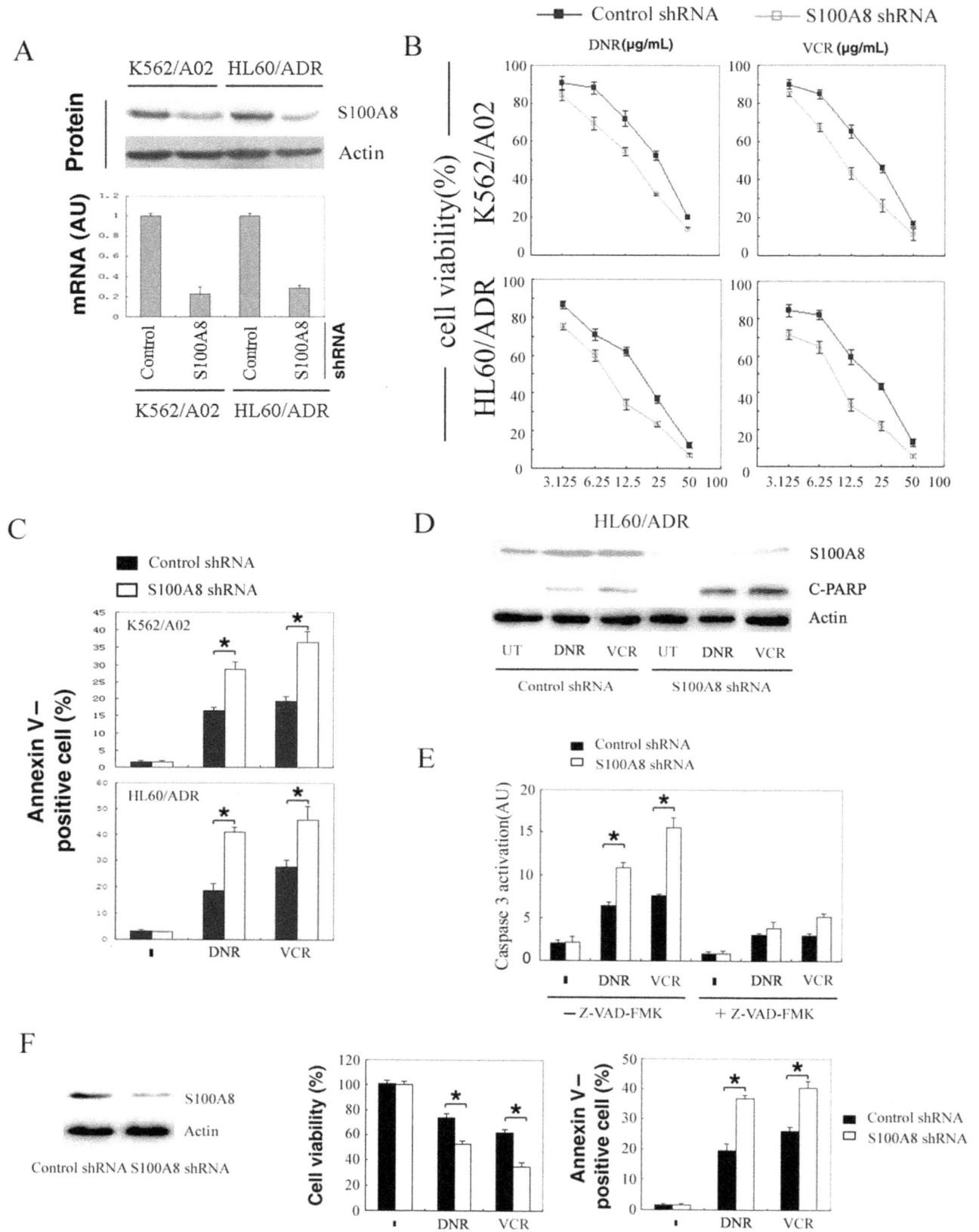

Figure 2. Suppression of S100A8 sensitized drug resistance leukemia cells to chemotherapy. (A) HL60/ADR and K562/A02 cells were transfected with control shRNA or S100A8 shRNA for 48 hours. Protein and mRNA level of S100A8 was assayed by Western blot and real time RT-PCR, respectively. (B) HL60/ADR and K562/A02 cells were transfected with control shRNA or S100A8 shRNA for 48 hours, then treated with adriamycin

(ADR) and vincristine (VCR) for an additional 24 hours. Cell viability was analyzed by MTT. (**C and D**) HL60/ADR and K562/A02 cells were transfected with control shRNA or S100A8 shRNA for 48 hours, treated with ADR (12.5 μg/mL), VCR (12.5 μg/mL) for additional 24 hours. Apoptosis was analyzed by measuring positive percentage of Annexin V cells via flow cytometry (**C**; n = 3; $^{*}P<0.05$); cleaved PARP was analyzed by Western blotting (**D**). (**E**) HL60/ADR and K562/A02 cells were transfected with control shRNA or S100A8 shRNA for 48 hours, and then treated with ADR (12.5 μg/mL), VCR (12.5 μg/mL) for additional 24 hours with or without ZVAD-FMK (20 μmol/L). Activation of caspase-3 was analyzed (n = 3; $^{*}P<0.05$). (**F**) HL60/ADR cells were transfected with control shRNA or S100A8 shRNA (from Gene Pharma, China) for 48 hours and then treated with ADR (12.5 μg/mL), VCR (12.5 μg/mL) for 24 hours. S100A8 protein was determined by Western blot; Cell viability was analyzed by MTT; apoptosis was analyzed by flow cytometry (n = 3; $^{*}P<0.05$).

Cell viability assay

Cell viability was assessed by MTT assay. Briefly, leukemia cells were seeded in 96-well plates (4000 cells/well) the day before treatment. Following treatment with ADR for 72 h, 25 μL MTT [3-(4,5-dimethylthiazol–2-yl)- 2,5-diphenyltetrazolium bromide; Sigma] was added to each well and incubated for 3.5 h, followed by the addition of 100 μL of N,Ndimethylformamide (D4551; Sigma). The plates were left at room temperature overnight to allow complete lysis of the cells, and read at 450 nm the following day. Half-maximal inhibitory concentration (IC50) was calculated using MS Excel, as previously described [15].

Western blot analysis

Cell lysates were prepared with cell lysis buffer [20 mmol/L Tris-HCl, pH 7.5; 150 mmol/L NaCl; 1 mmol/L Na2EDTA; 1 mmol/L EGTA; 1% Triton; 2.5 mmol/L sodium pyrophosphate; 1 mmol/L b-glycerophosphate; 1 mmol/L Na3VO4; 1 mg/mL leupeptin; 1 mmol/L phenylmethylsulfonylfluoride (PMSF); and 1 mmol/L PMSF], and cleared by centrifugation. Total protein concentration was determined with the bicinchoninic acid assay Kit (Bio-Rad). Proteins were resolved on a denaturing 10% SDS-PAGE gel and subsequently transferred to polyvinylidene fluoride membranes *via* semidry transfer. The membrane was blocked with 5% dried milk or 3% bovine serum albumin in Tris-buffered saline and Tween 20 (10 mmol/L Tris, pH 7.5; 100 mmol/L NaCl; and 0.1% Tween20), incubated with primary antibodies, and then with horseradish peroxidase–conjugated secondary antibodies. The signals were visualized by enhanced chemiluminescence.

Quantitative real-time PCR

Total RNA was extracted using TRIzol (Invitrogen, USA) according to the manufacturer's instructions. Reverse transcription (RT) was performed with 2 μg of total RNA with HiFi-MMLV Enzyme Mix (CWbio, China). Twenty ng cDNA was subjected to real-time quantitative PCR (TaqMan probes) for the evaluation of the relative S100A8 mRNA, with beta actin as an internal control with gene specific primers and fluorogenic probes (S100A8: forward primer 5′- CCTAACCGCTATAAAAGGAG -3′, reverse primer 5′- ATGATGCCCACGGACTTGCC -3, probe 5′ FAM-CCTCTCAGCCCTGCATGTCTCTT -TAMRA 3′; ACTB: forward primer 5′- GGCACCCAGCACAATGAAGA-3, reverse primer 5′-CGTCATACTCCTGCTTGCTG-3′, probe 5′FAM-CTGGAAGGTGGACAGCGAGGC-TAMRA 3′.) in an LightCycler 480 **System** (Roche). Quantification was determined by the standard curve and 2-ΔΔCt methods [15].

Immunoprecipitation analysis

Cells were lysed at 4°C in ice-cold radioimmunoprecipitation assay lysis buffer (Millipore, Billerica, MA, USA). Cell lysates were cleared by a brief centrifugation (12,000 g, 10 min). Protein concentration in the supernatant was determined by bicinchoninic acid assay. Before immunoprecipitation, equal amounts of proteins were pre-cleared with Protein A or protein G agarose/sepharose

(Millipore) at 4°C for 3 h and subsequently incubated with various irrelevant immunoglobulin-G or specific antibodies (5 μg/ml) in the presence of protein A or G agarose/sepharose beads for 2 h or overnight at 4°C with gently shaking. Following incubation, agarose/sepharose beads were washed extensively with phosphate buffered saline. Proteins were eluted by boiling in 2×SDS sample buffer before SDS–polyacrylamide gel electrophoresis and immunoblot analysis, as previously described [15,16].

Gene transfection and RNAi

Cells were transfected with S100A8 pLPCX constructs by square-pulse electroporation at 600 V for 2 msec and cultured under selection of neomycin (1 mg/ml; Gibco BRL, USA) and puromycin (10 mg/ml; Sigma) in order to obtain a pure population of transfected cells [13]. Lipofectamine 2000 Transfection Reagent (Invitrogen) was used to transfect S100A8-shRNA, BECN1-shRNA, PI3KC3-shRNA, ULK1-shRNA, RAGE-shRNA, TLR4-shRNA and Atg7 shRNA (Sigma) [16]. As a control experiment, another S100A8-shRNA was obtained from Gene Pharma (Shanghai, China).

Apoptosis assays

Apoptosis was assessed using the FITC Annexin V Apoptosis Detection kit, which involves staining cells with Annexin V-FITC (a phospholipid-binding protein that binds to disrupted cell membranes) in combination with PI (a vital dye that binds to DNA penetrating into apoptotic cells). Flow cytometric analysis (FACS) was performed to determine the percentage of apoptotic cells (Annexin V^{+}/PI).

Electron microscopy

Leukemia cells were collected and fixed in 2.5% glutaraldehyde for at least 3 h. Then cells were treated with 2% paraformaldehyde at room temperature for 60 min, 0.1% glutaraldehyde in 0.1 M sodium cacodylate for 2 h, post-fixed with 1% OsO4 for 1.5 h, dehydrated with graded acetone, and embedded in Quetol 812. Ultrathin sections were observed using a Hitachi H7500 electron microscope (Tokyo, Japan) [17].

Immunofluorescence and confocal microscopy

Cells were collected, fixed and permeabilized with 0.3% triton X-100 for 10 min, incubated with anti-LC3 for 1 h and then FITC-conjugated Anti-LC3A/B antibody (Abcam, ab58610) for 1 h at room temperature. Cell nuclei were stained using ProLong Gold Antifade Reagent with DAPI (Life Technologies). Samples were examined under an Olympus FV1000 confocal microscope. For evaluating tandem fluorescent LC3 puncta, cells were washed with PBS, fixed with 4% paraformaldehyde, mounted with DAPI and viewed under a confocal microscope [17].

Autophagy assays

To analyze autophagic flux, we monitored the formation of autophagic vesicles by the mRFP–GFP–LC3 method (Invitrogen). Due to the quenching of GFP in the acidic lysosomal environment

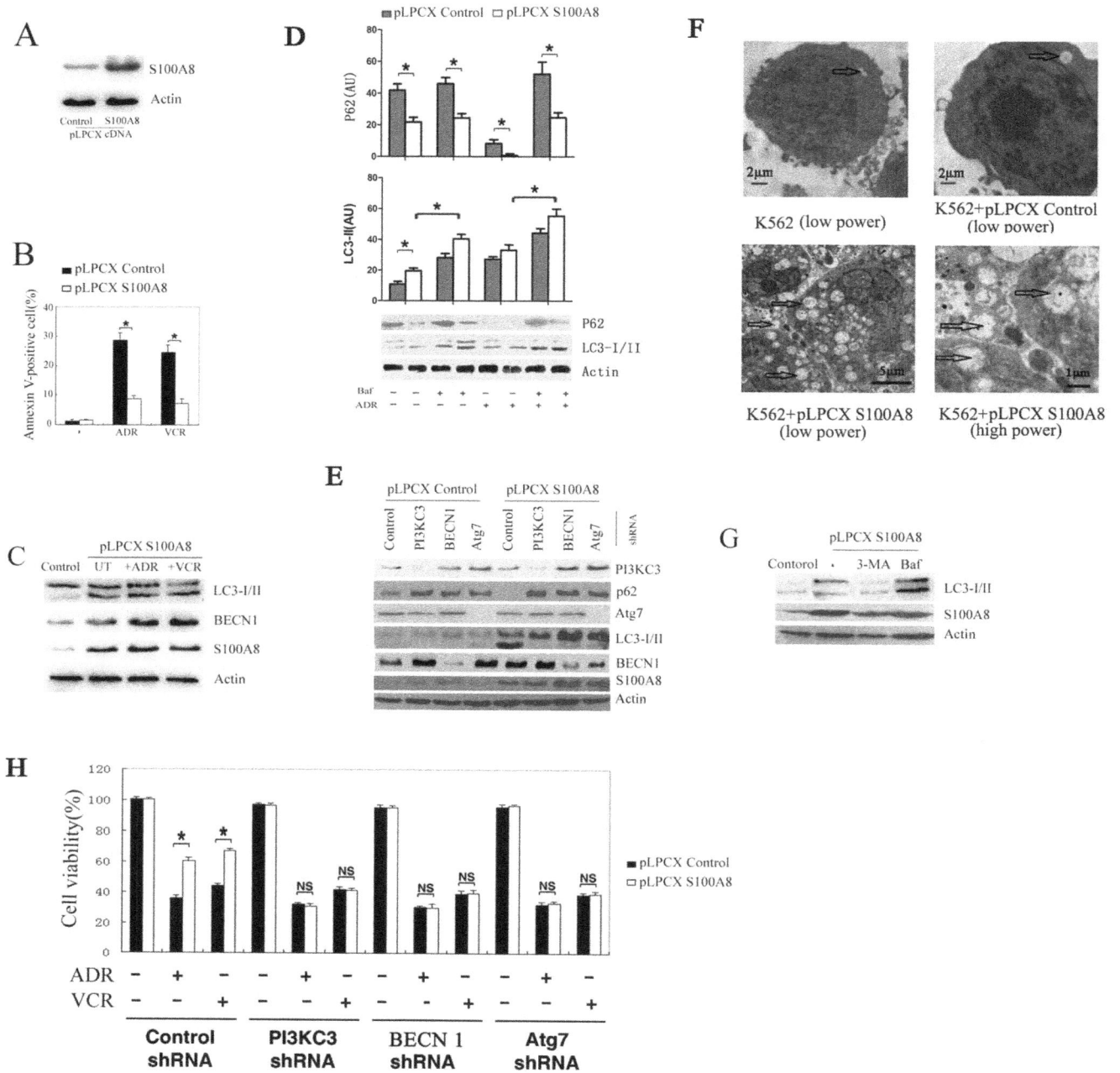

Figure 3. Overexpression of S100A8 increased the resistance of leukemia cells to chemotherapy. (A) K562 cells were transfected with control pLPCX or pLPCX-S100A8 plasmids. Protein level of S100A8 was assayed by Western blot. (B) K562 cells transfected with control pLPCX or pLPCX-S100A8 plasmids were treated with ADR (1 µg/mL) or VCR (1 µg/mL) for 24 hours. Apoptosis was analyzed by measuring Annexin V–positive cells with flow cytometry (n = 3; *P<0.05). (C) K562 cells were treated as B, LC3-I/II and BECN1 levels were assayed by Western blot analysis. UT, untreated group of K562 cells transfected with S100A8 plasmids. Control, K562 cells were transfected with control pLPCX plasmids. (D) K562 cells were transfected with pLPCX control or pLPCX -S100A8 cDNA for 48 hours and then treated with ADR (1 µg/mL) for 24 hours in the presence or absence of bafilomycin A1 (Baf; 100 nmol/L). The protein levels of LC3 and p62 were assayed by Western blot. (E) K562 cells were transfected pLPCX or pLPCX-S100A8 cDNA with or without the indicated shRNA for 48 hours. Protein levels of S100A8, PI3KC3, BECN1, Atg7, LC3, and p62 were assayed by Western blots. (F) K562 cells transfected with control pLPCX or pLPCX-S100A8 cDNA were subjected to TEM analysis. Autophagosomes were highlighted by arrows. (G) K562 cells transfected with PLPCX-S100A8 cDNA were treated with bafilomycin A1 (Baf; 100 nmol/L) or 3-methyladenine (3-MA; 10 mmo/L) for 12 hours. LC3 were assayed by Western blot. Control, K562 cells were transfected with control pLPCX. (H) K562 cells transfected the indicated shRNA were treated with ADR (1 µg/mL) and VCR (1 µg/mL) for 24 hours. Cell viability was analyzed by MTT assay (n = 3; *P<0.05). NS, not significant.

[17], we could distinguish the autophagosomes and autolysosomes through detecting both mRFP and GFP signals, followed by only the mRFP signal. K562 cells were transfected with mRFP-GFP-LC3 expressing pLenti6 lentivirus (Nanjing Mergene Life Science, Nanjing, China). Autophagic flux was determined by evaluating the punctuated pattern of GFP and mRFP (punctae/cell were

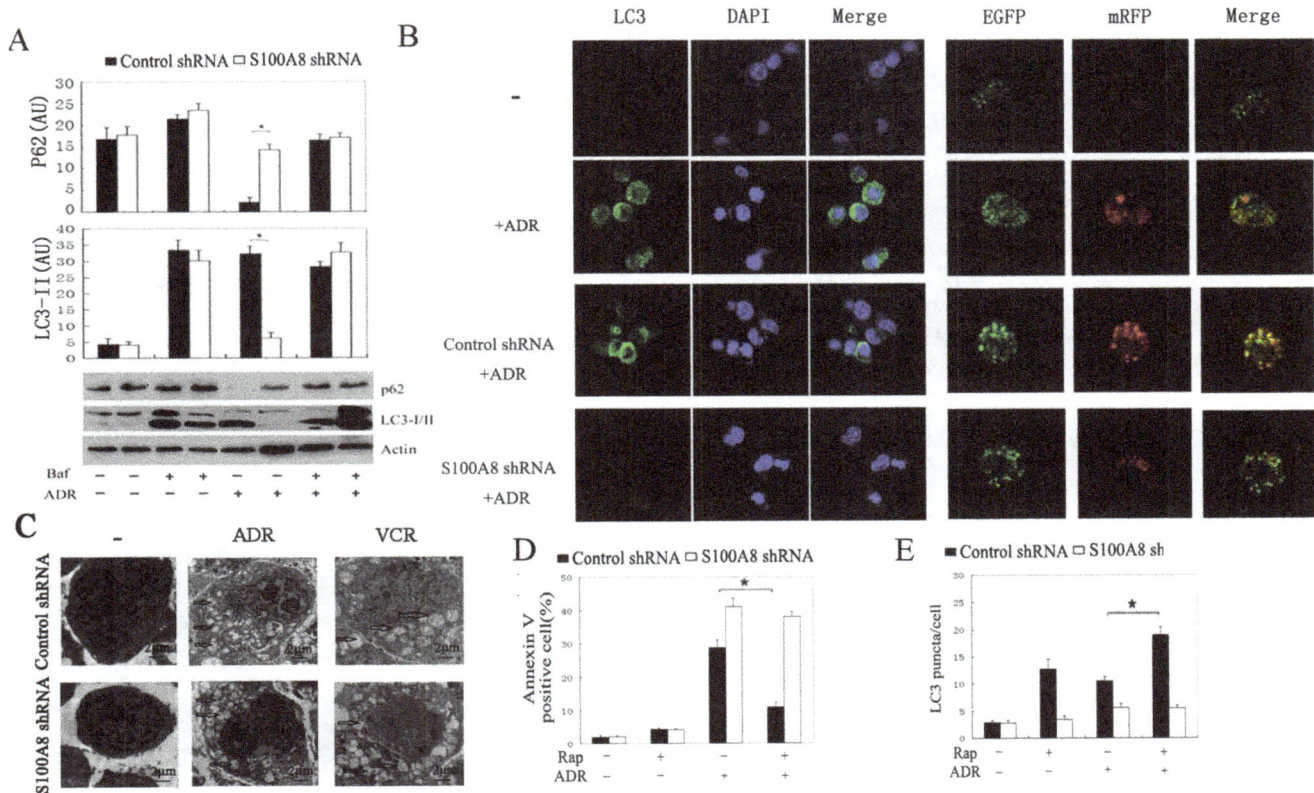

Figure 4. S100A8 regulated the chemotherapy–induced autophagy in leukemia cells. (A and B) K562 cells were transfected with control shRNA or S100A8 shRNA for 48 hours and then treated with ADR (1 µg/mL) and VCR (1 µg/mL) for 24 hours in the presence or absence of bafilomycin A1 (Baf; 100 nmol/L). The protein levels of LC3 and p62 were assayed by Western blot (**A**); LC3 puncta were analyzed by LC3 antibody or mRFP–GFP–LC3 (Magnification is 10×60 oil) (**B**) (n = 3; *P<0.05). (**C**) K562 cells were transfected with control shRNA or S100A8 shRNA for 48 hours and then treated with ADR (1 µg/mL) and VCR (1 µg/mL) for 24 hours. Autophagosome-like structures (indicated by the red arrows) were assayed by TEM (n = 3; *P<0.05). Bar = 2 µm. (**D and E**) K562/A02 cells were transfected with control shRNA or S100A8 shRNA for 48 hours. After pretreatment with rapamycin (Rap; 100 nmol/L) for 6 hours, cells were treated with ADR (1 µg/mL) for 24 hours. Apoptosis was analyzed by measuring Annexin V–positive cells with flow cytometry (**D**). Autophagy was analyzed by measuring LC3 puncta formation (**E**; n = 3; *P<0.05).

counted). Fluorescence was analyed on an Olympus (Aartselaar, Belgium) cell imaging station using Cell M software. The protein levels of LC3 and p62 were determined by Western blotting. Transmission electron microscopic (TEM) assessment of autophagosomes-like structures was performed as previously described [7].

Statistical analysis

All experiments were performed in at least triplicates per group, and data are reported as mean±SEM, unless otherwise indicated. Data were analyzed by 2-tailed Student t-test or ANOVA least significant difference test, and P<0.05 was considered significant.

Results

S100A8 was overexpressed in drug resistance leukemia cells and anticancer agents increased S100A8 expression in leukemia cells

S100A8 was differentially expressed in different cell lines, with relatively low S100A8 in Jurkat cells. We found that S100A8 protein was significantly increased in the drug resistance leukemia cell line K562/A02, relative to the nondrug resistant cell line K562 (Fig. 1A). Elevated S100A8 protein level was also observed in the drug resistance HL-60/ADR cells compared to HL-60 cells (Fig. 1A). Furthermore, there were relatively high levels of S100A8

mRNAs in HL-60, K562 and MV4-11 cells in comparison to Jurkat cells (Fig. 1B), and significantly increased S100A8 mRNAs in K562/A02 and HL-60/ADR compared with K562 and HL-60, respectively (Fig. 1C). These results showed that drug-resistant leukemia cells overexpress S100A8.

At the same time, we found the basal authophagy level in the drug resistant leukemia cells was higher compared to the non-drug resistant cell lines. We evaluated basal authophagy in leukaemia cells and compared the levels of autophagy with S100A8 expression. Basal authophagy in leukaemia cells was low. Moreover, we found there were no significant difference in levels of LC3-II/LC-I in HL-60, K562 and MV4-11 cells in comparison to Jurkat cells. However, the authophagy level were increased in K562/A02 relative to K562, and HL-60/ADR compared to HL-60 (Fig. 1D).

To explore the functions of S100A8 in drug resistance, we next analyzed the relationship between the IC50 of adriamycin and the expression level of S100A8. Increased expression of S100A8 was correlated with higher IC50 of adriamycin (Fig. 1E). Overexpression of S100A8 in K562/A02 and HL-60/ADR cells was coincident with dramatic increase in IC50 of adriamycin (Fig. 1F), indicating that S100A8 plays an important role in the drug resistance of leukemia cells.

It was reported that chemotherapeutic drugs induce S100A8 in the supernatants of cell cultures [14]. To further determine the

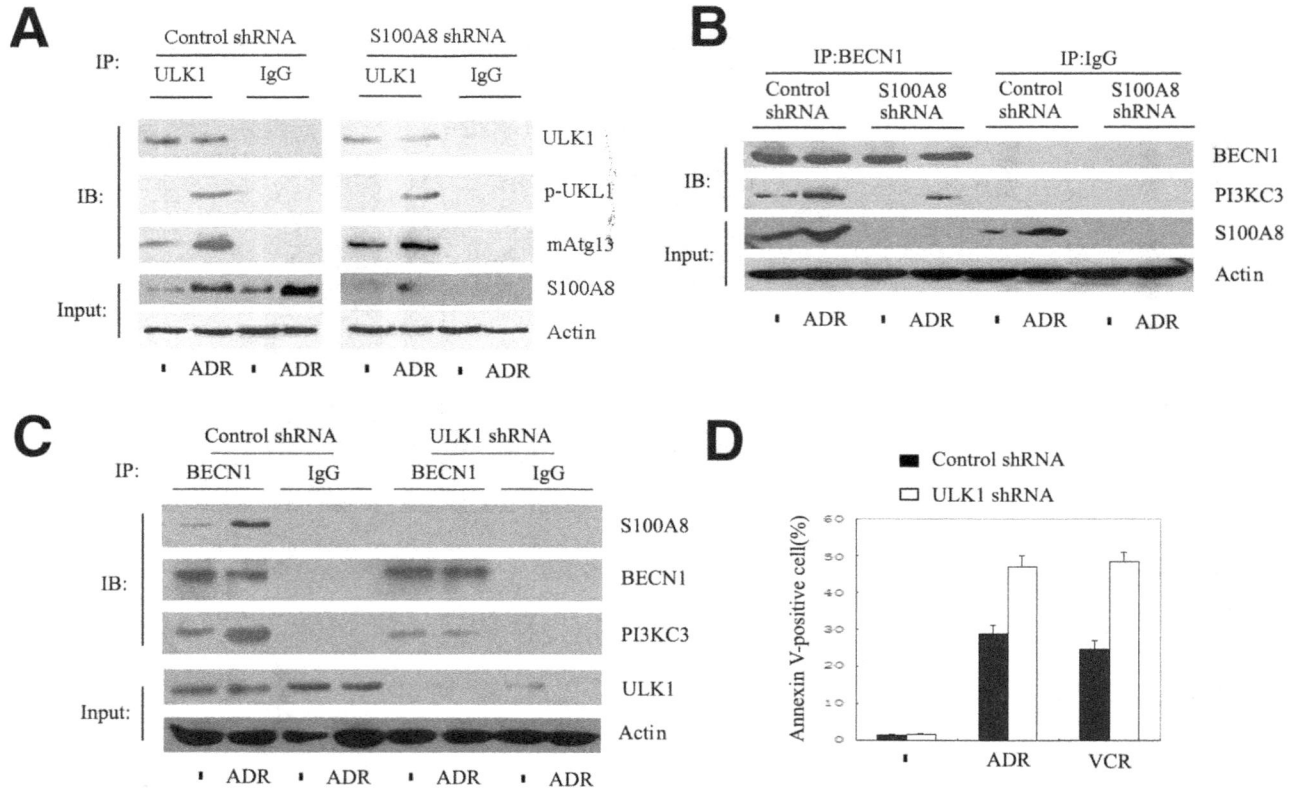

Figure 5. ULK1-mAtg13 regulated the fomation of S100A8-BECN1 complex formation in leukemia cells. (A-C) K562 cells were transfected with S100A8 shRNA (A and B) or ULK1 shRNA (C) for 48 hours and then were treated with ADR (1 μg/mL) for 24 hours. Cells were then processed for immunoprecipitation (IP) or Western blotting (IB) as described in Materials and Methods. All data are representative of 3 experiments. **(D)** K562 cells transfected with S100A8 shRNA (A and B) or ULK1 shRNA (C) for 48 hours were treated with ADR (1 μg/mL) or VCR (1 μg/mL) for 24 hours. Apoptosis was analyzed by measuring Annexin V–positive cells with flow cytometry (n = 3; $^*P<0.05$).

potential role of S100A8 in leukemia in response to chemotherapy, we quantified S100A8 of leukemia cells following treatment with vincristine (VCR, 1 μg/ml), adriamycin (ADR, 1 μg/ml), and arsenic trioxide (As2O3, 5 μM), which are widely used for the treatment of hematological malignancies. Treatment of K562, HL-60, Jurkat and MV4-11 cells with VCR, ADR and As2O3 for 24 h led to significant upregulation of S100A8 protein (Fig. 1G) and mRNA (Fig. 1H).

Suppression of S100A8 rescued the chemotherapy sensitivity in drug resistance leukemia cells

To evaluate whether overexpression of S100A8 results in drug resistance, we knocked down S100A8 by shRNA in HL60/ADR and K562/A02. S100A8 shRNA transfection led to a significant decrease of both S100A8 protein and mRNA in these cells (Fig. 2A). Knockdown of S100A8 significantly sensitized these cells to adriamycin and Vincristine (Fig. 2B), accompanied with high levels of apoptotic cell death (Fig. 2C) and an increase in cleaved PARP1 (Fig. 2D). Moreover, S100A8 knockdown increased the activation of the proapoptotic protein caspase-3 by both adriamycin and Vincristine, which was abolished by addition of the pan-caspase inhibitor Z-VAD-FMK (Fig. 2E). In addition, knockdown of S100A8 in HL60/ADR cells by another S100A8 shRNA from Gene Pharma also increased the sensitivity to DRN- and VCR-induced suppression of cell proliferation, and apoptosis (Fig. 2F). These data demonstrated that S100A8 increased the resistance of leukemia cells to cytotoxic agents and knockdown of S100A8 restored the sensitivity of K562/A02 and HL60/ADR cells to adriamycin and vincristine.

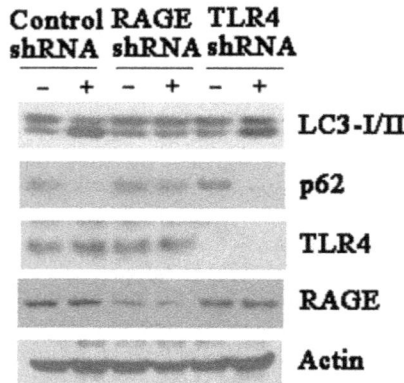

Figure 6. Exogenous S100A8 regulate autophagy through RAGE receptor. K562 cells were transfected with control shRNA, RAGE shRNA or TLR4 shRNA for 48 hours, and then treated with S100A8 protein (1 μg/ml) for 24 hours. LC3, p62, RAGE and TLR4 were assayed by Western blot. All data were representatives of 3 independent experiments.

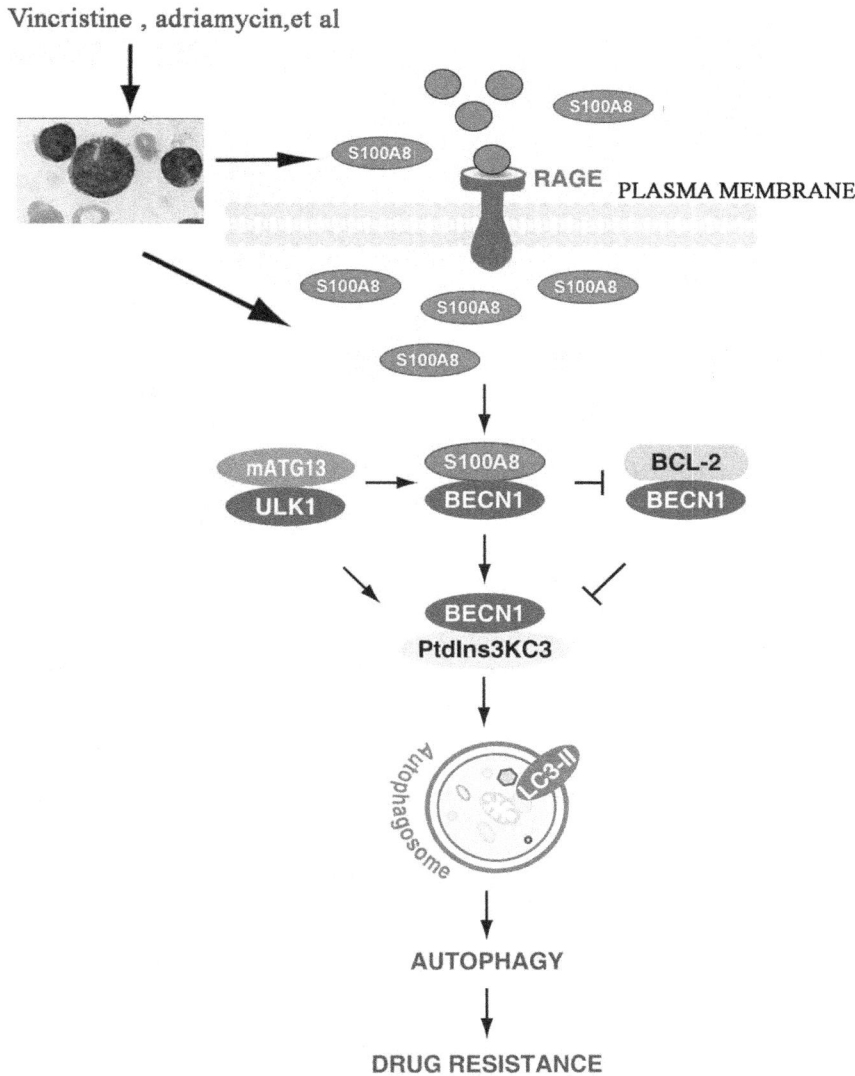

Figure 7. Scheme of S100A8-mediated autophagy promoting drug resistance in leukemia. Leukemia is the most common type of cancer occurs in childhood. Vincristine and adriamycin are the commonly used cytotoxic anticancer drugs in the treatment of patients with Leukemia. These drugs increase endogenous mRNA and protein expression of S100A8 in Leukemia cells by an unknown mechanism. Upregulated S100A8 competes with BCL-2 to bind BECN1, which increases the formation of the BECN1-PtdIns3KC3 complex and stimulates autophagosome maturation and autophagy. As an upstream signal, activation of the ULK1-mATG13 complex is required for the interaction between S100A8 and BECN1. Knockdown of S100A8 or inhibition of autophagy increase apoptosis, and reverses drug resistance in leukemia cells. Furthermore, exogenous S100A8 regulates autophagy through the RAGE receptor. Thus S100A8-mediated autophagy is a potential therapeutic target for leukemia.

Overexpression of S100A8 increases the resistance of leukemia cells to chemotherapy

To further determine the role of S100A8 in leukemia cells after chemotherapy, we transfected K562 leukemia cells with a plasmid containing full-length human S100A8 cDNA (Fig. 3A). Ectopic overexpression of S100A8 in K562 cells promoted resistance to apoptosis induced by adriamycin and vincristine (Fig. 3B). Autophagy and apoptosis can be triggered simultaneously by common upstream signals [18]. During autophagy, microtubule-associated protein light chain 3 (LC3) is processed post-translationally into soluble LC3-I, and subsequently converted to membrane-bound LC3-II, a marker for autophagosome [19]. Overexpression of S100A8 increased LC3-II following treatment with either ADR or VCR in K562 cells (Fig. 3C). Meanwhile, BECN1, which is necessary for the formation of autophagosomes

during the autophagic sequestration process [20], was significantly increased in S100A8 expressing leukemia cells treated with adriamycin or vincristine for 24 h compared with the untreated and control groups (Fig. 3C,D). The polyubiquitin-binding protein SQSTM1/aequestosome 1 (p62) has LC3 binding domains, which target p62 for incorporation into the autophagosomes, thus serving as a selective substrate of autophagy [21]. We found that overexpression of S100A8 increased LC3-II but decreased p62, indicating that p62 degradation is dependent on S100A8-induced autophagy (Fig. 3D,E). Electron microscopy analysis demonstrated that there was increased number of multiple autophagosome-like vacuoles with double-membrane structures in the S100A8 overexpressing cells compared with that of the control group (Fig. 3F).

We further found that increase of S100A8 during anticancer therapy could induce autophagic flux in leukaemia cells. Accumulation of LC3-II was observed in the presence of bafilomycin A1 (an inhibitor of late phase autophagy) in k562 cells both before and after treatment with adriamycin for 24 h compared with the absence of bafilomycin A1 (Fig. 3D). At the same time, overexpression of S100A8 induced autophagic p62 degradation (Fig. 3D).

Bafilomycin A1 increased the induction of LC3-II by S100A8 (Fig 3D), whereas 3-methyladenine, an inhibitor of early-phase autophagy [19], inhibited S100A8-induced LC3-II expression (Fig. 3G). PI3KC3, BECN1 (the mammalian ortholog of yeast Vps30/Atg6), and ATG7 are key regulators of the classical autophagy pathway in mammalian cells [22]. To extend our observation that S100A8 promotes anticancer drug resistance by enhancing autophagy, we knocked down PI3KC3, BECN 1, and Atg7 by shRNA and found that silencing of these genes inhibited LC3-II formation and prevented autophagic p62 degradation in S100A8 overexpressing K562 cells (Fig. 3E). Moreover, downregulation of these genes reversed S100A8-induced protection against chemotherapy (Fig. 3H). These findings indicate that autophagy is required for S100A8-mediated resistance to anticancer agents.

S100A8 regulates autophagy during chemotherapy in leukemia cells

S100A8 is required for the initiation of As2O3-reduced autophagy in leukemia cells [14]. To further explore the mechanism by which S100A8 regulates autophagy in leukemia cells, we detected LC3-I to LC3-II conversion by immunoblot analysis and LC3 puncta formation by fluorescent imaging analysis. Knockdown of S100A8 inhibited ADR-induced LC3-II (Fig. 4A). LC3 is lipidated and recruited to the autophagosomal membrane following autophagosome formation. Accordingly, accumulation of LC3-II was observed in the presence of bafilomycin A1 (Fig. 4A). Moreover, knockdown of S100A8 inhibited the accumulation of LC3 puncta in leukemia cells as detected by immunofluorenscence with a LC3 antibody (Fig. 4B). In addition, ultrastructural analysis revealed that cells transfected with S100A8 shRNA exhibited fewer autophagosomes during chemotherapy compared with cells transfected with control shRNA (Fig. 4C). To test whether S100A8 influences autophagic flux, we evaluated the expression of p62. Indeed, knockdown of S100A8 inhibited autophagic p62 degradation (Fig. 4A). These findings further support a critical role for S100A8 in the regulation of autophagy in leukemia cells.

Rapamycin induces autophagy by inhibiting the mammalian target of rapamycin complex 1 (mTORC1) [23]. Rapamycin pretreatment prevented ADR from inducing apoptosis in K562/A02 cells (Fig. 4D). However, rapamycin conferred less protection in K562/A02 cells transfected with S100A8 shRNA probably due to diminished autophagic capacity (Fig. 4E). These results suggest that S100A8 is an important regulator of autophagy-mediated leukemia cell survival.

S100A8 regulates the formation of BECN1–PI3KC3 complex but not ULK1–mAtg13 complex

Mammalian autophagy is a multi-step process including initiation, nucleation, elongation, closure, maturation, and finally degradation or extrusion, and regulated by a core family of ATG proteins [1,24]. To explore the underlying molecular mechanism of S100A8-mediated autophagy, we analyzed the early autophagic signaling event of ULK1 complex formation. ULK1 is essential for autophagy induction and is comprised of a large complex that includes a mammalian homologue of Atg13 (mAtg13). Knockdown of S100A8 did not affect the formation of ULK1-mAtg13 complex and phosphorylation of ULK1 at Ser55 following ADR treatment (Fig. 5A). However, S100A8 knockdown significantly reduced the formation of the BECN1-PI3KC3 complex (Fig. 5B), which mediates vesicle nucleation during autophagy. Consistent with the previous studies [14], S100A8 formed a complex with BECN1 in leukemia cells (Fig. 5C). Moreover, knockdown of ULK1 inhibited the interaction between S100A8 and BECN1 (Fig. 5C) and potentiated anticancer agent-induced cell apoptosis (Fig. 5D). These data suggest that S100A8 is a downstream signaling molecule from the ULK1-mAtg13 complex and facilitates autophagy in leukemia cells by interacting with BECN1.

RAGE was involved in exogenous S100A8-induced autophagy. To investigate whether extracellular S100A8 induce autophagy in leukemia cells, we treated K562 cells with 1 μg/ml S100A8 protein for 24 h and detected LC3-I/LC3-II and P62 by immunoblot analysis. We found that S100A8 treatment increased the expression of LC3-II, and decreased the expression of p62. To test the role of RAGE and TLR4 in S100A8-induced autophagy, we knocked down RAGE and TLR4 by shRNA in K562 cells. We found that silencing RAGE inhibited LC3-II formation and prevented autophagic p62 degradation. In contrast, knock down of TLR4 did not influence S100A8-induced autophagic flux. These findings indicate that RAGE is involved in exogenous S100A8-induced autophagy (Fig. 6)

Discussion

Chemotherapy is the major treatment strategy for nearly all types of childhood leukemia [25,26]; however, drug resistance often renders chemotherapy ineffective and negatively impacts long-term event-free survival [27]. Multidrug resistance results from multiple mechanisms including dysfunctional membrane transport, resistance to apoptosis, and the persistence of stem cell-like leukemia cells. Thus, attenuating drug resistance is a current challenge for the treatment of leukemia.

S100A8 is expressed in a wide variety of cell types and abundant in myeloid cells. Elevated expression of S100A8 has been found in disorders including rheumatoid arthritis, inflammatory bowel disease, and vasculitis [28]. S100A8 and HMGB1 are the ligands of receptor for advanced glycation endproducts (RAGE). RAGE/RAGE ligand interaction is associated with survival of cells expressing this receptor, and is involved in the development and progression of cancer [29]. Inhibition of RAGE interaction with S100p enhanced the anti-tumor activity of conventional chemotherapy in a xenograft model of pancreatic cancer [30]. We previously found that HMGB1-induced autophagy enhances chemotherapy resistance in leukemia cells [16]. It was reported that S100A8 protein balances tumor cell growth and apoptosis in a concentration-dependent manner [31]. Furthermore, variation of S100A8 transcripts has been found in AMLs and correlates with the FAB (French-American-British classification) subtype, or the differentiation of AML [32]. Nevertheless, the role of S100A8 in the pathogenesis of leukemia is unknown.

A number of anticancer therapies, including DNA-damaging chemotherapeutic drugs, induce the accumulation of autophagosomes in tumor cell lines, while pharmacologic inhibition of autophagy or genetic knockdown of phylogenetically conserved autophagy-related genes, such as Atg5 and Atg7, enhanced drug-induced cytotoxicities [33]. The ability to affect chemotherapy sensitivity by regulating autophagy in leukemia cells is a novel function of S100A8 [14]. In this study, we showed that A100A8-mediated autophagy is a significant contributor to drug resistance in leukemia. We found that S100A8 level was elevated in drug resistance leukemia cells relative to the nondrug resistant cells, and vincristine, adriamycin and arsenic trioxide enhanced the expression of S100A8 in human leukemia cells. Further, inhibition of S100A8 or autophagy increased the drug sensitivity of leukemia cells, and knockdown of S100A8 by shRNA increased cell death and suppressed leukemia cell growth. As a member of DAMPs, S100A8 demonstrate an anti-inflammatory, anti-oxidative, and protective effect on cells [34,35]. The expression of S100A8 in AML patients is associated with worse prognosis and a predictor of poor survival [12]. Thus, it is intriguing to propose that release of S100A8 by dying leukemia cells may help process and present leukemia antigens to immune effector cells.

Cancer cells respond to chemotherapy in a variety of ways, ranging from the activation of survival pathways to the initiation of cell death. Increased autophagy is observed in leukemia cells when exposed to chemotherapy drugs [5,36]. In general, autophagy is a "programmed cell survival" mechanism to prevent the accumulation of damaged or unnecessary components, but also functions to facilitate the recycling of these components to sustain homoeostasis. Therefore, autophagy functions as a double-edged sword in cancer development and progression by inducing both tumor cell survival and death. In tumor cells, the role of autophagy may depend on the type of tumors and the stage of tumorigenesis [37]. We found that inhibition of autophagy increases leukemia cell death and reverses S100A8-mediated drug resistance. A systematic study on cells exposed to many compounds showed that no single cytotoxic agent can induce cell death by autophagy [38], supporting the observation that autophagy is mostly a cytoprotective mechanism. Here, we found that knockdown of S100A8

decreased LC3 II formation and p62 degradation, which was associated with a decreased number of membrane-bound autophagosomes, as detected by TEM in leukemia cells.

We previously found that S100A8 interacts with BECN1 and displaces Bcl-2 [14]. In the current study, we found that the ULK1-mAtg13 complex is required for the interaction between S100A8 and BECN1, which promotes BECN1-PI3KC3 complex formation. However, the assembly of the BECN1 complexes is complicated and seems to differ in a cell- or tissue-dependent manner [39]. AMP-activated protein kinase (AMPK) is a key molecular player in energy homeostasis and important for the activation of ULK1 [40]. Further studies are needed to test whether AMPK or other kinases are involved in regulating the interaction between S100A8 and BECN1. Finally, we and found that exogenous S100A8 regulates autophagy through its receptor, RAGE, but not TLR4.

In conclusion, we showed that chemotherapy-induced S100A8 expression in leukemia cells promoted autophagy, which in turn inhibited apoptosis and increased drug resistance, indicating that S100A8 is an important regulator of autophagy. Moreover, suppression of S100A8 expression significantly increased drug sensity of leukemia cells, suggesting that S100A8 may be a novel target for leukemia therapy. (Fig 7).

Author Contributions

Conceived and designed the experiments: MY LC. Performed the experiments: MY PZ RK YY LY DT. Analyzed the data: MY DT LC. Wrote the paper: MY LC.

References

1. Yang Z, Klionsky DJ (2010) Eaten alive: a history of macroautophagy. Nat Cell Biol 12: 814–822.
2. Kroemer G, Marino G, Levine B (2010) Autophagy and the integrated stress response. Mol Cell 40: 280–293.
3. Helgason GV, Karvela M, Holyoake TL (2011) Kill one bird with two stones: potential efficacy of BCR-ABL and autophagy inhibition in CML. Blood 118: 2035–2043.
4. Zhu S, Cao L, Yu Y, Yang L, Yang M, et al. (2013) Inhibiting autophagy potentiates the anticancer activity of @/IFNalpha in chronic myeloid leukemia cells. Autophagy 9: 317–327.
5. Han W, Sun J, Feng L, Wang K, Li D, et al. (2011) Autophagy inhibition enhances daunorubicin-induced apoptosis in K562 cells. PLoS One 6: e28491.
6. Yu Y, Yang L, Zhao M, Zhu S, Kang R, et al. (2012) Targeting microRNA-30a-mediated autophagy enhances imatinib activity against human chronic myeloid leukemia cells. Leukemia 26: 1752–1760.
7. Liu L, Yang M, Kang R, Wang Z, Zhao Y, et al. (2011) DAMP-mediated autophagy contributes to drug resistance. Autophagy 7: 112–114.
8. Schafer BW, Heizmann CW (1996) The S100 family of EF-hand calcium-binding proteins: functions and pathology. Trends Biochem Sci 21: 134–140.
9. Foell D, Wittkowski H, Vogl T, Roth J (2007) S100 proteins expressed in phagocytes: a novel group of damage-associated molecular pattern molecules. J Leukoc Biol 81: 28–37.
10. Ghavami S, Kerkhoff C, Chazin WJ, Kadkhoda K, Xiao W, et al. (2008) S100A8/9 induces cell death via a novel, RAGE-independent pathway that involves selective release of Smac/DIABLO and Omi/HtrA2. Biochim Biophys Acta 1783: 297–311.
11. Cross SS, Hamdy FC, Deloulme JC, Rehman I (2005) Expression of S100 proteins in normal human tissues and common cancers using tissue microarrays: S100A6, S100A8, S100A9 and S100A11 are all overexpressed in common cancers. Histopathology 46: 256–269.
12. Nicolas E, Ramus C, Berthier S, Arlotto M, Bouamrani A, et al. (2011) Expression of S100A8 in leukemic cells predicts poor survival in de novo AML patients. Leukemia 25: 57–65.
13. Spijkers-Hagelstein JA, Schneider P, Hulleman E, de Boer J, Williams O, et al. (2012) Elevated S100A8/S100A9 expression causes glucocorticoid resistance in MLL-rearranged infant acute lymphoblastic leukemia. Leukemia 26: 1255–1265.
14. Yang L, Yang M, Zhang H, Wang Z, Yu Y, et al. (2012) S100A8-targeting siRNA enhances arsenic trioxide-induced myeloid leukemia cell death by down-regulating autophagy. Int J Mol Med 29: 65–72.
15. Yang MH, Zhao MY, Wang Z, Kang R, He YL, et al. (2011) WAVE1 regulates P-glycoprotein expression via Ezrin in leukemia cells. Leuk Lymphoma 52: 298–309.
16. Liu L, Yang M, Kang R, Wang Z, Zhao Y, et al. (2011) HMGB1-induced autophagy promotes chemotherapy resistance in leukemia cells. Leukemia 25: 23–31.
17. Klionsky DJ, Abdalla FC, Abeliovich H, Abraham RT, Acevedo-Arozena A, et al. (2012) Guidelines for the use and interpretation of assays for monitoring autophagy. Autophagy 8: 445–544.
18. Maiuri MC, Zalckvar E, Kimchi A, Kroemer G (2007) Self-eating and self-killing: crosstalk between autophagy and apoptosis. Nat Rev Mol Cell Biol 8: 741–752.
19. Mizushima N, Yoshimori T, Levine B (2010) Methods in mammalian autophagy research. Cell 140: 313–326.
20. Kihara A, Kabeya Y, Ohsumi Y, Yoshimori T (2001) Beclin-phosphatidylinositol 3-kinase complex functions at the trans-Golgi network. EMBO Rep 2: 330–335.
21. Pankiv S, Clausen TH, Lamark T, Brech A, Bruun JA, et al. (2007) p62/SQSTM1 binds directly to Atg8/LC3 to facilitate degradation of ubiquitinated protein aggregates by autophagy. J Biol Chem 282: 24131–24145.
22. Levine B, Kroemer G (2008) Autophagy in the pathogenesis of disease. Cell 132: 27–42.
23. Ravikumar B, Vacher C, Berger Z, Davies JE, Luo S, et al. (2004) Inhibition of mTOR induces autophagy and reduces toxicity of polyglutamine expansions in fly and mouse models of Huntington disease. Nat Genet 36: 585–595.
24. Klionsky DJ, Cregg JM, Dunn WA, Jr., Emr SD, Sakai Y, et al. (2003) A unified nomenclature for yeast autophagy-related genes. Dev Cell 5: 539–545.
25. Pui CH, Robison LL, Look AT (2008) Acute lymphoblastic leukaemia. Lancet 371: 1030–1043.
26. Rubnitz JE, Inaba H (2012) Childhood acute myeloid leukaemia. Br J Haematol 159: 259–276.
27. Norgaard JM, Olesen LH, Hokland P (2004) Changing picture of cellular drug resistance in human leukemia. Crit Rev Oncol Hematol 50: 39–49.
28. Nacken W, Roth J, Sorg C, Kerkhoff C (2003) S100A9/S100A8: Myeloid representatives of the S100 protein family as prominent players in innate immunity. Microsc Res Tech 60: 569–580.
29. Chavakis T, Bierhaus A, Nawroth PP (2004) RAGE (receptor for advanced glycation end products): a central player in the inflammatory response. Microbes Infect 6: 1219–1225.

30. Arumugam T, Ramachandran V, Logsdon CD (2006) Effect of cromolyn on S100P interactions with RAGE and pancreatic cancer growth and invasion in mouse models. J Natl Cancer Inst 98: 1806–1818.

31. Ghavami S, Rashedi I, Dattilo BM, Eshraghi M, Chazin WJ, et al. (2008) S100A8/A9 at low concentration promotes tumor cell growth via RAGE ligation and MAP kinase-dependent pathway. J Leukoc Biol 83: 1484–1492.

32. Cui JW, Wang J, He K, Jin BF, Wang HX, et al. (2004) Proteomic analysis of human acute leukemia cells: insight into their classification. Clin Cancer Res 10: 6887–6896.

33. Eisenberg-Lerner A, Bialik S, Simon HU, Kimchi A (2009) Life and death partners: apoptosis, autophagy and the cross-talk between them. Cell Death Differ 16: 966–975.

34. Sun Y, Lu Y, Engeland CG, Gordon SC, Sroussi HY (2013) The anti-oxidative, anti-inflammatory, and protective effect of S100A8 in endotoxemic mice. Mol Immunol 53: 443–449.

35. Yonekawa K, Neidhart M, Altwegg LA, Wyss CA, Corti R, et al. (2011) Myeloid related proteins activate Toll-like receptor 4 in human acute coronary syndromes. Atherosclerosis 218: 486–492.

36. Evangelisti C, Ricci F, Tazzari P, Tabellini G, Battistelli M, et al. (2011) Targeted inhibition of mTORC1 and mTORC2 by active-site mTOR inhibitors has cytotoxic effects in T-cell acute lymphoblastic leukemia. Leukemia 25: 781–791.

37. Dikic I, Johansen T, Kirkin V (2010) Selective autophagy in cancer development and therapy. Cancer Res 70: 3431–3434.

38. Shen S, Kepp O, Michaud M, Martins I, Minoux H, et al. (2011) Association and dissociation of autophagy, apoptosis and necrosis by systematic chemical study. Oncogene 30: 4544–4556.

39. Kang R, Zeh HJ, Lotze MT, Tang D (2011) The Beclin 1 network regulates autophagy and apoptosis. Cell Death Differ 18: 571–580.

40. Kim J, Kundu M, Viollet B, Guan KL (2011) AMPK and mTOR regulate autophagy through direct phosphorylation of Ulk1. Nat Cell Biol 13: 132–141.

16

An A91V SNP in the *Perforin* Gene Is Frequently Found in NK/T-Cell Lymphomas

Rebeca Manso[1], Socorro María Rodríguez-Pinilla[1,2]*, Luis Lombardia[3], Gorka Ruiz de Garibay[2,4], Maria del Mar López[2,5], Luis Requena[6], Lydia Sánchez[7], Margarita Sánchez-Beato[2,8], Miguel Ángel Piris[2,9]

1 Pathology Department, Fundación Jiménez Díaz, Madrid, Spain, **2** Molecular Pathology Programme, Lymphoma Group, CNIO, Madrid, Spain, **3** Clinical Research Programme, Molecular Diagnostics Clinical Research Unit, CNIO, Madrid, Spain, **4** Clinical Immunology Department, Hospital Clínico de San Carlos, Madrid, Spain, **5** Biotechnology Programme, Monoclonal Antibodies Unit, CNIO, Madrid, Spain, **6** Dermatology Department, Fundación Jimenez Díaz, Madrid, Spain, **7** Biotechnology Programme, Immunohistochemistry Unit, CNIO, Madrid, Spain, **8** Oncology-Haematology Area, Instituto Investigación Sanitaria, Hospital Universitario Puerta de Hierro-Majadahonda, Madrid, Spain, **9** Pathology Department, Hospital Universitario Marqués de Valdecilla, Universidad de Cantabria, IFIMAV, Santander, Spain

Abstract

NK/T-cell lymphoma (NKTCL) is the most frequent EBV-related NK/T-cell disease. Its clinical manifestations overlap with those of familial haemophagocytic lymphohistiocytosis (FHLH). Since *PERFORIN* (*PRF1*) mutations are present in FHLH, we analysed its role in a series of 12 nasal and 12 extranasal-NKTCLs. 12.5% of the tumours and 25% of the nasal-origin cases had the well-known g.272C>T(p.Ala91Val) pathogenic SNP, which confers a poor prognosis. Two of these cases had a double-CD4/CD8-positive immunophenotype, although no correlation was found with perforin protein expression. p53 was overexpressed in 20% of the tumoral samples, 80% of which were of extranasal origin, while none showed *PRF1* SNVs. These results suggest that nasal and extranasal NKTCLs have different biological backgrounds, although this requires validation.

Editor: Ken Mills, Queen's University Belfast, United Kingdom

Funding: This study was supported by grants from the Ministerio de Ciencia e Innovación, Spain (RETICC, SAF2008-03871, FIS 08/0856) and the Spanish Association Against Cancer (AECC). MSB is supported by a Miguel Servet Contract (CP11/00018) from the Fondo de Investigaciones Sanitarias. RM is supported by the Conchita Rábago Foundation. The funders had no role in study design, data collection and analysis, decision to publish, or preparation of the manuscript.

Competing Interests: The authors have declared that no competing interests exist.

* E-mail: smrodriguez@fjd.es

Introduction

Extranodal NK/T-cell lymphomas (NKTCLs) are the main group of EBV-positive neoplasms that affect TNK cells, according to the recently revised WHO classification, which also includes aggressive NK cell leukaemia, chronic active EBV disease (CAEBV), severe mosquito bite allergy and hydroa vacciniforme. The precise role of EBV in the aetiology of the disease is poorly understood, although the incidence of NKTCL and the other EBV-associated lymphoproliferative disorders (LPDs) parallels the geographic distribution of EBV infection (in Asian and Central and South American populations) [1]. Most NKTCLs probably originate from mature NK cells, while a small proportion of cases, which express $\alpha\beta$ or $\gamma\delta$ TCR, appear to derive from cytotoxic T-lymphocytes (CTLs). They usually arise as tumours or destructive lesions in the nasal cavity, maxillary sinuses or palate. More rarely, they can appear in other extranodal sites, such as the skin, testis, lung or gastrointestinal tract. Despite their localised presentation in most patients, NKTCL is an aggressive lymphoma associated with a median survival for advanced-stage disease of only 6–12 months. NKTCL has a wide cytological spectrum and is characterised by angioinvasion and angiodestruction, leading to coagulative necrosis. Tumoral cells usually express cytoplasmic CD3, CD2 and, less frequently, CD56, and strongly express cytotoxic markers, including TIA-1, granzyme B and perforin [2,3,4].

Perforin is a 67-kDa pore-forming protein that, in mammals, is uniquely expressed in CTL [5,6]. The complete absence of *PRF1* function typically results in an aggressive, fatal immunoregulatory disorder of early childhood known as type 2 familial haemophagocytic lymphohistiocytosis (FHLH). The overall frequency of *PRF1* mutations in FHLH is between 15% and 50% and depends on the geographical and ethnic origin of the patients [7]. FHLH and EBV-associated haemophagocytic lymphohistiocytosis (EBV-HLH) have overlapping clinical manifestations, whereby CAEBV is often associated with EBV-HLH and some EBV-associated LPD patients eventually evolve into proper NKTCL cases [8,9]. Interestingly, a case of CAEBV with a mutated *PRF1* gene has been described [10], and a girl initially diagnosed with EBV-HLH carrying a *PRF1* gene mutation (S168N) finally developed an NKTCL [11].

The aim of the study reported in this paper was to establish whether *PRF1* mutations are present in NKTCLs. We analysed a series of 24 consecutive NKTCLs, 12 each of nasal and extranasal origin, and found two *PRF1* single-nucleotide variations (SNVs) in 16.6% of the cases. These SNVs were the well-known pathogenic SNP g.272C>T(p.Ala91Val) and the hitherto unreported c.289G>A(p.Ala97Thr). The p.Ala91Val SNV was present in 12.5% of all cases analysed, which is twice the percentage of cases expected for a Caucasian population (3% in heterozygosity according to http://www.ncbi.nlm.nih.gov/SNP/snp;rs = rs35947132). These data are remarkable, since NKTCLs account for no more than 1% of all lymphomas in Europe. Furthermore, all positive cases were of nasal origin (33.3%), had a peculiar CD4/CD8-positive phenotype, exhibited no correlation with perforin expression, and conferred a poor prognosis on patients (median overall survival of 9.5 months compared with 25.54 and 10.6 months for nasal and extranasal-NKTCLs, respectively). Interestingly, in the present series, p53 was overexpressed in 20% of the tumoral samples, of which 80% were of extranasal origin, and none exhibited *PRF1* SNVs. These data suggest a specific background susceptibility to the development of this subgroup of tumours, at least in the Spanish population. However, a larger series of patients are needed to validate this finding.

Materials and Methods

Tissue samples

We analysed a series of 24 consecutive NKTCL cases submitted for diagnosis or a second opinion to the CNIO Pathology Laboratory between 2000 and 2010. Criteria for the diagnosis of NKTCLs were based on the WHO classification [12]. Complete clinical data were obtained from 21 patients. All patients who were alive at the end of the study or the direct relatives of deceased patients provided their written consent to participate. This specific project was supervised and approved by the Ethical Committee of the Hospital Carlos III, Madrid, and Hospital Universitario Marqués de Valdecilla, Santander.

Tissue microarray construction

Representative areas from formalin-fixed, paraffin-embedded lymphomas were carefully selected on H&E-stained sections and two 1-mm-diameter tissue cores were obtained from each specimen. The tissue cores were precisely arrayed into a new paraffin block using a tissue microarray (TMA) workstation (Beecher Instruments, Silver Spring, MD), following previously described methods [13].

Immunohistochemistry

TMA sections were immunohistochemically stained using the Endvision method with a heat-induced antigen-retrieval step. Sections were immersed in boiling 10 mM sodium citrate at pH 6.5 for 2 min in a pressure cooker. A panel of eight antibodies (CD3, CD4, CD8, CD56, p53, CD117, beta-catenin and perforin) were analysed (Table 1). Cases were considered positive whether the protein was present in more than 10% of the neoplastic cells. Perforin was analysed with respect to the presence or absence of the protein, the intensity of staining and the pattern of distribution of the granules. Three categories were created based on the intensity of staining: low, intermediate and high. Two groups were recognised, based on the distribution of the granules: a granular pattern limited to the Golgi region or one diffusely distributed throughout the cytoplasm. EBER-positive cells were considered to be neoplastic. Consecutive EBER-positive sections of each case were evaluated to quantify perforin staining. Reactive tonsil tissue was included as a control. The primary antibodies were omitted to provide negative controls.

EBV *in situ* hybridisation (EBER)

The presence of EBV RNA was established by non-isotopic *in situ* hybridisation with EBV-encoded RNA (EBER) 1 and 2 oligonucleotide probes (Dakocytomation) in paraffin-embedded tissue sections, as previously described [14].

PRF1 gene sequencing

Exons 2 and 3 of the *PRF1* gene have been amplified and sequenced with the primer sets shown in Table 2. Tissue sections from all cases contained between 50% and 80% tumoral cells. The 50-µl PCR reaction volume contained 0.2 mM of each dNTP, 1 unit Taq full DNA polymerase (Clontech Laboratories, Inc.), 0.2 µM of each of the forward and reverse primers and 100 ng of genomic DNA. After initial denaturation at 94°C for 2 min, 35 cycles of 15 s at 94°C, 30 s at 60°C and 30 s at 72°C were run in an MBS Satellite Thermal Cycler (Thermo Scientific). The expected size of the amplified PCR products (Table 2) was determined on an agarose gel with a 100-bp high-range ladder DNA size standard, and the amplified fragments were purified using the MSB Spin PCRapace (Invitek) system and sequenced by means of the dideoxy procedure with the BigDye Terminator v3.1 Cycle Sequencing kit (Life Technologies) and the same primers as for PCR, and analysed with a 3130XL ABI Genetic Analyzer and SeqScape v2.5 software (Life Technologies). PCR products from all cases were sequenced in duplicate from both strands and only cases with changes in both were considered as positive for each different SNV.

Results

Clinical features

There were 11 males and 13 females, with a median age at diagnosis of 56.6 years (range, 31–89 years). In 12 cases the lesion was initially nasal, two cases each had oropharyngeal tumours or involvement of the gastrointestinal tract, six cases involved skin and subcutis, and one case each affected pleura and testis, respectively. We obtained complete clinical data from 21 cases, whose median follow-up was of 18.4 months (range, 1–121 months). None of the patients was referred with haemophagocytic syndrome or leukaemic involvement of the peripheral blood. One patient had previously had a renal transplant, one was HIV-positive and another was HCV-positive. At initial diagnosis the Ann Arbor Stage was low (I–II) in seven and two, and high (III–IV) in five and six nasal and extranasal lymphoma patients, respectively. The frequencies of IPI classes for nasal and extranasal cases at diagnosis were: low (four and two patients, respectively), low-intermediate (four and one), intermediate-high (zero and three) and high (two and two). The frequency across PIT classes at presentation was low (eight nasal and three extranasal cases), low-intermediate (one and four), intermediate-high (one and one) and high (zero and zero). First-line therapy was with CHOP or CHOP-like regimens (CHOP-14, CHOP-21, Mega-CHOP) in 18 patients, followed by local radiotherapy in four patients. Three patients received radiotherapy alone and another one underwent local excision and was administered steroids. Two patients received further autologous stem cell transplantation, and in five cases other second line chemotherapeutic regimens, such as SMILE, alemtuzumab, HPER-CVAD, ESHAP and IEV, were also applied. Seventeen patients died of the disease (nine of nasal and eight of extranasal origin) while four remained alive at last follow-up. The median overall survival for patients with nasal and extranasal NKTCLs was 25.54 (range, 2–121) and 10.6 (range, 1–80) months, respectively (Table 3).

Immunohistochemical and *in situ* hybridisation characteristics

EBER and CD3 were positive in all cases, 75% expressed CD56 and there were six CD8-positive, two double-CD8/CD4-positive and 14 double-CD8/CD4-negative cases. Perforin was expressed in 23 (95.8%) of the 24 cases, the intensity of staining being strong in 26.1%, moderate in 43.5% and low in 30.4% of them. Neither CD117 nor beta-catenin was positive in any of the cases, while p53

Table 1. Antibodies used in this series.

Antibody	Clone	Source	Dilution	Method (Automated)	Antigen Retrieval
CD3 FLEX	Polyclonal Rabbit	Dako	Ready to use	AUTOSTAINER (Dako Cytomation)	TRIS EDTA, 20 MIN
CD4 FLEX	4b12	Dako	Ready to use	AUTOSTAINER (Dako Cytomation)	TRIS EDTA, 20 MIN
CD8 FLEX	C8/144b	Dako	Ready to use	AUTOSTAINER (Dako Cytomation)	TRIS EDTA, 20 MIN
CD56 FLEX	1b6	Dako	Ready to use	AUTOSTAINER (Dako Cytomation)	TRIS EDTA, 20 MIN
PERFORINA	5d10	Novocastra	1:25	AUTOSTAINER (Dako Cytomation)	TRIS EDTA, 20 MIN
P53	Do7 (mouse)	Dako	Ready to use	AUTOSTAINER (Dako Cytomation)	TRIS EDTA, 20 MIN
BETA-CATENIN	Beta-catenin-1 (mouse)	Dako	Ready to use	AUTOSTAINER (Dako Cytomation)	TRIS EDTA, 20 MIN
CD117 (C-KIT)	Rabbit polyclonal	Dako	1/200	AUTOSTAINER (Dako Cytomation)	CITRATE, 20 MIN

was intensively positive in five of 22 (22.7%) cases (Table 3 and Figure 1).

Mutational studies

Three cases were heterozygous for the g.272C>T, p.Ala91Val SNV (12.5%). This is a well-known SNP and the most common base substitution identified in the *PRF1* gene [5]. Interestingly, the substitution of c.289G>A resulting in the amino acid residue change p.Ala97Thr in the *PRF1* gene was found in one other case (2.16%). This SNV was not found in any of the SNP databases (dbSNP137; Hapmap; 1000 genomes) or in the COSMIC database (Table 3). Unfortunately, we did not have normal DNA of the patient to rule out the possibility of it being present in the germline. Additionally, 25% of patients showed other SNPs; four patients had the c822C>T; pAla274Ala SNV (all heterozygous), while six showed the g.900C>T; p.His300His SNV (five heterozygous and one homozygous).

All cases with potential pathological *PRF1* SNVs were of nasal origin, representing 25% (3 of 12) of all nasal cases, or 33.3% when considering all the *PRF1* SNVs. Moreover, three of the four cases with *PRF1* SNV died of the disease, following an overall survival of 9.5 months (range, 2–21 months). These data are more in accordance with the outcome of extranasal than with nasal patients. Two of these cases were those that were double-positive

Table 2. Primers used to amplify most of the exon 2 and 3 coding regions of the *PRF1* gene.

EXON 2	Primer Name	Sequence 5'-3'	Amplicon Length (bp)
	PRF_1_F	CATCCTTCTCCTGCTGCTG	221
	PRF_1_R	CCTCCTGTAGGGCATTTTCA	
	PRF_2_F	GCTCCTTCCCAGTGGACA	265
	PRF_2_R	ACATGCACATTGCTGGTG	
	PRF_3_F	ATCCGCAACGACTGGAAG	241
	PRF_3_R	CTTTCCAGGGCTCCTAGACC	
EXON 3	PRF_4_F	TCTCTCTCTTCTCGCAGTTTCC	231
	PRF_4_R	GTCCGTGAGCCCTTCCAG	
	PRF_5_F	CATATCGGCCCTCACTGC	248
	PRF_5_R	GCAGGTCGTTAATGGAGGTG	
	PRF_6_F	GCCTCCTTCCACCAAACCTA	248
	PRF_6_R	GCCCTGTCCGTCAGGTACT	

for CD4 and CD8, and one appeared in the tumoral tissue of the renal posttransplant patient. Neither intensity of staining nor the pattern of granule distribution was related to the presence of *PRF1* SNVs.

On the other hand, none of the p53-positive cases showed *PRF1* SNVs, and 80% were of extranasal origin. All cases were double-CD4/CD8-negative, and mainly had a cytoplasmic pattern of perforin expression. All these patients died after a median period of 4.2 months (Table 3).

Discussion

We report for the first time the presence of the g.272C>T, p.Ala91Val SNV of the *PRF1* gene in NKTCLs. We found it in 12.5% of our cases, which is more than twice the percentage of cases expected in a Caucasian population (3% in heterozygosity according to http://www.ncbi.nlm.nih.gov/SNP/snp;rs = rs35947 132). These frequencies are remarkable, since NKTCLs account for no more than 1% of all lymphomas in Europe.

The pathogenic role of the g.272C>T variant has long been controversial [15,16], although it is accepted that this SNV leads to reduced cytotoxic activity of the perforin protein due to incorrect folding that decreases its cleavage to the active form and increases its degradation [5,7,17,18,19]. Such a reduction in the level of activity could predispose an individual to late or atypical FHLH, and the development of anaplastic large cell lymphomas, B- and T-cell lymphomas and acute childhood lymphoblastic leukaemia carrying the BCR-ABL fusion gene [7,20,21,22,23]. Except for the ALCL cases described by Cannella et al [21] none of the other T-cell lymphoma cases exhibiting A91V SNV have been correctly categorised according to the current WHO classification. Cannella et al [21] described this SNV in heterozygosity in eight of the 12 patients in which they found other *PRF1* gene mutations. Clementi et al reported a series of eight cases with equal numbers showing *PRF1* gene mutations in homozygosis and heterozygosity. A91V SNV was heterozygous in three of them, one of the cases being a T-cell non-Hodgkin lymphoma (NHL) [24]. Moreover, a *PRF1* gene mutation was described in two cases of subcutaneous panniculitis-like T-cell lymphoma [24,25]. One patient presented the 1168C>T (Arg390stop) in a single allele and the other had two mutations, the 272C>T (A91V) and the 1262G>T (Phe 421Cys), in heterozygosity. Both patients suffered from HLH, a widely described phenomenon in both subcutaneous panniculitis αβ and γδ T-cell lymphomas [26].

Except for the double-CD4/CD8 positivity of two cases, which is rare [25,27], all other immunophenotypes of the cases presented

Table 3. Most relevant immunohistochemical and clinical data of these series.

CASE	MUTATION	SEX	AD	LDD	P53	CD56	CD8	CD4	PI	PG	STATUS	OS (months)
1	NMF	M	77	Nasal tissue	N	HI	N	N	N	NP	A	121
2	NMF	M	50	Skin	N	HI	HI	N	Mo	GR	NK	NK
3	NMF	M	57	Nasal tissue	N	LI	N	N	L	GR	D	10
4	g.272C>T; Ala91Val	M	71	Nasal tissue	N	N	HI	P	Mo	GR	D	2
5	NMF	M	47	Skin	N	N	LI	N	L	GR	A	80
6	NMF	F	75	Nasal tissue	N	N	N	N	Mo	GR	D	45
7	NMF	M	46	Testis	N	LI	N	N	Mo	TC	D	1
8	NMF	M	53	Nasal tissue	NV	HI	NV	N	Mo	TC	NK	NK
9	NMF	F	69	Pleura	P	HI	N	N	Mo	TC	D	2
10	NMF	F	31	Pharynx	N	HI	N	N	H	GR	NK	NK
11	NMF	F	53	Nasal tissue	N	N	N	N	L	GR	D	10
12	NMF	F	43	Nasal tissue	P	HI	N	N	H	TC	D	6
13	NMF	F	68	Skin	P	HI	N	N	Mo	TC	D	6
14	NMF	M	78	Nasal tissue	N	HI	N	N	H	GR	A	32
15	NMF	F	34	Intestine	NV	N	N	NV	H	GR	D	3
16	NMF	F	31	Stomach	P	HI	N	N	Mo	TC	D	4
17	NMF	F	89	Soft tissues	P	HI	N	N	Mo	GR	D	3
18	NMF	F	62	Oral cavity	N	N	HI	N	L	GR	D	1
19	NMF	M	78	Skin	N	LI	HI	N	L	GR	D	5
20	g.272C>T; Ala91Val	F	48	Nasal tissue	N	HI	HI	N	M	TC	A	21
21	c.289G>A; pAla97Thr	M	64	Nasal tissue	N	HI	N	N	M	GR	D	13
22	NMF	F	27	Skin	N	HI	N	N	M	TC	D	1
23	g.272C>T; Ala91Val	F	52	Nasal tissue	N	HI	LI	P	H	GR	D	2
24	NMF	M	57	Nasal tissue	N	HI	HI	N	H	GR	D	19

NMF:No mutation found; M:Male; F:F; AD:Age at Diagnosis; LDD:Location of the disease at Diagnosis; N:Negative; P:Positive; NV: Not evaluable; HI: High-Intensity; LI:Low-Intensity; L:Low; Mo:Moderate; NP: Not present; NK: Not Known; PI:Perforin Intensity; PG: Perforin Granules; GR: Golgi Region; TC: Throughout the cytoplasm; A: Alive; D:Dead; OS: Overall Survival.

here were in accordance with previous reports [4,28,29]. Interestingly, these two double-CD4/CD8-positive cases carried the A91V SNV. In the present study, perforin was present in all but one (95.8%) case, although the pattern and intensity of expression varied from case to case. In the various series reported, perforin-positive cases account for 65–86% of NKTCLs [27,30,31,32], perforin losses being related to poor outcome [27]. In the present study, neither intensity of staining nor the pattern of granule distribution was associated with the presence of the A91V SNV.

The expression of other genes frequently found mutated in cancer and NKTCLs were also investigated in these series. Intense p53 staining was found in 22.7% of cases, while none of them expressed either CD117 or beta-catenin. Interestingly, none of the p53-positive cases showed *PRF1* SNVs, all were double-CD4/CD8-negative, and mainly had a cytoplasmic pattern of perforin expression.

The frequencies of mutations of *p53*, *KIT* and *CTNNB1* genes in NKTCLs varied between Asian countries and the rest of the world, suggesting that the development of these mutations is influenced by geographical, environmental and ethnic differences, as has been discussed by many authors [33,34,35,36,37,38]. Moreover, there is a well-known discrepancy in the positive rates between mutational and expression studies [33,34,35,36,37,38,39]. The highest percentages of cases with mutated *KIT* and

CTNNB1 genes have been found in China (11.1%) and Japan (30.0%). Recently, Huang et al were unable to demonstrate nuclear beta-catenin expression, a result that accords with our findings [40]. The highest known rates for p53 mutation are those for Japan and Indonesia, where it was found in 62% and 63% of cases, respectively. The lowest mutation rates have been found in Korea (31% of cases) and Mexico (24%) [3]. Moreover, Quintanilla et al showed that the *p53* mutation is related to large cell morphology and advanced disease stage [35]. Quintanilla et al reported 60% and 86% of p53-positive cases in Mexican and Peruvian populations, respectively [35,41]. Pongpruttipan et al [29] found 68% of their cases from the Thai population to be positive, while Ye et al [42] found 33.3% of cases to be positive in the Chinese population. The latter two groups exhibited close correlation between p53 expression and both prognosis and advanced disease stage. This and all previously reported studies were done with the same Dako antibody for p53 and using the same cut-off value (>10% positive tumoral cells) to define positivity, with the exception of Ye et al, who used a value of 5%. However, the Quintanilla et al study included exclusively nasal NKTCLs while the others combined nasal and extranasal NKTCL cases in their analyses. In the present series, only one of the five positive cases was of nasal origin, representing 8.3% (one out of 12) of them, while 33.3% of those NKTCLs of extranasal origin (four out of 12) had p53 expression. These data suggest that

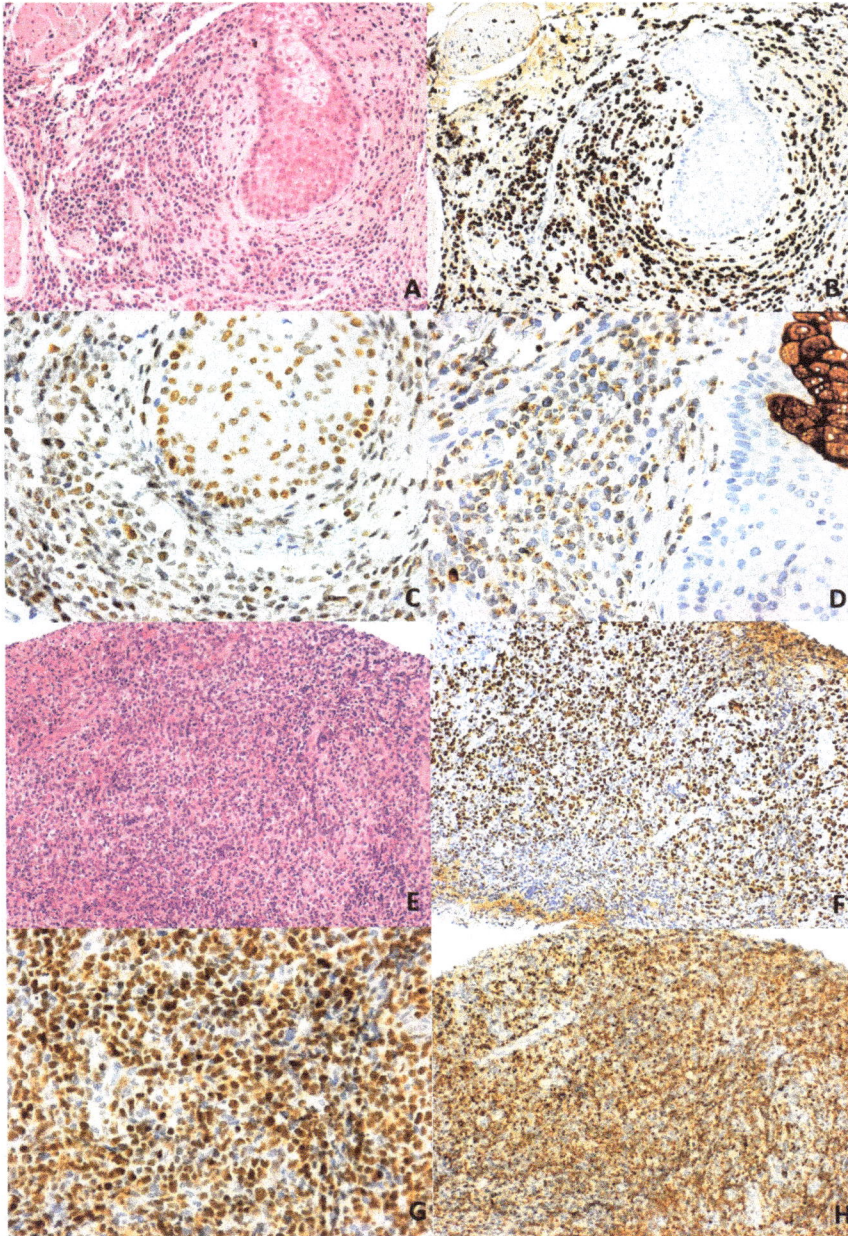

Figure 1. An A91V SNV-positive case (A-HE, staining, B-EBER-positive) showing negativity for p53 (C) and low-level of perforin expression (D). An A91V SNV-negative case (E-HE, staining, F-EBER-positive) showing intense expression of p53 (G) and perforin (H).

p53 expression in NKTCLs in the Spanish population is also different from that in other regions of the world. Nevertheless, in considering all the data from the present study, all of the positive cases were III/IV stage patients, while 52.9% and 29.4% of the negative cases were high- and low-stage patients, respectively.

We found the *PRF1* gene A91V SNV in 25% of nasal NKTCLs but in none of the extranasal ones, while 80% of p53-positive cases were extranasal in origin. Several papers have concluded that the clinical features and treatment response of extranasal and nasal NKTCLs are different [43,44,45,46,47,48], consistent with the results we present herein. Nevertheless, the underlying features responsible for these differences remain to be determined. On the other hand, some authors have suggested that nasal and extranasal

NKTCLs behave alike at the same stage of the disease [46,47]. One publication addressing this subject has suggested that there are different genetic alterations in the two subgroups [49]. Nasal NKTCL patients with *PRF1* SNVs seem to behave more aggressively than those without it. The median overall survival of nasal NKTCL patients in our series was 25.5 months, while that of patients carrying *PRF1* SNVs was 9.5 months. On the other hand, p53-positive patients died after a median period of 3.7 months (4.2 months when nasal cases were included), while the value for the entire subgroup of extranasal NKTCLs was 10.6 months. Interestingly, only one of the three nasal NKTCLs carrying the *PRF1* SNVs for whom complete clinical data were available had stage IV disease, while the others were stage I and II.

In addition, the nasal case and three of the four cases positive for p53 for whom clinical data were complete were stage III and IV, respectively.

The pathogenic role of this *PRF1* SNV has been demonstrated and p53 expression is in most cases a surrogate marker for the *P53* gene mutation. The fact that none of the cases carrying *PRF1* SNVs showed p53 expression suggests the role of different pathways in the two diseases. Considering these findings together, leads us to conclude that nasal and extranasal NKTCLs may have different biological backgrounds. Our series was too short to warrant statistical analysis, so a larger series of patients is needed to confirm our findings.

In conclusion, we suggest that the g.272C>T *PRF1* gene SNV in combination with other gene alterations could increase the risk of developing nasal NKTCL, at least in a subgroup of the Spanish population. Moreover, the presence of p53 in 80% of extranasal

NKTCLs not carrying the *PRF1* gene SNV suggests there is a different biological background in nasal and extranasal NKTCLs. However, a larger series of patients, stratified by origin and stage of disease and treated in a uniform way needs to be studied to validate our preliminary findings.

Acknowledgments

We thank IFIMAV and the staff of the CNIO Tumour Bank, especially Laura Cereceda and Maria Jesús Artiga.

Author Contributions

Conceived and designed the experiments: SMRP MSB MAP. Performed the experiments: RM GRG LL LS MML. Analyzed the data: RM SMRP LL MAP MSB. Contributed reagents/materials/analysis tools: LS LL LR. Wrote the paper: RM GRG SMRP MSB MAP.

References

1. Swerdlow SH CE, Harris NL, Jaffe ES (2008) WHO Classification of Tumours of Haematopoietic and Lymphoid Tissues. Mature T and NK-cell Neoplasm. Lyon: IARC Press.
2. Lee J, Kim WS, Park YH, Park SH, Park KW, et al. (2005) Nasal-type NK/T cell lymphoma: clinical features and treatment outcome. Br J Cancer 92: 1226–1230.
3. Aozasa K, Takakuwa T, Hongyo T, Yang WI (2008) Nasal NK/T-cell lymphoma: epidemiology and pathogenesis. Int J Hematol 87: 110–117.
4. Li S, Feng X, Li T, Zhang S, Zuo Z, et al. (2013) Extranodal NK/T-cell lymphoma, nasal type: a report of 73 cases at MD Anderson Cancer Center. Am J Surg Pathol 37: 14–23.
5. Brennan AJ, Chia J, Trapani JA, Voskoboinik I (2010) Perforin deficiency and susceptibility to cancer. Cell Death Differ 17: 607–615.
6. Pipkin ME, Rao A, Lichtenheld MG (2010) The transcriptional control of the perforin locus. Immunol Rev 235: 55–72.
7. Voskoboinik I, Trapani JA (2006) Addressing the mysteries of perforin function. Immunol Cell Biol 84: 66–71.
8. Isobe Y, Aritaka N, Setoguchi Y, Ito Y, Kimura H, et al. (2012) T/NK cell type chronic active Epstein-Barr virus disease in adults: an underlying condition for Epstein-Barr virus-associated T/NK-cell lymphoma. J Clin Pathol 65: 278–282.
9. Kimura H, Ito Y, Kawabe S, Gotoh K, Takahashi Y, et al. (2012) EBV-associated T/NK-cell lymphoproliferative diseases in nonimmunocompromised hosts: prospective analysis of 108 cases. Blood 119: 673–686.
10. Katano H, Ali MA, Patera AC, Catalfamo M, Jaffe ES, et al. (2004) Chronic active Epstein-Barr virus infection associated with mutations in perforin that impair its maturation. Blood 103: 1244–1252.
11. Lu G, Xie ZD, Zhao SY, Ye LJ, Wu RH, et al. (2009) Clinical analysis and follow-up study of chronic active Epstein-Barr virus infection in 53 pediatric cases. Chin Med J (Engl) 122: 262–266.
12. Chan KC Q-ML, Ferry JA, Peh SC (2008) Extranodal NK/T-cell lymphoma, nasal type. In: Swerdlow SH, Campo E, Harris NL, et al, eds. WHO Classification of Tumours of Haematopoietic and lymphoid Tissues. Lyon: IARC Press.
13. Garcia JF, Camacho FI, Morente M, Fraga M, Montalban C, et al. (2003) Hodgkin and Reed-Sternberg cells harbor alterations in the major tumor suppressor pathways and cell-cycle checkpoints: analyses using tissue microarrays. Blood 101: 681–689.
14. Kanavaros P, Lescs MC, Briere J, Divine M, Galateau F, et al. (1993) Nasal T-cell lymphoma: a clinicopathologic entity associated with peculiar phenotype and with Epstein-Barr virus. Blood 81: 2688–2695.
15. Molleran Lee S, Villanueva J, Sumegi J, Zhang K, Kogawa K, et al. (2004) Characterisation of diverse PRF1 mutations leading to decreased natural killer cell activity in North American families with haemophagocytic lymphohistiocytosis. J Med Genet 41: 137–144.
16. Zur Stadt U, Beutel K, Weber B, Kabisch H, Schneppenheim R, et al. (2004) A91V is a polymorphism in the perforin gene not causative of an FHLH phenotype. Blood 104: 1909; author reply 1910.
17. Voskoboinik I, Thia MC, Trapani JA (2005) A functional analysis of the putative polymorphisms A91V and N252S and 22 missense perforin mutations associated with familial hemophagocytic lymphohistiocytosis. Blood 105: 4700–4706.
18. Trambas C, Gallo F, Pende D, Marcenaro S, Moretta L, et al. (2005) A single amino acid change, A91V, leads to conformational changes that can impair processing to the active form of perforin. Blood 106: 932–937.
19. Risma KA, Frayer RW, Filipovich AH, Sumegi J (2006) Aberrant maturation of mutant perforin underlies the clinical diversity of hemophagocytic lymphohistiocytosis. J Clin Invest 116: 182–192.
20. Santoro A, Cannella S, Trizzino A, Lo Nigro L, Corsello G, et al. (2005) A single amino acid change A91V in perforin: a novel, frequent predisposing factor to childhood acute lymphoblastic leukemia? Haematologica 90: 697–698.
21. Cannella S, Santoro A, Bruno G, Pillon M, Mussolin L, et al. (2007) Germline mutations of the perforin gene are a frequent occurrence in childhood anaplastic large cell lymphoma. Cancer 109: 2566–2571.
22. Chia J, Yeo KP, Whisstock JC, Dunstone MA, Trapani JA, et al. (2009) Temperature sensitivity of human perforin mutants unmasks subtotal loss of cytotoxicity, delayed FHL, and a predisposition to cancer. Proc Natl Acad Sci U S A 106: 9809–9814.
23. Yang L, Liu H, Zhao J, Da W, Zheng J, et al. (2011) Mutations of perforin gene in Chinese patients with acute lymphoblastic leukemia. Leuk Res 35: 196–199.
24. Clementi R, Locatelli F, Dupre L, Garaventa A, Emmi L, et al. (2005) A proportion of patients with lymphoma may harbor mutations of the perforin gene. Blood 105: 4424–4428.
25. Chen RL, Hsu YH, Ueda I, Imashuku S, Takeuchi K, et al. (2007) Cytophagic histiocytic panniculitis with fatal haemophagocytic lymphohistiocytosis in a paediatric patient with perforin gene mutation. J Clin Pathol 60: 1168–1169.
26. Willemze R, Jansen PM, Cerroni L, Berti E, Santucci M, et al. (2008) Subcutaneous panniculitis-like T-cell lymphoma: definition, classification, and prognostic factors: an EORTC Cutaneous Lymphoma Group Study of 83 cases. Blood 111: 838–845.
27. Pongpruttipan T, Kummalue T, Bedavanija A, Khuhapinant A, Ohshima K, et al. (2011) Aberrant antigenic expression in extranodal NK/T-cell lymphoma: a multi-parameter study from Thailand. Diagn Pathol 6: 79.
28. Ng SB, Lai KW, Murugaya S, Lee KM, Loong SL, et al. (2004) Nasal-type extranodal natural killer/T-cell lymphomas: a clinicopathologic and genotypic study of 42 cases in Singapore. Mod Pathol 17: 1097–1107.
29. Pongpruttipan T, Sukpanichnant S, Assanasen T, Wannakrairot P, Boonsakan P, et al. (2012) Extranodal NK/T-cell lymphoma, nasal type, includes cases of natural killer cell and alphabeta, gammadelta, and alphabeta/gammadelta T-cell origin: a comprehensive clinicopathologic and phenotypic study. Am J Surg Pathol 36: 481–499.
30. Elenitoba-Johnson KS, Khorsand J, King TC (1998) Splenic marginal zone cell lymphoma associated with clonal B-cell populations showing different immunoglobulin heavy chain sequences. Mod Pathol 11: 905–913.
31. Gaal K, Sun NC, Hernandez AM, Arber DA (2000) Sinonasal NK/T-cell lymphomas in the United States. Am J Surg Pathol 24: 1511–1517.
32. Schwartz EJ, Molina-Kirsch H, Zhao S, Marinelli RJ, Warnke RA, et al. (2008) Immunohistochemical characterization of nasal-type extranodal NK/T-cell lymphoma using a tissue microarray: an analysis of 84 cases. Am J Clin Pathol 130: 343–351.
33. Li T, Hongyo T, Syaifudin M, Nomura T, Dong Z, et al. (2000) Mutations of the p53 gene in nasal NK/T-cell lymphoma. Lab Invest 80: 493–499.
34. Petit B, Leroy K, Kanavaros P, Boulland ML, Druet-Cabanac M, et al. (2001) Expression of p53 protein in T- and natural killer-cell lymphomas is associated with some clinicopathologic entities but rarely related to p53 mutations. Hum Pathol 32: 196–204.
35. Quintanilla-Martinez L, Kremer M, Keller G, Nathrath M, Gamboa-Dominguez A, et al. (2001) p53 Mutations in nasal natural killer/T-cell lymphoma from Mexico: association with large cell morphology and advanced disease. Am J Pathol 159: 2095–2105.
36. Hoshida Y, Hongyo T, Jia X, He Y, Hasui K, et al. (2003) Analysis of p53, K-ras, c-kit, and beta-catenin gene mutations in sinonasal NK/T cell lymphoma in northeast district of China. Cancer Sci 94: 297–301.
37. Hongyo T, Hoshida Y, Nakatsuka S, Syaifudin M, Kojya S, et al. (2005) p53, K-ras, c-kit and beta-catenin gene mutations in sinonasal NK/T-cell lymphoma in Korea and Japan. Oncol Rep 13: 265–271.
38. Kurniawan AN, Hongyo T, Hardjolukito ES, Ham MF, Takakuwa T, et al. (2006) Gene mutation analysis of sinonasal lymphomas in Indonesia. Oncol Rep 15: 1257–1263.

39. Takahara M, Kishibe K, Bandoh N, Nonaka S, Harabuchi Y (2004) P53, N-and K-Ras, and beta-catenin gene mutations and prognostic factors in nasal NK/T-cell lymphoma from Hokkaido, Japan. Hum Pathol 35: 86–95.

40. Huang Y, de Reynies A, de Leval L, Ghazi B, Martin-Garcia N, et al. (2010) Gene expression profiling identifies emerging oncogenic pathways operating in extranodal NK/T-cell lymphoma, nasal type. Blood 115: 1226–1237.

41. Quintanilla-Martinez L, Franklin JL, Guerrero I, Krenacs L, Naresh KN, et al. (1999) Histological and immunophenotypic profile of nasal NK/T cell lymphomas from Peru: high prevalence of p53 overexpression. Hum Pathol 30: 849–855.

42. Ye Z, Cao Q, Niu G, Liang Y, Liu Y, et al. (2013) p63 and p53 expression in extranodal NK/T cell lymphoma, nasal type. J Clin Pathol 66: 676–680.

43. Li YX, Fang H, Liu QF, Lu J, Qi SN, et al. (2008) Clinical features and treatment outcome of nasal-type NK/T-cell lymphoma of Waldeyer ring. Blood 112: 3057–3064.

44. Au WY, Weisenburger DD, Intragumtornchai T, Nakamura S, Kim WS, et al. (2009) Clinical differences between nasal and extranasal natural killer/T-cell lymphoma: a study of 136 cases from the International Peripheral T-Cell Lymphoma Project. Blood 113: 3931–3937.

45. Li YX, Liu QF, Fang H, Qi SN, Wang H, et al. (2009) Variable clinical presentations of nasal and Waldeyer ring natural killer/T-cell lymphoma. Clin Cancer Res 15: 2905–2912.

46. Suzuki R, Suzumiya J, Oshimi K (2009) Differences between nasal and extranasal NK/T-cell lymphoma. Blood 113: 6260–6261; author reply 6261–6262.

47. Li YX, Liu QF, Wang WH, Jin J, Song YW, et al. (2011) Failure patterns and clinical implications in early stage nasal natural killer/T-cell lymphoma treated with primary radiotherapy. Cancer 117: 5203–5211.

48. Jo JC, Yoon DH, Kim S, Lee BJ, Jang YJ, et al. (2012) Clinical features and prognostic model for extranasal NK/T-cell lymphoma. Eur J Haematol 89: 103–110.

49. Berti E, Recalcati S, Girgenti V, Fanoni D, Venegoni L, et al. (2010) Cutaneous extranodal NK/T-cell lymphoma: a clinicopathologic study of 5 patients with array-based comparative genomic hybridization. Blood 116: 165–170.

17

Rate of Primary Refractory Disease in B and T-Cell Non-Hodgkin's Lymphoma: Correlation with Long-Term Survival

Corrado Tarella[1,2]*, **Angela Gueli**[1,2], **Federica Delaini**[3], **Andrea Rossi**[3], **Anna Maria Barbui**[3], **Giuseppe Gritti**[3], **Cristina Boschini**[3], **Daniele Caracciolo**[1,4], **Riccardo Bruna**[1,2], **Marco Ruella**[1,2], **Daniela Gottardi**[1,2], **Roberto Passera**[5], **Alessandro Rambaldi**[4]

1 Department of Biotechnology and Life Sciences, University of Torino, Torino, Italy, 2 Hematology and Cell Therapy Division, Mauriziano Hospital, Torino, Italy, 3 Hematology and Bone Marrow Transplant Units, A. O. Papa Giovanni XXIII, Bergamo, Italy, 4 Division of Hematology I, A. O. Città della Salute, Torino, Italy, 5 Division of Nuclear Medicine, University of Torino, Torino, Italy

Abstract

Background: Primary refractory disease is a main challenge in the management of non-Hodgkin's Lymphoma (NHL). This survey was performed to define the rate of refractory disease to first-line therapy in B and T-cell NHL subtypes and the long-term survival of primary refractory compared to primary responsive patients.

Methods: Medical records were reviewed of 3,106 patients who had undergone primary treatment for NHL between 1982 and 2012, at the Hematology Centers of Torino and Bergamo, Italy. Primary treatment included CHOP or CHOP-like regimens (63.2%), intensive therapy with autograft (16.9%), or other therapies (19.9%). Among B-cell NHL, 1,356 (47.8%) received first-line chemotherapy with rituximab. Refractory disease was defined as stable/progressive disease, or transient response with disease progression within six months.

Results: Overall, 690 (22.2%) patients showed primary refractory disease, with a higher incidence amongst T-cell compared to B-cell NHL (41.9% vs. 20.5%, respectively, p<0.001). Several other clinico-pathological factors at presentation were variably associated with refractory disease, including histological aggressive disease, unfavorable clinical presentation, Bone Marrow involvement, low lymphocyte/monocyte ration and male gender. Amongst B-cell NHL, the addition of rituximab was associated with a marked reduction of refractory disease (13.6% vs. 26.7% for non-supplemented chemotherapy, p<0.001). Overall, primary responsive patients had a median survival of 19.8 years, compared to 1.3 yr. for refractory patients. A prolonged survival was consistently observed in all primary responsive patients regardless of the histology. The long life expectancy of primary responsive patients was documented in both series managed before and after 2.000. Response to first line therapy resulted by far the most predictive factor for long-term outcome (HR for primary refractory disease: 16.52, p<0.001).

Conclusion: Chemosensitivity to primary treatment is crucial for the long-term survival in NHL. This supports the necessity of studies aimed to early identify refractory disease and to develop different treatment strategies for responsive and refractory patients.

Editor: Francesco Bertolini, European Institute of Oncology, Italy

Funding: This work was supported in part by grants from Associazione Italiana per la Ricerca contro il Cancro (AIRC), Associazione Italiana Lotta alla Leucemia (AIL), Ministero dell'Istruzione, dell'Università e della Ricerca (MIUR) and Regione Piemonte (Ricerca Finalizzata and the Piedmont Regional Government). The funders had no role in study design, data collection and analysis, decision to publish, or preparation of the manuscript.

Competing Interests: The authors have declared that no competing interests exist.

* Email: corrado.tarella@unito.it

Introduction

Despite improvements in the efficacy of the available treatments, there is a variable proportion of non-Hodgkin's Lymphoma (NHL) patients displaying very poor or transient response to primary treatment. [1–3] These patients have primary refractory disease. At present, primary refractoriness remains a challenge in the management of malignant lymphoma. [4,5] In fact, several studies are investigating molecular markers that may be associated with refractory disease. [6–11] These markers might allow for early diagnosis, as well as the identification of novel therapeutic targets. [12–14] Moreover, alternative treatment options are sought in order to improve the usually poor outcome for refractory lymphoma patients. [15–17].

Although response to primary treatment has relevant clinical implications, there are several open issues regarding primary refractory disease. In particular, it has to be determined: (i) the real proportion of refractory patients amongst the various lymphoma subgroups; (ii) the influence of the presently available treatments on the rate of refractory disease; (iii) the actual long-term survival of primary responsive compared to primary refractory patients.

To address these issues, we performed a long-term, retrospective survey on 3,106 NHL patients that had been managed over the last three decades. Aims of the study were to define the rate of responsiveness among patients requiring primary systemic treatment for their newly diagnosed malignant lymphoma, and to outline the impact of the response to primary treatment on the overall survival.

Methods

Data sources, patient population, and clinical procedures

The retrospective review was performed on newly diagnosed, NHL patients, admitted and managed at the University Hematology of Torino (S. Giovanni Battista and Mauriziano Hospitals) and at the Hematology Division of Ospedali Riuniti of Bergamo, Italy, during the last three decades (1982–2012). An electronic database has been used since early 1980 s at the Hematology Division of Bergamo. [18] A similar database has been used since 2000 at the University Department of Hematology in Torino. [19] Based on these registries, data have been collected of 3,393 NHL patients requiring systemic therapy. The retrospective analysis was approved by our local Ethical Committee (Ospedale Infantile Regina Margherita [O.I.R.M.]/Sant'Anna - Ordine Mauriziano, Torino) (prot.No. 100355/A210). The Ethical Committee did not require a written informed consent form for the patients included in the analysis. However, patient information was anonymized in the recorded files.

All patients underwent common diagnostic procedures, in order to define the type of lymphoma and disease extension, and then to evaluate response to treatment. A total of 3,393 patients entered in our data base, however information on response to primary treatment was lacking for 78 (2.3%) of them and overall 3,315 could be considered for the analysis. In addition, 209 patients (6.3%), with a median age of 69 (range, 20–98), died early (within 8 months) during or before any treatment was given, and could not be properly evaluated for response. Causes of early death were: i. early, treatment related toxicities (n = 163, 4.9% of the whole series), including cardiac, hepatic, renal, pulmonary or infectious causes; ii. other cancers (n = 8, 0.2%); iii. unknown reasons (n = 17, 0.5%); iv. probable but not formally proven lymphoma progression (n = 21, 0.6%). Thus, we were able to complete an extensive analysis on response to primary systemic treatment on 3,106 patients.

All patients received chemotherapy, with or without rituximab, depending on the time of diagnosis in relationship to the time of rituximab availability in the clinical setting. [20,21] Overall, patients were managed with three main treatment strategies: (i) CHOP or CHOP-like schedules, including MACOP-B, VACOP, ACOP, CNOP, COMP, and CHOEP; [22,23] (ii) high-dose sequential program with autograft (HDS regimen); [19] (iii) a miscellaneous group of other therapies, mostly including the different schedules that are variously employed for low-grade lymphoma, such as single-agents, Chlorambucil, Fludarabine, Cladribine, Mechlorethamine, Cyclophosphamide, Bendamustine, or combination schedules, such as CVP, FND, DHAP, MINE, or intensive programs (BFM or Magrath-schedule) for Burkitt's or Burkitt-like lymphoma. [1,4,24–26].

Study outcomes

The main objectives of the study were: (i) to define the rate of primary refractory disease; (ii) to evaluate the clinical and therapeutic factors associated with refractory disease; and (iii) to investigate the overall survival (OS) of refractory vs. responsive patients, according to Cheson criteria. [27] Refractory disease was defined as:

i. stable or progressive disease (fully refractory), following front-line therapy, either completed or discontinued in order to shift to an intensified salvage program;

ii. transient response with disease progression within six months (early progression), following first-line chemotherapy.

Statistical analysis

Patient characteristics were tested using the Fisher's exact test for categorical variables and the Mann-Whitney test for continuous ones. For univariate survival analyses, the OS curves were first estimated by the Kaplan-Meier method, and compared using the log-rank test, then the Cox proportional hazards model was used to compare risk factors by the Wald test [28,29]. Comparison included the following parameters: gender, age at diagnosis (>60 vs. ≤60 yrs), histological subtypes, IPI score (3–5 vs. 0–2), bone marrow (BM) involvement, rituximab administration, lymphocyte to monocyte ratio at diagnosis (≤2.6 vs.>2.6) [30], presence and type of primary refractory disease, and the administration of HDS front-line. The multivariate Cox model was also used to assess the effects of these risk factors on OS; all the above-mentioned covariates, except gender, were treated as time-dependent variables, similar to the univariate ones. At last, the same predictors were used as independent variables in different univariate and multivariate binary logistic regression models, in order to identify the possible risk factors for the status of refractoriness (dependent variable); these results are presented as OR and 95% CIs. The diagnostic performances of these models are expressed as accuracy, sensitivity, specificity, and positive/negative predictive values. All reported p-values were two-sided, at the conventional 5% significance level. Data were analyzed as of October 2013, using IBM SPSS 21.0.0 and R 3.0.0. At the time of analysis, there were 1,864 (60%) patients known to be alive: 1,508 (80.9%) of them had been seen in the clinic or had been contacted by phone at least once over the last 18 mos., whereas 356 (19.1%) patients had been followed for a median of 6.5 years (range 0.5–29 years), afterwards they discontinued the follow up.

Results

The main clinical characteristics of the whole series of 3,315 patients that were analyzed are summarized in **Table 1**. There were no significant differences in the distribution of the main clinical parameters between the Bergamo and Torino Centers. All patients who had undergone primary systemic treatment were considered eligible for the study, including patients with very advanced age. Indeed, there were 148 patients (4.5%) over 80 years old. Among initial 3,315 patients, 209 patients had an early death, mainly due to toxicity (see Patients and Methods and Table 1). Thus, the rate of response to first line therapy could be properly determined in 3,106 patients.

Raw incidence of refractory disease

As reported in **Table 2**, 690 (22.2%) out of 3,106 assessable patients showed refractory disease, with similar frequencies in Bergamo and Torino Centers. A markedly higher raw incidence of

Table 1. Characteristics of the Study Cohort.

Characteristic	Patients *(N=3,315)*[1]
Age – *yr* median (range)	59 (15–98)
Male sex – *no. (%)*	1,808 (54.5)
Histology - *no. (%)*	
• B cell	3,066(92.5)
• T cell	249(7.5)
B-cell subtypes[2]– *no. (%)*	
• DLB-CL	1,694 (55.3)
• FL	607 (19.8)
• MCL	196 (6.4)
• Miscellaneous	569(18.5)
Histological grade[3] - *no. (%)**	
• low grade	992 (29.9)
• intermediate/high grade	2,322 (70.1)
Ann Arbor Stage - *no. (%)***	
• I–II	1,070 (33)
• III–IV	2,172 (67)
BM involvement - *no. (%)****	
• NO	1,818 (65.2)
• YES	971 (34.8)
LDH serum level - *no. (%)*[†]	
• normal	1,657 (58.7)
• high	1,167 (41.3)
IPI score[4] - *no. (%)*[††]	
• 0–2	1,448 (58)
• 3–5	1049 (42)
LM ratio[5] - *no. (%)*[‡]	
• >2.6	1,281 (59.3)
• ≤2.6	879 (40.7)
Chemotherapy schedule[6] - *no. (%)*[†††]	
• CHOP or CHOP-like	2,089 (64)
• HDT and autograft	529 (16.2)
• other schemes	648 (19.8)
Rituximab addition among B-cell subtypes - *no. (%)*[§]	
• NO	1,595(53.2)
• YES	1,405(46.8)
Referral Center	
• Torino	840(25.3)
• Bergamo	2,475(74.7)

[1]Among 3,315 assessable patients in our data base, 209 died early, due to early toxic death (n = 163, 4.9%), other cancers (n = 8, 0.2%), unknown reasons (n = 17), probable but not formally proven lymphoma progression (n = 21); overall, 3,106 could be properly evaluated for response to therapy;[2]B-cell lymphoma was classified into four groups, i.e.: Diffuse Large B-Cell Lymphoma (DLB-CL), Follicular Lymphoma (FL), Mantle-Cell Lymphoma (MCL), and miscellaneous histologies, including marginal-zone (MZL), small lymphocytic (SL), and Burkitt's and lymphoblastic lymphoma; [3]low-grade lymphoma included FL-MZL-SL-low-grade T-cell lymphoma, all remaining subtypes, i.e. MCL, DLCL, transformed-FL, high-grade peripheral T-cell NHL, other aggressive histotypes (Burkitt's and Burkitt-like NHL, Lymphoblastic lymphoma) were included among intermediate/high-grade histologies; [4]IPI: International Prognostic Index: assessed in all diffuse large-cell lymphoma, and low-grade lymphoma; [5]the Lymphocyte to Monocyte (LM) ratio was assessed at diagnosis by automatic blood count; [6]Chemotherapy was delivered to all patients, according to various schedules, as detailed in the text.
missing values: * = 1; ** = 73 (2.2%); *** = 526 (15.9%); [†] = 491 (14.8%); [††] (including cases where IPI was NA) = 818 (24.7%); [‡] = 1,155 (34.8%); [†††] = 49 (1.5%); [§] = 66 (2.1%).

refractory disease was observed amongst T-cell compared to B-cell NHL (41.9% vs. 20.5%, respectively, *p*<0.001). In addition, aggressive disease, defined in terms of either histology or clinical prognostic presentation, was associated with significantly increased incidence of refractory disease. Female patients were slightly, but significantly, more responsive than male patients. By contrast, the overall frequency of refractory patients was not significantly influenced by age (23.1%, above 60 years, vs. 21.5%, 60 or

Table 2. Raw Incidence of Primary Responsive vs Primary Refractory Disease, According to Main Clinical and Therapeutic Factors, Among 3,106 Patients Evaluable for Response to First Line Therapy.

Parameter	Responsive n = (%)	Fully refractory n = (%)	Early progression n = (%)	p =
all patients	2,416 (77.8)	386 (12.4)	304 (9.8)	–
Center				
• Bergamo	1,780 (78.3)	274 (12.0)	220 (9.7)	0.509
• Torino	636 (76.4)	112 (13.5)	84 (10.1)	
Gender				
• Female	1,138 (80.9)	148 (10.5)	121 (8.6)	0.001
• Male	1,278 (75.2)	238 (14.0)	183 (10.8)	
Age				
• ≤60 yrs.	1,335 (78.5)	204 (12.0)	161 (9.5)	0.547
• >60 yrs.	1,081 (76.9)	182 (12.9)	143 (10.2)	
Main histology I.				
• B-cell	2,272 (79.5)	317 (11.1)	269 (9.4)	<0.001
• T-cell	144 (58.1)	69 (27.8)	35 (14.1)	
Main histology II.				
• int/high-grade	1,605 (75.0)	310 (14.5)	224 (10.5)	<0.001
• low-grade	810 (83.9)	76 (7.9)	80 (8.3)	
Ann Arbor Stage				
• I–II	900 (87.3)	69 (6.7)	62 (6.0)	<0.001
• III–IV	1,485 (73.3)	302 (14.9)	239 (11.8)	
IPI				
• 0–2	1,241 (87.4)	92 (6.5)	87 (6.1)	<0.001
• 3–5	669 (67.8)	186 (18.9)	131 (13.3)	
LM ratio				
• >2.6	1,023 (83.7)	101 (8.3)	98 (8.0)	0.311
• ≤2.6	625 (77.5)	115 (14.3)	66 (8.2)	
BM involvement				
• NO	1,434 (82.5)	168 (9.7)	135 (7.8)	0.001
• YES	673 (73.6)	133 (14.6)	108 (11.8)	
Chemotherapy schedule				
• Conventional chemotherapy	1,961 (77.3)	331 (13.0)	245 (9.7)	0.012
• HDT and autograft	425 (81.0)	44 (8.4)	56 (10.7)	

younger). Lastly, an intensive primary therapy with autograft was associated with a significantly higher response compared to conventional chemotherapy regimens (overall refractory disease: 19% vs. 22.7%, respectively, $p = 0.012$).

Among B-cell NHL, patients receiving rituximab-supplemented chemotherapy (n = 1,356) had a marked reduction of overall refractory disease (13.6%, including 8.8% of fully refractory and 4.7% of early progression) compared to patients receiving non-supplemented chemotherapy (n = 1,481), where refractory disease resulted of 26.7%, including 8.8% of fully refractory and 4.7% of early progression ($p<0.001$). As shown in **Figure 1**, the overall rate of primary refractory disease was significantly reduced in all B-cell subtypes when chemotherapy was given with rituximab addition compared to non-supplemented chemotherapy.

When assayed in multivariate binary logistic regression analysis, several clinical and therapeutic factors maintained their independent association with either fully refractory disease or early progression or both, as detailed in **Table 3**.

Long-term outcome

The overall survival curve for the whole series of 3,315 patients is reported in Figure 2.

The long-term outcome has been then evaluated in the 3,106 patients assessable for response to primary treatment. As of October 2013, 1,864 (60.0%) were known to be alive, and at a median follow-up of 7.5 yrs, the 5, 10 and 15 yr. survival projections were 69.9%, 57.9% and 49.2%, respectively, with a median survival of 14.6 yrs. Patients with B-cell lymphoma had a much longer overall survival than those with T-cell subtypes, with median survival of 15.0 and 6.4 yrs, respectively. Among B-cell subtypes, the median survival was 25.0, 15.0, and 5.7 yrs, for FL, DLB-CL, and MCL, respectively (P<0.001). Moreover, B-cell NHL had a marked survival improvement since the addition of rituximab to chemotherapy, with a median survival of 11.4 yrs for patients treated without rituximab, whereas the median survival has not yet been reached for patients treated with chemotherapy plus rituximab. For these latter patients, the 5, 10 and 15 yr

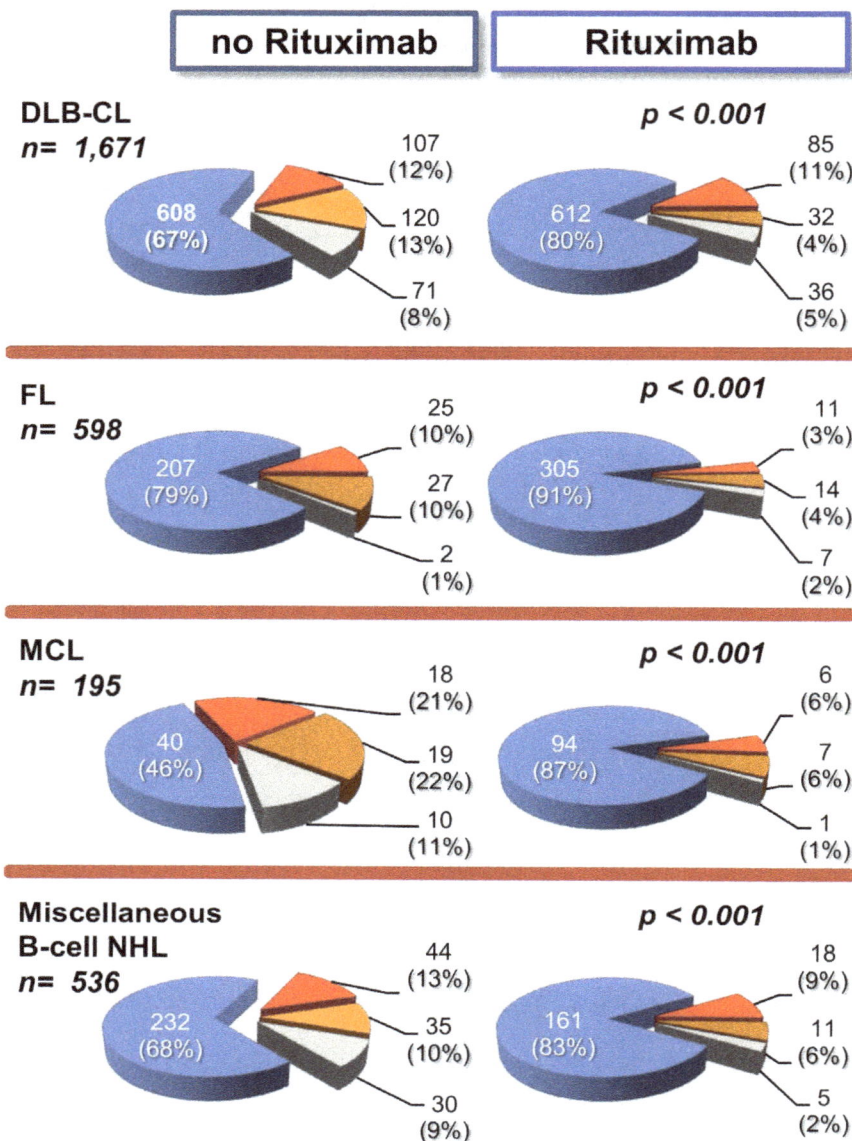

Figure 1. Raw Incidence of Primary Responsive vs Primary Refractory Patients Among Main B-Cell Lymphoma Subtypes, According to Rituximab Administration. Blue = responsive, red = fully refractory, brown = early progression, grey = early death. No Rituximab = Chemotherapy without Rituximab; Rituximab = chemotherapy supplemented with Rituximab. DLB-CL: Diffuse Large B-Cell Lymphoma; FL: Follicular Lymphoma; MCL: Mantle-Cell Lymphoma; Miscellaneous B-cell NHL: marginal-zone, small lymphocytic, Burkitt's and lymphoblastic lymphoma. Data on Rituximab administration were lacking on 21 out of 2,858 B-cell lymphoma patients. *p values* were calculated for responsive/refractory ratio in No Rituximab compared to Rituximab.

survival projections are 79.3%, 70.0% and 63.0%, respectively (data not shown).

Overall, primary responsive patients had a very prolonged life expectancy, with a median survival of 19.8 yrs., whereas patients with primary refractory disease had a markedly short survival, as shown in **Figure 3A**. Indeed, fully refractory patients had an even shorter median survival of 10.8 mos., compared to 1.9 yrs for early progression patients. The favorable outcome of primary responsive compared to primary refractory patients was reliably recorded both among patients registered up to 1,999 (**Figure 3B**) and those included after 2,000 (**Figure 3C**). A slight though significant improvement in life expectancy was observed by comparing patients registered in the period up to 1,999 vs. those

diagnosed and treated after 2,000, both among primary responsive patients (median survival 18,2 yrs vs. not reached, respectively) and early progression patients (median survival 1.75 yrs vs. 2.4 yrs., respectively), whereas no significant differences were seen among fully refractory patients (median survivals of 0.86 and 0.95 yr, prior and after 2,000, respectively).

The very prolonged survival of responsive patients was equally observed in B-cell and T-cell subtypes (median survivals: 19.3 yrs and not reached, for B-cell and T-cell, respectively), as shown in **Figure 4**.

The marked difference in survival between primary responsive and primary refractory patients was consistently observed in all subtypes, with distinct OS curves according to histology.

Table 3. Multivariate Binary Logistic Regression Analyses on Factors Associated with Refractory Disease.

Parameters associated with:	All evaluable patients (n = 3,106)			B-cell subtype (n = 2,858)		
	O R[1]	95% C.I.	p =	O R[1]	95% C.I	p =
➢ *Fully refractory vs responsive disease:*						
T-cell vs. B-cell histology	1.86	1.06–3.28	0.030	NA	NA	NA
Int/high vs. low grade histology	1.74	1.09–2.78	0.019	1.71	1.07–2.72	0.024
IPI score 3–5 vs. 0–2	4.18	2.94–5.96	<0.001	3.74	2.57–5.44	<0.001
Rituximab adm. Yes vs. No	0.43	0.30–0.62	<0.001	0.43	0.30–0.62	<0.001
HDT &autograft Yes vs. No	0.41	0.24–0.72	0.002	0.41	0.22–0.76	0.005
Gender F vs. M	0.74	0.53–1.04	0.085	0.69	0.48–0.99	0.044
LM ratio ≤2.6 vs>2.6	1.57	1.11–2.23	0.011	1.79	1.24–2.59	0.002
➢ *early progression vs responsive disease:*						
Int/high vs. low grade histology	1.64	0.92–2.90	0.092	1.68	0.94–3.03	0.082
IPI score 3–5 vs. 0–2	2.24	1.36–3.70	0.002	1.99	1.15–3.43	0.014
Rituximab adm. Yes vs. No	0.15	0.09–0.24	<0.001	1.16	0.10–0.27	<0.001
BM involvement Yes vs. No	2.26	1.35–3.80	0.002	2.79	1.60–4.87	<0.001
LM ratio ≤2.6 vs>2.6	1.47	0.93–2.31	0.099	1.30	0.79–2.15	0.300
HDT &autograft Yes vs. No	0.50	0.24–1.05	0.066	0.46	0.19–1.09	0.078
Gender F vs. M	0.71	0.46–1.11	0.135	0.58	0.35–0.94	0.028

Figures 5 shows the survival curves of the two most representative main histological subgroups, i.e. intermediate/high and low-grade lymphoma (see Table 1 for details), according to the two main periods of patient registration. As shown in Figure 5 A and B, primary responsive intermediate/high grade lymphoma patients had a very prolonged survival, with median survival of 17.7 yrs and not reached, for the series up to 1,999 and since 2,000, respectively. The outcome was very poor for primary refractory patients, with median survival of 1.5 and 2.0 for early

progression patients and 0.7 and 0.9 yrs for fully refractory patients, in the up to 1,999 and since 2,000 series, respectively. Figure 5 C and D show the long-term outcome of low-grade lymphoma patients: again, primary responsive patients had a prolonged survival, both in the series registered up to 1,999 and since 2,000, with median survival of 20.8 yrs and not reached, respectively. Among refractory patients, median survival was of was 5.2 and 5.6 for early progression patients and 3.0 and 2.7 yrs

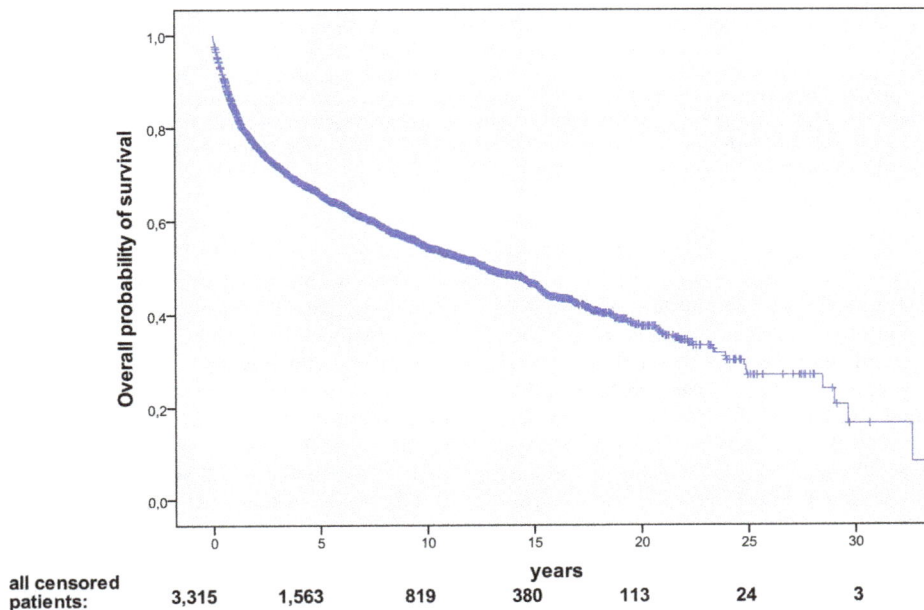

all censored patients:	3,315	1,563	819	380	113	24	3

Figure 2. Overall Survival of 3,315 Non-Hodgkin's Lymphoma (NHL) Patients following first line therapy. At a median follow-up of 7.3 years., the median survival for the entire cohort was of 12.7 yrs. (range: 0–32.6yrs).

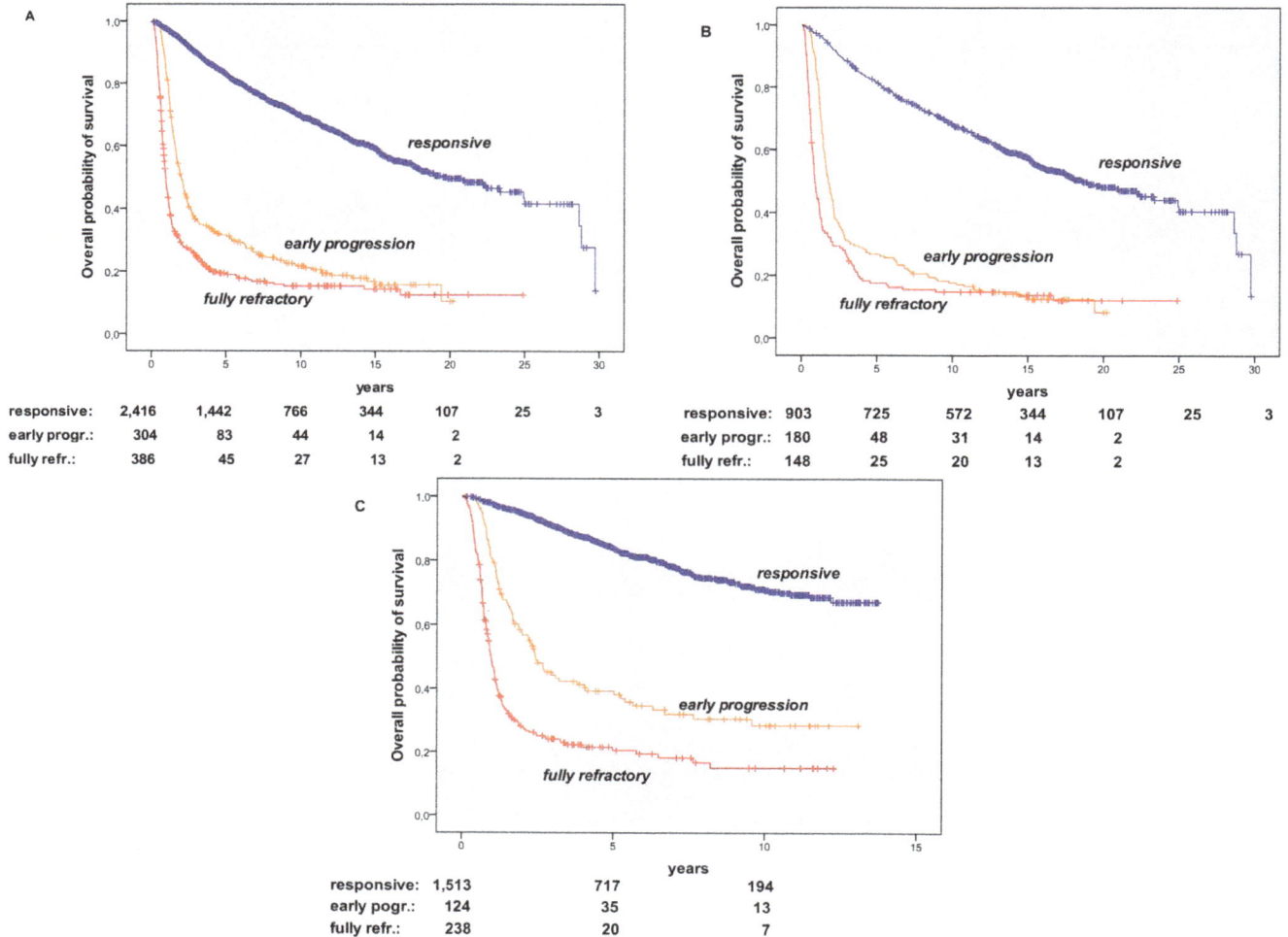

Figure 3. Overall Survival in Non-Hodgkin's Lymphoma (NHL) Patients according to response to primary therapy. A. Overall survival (OS) of 3,106 NHL patients diagnosed and managed during the period 1982–2012. The OS projections are of 82.8%, 69.5%, and 59.2%, for responsive patients, 31.5%, 21.6%, and 15.7% for early progression, 18.9%, 15.2%, and 14.2% for fully refractory patients, at 5, 10, and 15 years, respectively (responsive vs. refractory: p<0.001). Median follow-up for the whole series is 7.5 yrs (range, 0.6–31.2). B. OS of 1,231 NHL patients diagnosed and managed up to 1,999. The OS projections are of 81.4%, 68.1%, and 57.6%, for responsive patients, 26.7%, 17.7%, and 12.4% for early progression, 17.6%, 14.8%, and 13.8% for fully refractory patients, at 5, 10, and 15 years, respectively (responsive vs. refractory: p<0.001). Median follow-up for the whole series is 16 yrs (range, 0.6–31.2) C. OS of 1,875 NHL patients diagnosed and managed since 2,000. The OS projections are of 83.8% and 70.7%, for responsive patients, 39.1% and 28.4%, for early progression, 20.4% and 14.9%, for fully refractory patients, at 5 and 10 years, respectively (responsive vs. refractory: p<0.001). Median follow-up for the whole series is 5.1 yrs (range, 0.6–13.7).

for fully refractory patients, in the up to 1,999 and since 2,000 series, respectively.

Table 4 specifies the main parameters that have independent prognostic value on overall survival. Primary refractoriness was the strongest risk factor, with a higher risk for fully refractory disease compared to early progression. The multivariate Cox proportional hazard regression analysis on factors affecting the OS was also performed on the three main B-cell subgroups, DLB-CL, FL, and MCL. In all subgroups, the high predictive value of primary refractory disease was confirmed (HR 15.2, 13.7, and 21.5, for DLB-CL, FL, and MCL, respectively).

Discussion and Conclusions

The availability of databases containing large volumes of data on lymphoma patients, managed over the last three decades, allowed us to investigate the role of response to primary treatment

on long-term survival. [18,19,31] A variable proportion of patients refractory to primary treatment were observed in all lymphoma subgroups, with the highest frequency amongst T-cell subtypes. Amongst B-cell lymphoma, a marked reduction in the frequency of primary refractory disease occurred since the introduction of rituximab to chemotherapy. Overall, response to primary treatment resulted as the key factor for long-term outcome, with a median overall survival of 19.8 years for primary responsive patients, compared to 1.3 years for primary refractory patients.

The series included all evaluable, adult patients that were managed at the Hematology Centers of Torino and Bergamo over the last three decades. Our analysis was performed on an unselected patient population, including all patients older than 14 years, requiring systemic treatment for lymphoma. These patients represent the common lymphoma population that is managed with systemic chemotherapy or chemo-immunotherapy in a hematology Center. [32] B-cell lymphoma was, by far, the

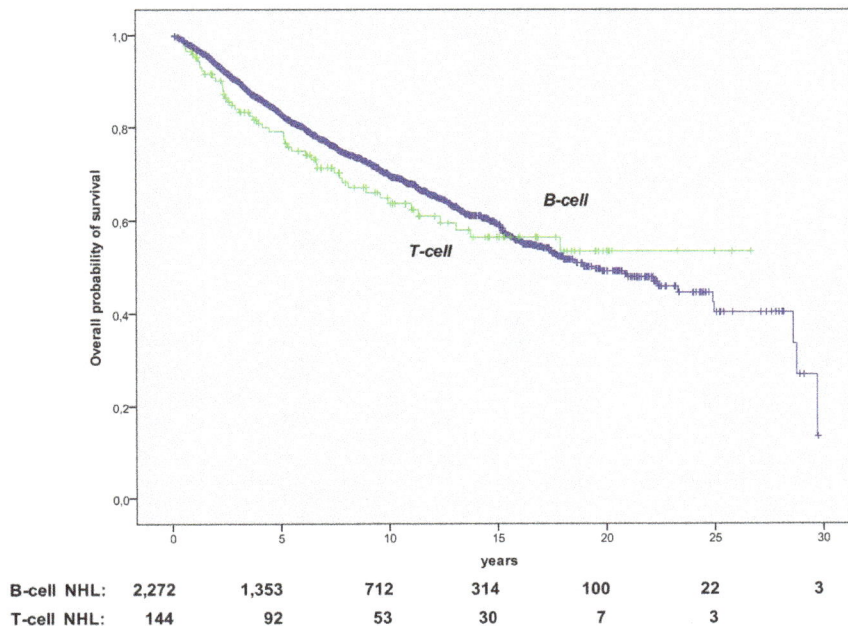

Figure 4. OS in responsive lymphoma, according to T-cell vs. B-cell subtype. The OS projections are of 78.9%, 62.5%, and 55.2%, for T-cell lymphoma patients (median follow up: 10.1 yrs, range, 0.9–26.7), and 83.1%, 69.9%, and 59.5%, for B-cell lymphoma patients (median follow up: 7.5 yrs, range, 0.6–31.2), at 5, 10, and 15 years, respectively (p = 0.326).

most frequent histological form. In particular, there was a marked prevalence in the DLB-CL subtype, followed by FL. Thus, the present analysis reflects the common situations that a hemato-oncologist faces whenever a patient needs treatment for his newly diagnosed lymphoma.

Patients showing stable or progressive disease following primary treatment, or with transient response soon followed by disease progression within six months since therapy completion, are usually classified as primary refractory patients. [4,5,13,27,33] All lymphoma subtypes showed the presence of a variable proportion of refractory patients, indicating that chemotherapy resistance is a feature that can occur in both aggressive and indolent lymphoma. The highest raw incidence of primary refractory disease was found in the T-cell lymphoma subgroup, with a percentage of refractory patients as high as 41.9%, confirming that the main problem in the management of T-cell lymphoma remains the reduced CR/PR achievement following induction therapy. [2,34,35] Indeed, no significant differences were observed between T-cell and B-cell subtypes in the survival curves when the analysis was restricted to responsive patients. Other clinic-pathological variables that were associated with either fully refractory disease or early progression or both were intermediate/high-grade histology, advanced disease presentation, male gender, BM involvement and low lymphocyte/monocyte ratio. Interestingly, advanced age over 60 years was not associated with therapy-resistance. Thus, factors other than disease refractoriness are likely to be responsible for the poorer outcome of elderly lymphoma patients compared to patients younger than 60 years.

Among B-cell types, the addition of rituximab brought a marked fall of refractory disease. This effect was consistently observed in each histological subtype. Since the introduction of rituximab in clinical practice, the chemotherapeutic programs have also been modified, particularly in FL and MCL. [3,10,24,25] Thus the reduction of refractory disease might be ascribed to both the high anti-lymphoma activity of rituximab and

to chemotherapy schemes with improved therapeutic efficacy. However, the treatment schedule for aggressive lymphoma has not changed remarkably over the last 20 years, as it remains largely based on the CHOP or CHOP-like schedules.[21-23] Thus, at least in the most frequent DLB-CL subtype, rituximab is mainly responsible for the reduction of refractory disease, falling from 27.2% to 16.0%, confirming that rituximab front-line is crucial and may overcome some tumor-associated drug-resistance. [36,37].

The front-line use of intensive chemotherapy with autograft was associated with a significant reduction of refractory disease. However, this had no significant impact on the overall survival when front-line autograft was evaluated in the multivariate Cox analysis. The early and late fatal toxicities may have offset the increased anti-tumor efficacy of autograft-based front-line therapy. [38] An intensified rescue program with either autologous or allogeneic transplantation should be early considered in those patients showing poor response to standard chemo- or chemo-immunotherapy. At present, there are inadequate data to define which might be the optimal choice, i.e. autologous vs. allogeneic transplantion, for patients with chemorefractory disease. Meanwhile, studies are needed in order to develop novel and effective treatment strategies with reduced toxicity to be employed front-line in those patients at high risk of primary refractory disease.

The prolonged survival of primary responsive patients is an impressive, and somewhat unexpected, finding. Both the analysis of a large patient population and the long-term follow-up have allowed the first documentation that primary responsive lymphoma patients have a global median survival around 19 years. The median survivals of 25 yrs. for responsive FL and 15 yrs. for responsive DLB-CL are definitely unanticipated. The long-term survival is expected to further improve for responsive patients receiving first-line therapy with rituximab. In fact, patients managed since 2,000 show survival projections longer compared to the cohort treated in the period up to 1,999. The survival

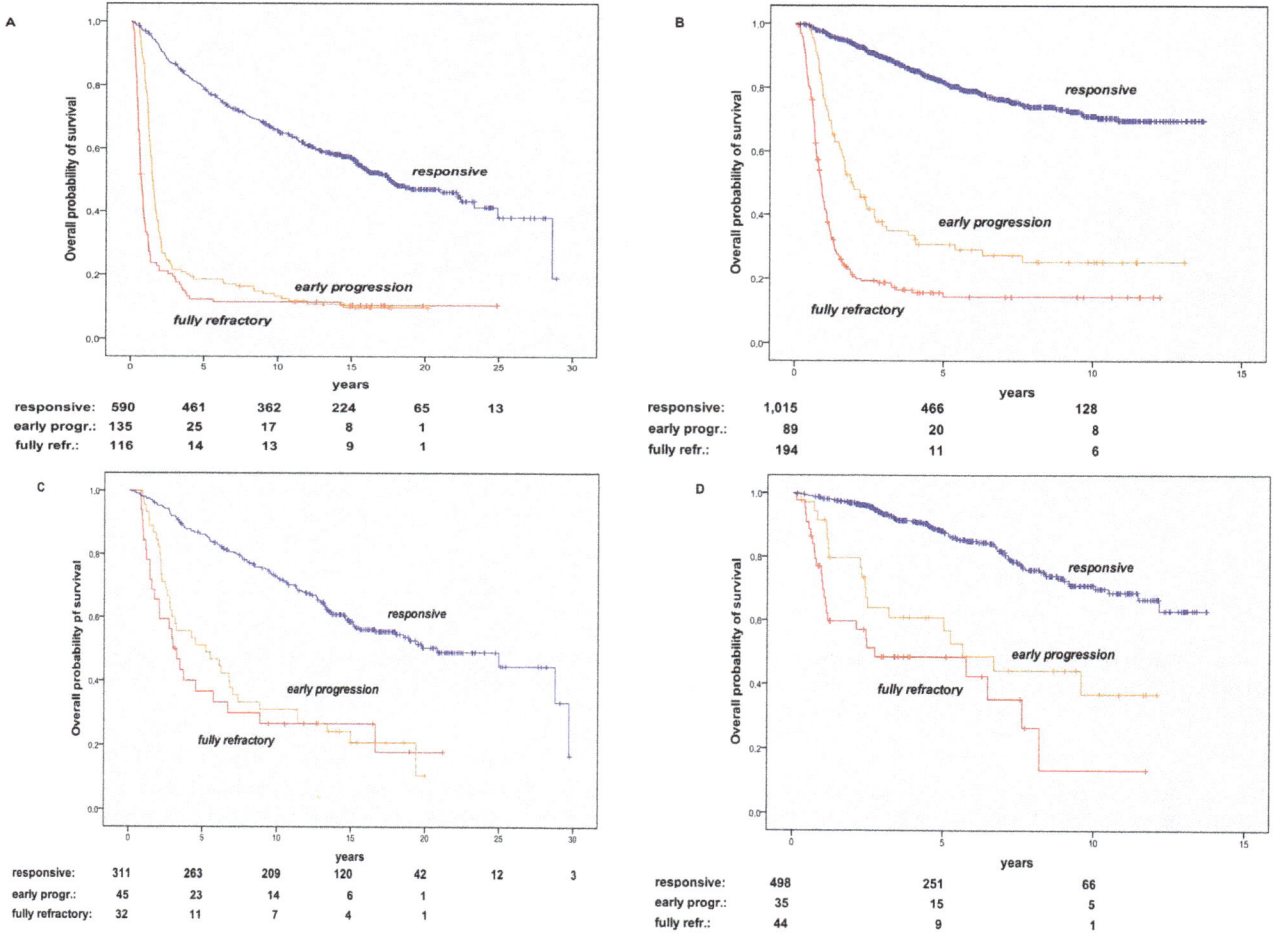

Figure 5. OS in Low-grade and Intermediate/High-grade NHL subtypes according to response to primary therapy. A. OS of 842 Intermediate/High-grade NHL patients diagnosed and managed up to 1,999. The OS projections are of 78.9%, 65.6%, and 57.2%, for responsive patients, 18.5%, 13.2%, and 9.7% for early progression, 12.3%, 11.4%, and 10.4% for fully refractory patients, at 5, 10, and 15 years, respectively. Median follow-up for the whole series is 15.9 yrs (range, 0.6–28.9) B. OS of 1,301 Intermediate/High-grade NHL patients diagnosed and managed since 2,000. The OS projections are of 81.6% and 71.1%, for responsive patients, 30.7% and 25.2% for early progression, 14.3% and 14.3% for fully refractory patients, at 5 and 10 years, respectively. Median follow-up for the whole series is 5.0 yrs (range, 0.6–13.7) C. OS of 388 Low-grade NHL patients diagnosed and managed up to 1,999. The OS projections are of 78.0%, 64.0%, and 51.8%, for responsive patients, 51.1%, 31.1%, and 20.8% for early progression, 36.7%, 26.7%, and 26.7% for fully refractory patients, at 5, 10, and 15 years, respectively. Median follow-up for the whole series is 16.3 yrs (range, 1.7–31.2) D. OS of 574 Low-grade NHL patients diagnosed and managed since 2,000. The OS projections are of 83.5% and 64.2%, for responsive patients, 60.7% and 36.8% for early progression, 48.4% and 13.2% for fully refractory patients, at 5 and 10 years, respectively. Median follow-up for the whole series is 5.1 yrs (range, 0.5–13.7). (responsive vs. refractory: $p<0.001$, in all series).

Table 4. Multivariate Cox Proportional Hazard Regression Analysis on Factors Affecting the Overall Survival.

Parameter associated with survival*	All evaluable patients n = 3,106			B-cell subtype n = 2,858		
	H R^2	95% C.I.	p =	H R^2	95% C.I	p =
Age>60 yrs	1.66	1.27–2.18	<0.001	1.76	1.31–2.35	0.001
high vs. low grade histology	2.45	1.76–3.42	<0.001	2.46	1.76–3.44	<0.001
IPI score 3–5 vs. 0–2	1.57	1.28–1.92	<0.001	1.55	1.25–1.91	<0.001
Rituximab adm. Yes vs. No	0.60	0.49–0.73	<0.001	0.60	0.49–0.74	<0.001
Primary Refr.						
• fully refr	26.73	18.10–39.47	<0.001	27.03	17.89–40.84	<0.001
• Early progr	10.22	7.20–14.50	<0.001	10.92	7.55–15.81	<0.001

*treated as time-dependent variables.

improvements might be ascribed either to the use of rituximab or to the effective salvage treatments developed in the last decade, or, possibly, to both of these factors. [1,4,12,26,33] Nevertheless, the analysis demonstrates that primary responsive patients have a very favorable outcome. Currently, patients presenting with advanced-stage B-cell lymphoma have a life expectancy longer than 10 years if they are responsive to their rituximab-containing, first-line chemotherapy.

Since 2,000 when rituximab was introduced in the clinical practice, survival improvements have also been observed for refractory patients, particularly those with initial, though transient, response. The current practice is to shift early to intensive treatments, including autologous or allogeneic transplantation, as soon as therapy resistance is clinically identified. [4,5,15,17,19,26,39] These measures are likely responsible for the improved survival of refractory patients treated in the last 13 years. Nevertheless, the long-term outcome of primary refractory patients remains poor, particularly those with intermediate/high grade histology and fully refractory disease. In addition, the Cox

multivariate analysis on the whole series of 3,106 patients indicates refractory disease as the most predictive factor for the long-term outcome, with the highest risk associated with fully refractory disease. The markedly unfavorable prognostic value of primary unresponsive disease was consistently observed in all subtypes, including low-grade lymphoma. Thus, achievement of persistent CR or PR at the initial treatment is the most important prognostic factor in the management of any lymphoma patient. This finding has several implications for any future investigation concerning novel drugs or biosimilar drugs, such as their possible inclusion in first-line treatment for lymphoma patients. [40].

Author Contributions

Conceived and designed the experiments: CT A. Rambaldi. Performed the experiments: AG FD A. Rossi RB. Analyzed the data: CT A. Rambaldi RP CB. Contributed reagents/materials/analysis tools: CT AG FD RB RP A. Rambaldi. Wrote the paper: CT A. Rambaldi. Management of the patients: CT AG A. Rossi AMB GG DC RB MR DG A. Rambaldi. Full access to all of the data: CT AG FD RP CB A. Rambaldi.

References

1. Mahadevan D, Fisher RI (2011) Novel therapeutics for aggressive non-Hodgkin's lymphoma. J Clin Oncol 29: 1876–1884.
2. Armitage JO (2012) The aggressive peripheral T-cell lymphomas: 2012 update on diagnosis, risk stratification, and management. Am J Hematol 87: 511–519.
3. Tan D, Horning SJ, Hoppe RT, Levy R, Rosenberg SA, et al. (2013) Improvements in observed and relative survival in follicular grade 1–2 lymphoma during 4 decades: the Stanford University experience. Blood 122: 981–987.
4. Cabanillas F (2011) Non-Hodgkin's lymphoma: the old and the new. Clin Lymphoma Myeloma Leuk 11 Suppl 1: S87–90.
5. Moskowitz C (2012) Diffuse large B cell lymphoma: how can we cure more patients in 2012? Best Pract Res Clin Haematol 25: 41–47.
6. Rosenwald A, Wright G, Chan WC, Connors JM, Campo E, et al. (2002) The use of molecular profiling to predict survival after chemotherapy for diffuse large-B-cell lymphoma. N Engl J Med 346: 1937–1947.
7. Dave SS, Wright G, Tan B, Rosenwald A, Gascoyne RD, et al. (2004) Prediction of survival in follicular lymphoma based on molecular features of tumor-infiltrating immune cells. N Engl J Med 351: 2159–2169.
8. Snuderl M, Kolman OK, Chen YB, Hsu JJ, Ackerman AM, et al. (2010) B-cell lymphomas with concurrent IGH-BCL2 and MYC rearrangements are aggressive neoplasms with clinical and pathologic features distinct from Burkitt lymphoma and diffuse large B-cell lymphoma. Am J Surg Pathol 34: 327–340.
9. Aukema SM, Siebert R, Schuuring E, van Imhoff GW, Kluin-Nelemans HC, et al. (2011) Double-hit B-cell lymphomas. Blood 117: 2319–2331.
10. Royo C, Salaverria I, Hartmann EM, Rosenwald A, Campo E, et al. (2011) The complex landscape of genetic alterations in mantle cell lymphoma. Semin Cancer Biol 21: 322–334.
11. Piccaluga PP, Fuligni F, De Leo A, Bertuzzi C, Rossi M, et al. (2013) Molecular profiling improves classification and prognostication of nodal peripheral T-cell lymphomas: results of a phase III diagnostic accuracy study. J Clin Oncol 31: 3019–3025.
12. Sawas A, Diefenbach C, O'Connor OA (2011) New therapeutic targets and drugs in non-Hodgkin's lymphoma. Curr Opin Hematol 18: 280–287.
13. Cheson BD, Bartlett NL, Vose JM, Lopez-Hernandez A, Seiz AL, et al. (2012) A phase II study of the survivin suppressant YM155 in patients with refractory diffuse large B-cell lymphoma. Cancer 118: 3128–3134.
14. Leskov I, Pallasch CP, Drake A, Iliopoulou BP, Souza A, et al. (2013) Rapid generation of human B-cell lymphomas via combined expression of Myc and Bcl2 and their use as a preclinical model for biological therapies. Oncogene 32: 1066–1072.
15. Cuccuini W, Briere J, Mounier N, Voelker HU, Rosenwald A, et al. (2012) MYC+ diffuse large B-cell lymphoma is not salvaged by classical R-ICE or R-DHAP followed by BEAM plus autologous stem cell transplantation. Blood 119: 4619–4624.
16. Wilson WH, Jung SH, Porcu P, Hurd D, Johnson J, et al. (2012) A Cancer and Leukemia Group B multi-center study of DA-EPOCH-rituximab in untreated diffuse large B-cell lymphoma with analysis of outcome by molecular subtype. Haematologica 97: 758–765.
17. d'Amore F, Relander T, Lauritzsen GF, Jantunen E, Hagberg H, et al. (2012) Up-front autologous stem-cell transplantation in peripheral T-cell lymphoma: NLG-T-01. J Clin Oncol 30: 3093–3099.
18. Galli M, Nicolucci A, Valentini M, Belfiglio M, Delaini F, et al. (2005) Feasibility and outcome of tandem stem cell autotransplants in multiple myeloma. Haematologica 90: 1643–1649.
19. Tarella C, Zanni M, Magni M, Benedetti F, Patti C, et al. (2008) Rituximab improves the efficacy of high-dose chemotherapy with autograft for high-risk follicular and diffuse large-B-cell lymphoma: a multicenter Gruppo Italiano Terapie Innnovative nei linfomi survey. J Clin Oncol 26: 3166–3175.
20. Coiffier B, Lepage E, Briere J, Herbrecht R, Tilly H, et al. (2002) CHOP chemotherapy plus rituximab compared with CHOP alone in elderly patients with diffuse large-B-cell lymphoma. N Engl J Med 346: 235–242.
21. Sehn LH, Donaldson J, Chhanabhai M, Fitzgerald C, Gill K, et al. (2005) Introduction of combined CHOP plus rituximab therapy dramatically improved outcome of diffuse large-B-cell lymphoma in British Columbia. J Clin Oncol 23: 5027–5033.
22. Fisher RI, Gaynor ER, Dahlberg S, Oken MM, Grogan TM, et al. (1993) Comparison of a standard regimen (CHOP) with three intensive chemotherapy regimens for advanced non-Hodgkin's lymphoma. N Engl J Med 328: 1002–1006.
23. Pfreundschuh M, Kuhnt E, Trümper L, Österborg A, Trneny M, et al. (2011) CHOP-like chemotherapy with or without rituximab in young patients with good-prognosis diffuse large-B-cell lymphoma: 6-year results of an open-label randomised study of the MabThera International Trial (MInT) Group. The Lancet Oncology 12: 1013–1022.
24. Lunning MA, Vose JM (2012) Management of indolent lymphoma: where are we now and where are we going. Blood Rev 26: 279–288.
25. Zinzani PL, Marchetti M, Billio A, Barosi G, Carella AM, et al. (2013) SIE, SIES, GITMO revised guidelines for the management of follicular lymphoma. Am J Hematol 88: 185–192.
26. Sweetenham JW (2008) Highly aggressive lymphomas in adults. Hematol Oncol Clin North Am 22: 965–978, ix.
27. Cheson BD, Pfistner B, Juweid ME, Gascoyne RD, Specht L, et al. (2007) Revised response criteria for malignant lymphoma. J Clin Oncol 25: 579–586.
28. Mantel N, Haenszel W (1959) Statistical aspects of the analysis of data from retrospective studies of disease. J Natl Cancer Inst 22: 719–748.
29. Cox DR (1972) Regression Models and Life-Tables. Journal of the Royal Statistical Society Series B (Methodological) 34: 187–220.
30. Li ZM, Huang JJ, Xia Y, Sun J, Huang Y, et al. (2012) Blood lymphocyte-to-monocyte ratio identifies high-risk patients in diffuse large B-cell lymphoma treated with R-CHOP. PLoS One 7: e41658.
31. Rambaldi A, Boschini C, Gritti G, Delaini F, Oldani E, et al. (2013) The lymphocyte to monocyte ratio improves the IPI-risk definition of diffuse large B-cell lymphoma when rituximab is added to chemotherapy. Am J Hematol 88: 1062–1067.
32. Surveillance, Epidemiology, and End Results (SEER) Program. SEER*Stat Database: Incidence-SEER Research Data (1973–2010). National Cancer Institute, DCCPS, Surveillance Research Program, Surveillance Systems Branch, released April 2013, based on the November 2012 submission. Available: http://seer.cancer.gov/data/.
33. Elstrom RL, Andemariam B, Martin P, Ruan J, Shore TB, et al. (2012) Bortezomib in combination with rituximab, dexamethasone, ifosfamide, cisplatin and etoposide chemoimmunotherapy in patients with relapsed and primary refractory diffuse large-B-cell lymphoma. Leuk Lymphoma 53: 1469–1473.
34. Gisselbrecht C, Gaulard P, Lepage E, Coiffier B, Brière J, et al. (1998) Prognostic Significance of T-Cell Phenotype in Aggressive Non-Hodgkin's Lymphomas. Blood 92: 76–82.

35. Gallamini A, Zaja F, Patti C, Billio A, Specchia MR, et al. (2007) Alemtuzumab (Campath-1H) and CHOP chemotherapy as first-line treatment of peripheral T-cell lymphoma: results of a GITIL (Gruppo Italiano Terapie Innovative nei Linfomi) prospective multicenter trial. Blood 110: 2316–2323.

36. Mounier N, Briere J, Gisselbrecht C, Emile JF, Lederlin P, et al. (2003) Rituximab plus CHOP (R-CHOP) overcomes bcl-2–associated resistance to chemotherapy in elderly patients with diffuse large B-cell lymphoma (DLBCL). Blood 101: 4279–4284.

37. Muller C, Murawski N, Wiesen MH, Held G, Poeschel V, et al. (2012) The role of sex and weight on rituximab clearance and serum elimination half-life in elderly patients with DLBCL. Blood 119: 3276–3284.

38. Tarella C, Passera R, Magni M, Benedetti F, Rossi A, et al. (2011) Risk factors for the development of secondary malignancy after high-dose chemotherapy and autograft, with or without rituximab: a 20-year retrospective follow-up study in patients with lymphoma. J Clin Oncol 29: 814–824.

39. Maloney D (2008) Allogeneic transplantation following nonmyeloablative conditioning for aggressive lymphoma. Bone Marrow Transplant 42 Suppl 1: S35–S36.

40. Schneider CK, Vleminckx C, Gravanis I, Ehmann F, Trouvin JH, et al. (2012) Setting the stage for biosimilar monoclonal antibodies. Nat Biotechnol 30: 1179–1185.

18

ELMO1 is Upregulated in AML CD34+ Stem/Progenitor Cells, Mediates Chemotaxis and Predicts Poor Prognosis in Normal Karyotype AML

Marta E. Capala, Edo Vellenga, Jan Jacob Schuringa*

Department of Experimental Hematology, Cancer Research Center Groningen (CRCG), University Medical Center Groningen, University of Groningen, Groningen, the Netherlands

Abstract

Both normal as well leukemic hematopoietic stem cells critically depend on their microenvironment in the bone marrow for processes such as self-renewal, survival and differentiation, although the exact pathways that are involved remain poorly understood. We performed transcriptome analysis on primitive $CD34^+$ acute myeloid leukemia (AML) cells (n = 46), their more differentiated $CD34^-$ leukemic progeny, and normal $CD34^+$ bone marrow cells (n = 31) and focused on differentially expressed genes involved in adhesion and migration. Thus, Engulfment and Motility protein 1 (ELMO1) was identified amongst the top 50 most differentially expressed genes. ELMO1 is a crucial link in the signaling cascade that leads to activation of RAC GTPases and cytoskeleton rearrangements. We confirmed increased ELMO1 expression at the mRNA and protein level in a panel of AML samples and showed that high ELMO1 expression is an independent negative prognostic factor in normal karyotype (NK) AML in three large independent patient cohorts. Downmodulation of ELMO1 in human CB $CD34^+$ cells did not significantly alter expansion, progenitor frequency or differentiation in stromal co-cultures, but did result in a decreased frequency of stem cells in LTC-IC assays. In BCR-ABL-transduced human CB $CD34^+$ cells depletion of ELMO1 resulted in a mild decrease in proliferation, but replating capacity of progenitors was severely impaired. Downregulation of ELMO1 in a panel of primary $CD34^+$ AML cells also resulted in reduced long-term growth in stromal co-cultures in two out of three cases. Pharmacological inhibition of the ELMO1 downstream target RAC resulted in a severely impaired proliferation and survival of leukemic cells. Finally, ELMO1 depletion caused a marked decrease in SDF1-induced chemotaxis of leukemic cells. Taken together, these data show that inhibiting the ELMO1-RAC axis might be an alternative way to target leukemic cells.

Editor: Zoran Ivanovic, French Blood Institute, France

Funding: This work was supported by a grant from The Netherlands Organization for Scientific Research (NWO-VIDI 91796312) to JJS. The funders had no role in study design, data collection and analysis, decision to publish, or preparation of the manuscript.

Competing Interests: The authors have declared that no competing interests exist.

* Email: j.j.schuringa@umcg.nl

Introduction

Acute myeloid leukemia (AML) is a heterogeneous disease in which various molecular events lead to a block in differentiation along the myeloid lineage, resulting in an accumulation of immature cells termed leukemic blasts, as well as impaired normal hematopoiesis. The current classification of AML based on morphological, cytogenetic and molecular abnormalities does not cover the heterogeneity in response to treatment, especially in the intermediate risk group constituting the majority (60%) of AML cases [1,2]. Therefore, new markers that would allow a more accurate stratification of patients are needed to better guide treatment options. In recent years, several gene expression profiling (GEP) studies have been performed in order to identify leukemia-specific gene expression patterns and select a gene, or more likely a panel of genes, that could be used to better classify patients within the existing subgroups [3–8]. However, most of these studies were performed on the total mononuclear fraction (MNC) of AML samples, which contains mostly leukemic blasts.

It has been shown that leukemic stem cell (LSC) activity, similarly to normal hematopoietic stem cell (HSC) activity, is contained within the $CD34^+$ fraction of AML cells in the vast majority of cases [9–13]. LSCs are defined as the cells able to transplant leukemia into immunodeficient recipients. In patients, LSCs are thought to be responsible for the relapse of disease and treatment failure [9,14–16]. Therefore, we compared gene expression profiles of $CD34^+$ AML, their $CD34^-$ progeny and normal bone marrow (NBM) $CD34^+$ cells [17,18]. Here, we focused specifically on genes that might be involved in adhesion and/or migration properties and thus were able to identify Engulfment and Motility protein 1 (ELMO1) amongst the top 50 $CD34^+$ AML-specific genes. ELMO1 is known to be a crucial link in the signaling cascade leading to the activation of Rac GTPases [19–21]. We identified ELMO1 as an independent prognostic marker in the normal karyotype (NK) AML subgroup and showed that high expression of ELMO1 was associated with poor prognosis in three independent cohorts of patients. Knockdown of ELMO1 or inhibition one of its downstream protein RAC impaired long-term expansion of leukemic cells on stroma, and ELMO1 depletion decreased the migration potential of hematopoietic cells towards an SDF-1 gradient.

Materials and Methods

Primary cell isolation and culture conditions

Neonatal cord blood (CB) was obtained from healthy full-term pregnancies after informed consent in accordance with the Declaration of Helsinki from the obstetrics departments of the University Medical Centre Groningen (UMCG) and Martini Hospital Groningen, Groningen, The Netherlands. All protocols were approved by the Medical Ethical Committee of the UMCG. After separation of mononuclear cells with lymphocyte separation medium (PAA Laboratories, Coble, Germany), CD34+ cells were isolated using a magnetically activated cell sorting (MACS) CD34 progenitor kit (Miltenyi Biotech, Amsterdam, The Netherlands). For liquid cultures, CD34+ cells were expanded in human progenitor growth medium (HPGM; Cambrex, Verviers, Belgium) supplemented with 100 ng/ml stem cell factor (SCF), FLT3 Ligand (Flt3L; both from Amgen, Thousand Oaks, USA) and thrombopoietin (TPO; Kirin, Tokyo, Japan). For the MS5 co-culture experiments, cells were grown in Gartner's medium consisting of α-modified essential medium (α–MEM; Fisher Scientific Europe, Emergo, The Netherlands) supplemented with 12.5% heat-inactivated fetal calf serum (Lonza, Leusden, The Netherlands), 12.5% heat-inactivated horse serum (Invitrogen, Breda, The Netherlands), 1% penicillin and streptomycin, 2 mM glutamine (all from PAA Laboratories), 57.2 μM β-mercaptoethanol (Merck Sharp & Dohme BV, Haarlem, The Netherlands) and 1 μM hydrocortisone (Sigma-Aldrich Chemie B.V., Zwijndrecht, The Netherlands). AML blasts from peripheral blood cells or bone marrow cells from untreated patients with AML were obtained and studied after informed consent in accordance with the Declaration of Helsinki, and the protocol was approved by the Medical Ethical Committee. AML mononuclear cells were isolated by density gradient centrifugation, and CD34+ cells were stained using CD34-PE antibody (BD Biosciences, San Jose, CA, USA) and selected by sorting on a MoFLo (DakoCytomation, Carpinteria, CA, USA). AML co-cultures were expanded in Gartner's medium supplemented with 20 ng/mL interleukin 3 (IL-3; Gist-Brocades, Delft, The Netherlands), granulocyte-colony stimulating factor (G-CSF; Rhone-Poulenc Rorer, Amstelveen, The Netherlands) and TPO.

Cell lines and culture conditions

293T embryonic kidney cells (ACC-635 DSMZ, Braunschweig, Germany) and PG13 packaging cells (ATCC CRL-10686, Wesel, Germany) were grown in DMEM medium with 200 mM glutamine (BioWhittaker, Veries, Belgium) supplemented with 10% FSC and 1% penicillin and streptomycin. K562 myelogenous leukemia cells (ACC-10, DSMZ), TF-1 erythroleukemic cells (ACC-334, DSMZ) and THP-1 acute monocytic leukemia cells (ACC-16, DSMZ) were grown in RPMI medium with 200 mM glutamine (BioWhittaker) supplemented with 10% FCS, and 1% penicillin and streptomycin, and for TF-1 cells with 5 ng/ml granulocyte-macrophage colony stimulating factor (GM-CSF; Genetics Institute, Cambridge, MA, USA). MS-5 murine stromal cells (ACC-441, DSMZ) were grown in αMEM with 200 mM glutamine (BioWhittaker) supplemented with 10% FCS and 1% penicillin and streptomycin.

Immunoblotting

Western blot analysis was performed according to standard protocols and as described previously [22]. Briefly, 5×10^5 cells were lysed to prepare whole cell extract by boiling in Laemmli buffer for 5 min prior to separation on 12.5% SDS gels. After overnight transfer, membranes were blocked in phosphate-buffer saline (PBS) with 5% nonfat milk prior to incubating with antibodies. Binding of antibodies was detected by chemiluminescence, according to the manufacturer's instructions (Roche Diagnostics, Basel, Switzerland). Antibody against ELMO1 (ab2239) was obtained from Abcam (Abcam, Cambridge, UK) and was used at a dilution of 1:1000. Antibody against phosphoPAK (#2601) was obtained from Cell Signaling (Cell Signaling, Leiden, The Netherlands) and used at a dilution of 1:1000. Antibody against β-actin (#J2207, Santa Cruz Biotechnology, CA, USA) was used at a dilution of 1:4000. Secondary antibodies were purchased from Dako Cytomation (Dako Cytomation, Glosturp, Denmark) and used at 1:2500 dilutions.

RNA extraction and Real-time PCT analysis

ELMO1 expression was assessed by quantitative real-time PCR (qRT-PCR) as described previously [23]. Briefly, total RNA was isolated using an RNeasy kit (Qiagen, Venlo, The Netherlands) following the manufacturer's recommendations. After reverse transcription using M-MuLV reverse transcriptase (Fermentas, St Leon-Roth, Germany), according to manufacturer's instructions, aliquots of cDNA were real-time amplified using iQ SYBR Green mix (Bio-Rad, CA, USA) on a MyIQ thermocycler (Bio-Rad). ELMO1 primers (forward primer: CCGGATTGTGCTT-GAGAACA, reverse primer: CTCACTAGGCAACTCGCCCA) were obtained from Invitrogen. Expression was quantified using MyIQ software (Bio-Rad) and RPL27 expression was used to calculate relative expression levels of investigated genes according to the standard curve method. RPL27 was not differentially expressed in our AML versus NBM CD34+ cells (data not shown).

Retro- and lentivirus generation and transduction

Stable PG13 producer cell lines of BCR-ABL retroviral constructs were generated and used as published previously [24]. Supernatants from the PG13 cells were harvested after 8–12 hours of incubation in HPGM before the retroviral transduction rounds and passed through 0.45-mm filters (Sigma-Aldrich). Before the first transduction round, CD34+ CB cells were pre-stimulated for 48 hours in HPMG supplemented with 100 ng/mL of SCF, Flt3L and TPO. Three rounds of transduction were performed on retronectin-coated 24-well plates in the presence of the same cytokines as for pre-stimulation and 4 μg/mLpolybrene (Sigma-Aldrich). With the last round of transduction, lentiviral transduction with the constructs described below was performed.

Short hairpin RNA (shRNA) sequences targeting ELMO1 were derived from the literature [25,26] and ligated into pHR'trip vector using AcsI and SbfI restriction sites. For the control, scrambled (shSCR) shRNA sequence was used. 293T embryonic kidney cells were transfected using FuGENE6 (Roche, Almere, The Netherlands) with 3 μg pCMV Δ8.91, 0,7 μg VSV-G, and 3 μg of vector constructs (pHR'trip-Scrambled shRNA [shSCR], or -ELMO1 shRNA [shELMO1]). After 24 hours, medium was changed to HPGM and after 12 hours, supernatant containing lentiviral particles was harvested and either stored at −80°C or used fresh for transduction of target cells. K562, TF-1, THP-1, isolated CD34+ CB cells that were pre-stimulated for 12 hours, or BCR-ABL-transduced CD34+ CB cells were subjected to 1 round of transduction with lentiviral particles in the presence of prestimulation cytokines and 4 μg/mL polybrene (Sigma) on retronectin-coated 24-well plates (Takara, Tokyo, Japan). After transduction, transduced green fluorescent protein-positive (GFP-positive), truncated nerve growth factor receptor-positive (NGFR-positive) or double-positive cells were sorted on a MoFlo sorter (Dako Cytomation). AML CD34$^+$ cells were transduced as described previously [27]. Briefly, transductions were performed in 3 consecutive rounds of 8 to 12 hours with lentiviral supernatant supplemented with 10% FCS, IL-3, granulocyte-colony stimulating factor (G-CSF; Rhone-Poulenc Rorer, Amstelveen, The Netherlands) and TPO (20 ng/m each) and polybrene (4 µg/mL) on a retronectin-coated 24-wells plate. After washing away the virus supernatant, unsorted cells were used to initiate co-cultures.

Liquid cultures, long-term cultures on stroma, CAFC and CFC assay

For liquid cultures, 3×10^5 CD34$^+$ CB cells or BCR-ABL cells were plated in 1 mL IMDM medium supplemented with 20% FSC, 1% P/S and 20 gn/mL of SCF and IL-3. 10^5 CD34$^+$ CB cells, 5×10^3 BCR-ABL cells and 4×10^4 cells (AML sample 3), 7×10^4 cells (AML sample 1) or 12×10^4 cells (AML sample 2) were plated onto a T25 flask pre-coated with MS5 stromal cells (ACC-441, DSMZ) in 5 ml of Gartner's medium in duplicate. AML culture medium was supplemented with 20 ng/mL IL-3, G-CSF and TPO. Co-cultures were kept at 37°C and 5% CO$_2$ and cells were demi-depopulated weekly for analysis. For the inhibition of Rac activity, NSC2766 (NSC; Calbiochem, VWR, Amsterdam, The Netherlands) was added to the co-culture medium to the final concentration of 20 µM, 40 µM or 100 µM. CFC assays were performed as previously described [28]. 1000 CD34$^+$ CB or 500 BCR-ABL-transduced cells were plated in 1 mL of CFC assay medium consisting of MethoCult H4230 (StemCell Technologies, France), 1% penicillin and streptomycin, 19% IMDM (PAA Laboratories), IL-3, interleukin-6 (IL-6; Gist-Brocades), G-CSF, SCF (all 20 ng/mL) and 1 U/mL erythropoietin (EPO; Cilag; Eprex, Brussels, Belgium) in duplicate directly after transduction and 10^4 cells were used at later time points. After 14 days of culturing colony-forming unit granulocyte-macrophage (CFU-GM) and burst-forming unit erythroid (BFU-E) were scored. For CFC replate, colony cells were harvest after 14 days of culture, and 10^5 cells were plated in 1 ml fresh CFC assay medium in duplicate. For CAFC assay, CFC assay medium was added to the co-cultures after 5 weeks. CAFC were counted 2 weeks after the addition of CFC medium by microscopic evaluation of co-cultures.

Flow cytometry analysis and sorting

All fluorescence-activated cell sorter (FACS) analyses were performed on a FACScalibur (Becton-Dickinson [BD], Alpen a/d Rijn, the Netherlands) and data were analyzed using WinList 3D (Verity Software House, Topsham, USA). Cells were sorted on a MoFlo sorter. Antibodies: CD34-PE, NGFR-APC, CD14-PE, CD15-APC, CD71-APC and GPA-PE were obtained from BD. Viability was assessed using Annexin V APC (IQ Products, Groningen, The Netherlands) according to the manufacturer's recommendations. Briefly, cells were harvested, resuspended in 100 µL calcium buffer containing 5 µL Annexin V, and incubated for 20 min at 4°C in the dark, washed with 5 mL calcium buffer and binding of APC-conjugated Annexin V was measured by FACS.

Migration assay

Migration assays were performed in transwell plates with 8 µm pore size (Corning Costar, Cambridge, UK) towards the gradient of SDF-1 (100 ng/mL; R&D Systems, Abingdon, UK). TF-1 or THP-1 leukemic cell lines were transduced with either shSCR or shELMO1, sorted and plated in the upper chamber of the transwell. Migration was allowed for 4 hours, after which the cells were harvested from the bottom chamber and counted by FACS using TruCOUNT counting beads (BD).

Statistical analysis and transcriptome datasets used

Statistical analyses were performed with SPSS software (IBM, Amsterdam, The Netherlands), release 16.0. The association between the transcript level of ELMO1 and overall survival (OS) was tested in univariate Cox models. All values are expressed as means ± standard deviation (SD). Student's t test was used for all other comparisons. All tests were two tailed, and differences were considered statistically significant at $p < 0,05$.

We made use of various previously published transcriptome datasets in our studies here. For Figure 1A,B, C and D we used data generated by ourselves containing AML CD34$^+$ (n = 46) and NBM CD34$^+$ (n = 31) [18] deposited in GEO under GEO30029). For Figure 1H we used data of intermediate risk AML samples (total cohort of 525 patients of which 300 were intermediate risk) [6,29] deposited in GEO under GSE6891. At page 10 we describe data in two other NK AML datasets generated by the Bullinger lab indicating that high ELMO1 expression also predicts poor prognosis in these datasets and these data were already included in the Supplemental files of our previous paper [18]. Data for Figure S1B was derived from the HemaExplorer database (http://servers.binf.ku.dk/hemaexplorer/) [30]. For Figure S1C we used data from the Noverhstern lab [31].

Results

ELMO1 expression is increased in AML CD34$^+$ cells and predicts poor prognosis in normal karyotype AML patients

Recently, we identified AML CD34$^+$ leukemic stem cell-enriched transcriptomes by comparing gene expression profiles of paired AML CD34$^+$ and CD34$^-$ samples with those of normal BM CD34$^+$ cells [17,18]. Thus, 1677 AML CD34$^+$-specific genes were identified (Figure 1A). Based on Gene Ontology (GO) analysis for Cellular Component (CC) this list of 1677 genes could be annotated to several CCs such as plasma membrane (253), cytosol (136), mitochondrion (116), cytoskeleton (108) and extracellular space (46) (Figure 1B). Since leukemic stem cells critically depend on their microenvironment in the bone marrow for processes such as self-renewal and survival, we focused on differentially expressed genes involved in adhesion and migration and an overview of selected GO terms is shown in Figure 1C. Thus, Engulfment and Motility protein 1 (ELMO1) was identified. In prior analyses we looked for prognostic significance by univariate cox regression analyses using the continuous transcript levels of the top 50 CD34$^+$- specific genes and overall survival (OS) in a large series of de novo normal karyotype AML [18]. ELMO was present in this list, and could predict OS in 2 independent cohorts of patients (cohort 1: n = 163, p = 0.021, hazard ratio 1.782 and cohort 2: n = 218, p = 0.015, hazard ratio 1.657) [18]. ELMO1 is a crucial link in the signaling cascade that leads to activation of RAC GTPases and cytoskeleton rearrangements and therefore we decided to study its role in more detail. ELMO1 mRNA was significantly higher expressed in AML CD34$^+$ (n = 46) as compared to AML CD34$^-$ cells ($p < 0.0001$), as well as to NBM CD34$^+$ cells (n = 31) ($p < 0.0001$) (Figure 1D). Increased expression of ELMO1 was further confirmed by independent Q-PCRs, which showed a good correlation with the Illumina BeadArrays data

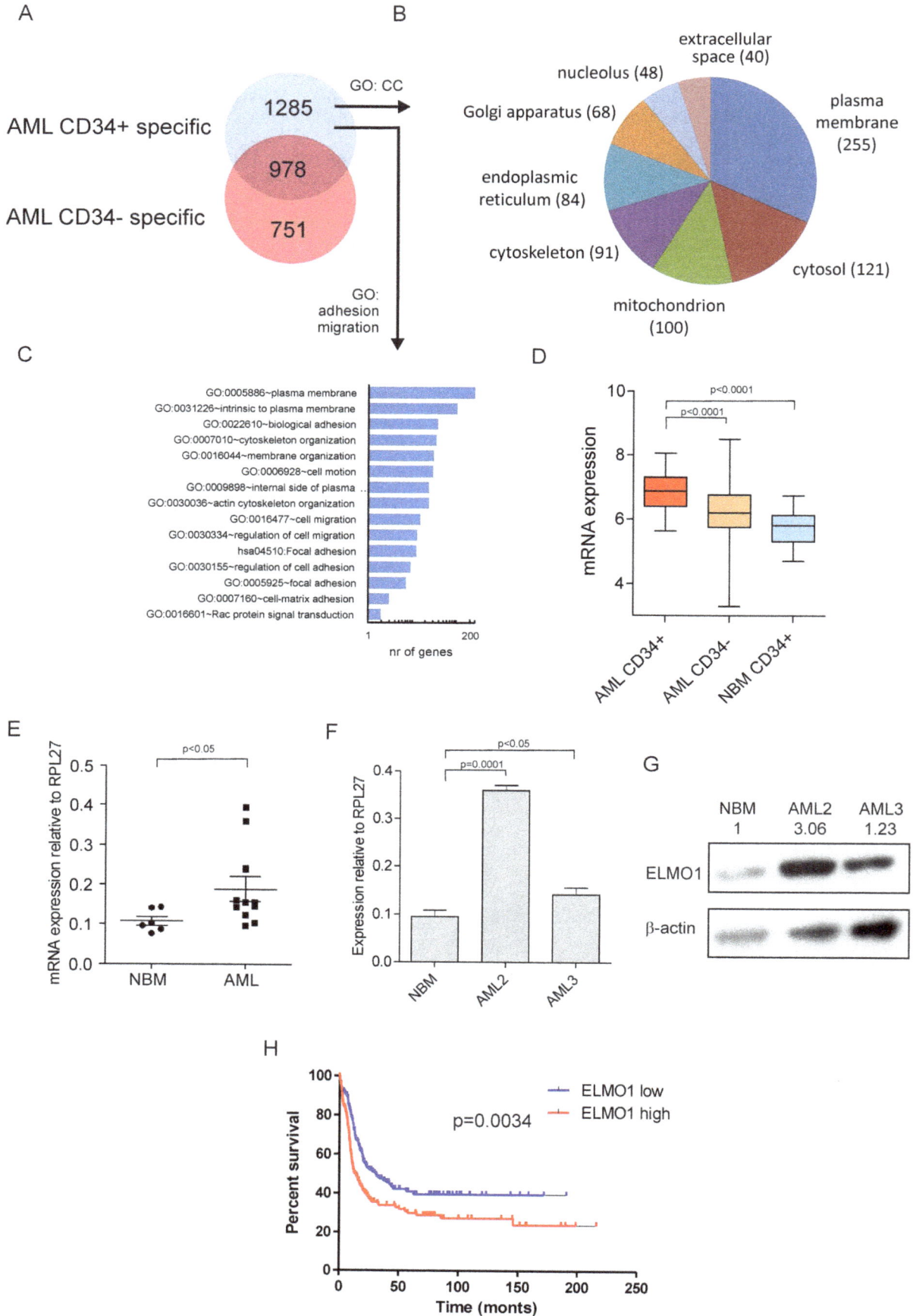

Figure 1. ELMO1 expression is increased in AML CD34$^+$ cells and predicts poor prognosis in normal karyotype AML patients. (A) VENN diagram displaying the overlap in AML CD34$^+$ specific and AML CD34$-$ specific transcriptomes compared to NBM CD34$^+$ cells [17,18]. (B) 1677 AML CD34$^+$-specific genes were subjected to Gene Ontology (GO) analysis for Cellular Component (CC) of which several CCs are shown. (C) 1677 AML CD34$^+$-specific genes were subjected to GO analysis for terms associated with adhesion and migration. (D) ELMO1 mRNA was significantly higher expressed in AML CD34$^+$ (n = 46) as compared to AML CD34$^-$ cells ($p<0.0001$), as well as to NBM CD34$^+$ cells (n = 31) ($p<0.0001$). (E) Increased expression of ELMO1 was further confirmed by independent Q-PCRs in a panel of 11 AML and 6 NBM samples. (F, G) The increase in ELMO1 mRNA was paralleled by increased protein levels in two representative cases. (H) High expression of ELMO1 predicts poor survival in a cohort of NK AML patients (based on [6,29]) ($p = 0.0034$).

(Figure 1E and Figure S1A). Moreover, elevated mRNA expression was paralleled by an increase on the protein level in two representative cases (Figure 1F,G). Increased ELMO1 expression in AML compared to normal stem/progenitor cells was also observed in the HemaExplorer dataset [30] (Figure S1B). Finally, we analyzed the expression of ELMO1 in a third independent cohort of NK AML patients [6,29], which again indicated that ELMO1 significantly predicts poor survival (p = 0.0034, Figure 1H).

ELMO1 downmodulation in human CB CD34$^+$ cells does not alter expansion, colony formation or differentiation, but results in a significant decrease in stem cell frequency

In a recent study by Novershtern *et al.*, gene expression profiling was performed comparing 38 distinct purified populations of human hematopoietic cells [31]. Analysis of the data generated in this study revealed that ELMO1 is significantly more highly expressed in the most primitive hematopoietic compartment (HSCs) as compared with more differentiated cells (Figure S1C). Therefore, we set out to investigate the effect of ELMO1 depletion in CD34$^+$ population of CB cells, enriched for hematopoietic stem and progenitor cells (HSPCs). In order to downregulate ELMO1 expression, lentiviral vectors containing ELMO1-targeting shRNA sequence were generated (shELMO1). The efficiency of downregulation was first tested in the K562 cell line, where transduction with shELMO1 significantly decreased ELMO1 expression both at the mRNA as well as protein level (Figure 2A). Subsequently, CB CD34$^+$ cells were transduced with control (shSCR), or shELMO1-containing vectors, with transduction efficiencies of 59% for shSCR and 46% for shELMO1 (Figure 2B). Transduced cells were then sorted and plated either in liquid culture, or in a co-culture on stromal MS5 cells. The growth of CB CD34$^+$ in liquid culture was followed for 28 days and within that time no significant differences were observed between the proliferation of ELMO1-depleted and control cells (Figure 2C). In contrast, the expansion of shELMO1-transduced cells during the 5-week co-culture on stroma was slightly lower than of the control cells (Figure 2D, E). We assessed cell differentiation along the myeloid lineage during the co-culture and saw that it was not affected by ELMO1 downregulation (Figure S2). Also the progenitor frequency and their self-renewal potential were not changed upon ELMO1 depletion. Of note, CFC cells from shELMO1-transduced group initiated slightly more colonies upon replate than the control, although this did not reach significance (Figure 2F). Finally, the LTC-IC frequency was assessed at the end of co-culture. In the shELMO1-transduced group significantly fewer colonies were observed (p = 0.042) indicative of the reduced stem cell frequency (Figure 2G). Overall, these data indicate that ELMO1 depletion did not significantly affect CB CD34$^+$ proliferation in liquid culture and co-culture, myeloid differentiation or progenitor cell frequencies, but did cause a reduction of the most primitive stem cells.

Depletion of ELMO1 results in a slight proliferative disadvantage and reduced replating capacity of BCR-ABL-transformed human CB CD34$^+$

Several studies have shown that RAC GTPases play an essential role in leukemic transformation mediated by BCR-ABL oncoprotein [32–37]. Since ELMO1 is involved in the activation of RAC proteins by the Dock180 family of GEFs, we hypothesized that depletion of ELMO1 would have a profound effect on the expansion of BCR-ABL-transformed cells. We performed a double transduction of CD34$^+$ CB cells with BCR-ABL-containing retroviral vectors, together with shSCR or shELMO1 shRNA-containing lentiviral vectors. Double-transduced cells were then sorted (Figure 3A) and plated either in liquid culture or in a co-culture on MS5 stromal cells. Somewhat contrary to our expectations, proliferation of BCR-ABL cells was not markedly affected by ELMO1 downregulation during the 34 days of liquid culture (Figure 3B). Moreover, ELMO1-depleted BCR-ABL cells initially showed an increased proliferation in MS5 co-culture, but upon replating shELMO1-transduced cells did expand significantly less than the control suggesting that self-renewal properties were affected (Figure 3C, D). No marked differences were observed in the differentiation potential (data not shown). In the colony forming assay, shELMO1-transduced cells initiated the same number of colonies at week 1 of the co-culture, however at week 2 the number of colonies arising from shELMO1-transduced cells was lower that the control (Figure 3E). Moreover, significantly fewer secondary colonies were observed upon ELMO1 downregulation, again suggesting that self-renewal properties might be affected (Figure 3E). Taken together, these data indicate that ELMO1 depletion does not markedly affect BCR-ABL-transduced CB CD34$^+$ cell proliferation in liquid culture and co-culture, but it decreases replating capacity of progenitor cells.

Effects of ELMO1 depletion on long-term expansion of primary AML CD34$^+$ cells on MS5 stroma

Next, we investigated the effect of ELMO1 downregulation in a panel of AML samples that showed high ELMO1 expression levels in the microarray profiling [18]. The following samples were used: 2003 022 (AML1), 2003 119 (AML2) and 2003 160 (AML3). The sample characteristics such as FAB classification, cytogenetic characteristics, risk group according to HOVON/SAKK protocols and FLT3/NPM mutation status are provided in Table 1. In order to downmodulate ELMO1, CD34$^+$ cells were sorted from the AML mononuclear fraction and transduced with shSCR- or shELMO1-containing lentiviral vectors. Directly after transduction cells were plated on MS5 stroma and their expansion and GFP expression were followed during the co-culture. Transduction efficiencies obtained with shRNA constructs were variable, ranging from 16% in AML3 to 40% in AML1 and above 60% in AML2. AML3 ceased to expand beyond day 26 and within that time no significant differences in proliferation between shSCR- and shELMO1-transduced cells were observed. However, AML1 and AML2 could expand for as long as 41 days and in those cultures ELMO1-depleted cells grew markedly less than the control cells (Figure 4).

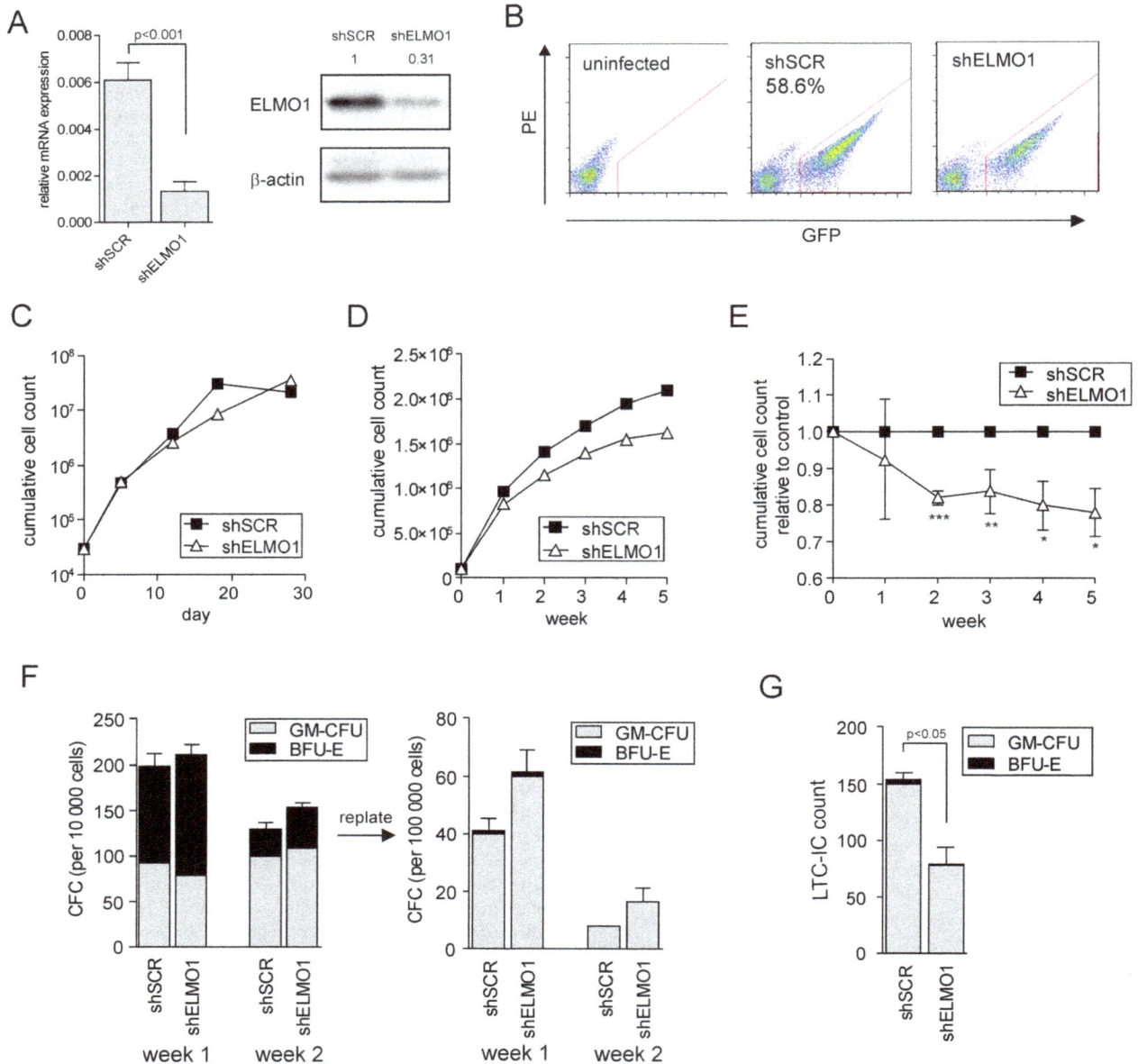

Figure 2. ELMO1 downmodulation in human CB CD34+ cells does not alter growth, colony formation or differentiation, but significantly decreases stem cell frequency. (A) K562 cells were transduced with control scrambled shRNA vector (shSCR) or with ELMO1-targeting shRNA vectors (shELMO1), sorted and used for RNA extraction. Quantitative PCR was performed to measure ELMO1 expression in transduced cells. ELMO1 mRNA levels were normalized against RPL27 mRNA expression. Alternatively, cells were used for Western blot analysis to determine ELMO1 protein levels. (B) FACS plots showing transduction efficiencies of cord blood (CB) CD34[+] stem/progenitor cells transduced with shSCR or shELMO1. (C) 3×10^5 transduced and sorted cells per group were plated in liquid culture and followed for thirty days. Cumulative cell count is showed representative of 3 independent experiments. (D) 10^5 transduced and sorted cells per group were plated on MS5 stromal cells and kept in the co-culture for 5 weeks; cultures were demi-depopulated weekly for analysis. Weekly cumulative cell growth is shown for a representative experiment of 3 independent experiments and the average of those 3 experiments is shown in (E). (F) Suspension cells from MS5 co-cultures as described in panel D were analyzed for progenitor frequency by CFC assay. 10^4 cells from each co-culture were plated in a CFC assay in methylcellulose in duplicate, and colonies were evaluated 2 weeks after plating. CFC cells were then harvested and 10^5 cells were re-plated to form secondary CFCs. CFU-GM and BFU-E numbers are shown from a representative of 3 independent experiments; error bars indicate standard deviation. (G) LTC-IC frequencies were determined in bulk on MS5 stromal cells. After 5 weeks of co-culture methylcellulose was added to and colonies were scored two weeks later. CFU -GM, colony-forming unit-granulocyte-macrophage; BFU-E, burst forming unit-erythroid. * $P<0.05$, ** $P<0.01$, *** $P< 0.001$.

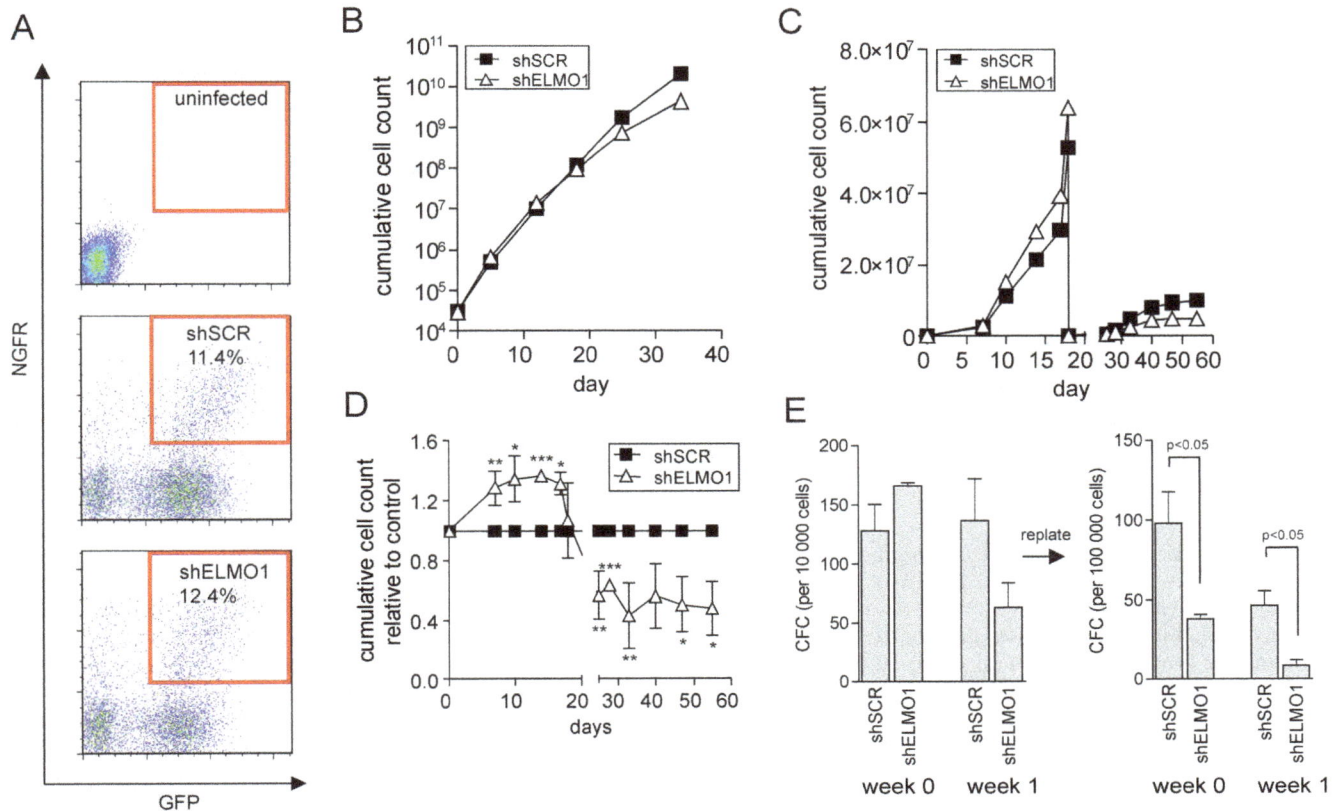

Figure 3. BCR-ABL-transformed human CB CD34⁺ show proliferative disadvantage and markedly reduced replating capacity upon ELMO1 depletion. (A) CB CD34⁺ stem/progenitor cells were double-transduced with BCR-ABL and either control scrambled shRNA vector (shSCR) or with ELMO1-targeting shRNA vector (shELMO1). FACS plots of transduction efficiency are shown. (B) 3×10^5 double-transduced cells per group were plated in liquid culture and followed for 35 day. Cumulative cell count is shown representative of 3 independent experiments. (C) 5×10^3 double-transduced cells were sorted per group and plated on MS5 stromal cells; cultures were demi-depopulated on indicated days for analysis and replated when stroma showed signs of detaching. Cumulative cell growth is shown for a representative experiment of 3 independent experiments and the average of those 3 experiments is shown in (D). (E) Suspension cells from MS5 co-cultures as described in panel B were analyzed for progenitor frequency by CFC assay. 10^3 freshly transduced cells or 10^4 cells from each co-culture were plated in a CFC assay in methylcellulose in duplicate, and colonies were evaluated 2 weeks after plating. CFC cells were harvested and 10^5 cells were replated to assess secondary CFC formation. Total CFC numbers are shown from a representative of 3 independent experiments; error bars indicate standard deviation. * $P<0.05$, ** $P< 0.01$, *** $P<0.001$.

Global inhibition of RAC activity severely impairs proliferation and survival of leukemic cells while ELMO1 depletion affects mostly cell migration

Subsequently, we investigated whether global inhibition of RAC activity, as a downstream target of ELMO1, would have an effect on the expansion of BCR-ABL-expressing leukemic cells. To this end, we used either BCR-ABL-transduced CD34⁺ CB cells, or primary blast crisis chronic myeloid leukemia (BC CML) cells. After plating on stroma, cells were allowed to expand and form cobblestones, after which the RAC inhibitor NSC23766 (NSC) was added to the co-cultures in concentrations of 20 µM to 100 µM. In BCR-ABL CB cells, inhibition of RAC activity caused a marked decrease in cell proliferation, apparent as early as 4 days after the addition of NSC. By day 9, cultures treated with 20 µM and 40 µM of NSC ceased to expand, while cells treated with

Table 1. Summary of clinical parameters of AML patients used in this study.

	2003 022	2003 119	2003 160
FAB classification	M5	M0	M1
Cytogenetic characteristics	NK	NK	complex karyotype
Risk group	intermediate	poor	poor
FLT3/NPM1	ITD/NPMc+	ITD/wt	wt/wt

Abbreviations: *FLT3*, fms-related tyrosine kinase 3; ITD, internal tandem duplication; NK, normal karyotype; *NPM1*, nucleophosmin 1; NPMc⁺, cytoplasmic dislocalization of NPM1; wt, wild type.

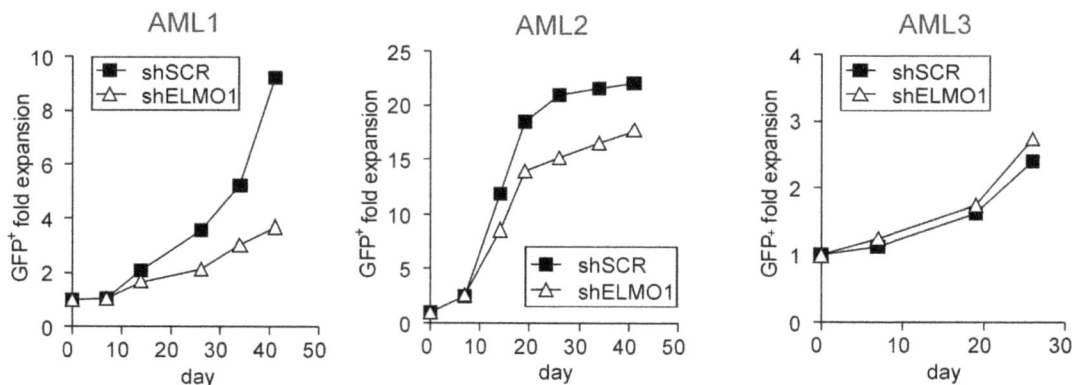

Figure 4. ELMO1 depletion in primary AML CD34⁺ cells impairs long-term expansion on stroma. AML CD34⁺ cells were transduced with control scrambled shRNA vector (shSCR) or with ELMO1-targeting shRNA vector (shELMO1). After washing away the virus all the cells were plated on MS5 stroma; cultures were demi-depopulated on indicated days for analysis. Cumulative cell growth is shown for each AML sample studied.

100 μM of inhibitor were depleted from the co-culture (Figure 5A). Analysis of phosphorylated PAK as a readout for RAC activity revealed that 40 μM of NSC23766 was sufficient to almost completely abolish RAC activity in the treated cells (Figure S3A). NSC-treated co-cultures showed an increased level of apoptotic cells, and the cells did not recover even after discontinuation of the treatment (Figure 5C and Figure S3B). Similarly, primary BC CML cells were highly sensitive to RAC inhibition. Co-cultures treated with the highest concentration of NSC did not survive past week 2, while cells treated with 20 μM or 40 μM of the inhibitor stopped expanding at were lost from the co-culture at week 3 (Figure 5B). The data are directly in line with our previously published data on the effects of the RAC inhibitor NSC on primary AML cells, where we also observed a strong reduction in long-term expansion on MS5 stromal cocultures [22].

Since global inhibition of RAC activity resulted in a much more severe phenotype than downregulation of ELMO1, we hypothesized that the activation via ELMO1-Dock180 pathway may be important for only some functions of RAC proteins. RAC GTPases have a well-described role in regulating migration and chemotaxis [38]; therefore we investigated the affected of ELMO1 depletion on the migratory potential of leukemic cells. To this end we transduced leukemic cell lines TF-1 and THP-1 with either shSCR- or shELMO1-containing lentiviral constructs. Depletion of ELMO1 resulted in an approximately 20% decrease of phospho-PAK activity and a slight proliferative disadvantage (Figure S4A, S4B). However, when we performed a transwell assay on either shSCR- or shELMO1-transduced leukemic cell lines we observed a marked decrease in the percentage of cells migrating towards the SDF-1 gradient upon ELMO1 downmodulation, indicative of a reduced chemotaxis (Figure 5D). Interestingly, treatment with RAC inhibitor resulted in a very pronounced apoptotic response in those cell lines, with virtually all cells dead within 3 days of treatment with 100 μM of NSC (Figure S4C, S4D). Therefore, while abolishing RAC activity was detrimental to the survival and proliferation of leukemic cells, inhibiting ELMO1-Dock180 activation pathway seemed to affect mostly their migratory potential.

Discussion

The current study shows that ELMO1 is more highly expressed in AML CD34⁺ cells as compared with NBM CD34⁺ cells, and that this high expression has a prognostic significance in the NK subset of AML patients. Depletion of ELMO1 modestly impaired expansion in the long-term cultures of oncogene-transduced or primary leukemic CD34⁺ cells, while chemotaxis towards an SDF-1 gradient was significantly reduced.

Analysis of the data generated in the study by Novershtern et al. revealed that ELMO1 was significantly higher expressed in the most primitive hematopoietic compartment (HSCs) as compared with the more differentiated cells [31]. Importantly, in a recent proteome analysis of the plasma membrane fractions of CB CD34⁺ cells, we have found ELMO1 to be specifically associated with the plasma membrane of CD34⁺/CD38⁻ HSCs (data not shown). Taken together, these results identified ELMO1 as a protein most abundant in the primitive compartment of the hematopoietic system and suggested that ELMO1 might contribute to the biology of HSCs. Although downregulation of ELMO1 in CB CD34⁺ cells did not significantly affect proliferation, differentiation or progenitor cell frequencies, depletion of ELMO1 did result in a significant decrease of stem cell frequencies as determined by LTC-IC assay. Considering that increased expression of ELMO1 was predominantly observed within the most primitive stem and progenitor cells it is conceivable that those cells are most affected by downregulation of ELMO1.

We identified ELMO1 to be an AML34⁺-specific gene in a recent transcriptome analysis of paired AML CD34⁺ and CD34⁻ samples, and BM CD34⁺ cells [17,18]. Although to date there is no data available on the involvement of ELMO1 in the hematopoietic malignancies, RAC proteins have been identified as crucial factors in the BCR-ABL- and MLL-AF9-induced leukemic transformation [32–37]. This led us to hypothesize that the increased expression of ELMO1 that we observed in leukemic cells may act by increasing RAC activity in these cells. ELMO1 downregulation in BCR-ABL-transduced CB CD34⁺ cells or in primary AML CD34⁺ cells initially did not strongly affect their long-term growth in stromal co-cultures, but upon serial replating of MS5 cocultures or upon serial replating of CFCs a significant reduction was observed. In two out of three AML cases a significant reduction in long-term growth on MS5 assays was also observed. Nevertheless, the effect of global RAC inhibition in BCR-ABL-expressing cells was far more pronounced than that of ELMO1 downregulation, both on the RAC activity levels and the cell proliferation and survival. These data are directly in line with our previously published data in primary AML cells, where we also observed a strong reduction in long-term expansion on MS5 stromal cocultures [22]. One possible explanation for differences

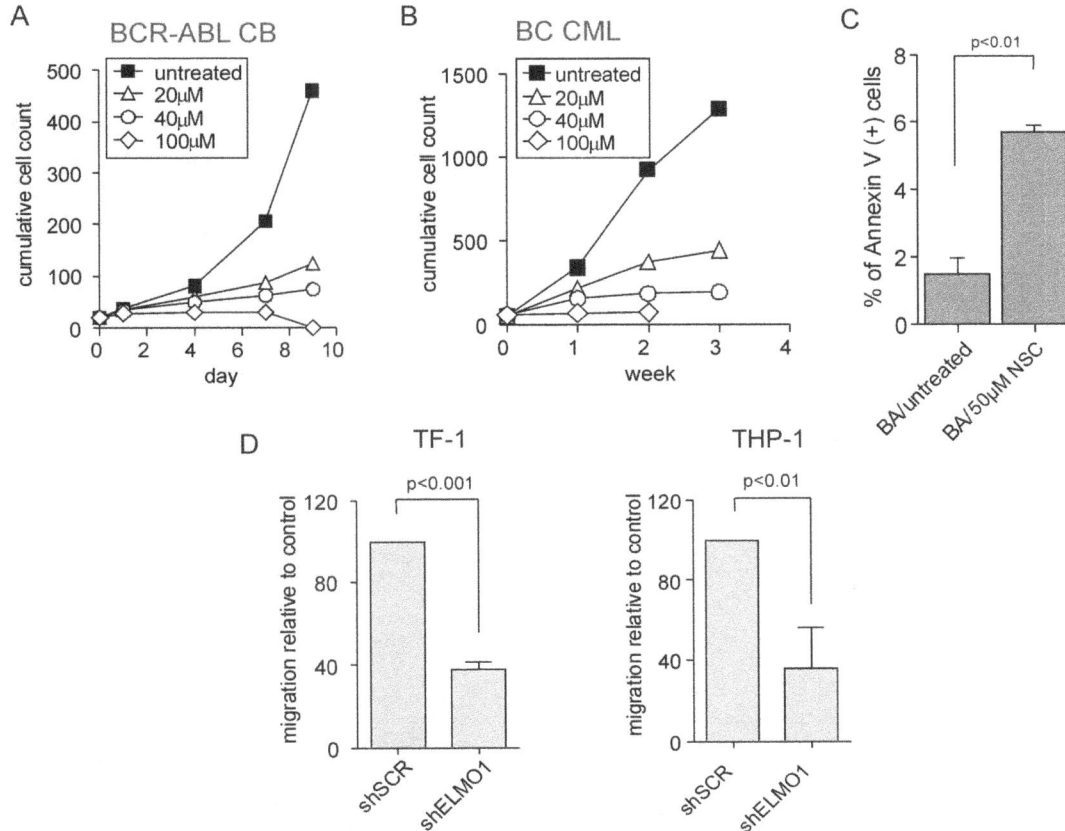

Figure 5. Global inhibition of RAC activity severely impairs proliferation and survival of leukemic cells while ELMO1 depletion strongly affects migration. (A) CB CD34$^+$ cells were transduced with BCR-ABL-expressing vector, sorted and plated on MS5 stroma. Cells were allowed to proliferate for 5 days after which RAC inhibitor was added to the following concentrations: 20 µM, 40 µM or 100 µM. Co-cultures were demi-depopulated on indicated days for analysis. Cumulative cell count is shown representative of 3 independent experiments. (B) CD34$^+$ cells were sorted from BC CML patient sample and plated on MS5 stroma. Cells were allowed to proliferate for 5 days after which RAC inhibitor was added to the following concentrations: 20 µM, 40 µM or 100 µM. Co-cultures were demi-depopulated on indicated days for analysis. Cumulative cell count is shown representative of 3 independent experiments. (C) BCR-ABL transduced cells as described in (A) were treated with 50 µM NSC for 3 days after which suspension cells were harvested and stained with Annexin V to assess apoptosis. (D) TF-1 and THP-1 cells were transduced with control scrambled shRNA vector (shSCR) or with ELMO1-targeting shRNA vector (shELMO1) and migration was evaluated in a transwell assay. The percentage of migrating cells relative to control is shown as an average of 3 independent experiments.

in sensitivity towards ELMO or RAC knockdown might be that the residual ELMO1 expression in the transduced cells was still sufficient to maintain RAC activity and function. Also, it is plausible that redundancy exists between other members of the ELMO family that would compensate for ELMO1 loss, or alternatively other pathways might have become dominant in activating RAC upon ELMO1 depletion. Further studies are required to resolve these issues.

Previous studies have shown that increased expression of ELMO1 was responsible for the malignant behavior of ovarian and breast cancer, as well as glioma cells [25,39–41]. In those cases, ELMO1 played a role in conferring the migratory and invasive properties of the malignant cells. Accordingly, when we assessed migratory potential of leukemic cell lines, we saw that it was reduced upon ELMO1 downmodulation. It is therefore possible that an increased expression of ELMO1 in LSCs confers migratory properties that contribute to the malignant phenotype and worse overall survival of AML patients.

Overall, we have shown that ELMO1 is more highly expressed in primitive leukemic cells and that it predicts prognosis in NK AML patients. Further studies using *in vivo* leukemia models are

necessary to assess whether ELMO1 depletion could affect LSC homing and long-term engraftment, and ultimately whether targeting ELMO1 might have therapeutic benefit in the treatment of leukemia patients.

Supporting Information

Figure S1 (A) Relative mRNA expression of ELMO1 was analyzed by Q-PCR in a panel of 11 AML samples and the correlation with Illumina BeadsArray expression data was assessed. Calculated r2 = 0.6. (B) Relative mRNA expression of ELMO1 (derived from HemaExplorer) was analyzed across different AML subtypes and compared to NBM populations. Number of samples per group: AML1-ETO n = 39; APL n = 37; inv16/t16 n = 28; t(11q23) n = 38; HSC_BM n = 7; HPC_BM n = 4. (C) Comparison of mRNA expression of ELMO1 in various human hematopoietic populations analyzed in the Novershtern dataset.

Figure S2 CD34$^+$ CB cells were transduced with either control shSCR or shELMO1 constructs, and 105 trans-

duced and sorted cells per group were plated on MS5 stromal cells and kept in the co-culture for 5 weeks. Cultures were demi-depopulated weekly and suspension cells were analyzed for differentiation along myeloid lineages. Percentage of CD14/CD15-double negative, CD14-positive and CD15-positive cells are shown.

Figure S3 (A) CB CD34$^+$ cells were transduced with BCR-ABL-expressing vector, sorted and plated on MS5 stroma. Cells were allowed to proliferate for 5 days after which RAC inhibitor NSC was added to the following concentrations: 20 μM, 40 μM or 100 μM. After 3 days of treatment suspension cells were collected and phospho-PAK levels were assessed by Western blot. Quantification of phospho-PAK levels relative to control is indicated above each lane. (B) BCR-ABL-expressing cells as 3 described in (A) were treated with 50 μM NSC and co-cultures were demi-depopulated on indicated days for analysis. After 20 days NSC was washed away from the culture and treated cells were culture for additional 13 days after which all the cells were harvested for analysis. Cell counts are shown representative of 3 independent experiments.

Figure S4 (A) THP-1 cells were transduced with either control shSCR or shELMO1 vector and sorted. After 5 days of culture expression of phospo-PAK in transduced cells was analyzed by Western blot. Quantification of phospho-PAK levels relative to control is indicated above each lane. (B) shSCR- or shELMO1-transduced THP-1 cells were cultured for 9 days and cells were counted on the indicated time points. Cumulative cell count is shown representative of 3 independent experiments. (C) THP-1 cells were treated with either 50 μM or 100 μM NSC for 3 days and then stained with Annexin V to assess apoptosis. FACS plots representative of 3 independent experiments are shown and quantification of Annexin V (+) cells is shown in (D).

Acknowledgments

The authors would like to thank Annet Brouwers-Vos for help with Illumina bead array experiments and all members of the Experimental Hematology lab for helpful discussions.

Author Contributions

Conceived and designed the experiments: MEC JJS. Performed the experiments: MEC JJS. Analyzed the data: MEC EV JJS. Wrote the paper: MEC JJS.

References

1. Byrd JC, Mrózek K, Dodge RK, Carroll AJ, Edwards CG et al. (2002) Pretreatment cytogenetic abnormalities are predictive of induction success, cumulative incidence of relapse, and overall survival in adult patients with de novo acute myeloid leukemia: results from Cancer and Leukemia Group B (CALGB 8461). Blood 100: 4325–4336.

2. Vardiman JW, Thiele J, Arber DA, Brunning RD, Borowitz MJ et al. (2009) The 2008 revision of the World Health Organization (WHO) classification of myeloid neoplasms and acute leukemia: rationale and important changes. Blood 114: 937–951.

3. Alcalay M, Tiacci E, Bergomas R, Bigerna B, Venturini E et al. (2005) Acute myeloid leukemia bearing cytoplasmic nucleophosmin (NPMc+ AML) shows a distinct gene expression profile characterized by up-regulation of genes involved in stem-cell maintenance. Blood 106: 899–902.

4. Bullinger L, Dohner K, Bair E, Frohling S, Schlenk RF et al. (2004) Use of gene-expression profiling to identify prognostic subclasses in adult acute myeloid leukemia. N Engl J Med 350: 1605–1616.

5. Radmacher MD, Marcucci G, Ruppert AS, Mrozek K, Whitman SP et al. (2006) Independent confirmation of a prognostic gene-expression signature in adult acute myeloid leukemia with a normal karyotype: a Cancer and Leukemia Group B study. Blood 108: 1677–1683.

6. Valk PJ, Verhaak RG, Beijen MA, Erpelinck CA, Barjesteh van Waalwijk van DoornKhosrovaniet al. (2004) Prognostically useful gene-expression profiles in acute myeloid leukemia. N Engl J Med 350: 1617–1628.

7. Wouters BJ, Lowenberg B, Delwel R (2009) A decade of genome-wide gene expression profiling in acute myeloid leukemia: flashback and prospects. Blood 113: 291–298.

8. Wouters BJ, Lowenberg B, Erpelinck-Verschueren CA, van Putten WL, Valk PJ et al. (2009) Double CEBPA mutations, but not single CEBPA mutations, define a subgroup of acute myeloid leukemia with a distinctive gene expression profile that is uniquely associated with a favorable outcome. Blood 113: 3088–3091.

9. Bonnet D, Dick JE (1997) Human acute myeloid leukemia is organized as a hierarchy that originates from a primitive hematopoietic cell. Nat Med 3: 730–737.

10. Lapidot T, Kollet O (2002) The essential roles of the chemokine SDF-1 and its receptor CXCR4 in human stem cell homing and repopulation of transplanted immune-deficient NOD/SCID and NOD/SCID/B2m(null) mice. Leukemia 16: 1992–2003.

11. Schuringa JJ, Schepers H (2009) Ex vivo assays to study self-renewal and long-term expansion of genetically modified primary human acute myeloid leukemia stem cells. Methods Mol Biol 538: 287–300.

12. van Gosliga D, Schepers H, Rizo A, van der Kolk D, Vellenga E et al. (2007) Establishing long-term cultures with self-renewing acute myeloid leukemia stem/progenitor cells. Exp Hematol 35: 1538–1549.

13. Warner JK, Wang JC, Takenaka K, Doulatov S, McKenzie JL et al. (2005) Direct evidence for cooperating genetic events in the leukemic transformation of normal human hematopoietic cells. Leukemia 19: 1794–1805.

14. Jordan CT, Upchurch D, Szilvassy SJ, Guzman ML, Howard DS et al. (2000) The interleukin-3 receptor alpha chain is a unique marker for human acute myelogenous leukemia stem cells. Leukemia 14: 1777–1784.

15. Lane SW, Scadden DT, Gilliland DG (2009) The leukemic stem cell niche: current concepts and therapeutic opportunities. Blood 114: 1150–1157.

16. Lapidot T, Sirard C, Vormoor J, Murdoch B, Hoang T et al. (1994) A cell initiating human acute myeloid leukaemia after transplantation into SCID mice. Nature 367: 645–648.

17. Bonardi F, Fusetti F, Deelen P, van GD, Vellenga E et al. (2013) A Proteomics and Transcriptomics Approach to Identify Leukemic Stem Cell (LSC) Markers. Mol Cell Proteomics 12: 626–637.

18. de Jonge HJ, Woolthuis CM, Vos AZ, Mulder A, van den BE et al. (2011) Gene expression profiling in the leukemic stem cell-enriched CD34(+) fraction identifies target genes that predict prognosis in normal karyotype AML. Leukemia 25: 1825–1833.

19. Gumienny TL, Brugnera E, Tosello-Trampont AC, Kinchen JM, Haney LB et al. (2001) CED-12/ELMO, a Novel Member of the CrkII/Dock180/Rac Pathway, Is Required for Phagocytosis and Cell Migration. Cell 107: 27–41.

20. Lu M, Kinchen JM, Rossman KL, Grimsley C, Hall M et al. (2005) A Steric-Inhibition Model for Regulation of Nucleotide Exchange via the Dock180 Family of GEFs. Current Biology 15: 371–377.

21. Lu M, Ravichandran KS (2006) Dock180-ELMO Cooperation in Rac Activation. Volume 406: 388–402.

22. Rozenveld-Geugien M, Baas IO, van Gosliga D, Vellenga E, Schuringa JJ (2007) Expansion of normal and leukemic human hematopoietic stem/progenitor cells requires rac-mediated interaction with stromal cells. Exp Hematol 35: 782–792.

23. Schepers H, van GD, Wierenga AT, Eggen BJ, Schuringa JJ et al. (2007) STAT5 is required for long-term maintenance of normal and leukemic human stem/progenitor cells. Blood 110: 2880–2888.

24. Rizo A, Horton SJ, Olthof S, Dontje B, Ausema A et al. (2010) BMI1 collaborates with BCR-ABL in leukemic transformation of human CD34+ cells. Blood 116: 4621–4630.

25. Jarzynka MJ, Hu B, Hui KM, Bar-Joseph I, Gu W et al. (2007) ELMO1 and Dock180, a Bipartite Rac1 Guanine Nucleotide Exchange Factor, Promote Human Glioma Cell Invasion. Cancer Research 67: 7203–7211.

26. Shimazaki A, Tanaka Y, Shinosaki T, Ikeda M, Watada H et al. (2006) ELMO1 increases expression of extracellular matrix proteins and inhibits cell adhesion to ECMs. Kidney Int 70: 1769–1776.

27. Schepers H, Wierenga AT, van Gosliga D., Eggen BJ, Vellenga E et al. (2007) Reintroduction of C/EBPalpha in leukemic CD34+ stem/progenitor cells impairs self-renewal and partially restores myelopoiesis. Blood 110: 1317–1325.

28. Schuringa JJ, Wu K, Morrone G, Moore MA (2004) Enforced activation of STAT5A facilitates the generation of embryonic stem-derived hematopoietic stem cells that contribute to hematopoiesis in vivo. Stem Cells 22: 1191–1204.

29. de Jonge HJ, Valk PJ, Veeger NJ, Ter EA, den Boer ML et al. (2010) High VEGFC expression is associated with unique gene expression profiles and predicts adverse prognosis in pediatric and adult acute myeloid leukemia. Blood 116: 1747–1754.

30. Bagger FO, Rapin N, Theilgaard-Monch K, Kaczkowski B, Jendholm J et al. (2012) HemaExplorer: a Web server for easy and fast visualization of gene expression in normal and malignant hematopoiesis. Blood 119: 6394–6395.

31. Novershtern N, Subramanian A, Lawton LN, Mak RH, Haining WN et al. (2011) Densely interconnected transcriptional circuits control cell states in human hematopoiesis. Cell 144: 296–309.

32. Muller LU, Schore RJ, Zheng Y, Thomas EK, Kim MO et al. (2008) Rac guanosine triphosphatases represent a potential target in AML. Leukemia 22: 1803–1806.

33. Nieborowska-Skorska M, Kopinski PK, Ray R, Hoser G, Ngaba D et al. (2012) Rac2-MRC-cIII-generated ROS cause genomic instability in chronic myeloid leukemia stem cells and primitive progenitors. Blood 119: 4253–4263.

34. Sengupta A, Arnett J, Dunn S, Williams DA, Cancelas JA (2010) Rac2 GTPase deficiency depletes BCR-ABL+ leukemic stem cells and progenitors in vivo. Blood 116: 81–84.

35. Skorski T, Wlodarski P, Daheron L, Salomoni P, Nieborowska-Skorska M et al. (1998) BCR/ABL-mediated leukemogenesis requires the activity of the small GTP-binding protein Rac. Proc Natl Acad Sci U S A 95: 11858–11862.

36. Thomas EK, Cancelas JA, Chae HD, Cox AD, Keller PJ et al. (2007) Rac guanosine triphosphatases represent integrating molecular therapeutic targets for BCR-ABL-induced myeloproliferative disease. Cancer Cell 12: 467–478.

37. Thomas EK, Cancelas JA, Zheng Y, Williams DA (2008) Rac GTPases as key regulators of p210-BCR-ABL-dependent leukemogenesis. Leukemia 22: 898–904.

38. Williams DA, Zheng Y, Cancelas JA (2008) Rho GTPases and Regulation of Hematopoietic Stem Cell Localization. Volume 439: 365–393.

39. Li H, Yang L, Fu H, Yan J, Wang Y et al. (2013) Association between Gai2 and ELMO1/Dock180 connects chemokine signalling with Rac activation and metastasis. Nat Commun 4: 1706.

40. Wang H, Linghu H, Wang J, Che Yl, Xiang Tx et al. (2010) The role of Crk/Dock180/Rac1 pathway in the malignant behavior of human ovarian cancer cell SKOV3. Tumor Biol 31: 59–67.

41. Wang J, Dai Jm, Che Yl, Gao Ym, Peng Hj et al. (2014) Elmo1 Helps Dock180 to Regulate Rac1 Activity and Cell Migration of Ovarian Cancer. International Journal of Gynecological Cancer 24.

19

High-Dose Cytarabine in Acute Myeloid Leukemia Treatment

Wei Li[1], Xiaoyuan Gong[1], Mingyuan Sun[1], Xingli Zhao[1], Benfa Gong[1], Hui Wei[1], Yingchang Mi[1], Jianxiang Wang[1,2]*

1 Leukemia Diagnosis and Treatment Center, Institute of Hematology and Blood Disease Hospital, Chinese Academy of Medical Sciences and Peking Union of Medical College, Tianjin, China, 2 State Key Laboratory of Experimental Hematology, Institute of Hematology and Blood Disease Hospital, Chinese Academy of Medical Sciences and Peking Union of Medical College, Tianjin, China

Abstract

The optimal dose, scheme, and clinical setting for Ara-C in acute myeloid leukemia (AML) treatment remain uncertain. In this study, we performed a meta-analysis to systematically assess the impact of high-dose cytarabine (HDAC) on AML therapy during the induction and consolidation stages. Twenty-two trials with a total of 5,945 *de novo* AML patients were included in the meta-analysis. Only patients less than 60 year-old were included in the study. Using HDAC in induction therapy was beneficial for RFS (HR = 0.57; 95% CI, 0.35–0.93; $P = 0.02$) but not so for CR rate (HR = 1.01; 95% CI, 0.93–1.09; $P = 0.88$) and OS (HR = 0.83; 95% CI, 0.66–1.03; $P = 0.1$). In consolidation therapy, HDAC showed significant RFS benefits (HR = 0.67; 95% CI, 0.49–0.9; $P = 0.008$) especially for the favorable-risk group (HR = 0.38; 95% CI, 0.21–0.69; $P = 0.001$) compared with SDAC (standard dose cytarabine), although no OS advantage was observed (HR = 0.84; 95% CI, 0.55–1.27; $P = 0.41$). HDAC treatment seemed less effective than auto-BMT/allo-BMT treatment (HR = 1.66, 95% CI, 1.3–2.14; $P<0.0001$) with similar OS. HDAC treatment led to lower relapse rate in induction and consolidation therapy than SDAC treatment, especially for the favorable-risk group. Auto-BMT/allo-BMT was more beneficial in prolonging RFS than HDAC.

Editor: Wilbur Lam, Emory University/Georgia Institute of Technology, United States of America

Funding: This study was supported by National Natural Science Foundation (81270635), National Public Health Grand Research Foundation (201202017), National Science & Technology Major Projects (201 1ZX09302-007-04) of China and Tianjin Major Science and Technology Project (12ZCDZSY17500). The funders had no role in study design, data collection and analysis, decision to publish, or preparation of the manuscript.

Competing Interests: In this article we declared that Jianxiang Wang acts as consultant of Novartis and Bristol Myers Squibb.

* Email: wangjx@ihcams.ac.cn

Introduction

Cytarabine (Ara-C) has been a major drug for acute myeloid leukemia (AML) treatment for more than three decades. Initially, the drug was used at 100–200 mg/m^2 for 7–10 days for standard treatment [1]. In recent years, multiple cycles of high-dose cytarabine (HDAC) therapy (at 3.0 g/m^2 every 12 hours) have been commonly used as the consolidation therapy in multicenter trials; it was observed to maximize Ara-C's anti-leukemia effect in AML patients, leading to improve disease- free-survival (DFS) [2,3]. After that, HDAC instead of standard-dose cytarabine multiagent chemotherapy has become a common practice in the treatment of AML, especially in patients younger than 60 years of age, either for remission induction or consolidation, based on the guidelines of the National Comprehensive Cancer Network (*VI.* 2013). However, recent randomized controlled trials with 781 patients have challenged the benefits of HDAC [4]. HDAC failed to show significant improvement in five-year relapse-free survival and five-year overall survival as compared with SDAC regimen in AML treatments, especially in the consolidation therapy. After these new studies, the dose and effect of HDAC during AML induction and consolidation therapies are open for new evaluation [5]. Therefore, a systematic analysis needs to be performed to

clarify these issues, which is the focus of this meta-analytical review. Specifically, this review study compared the effectiveness of HDAC versus SDAC as AML therapy in adult patients during the induction and consolidation phases, in order to shed lights on defining the optimal dose and scheme of Ara-C treatment with minimum possible toxicity. On the other hand, we assessed the effectiveness of HDAC compared with bone marrow transplantation (BMT) in order to explore the best therapy in the consolidation phase.

Methods

Literature Search

Independent reviewers (L.W and G. XY) systematically searched PubMed for relevant research papers published in English between January 1990 and March 2013 using the following query terms: acute myeloid leukemia, high-dose, and cytarabine. The titles and abstracts of the identified studies were reviewed to determine potential eligibility for meta-analysis. Relevant review and meta-analysis articles were included to identify additional studies that met the inclusion criteria. Further studies were referred by means of manual search of secondary

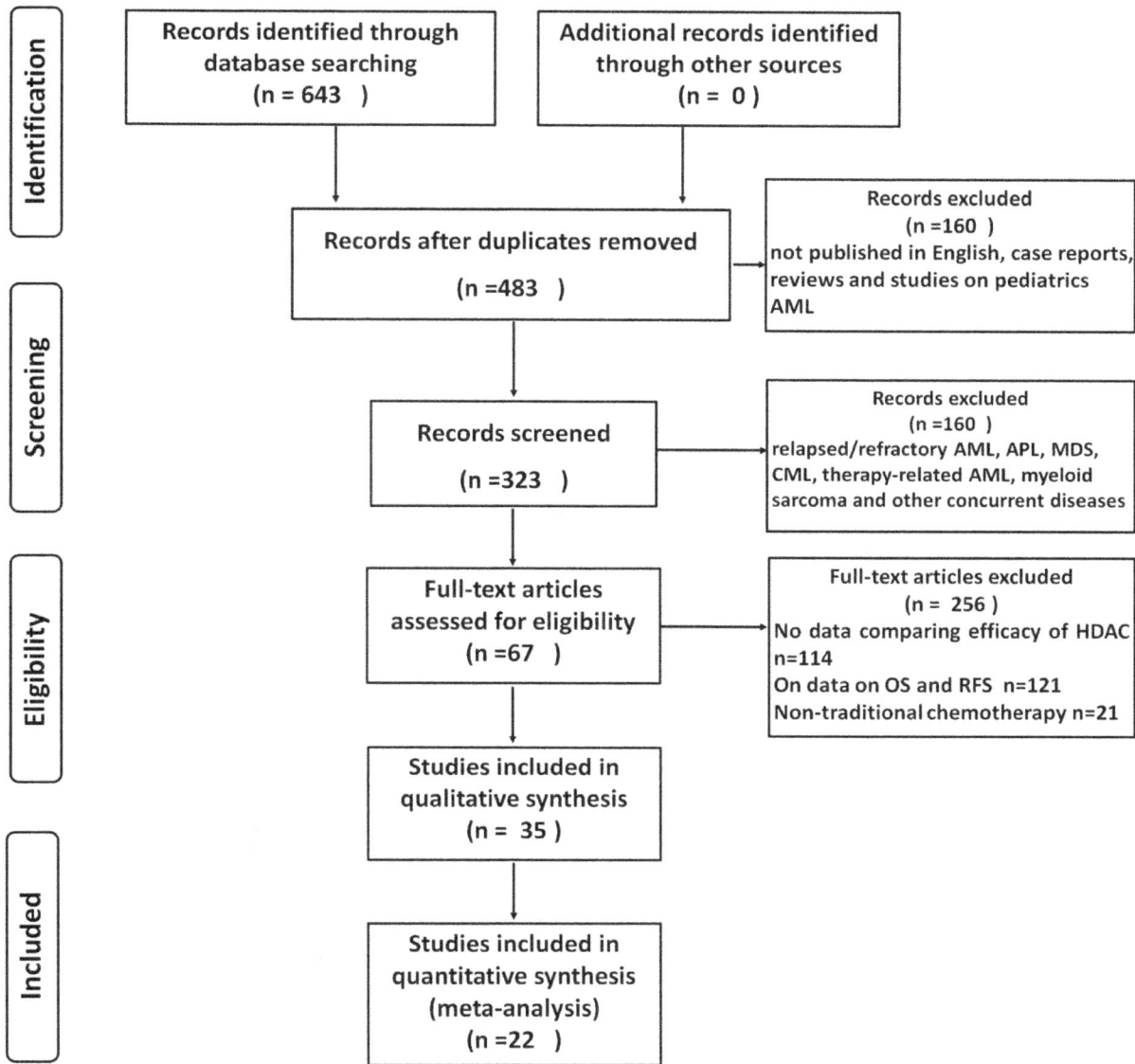

Figure 1. Flow chart explaining the selection of eligible studies included in the meta-analysis.

sources. Divergences among the reviewers must be resolved to reach a consensus after further discussion.

Inclusion and Exclusion Criteria

Identified articles were independently appraised according to the inclusion criteria by the same two reviewers (L.W and G. XY). All patients were required to have untreated acute myeloid leukemia, de novo AML, and patients with acute promyelocytic leukemia and translocation t(15;17) did not included this study. The included trials described the comparsion of HDAC (2.0–3.0 g/m^2) and standard-dose cytarabine (SDAC, ≤200 mg/m^2) in induction and consolidation therapy, or bone marrow transplantion (BMT) in consolidation therapy. new medicine research and phase II/III clinical trials were excluded. Studies reported hazard ratios (HRs) and 95% confidence intervals (CIs) for overall survival (OS)/relapse free survival (RFS) benefit, or those provided data to estimate HR by the method of Parmar *et al* [6]. If multiple articles were identified to report on the same study, the most recent one

was analyzed. Only randomized controlled trials (RCT) were included in the comparison of HDAC and SDAC, but observed study met the inclusion criteria for the study of BMT vs HDAC, because it was difficult to ensure that each patient had donor and even more difficult to complete RCT.

Data Extraction. Data were extracted in the standardized format by two independent reviewers. Data collected for each study included study name, name of first author, year of publication, period of enrollment, total number of subjects allocated to therapies, median patient age (years), chemotherapy regimens, number of events (death, relapse) in each group, and study end points of overall survival benefit, RFS benefit, or both. We used overall survival (OS) and relapse free survival (RFS) of individual studies. Discrepancies in data extraction were resolved by identifying consensus, referring back to the original article, or contacting study authors if necessary. When missing data were encountered, the authors were contacted to complete data analysis.

Table 1. Characteristics of included Studies for induction therapy.

Source	Study ID	Enrollment Period	Multi-center	No. of patients	RCTs	Study entry criteria	Induction therapy
J.P. Matthews et al, 2001 [7]	ALSG	1987–1991	Yes	248	Yes	de novo AML median age: 42 years	DEA (DNR+VP-16+Ara-c 100 mg/m^2/d×7d) / DEA (DNR+VP-16+Ara-c 3 g/m^2 q12 h d1,3,5,7d)
JK. Weick et al, 1996 [8]	SWOG	1986–1991	Yes	723	Yes	de novo or secondary AML M/F: 397/326 age range: 15–64 years WBC range: 0.4–416×10^9/L	DA (DNR+Ara-c 200 mg/m^2/d×7d) / DA (DNR+Ara-c 3 g/m^2 q12 h×6d)
T. Büchner et al, 2006 [9]▲	—	1999–2005	Yes	1770	Yes	de novo or secondary AML, age range: 16~85 years※	Double induction TAD (6-TG+DNR+Ara-c 100 mg/m^2/d×8d) + HAM (MTZ+Ara-c 3 g/m^2 q12 h×3d) / HAM+HAM (MTZ+Ara-c 3 g/m^2 q12 h×3d)
T. Büchner et al, 1999 [10]	CAMLCG	1985–1992	Yes	725	Yes	de novo AML, M/F: 336/389 median age: 44 (16–60) years WBC range: 0.1–405×10^9/L	Double induction TAD+TAD (6-TG+DNR+Ara-c100 mg/m^2/d×8d) / TAD (6-TG+DNR+Ara-c 100 mg/m^2/d×8d) + HAM (MTZ+Ara-c 3 g/m^2 q12 h×3d)
T. Büchner et al, 2009 [11]▲	CAMLCG	1993–2005	Yes	1284	Yes	de novo AML, years range: 16~85 years※ WBC range: 0.05–1017×10^9/L	Double induction TAD (6-TG+DNR+Ara-c 100 mg/m^2/d×8d) + HAM (MTZ+Ara-c 3 g/m^2 q12 h×3d) / HAM+HAM (MTZ+Ara-c 3 g/m^2 q12 h×3d)

Note: ▲ T. Büchner et al, 2009 repeated the same trial of T. Büchner et al, 2006.
※analyze <60 years patients in each trial.
Abbreviations: NR, not reported; IDA, idarubicin; Ara-c, cytarabin; VP-16, etoposide; DNR, daunorubicin.

A

Study or Subgroup	Experimental Events	Total	Control Events	Total	Weight	Risk Ratio M-H. Random. 95% CI
J.P. Matt hews(ALSG)2001	91	124	88	124	17.3%	1.03 [0.89, 1.21]
JK. Weick(SWOG) 1996	275	493	120	230	18.7%	1.07 [0.92, 1.24]
T. Bu¨chner(CAMLCG) 2006	336	473	307	451	34.4%	1.04 [0.96, 1.14]
T. Bu¨chner(CAMLCG)1999	234	360	260	365	29.6%	0.91 [0.83, 1.01]
Total (95% CI)		**1450**		**1170**	**100.0%**	**1.01 [0.93, 1.09]**
Total events	936		775			

Heterogeneity: Tau² = 0.00; Chi² = 5.15, df = 3 (P = 0.16); I² = 42%
Test for overall effect: Z = 0.15 (P = 0.88)

B

Study or Subgroup	log[Risk Ratio]	SE	Weight	Risk Ratio IV. Fixed. 95% CI
J.P. Matt hews(ALSG)2001	-0.78	0.33	11.8%	0.46 [0.24, 0.88]
JK. Weick(SWOG) 1996	-0.39	0.76	2.2%	0.68 [0.15, 3.00]
T. Bu¨chner(CAMLCG)1999	-0.09	0.16	50.3%	0.91 [0.67, 1.25]
T.Bu¨chner (CAMLCG)2009	-0.12	0.19	35.7%	0.89 [0.61, 1.29]
Total (95% CI)			**100.0%**	**0.83 [0.66, 1.03]**

Heterogeneity: Chi² = 3.79, df = 3 (P = 0.28); I² = 21%
Test for overall effect: Z = 1.67 (P = 0.10)

C

Study or Subgroup	log[Risk Ratio]	SE	Weight	Risk Ratio IV. Random. 95% CI
J.P. Matt hews(ALSG)2001	-1.39	0.34	20.8%	0.25 [0.13, 0.48]
JK. Weick(SWOG) 1996	-0.71	0.26	24.7%	0.49 [0.30, 0.82]
T. Bu¨chner(CAMLCG)1999	-0.27	0.19	28.3%	0.76 [0.53, 1.11]
T.Bu¨chner (CAMLCG)2009	-0.08	0.23	26.3%	0.92 [0.59, 1.45]
Total (95% CI)			**100.0%**	**0.57 [0.35, 0.93]**

Heterogeneity: Tau² = 0.18; Chi² = 12.13, df = 3 (P = 0.007); I² = 75%
Test for overall effect: Z = 2.25 (P = 0.02)

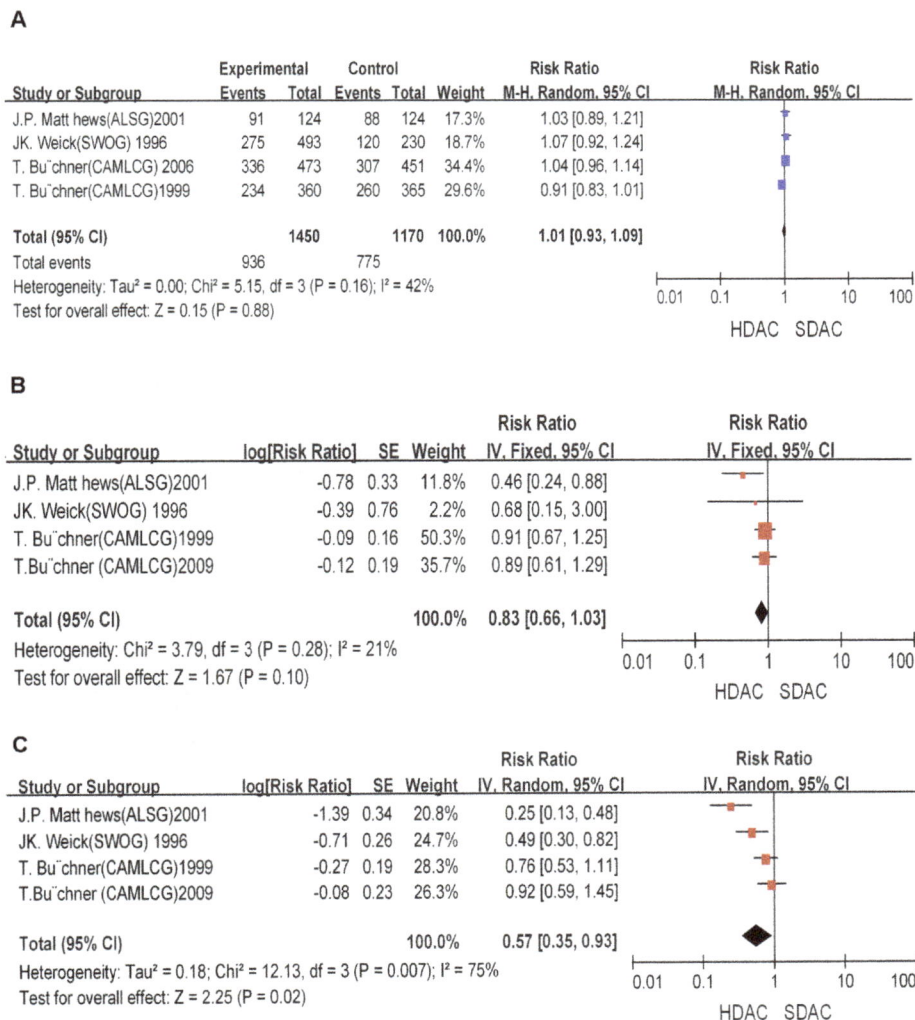

Figure 2. Effect of HDAC versus SDAC in induction therapy. A: Effect of HDAC versus SDAC in induction therapy on CR rate. **B**: Overall survival benefit of HDAC in induction therapy. **C**: Relapse free survival benefit of HDAC in induction therapy.

Assessment of methodological quality. Two reviewers assessed the methodological quality of each trial. The risk of bias in each trial was assessed according to Cochrane methodology by using the following criteria: considering random sequence generation, allocation concealment, the blinding of patients and personnel, incomplete outcome data, selective reporting, and Begg's funnel plots and Egger's test were used to reveal possible publication bias. Heterogeneity was assessed by forest plots and with a standard Chi² test and an inconsistency (I^2) statistic. Both the fixed-effect model and the random-effect model were initially used to calculate total HRs, and finally selected with regards to heterogeneity in the survival analyses. If the heterogeneity ($I^2 > 75\%$) was too great for a summary estimate to be calculated, subgroup analysis was needed.

Data synthesis. Data were synthesized using the Cochrane Statistics package RevMan (version 4.0.4). The threshold of significance was $P \leq 0.05$. A forest plot with combined HRs (with 95% CIs) for OS and RFS benefit of SDAC *vs.* HDAC, or HDAC *vs.* auto-BMT/allo-BMT was constructed using random-effects meta-analysis. We also performed additional analysis that stratified treatment options by cytogenetic characteristics. In such analysis,

patients were stratified into poor-, intermediate-, and favorable-risk groups by cytogenetic characteristics. OS and RFS benefits of HDAC for different cytogenetic risk groups were analyzed.

Results

Studies selected for meta-analysis

The initial search on MEDLINE (PubMed) database and the abstract review identified 643 articles. After the screening of titles and abstracts (by two reviewers L.W and G. XY), 160 non-relevant articles were excluded, which were those that were published in languages other than English, case reports, reviews, and studies on pediatrics AML. For the secondary search, the reference lists of review articles were manually examined to identify additional studies. The 483 selected articles were retrieved for further reviews in a structured format. As a result, 160 more articles were excluded, because those studies involved relapsed/refractory AML, APL, high-risk MDS, CML, therapy-related AML, myeloid sarcoma, or other concurrent diseases (including status of other concurrent tumors, definite MDS history) of AML that conflicted with the inclusion criteria. For the remaining 323

Table 2. Characteristics of Included Studies for consolidation therapy.

Source	Study ID	Enrollment Period	RCT	Multicenter	No. of patients	Median age/age range (years)	Consolidation therapy	follow-up (years)
JK. Weick et al. 1996 [8]	SWOG	1986–1991	Yes	Yes	287	45 (15–64)	DA (DNR+Ara-C 200 mg/m²/d×7) continuous 2 courses DA (DNR+Ara-C 3 g/m² q12 h×6) 1 course	4.3
K.F. Bradstock et al, 2005 [12]	ALLG	1995–2000	Yes	Yes	202	43 (15–60)	IcE (IDA+VP-16+Ara-c 100 mg/m²/d×5) continuous 2 courses ICE (IDA+VP-16+Ara-c 3 g/m² q12 h d1,3,5,7) 1 course	4
M. Fopp et al, 1997 [13]	SAKK	1985–1992	Yes	Yes	137	16–64	DA (DNR+Ara-C 100 mg/m²/d×7) 2 courses DA (DNR+Ara-C 3 g/m² q12 h×3) 1 course	6
PA. Cassileth et al, 1992 [14]	ECOG	1984–1988	Yes	Yes	170	15–65	TA (6-TG+Ara-c 60 mg/m²/d×5) AA (Amsa+Ara-c 3 g/m² h×3) (no courses in detail)	4
R.J.Mayer et al, 1994 [15]	CALGB	1985–1990	Yes	Yes	389	16–86★	SDAC (Ara-c 100 mg/m²/d×5) continuous 4 courses HDAC (Ara-c 3 g/m² q12 h×3) continuous 4 courses (no detail therapy)	4.3
S. Miyawaki et al, 2011b [4]▲	JALSG	2001–2005	Yes	Yes	781	15–64	DA, MA, AA, VEA (DNR, MTZ, Acl-a, VP-16, VCR+Ara-C200 mg/m²/dx5) continuous 4 courses HDAC (2 g/m² q12 h×5) continuous 3 courses	4
S, Ohtake et al, 2011a [16]▲	JALSG	2001–2005	Yes	Yes	781	15–64	DA, MA, AA, VEA (DNR, MTZ, Acl-a, VP-16, VCR+Ara-C200 mg/m²/dx5) continuous 4 courses HDAC (2 g/m² q12 h×5) continuous 3 courses	4
T. Büchner et al, 2003 [17]	CAMLCG	1992–1999	Yes	Yes	576	16–82★	TAD (6-TG, DNR, Ara-C200 mg/m²/dx5) continuous several courses HAM (MTZ+Ara-c 2 g/m² q12 h d1,2,8,9)	NR
CD. Bloomfield et al, 1998 [19]	CALGB	1985–1990	Yes	No	186	>16	Ara-C 100 mg/m²/dx5 continuous 4 courses Ara-c 3.0 g/m² q12 h d1,3,5 continuous 4 courses (no detail therapy)	5
X. Thomas et al, 2011 [20]	ALFA	1999–2006	Yes	Yes	237	15–50	AA (Amsa+Ara-C), TSC (MTZ+VP-16+Ara-C500 mg/m²/dx d8–10) continuous 2 course Ara-c 3.0 g/m² q12 h d1,3,5 continuous 4 courses	10
AM. Tsimberidu et al, 2003 [21]	HCG	1996–2000	No	No	120	15–60	Ara-c 3.0 g/m² q12 h d1,3,5 continuous 2 courses preparative regimen: BU+VP-16+CTX Allo-BMT/auto- SCT	5.3
JL. Harousseau et al, 1997 [22]	GOELAM	1987–1994	No	No	517	15–60	ICC (IDR+Ara-c 3.0 g/m² q12 h d1–4) continuous 2 courses preparative regimen: BU+CTX/TBI+CTX Allo-BMT/auto-SCT	8.5
PA. Cassileth et al, 1998 [23]	No	1990–1997	Yes	Yes※	808	16–55	Ara-c 3.0 g/m² q12 h d1–3 preparative regimen: CTX+BU Allo-BMT/auto-SCT	4
RA. Zittoun et al, 1995 [24]	GIMEMA	1986–1993	Yes	Yes※	623	33 (10–59)	AA (Amsa+Ara-c 2.0 g/m² d1–6) continuous 2 courses preparative regimen: CTX+TBI+/−BU Allo-BMT/auto-SCT	8
S. Brunet et al, 2004 [25]	Spain	1994–1999	No	No	200	15–60	Ara-c 3.0 g/m² q12 h d1–3 continuous 2 courses preparative regimen: CTX+TBI+/−BU Allo-BMT/auto-SCT	7
R. Bassan et al, 1998 [26]	Italy	1987–1993	No	No	108	15–60	Ara-c 2.0 g/m²/d d1–6 preparative regimen: Dox+TBI Allo-BMT/auto-SCT	>5
PA. Cassileth et al, 1992 [14]	ECOG	--	No	Yes※	534	44 (15–65)	Ara-c 3.0 g/m² q12 h d1–6 1 course preparative regimen: CTX+TBI Allo-BMT	6

Table 2. Cont.

Source	Study ID	Enrollment Period	RCT	Multicenter	No. of patients	Median age/age range (years)	Consolidation therapy	follow-up (years)
G.J. Schiller et al, 1992 [27]	----	1982–1990	No	No	103	16–45	MA, DA (MTZ, DNR+Ara-c 2.0–3.0 g/m² q12 h d1–4) 2–3 course preparative regimen: TBI+CTX/MTX/Ara-C Allo-BMT	8
J.L. Harousseau et al, 1991 [28]		1984–1987	No	Yes※	115	44 (13–65)	ICC (Amsa+Ara-c 3.0 g/m² q12 h d1–4) 2 course no preparative regimen Allo-BMT	7

Note: ▲ S. Miyawaki et al, 2011 repeated the same trial of S, Ohtake et al. 2011.
※BMT randomized trials were defined that if the patients didn't have donors, they were randomized into auto-BMT and high-dosed Ara-C groups.
★analyze analyze <60 years the patients in each trial.
Abbreviations: NR, not reported; IDA, idarubicin; Ara-c, cytarabin; VP-16, etoposide; DNR, daunorubicin MCT, multiagent chemotherapy; CTX, cyclophosphamide; MTZ, mitoxantrone; AZQ, diaziquone; 6-TG, thioguanine; AMS, amsacrine.

articles, full texts were further reviewed. A total of 256 articles were further excluded: 114 articles did not report data comparing the efficacy of HDAC on the OS and RFS of adult AML patients; 121 articles did not provide prospective data on OS and RFS outcome; and 21 articles used non-traditional chemotherapy regimens. The remaining 67 articles met the inclusion criteria. However, 22 articles were further excluded by experts, because the induction or consolidation therapy used in these studies were not consistent, along with confusing risk groups in some articles; 10 more articles were also excluded because only HDAC was used thus no comparison data available; and 4 articles were reporting the same trials [2,9,18,4]. As a result, a total of 22 articles passed through all examinations and were finally used for the meta-analysis in this study [Figure 1].

Quality Assessment

According to Cochrane methodology, the risk of bias of total RCT articles were assessed by Cochrane factors. The studies at low risk of bias had values (a quantitative index of the risk of bias, range 0–100%) of 64.3%, 64.3%, 0, 92.9%, 50%, 42.9%. (Figure S1).

HDAC versus SDAC in induction therapy

Four randomized controlled trials compared HDAC with SDAC in induction therapy [Table1]. In all 4 trials, the end points of CR, OS, and RFS were reported. Initial baseline characteristics between the treatment group and the control group were quite balanced. A total of 2,980 *de novo* AML patients enrolled from 1985 to 2005 were included. In the CAMLCG2009 and CAMLCG 2006 trials, the inclusion criteria for patient age were different from those of the rest of trials. Patients younger than 60 year-old were analyzed in the majority of trials. No significant differences in CR between patients received HDAC and those received SDAC [Figure 2] (HR = 1.01; 95% CI, 0.93–1.09; $P = 0.88$). The OS and RFS results were overall heterogeneous. In the trial ALSG 1996, OS and RFS were much longer in the HDAC group than those in the SDAC group. On the other hand, a larger number of patients receiving HDAC treatment showed shorter OS in the CAMLCG trial. Overall, no significant differences in OS were observed between HDAC and SDAC in the induction phase (HR = 0.83; 95% CI, 0.66–1.03; $P = 0.1$) [Figure 2]. Patients in the HDAC group showed similar OS as that of the SDAC group. However, a statistically significant difference in RFS was observed between HDAC and SDAC in the induction phase (HR = 0.57; 95% CI, 0.35–0.93; $P = 0.02$) [Figure 2]. Therefore, HDAC used in the induction therapy clearly improved RFS but not OS in AML patients.

HDAC versus SDAC in consolidation therapy

Nine trials were identified to contain the comparison of HDAC and SDAC in consolidation therapy [Table 2]. All 9 trials were randomized controlled studies, and 7 of them were multicenter trials. A total of 2,965 *de novo* AML patients enrolled from 1978 to 2005 were included, and the longest follow-up period of each trial was 10 years. Only patients younger than 60 year-old were analyzed. The initial baseline characteristics (age, sex, race, FAB classification, and cytogenetics) between two groups were similar, although detailed information about initial baseline characteristics in the ECOG1992 trial was not shown. In addition, only 1 course of HDAC was used in the SWOG1996 and SAKK1997 trials, different from all other trials. In 5 trials, HDAC was used concomitantly with other drugs, while 4 other trials only used single dose of Ara-C (2–3 g/m²), which may lead to heterogeneity among different trials. All the 9 trials reported end points of 4-year

A

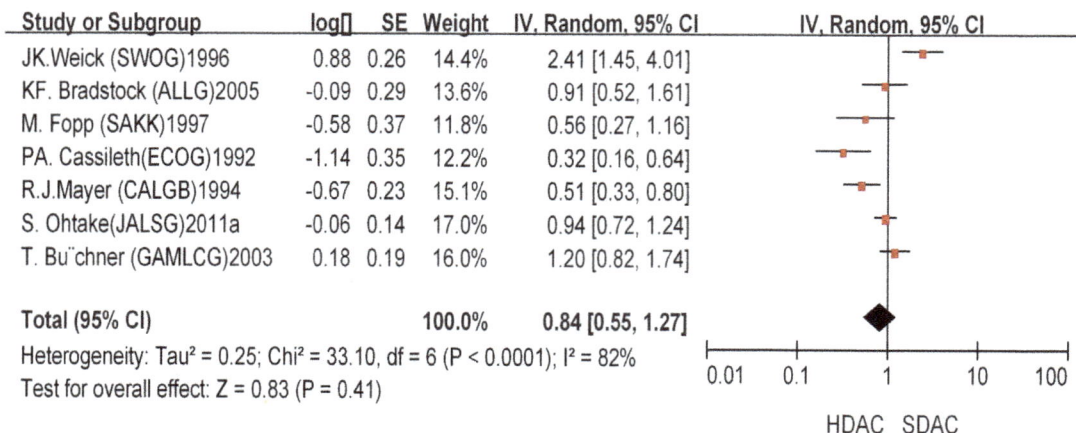

B

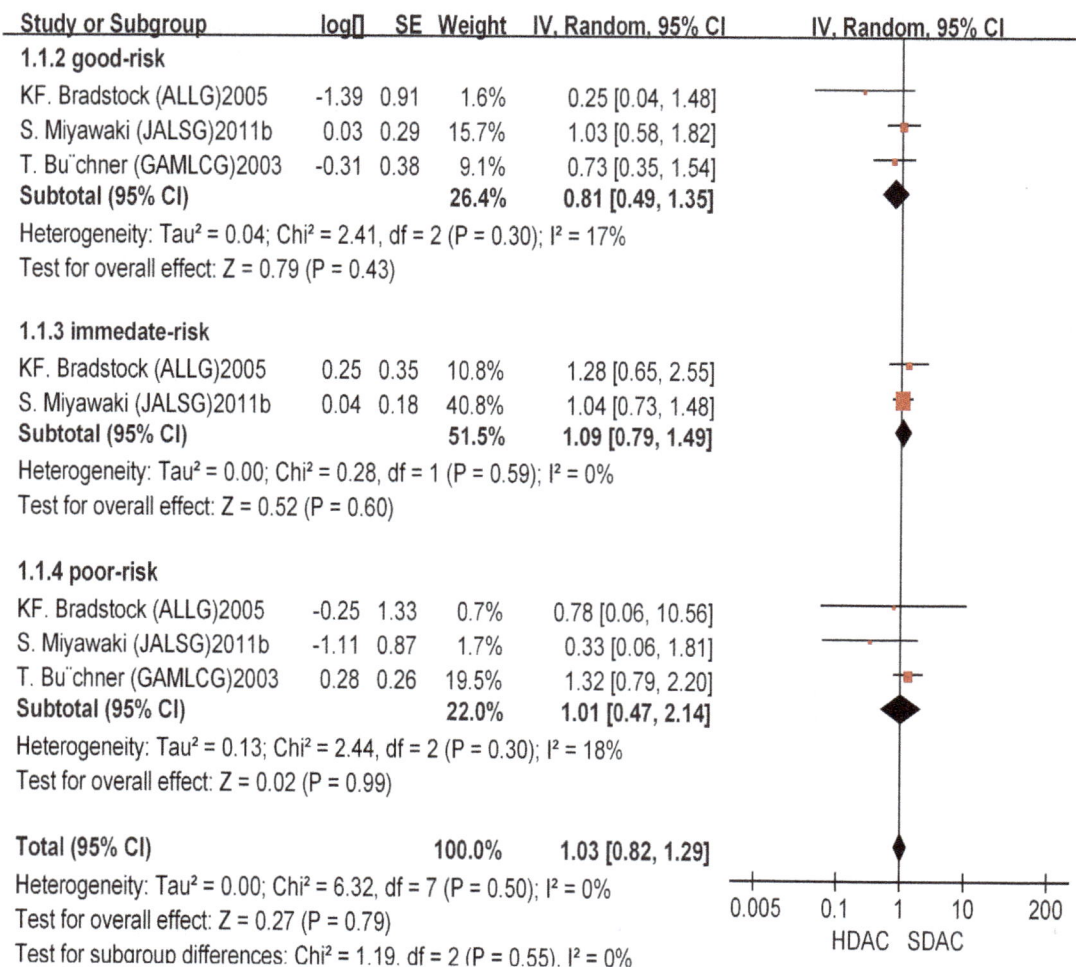

Figure 3. Overall survival benefit of HDAC in consolidation therapy. A: Total overall survival benefit of HDAC in consolidation therapy. **B**: Overall survival benefit of different subgroups of HDAC in consolidation therapy.

A

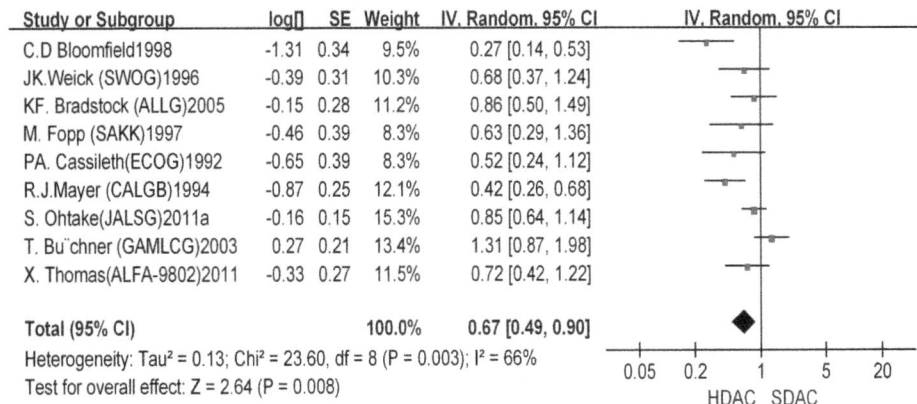

Study or Subgroup	log[]	SE	Weight	IV, Random, 95% CI
C.D Bloomfield1998	-1.31	0.34	9.5%	0.27 [0.14, 0.53]
JK.Weick (SWOG)1996	-0.39	0.31	10.3%	0.68 [0.37, 1.24]
KF. Bradstock (ALLG)2005	-0.15	0.28	11.2%	0.86 [0.50, 1.49]
M. Fopp (SAKK)1997	-0.46	0.39	8.3%	0.63 [0.29, 1.36]
PA. Cassileth(ECOG)1992	-0.65	0.39	8.3%	0.52 [0.24, 1.12]
R.J.Mayer (CALGB)1994	-0.87	0.25	12.1%	0.42 [0.26, 0.68]
S. Ohtake(JALSG)2011a	-0.16	0.15	15.3%	0.85 [0.64, 1.14]
T. Bu¨chner (GAMLCG)2003	0.27	0.21	13.4%	1.31 [0.87, 1.98]
X. Thomas(ALFA-9802)2011	-0.33	0.27	11.5%	0.72 [0.42, 1.22]
Total (95% CI)			100.0%	0.67 [0.49, 0.90]

Heterogeneity: Tau² = 0.13; Chi² = 23.60, df = 8 (P = 0.003); I² = 66%
Test for overall effect: Z = 2.64 (P = 0.008)

B

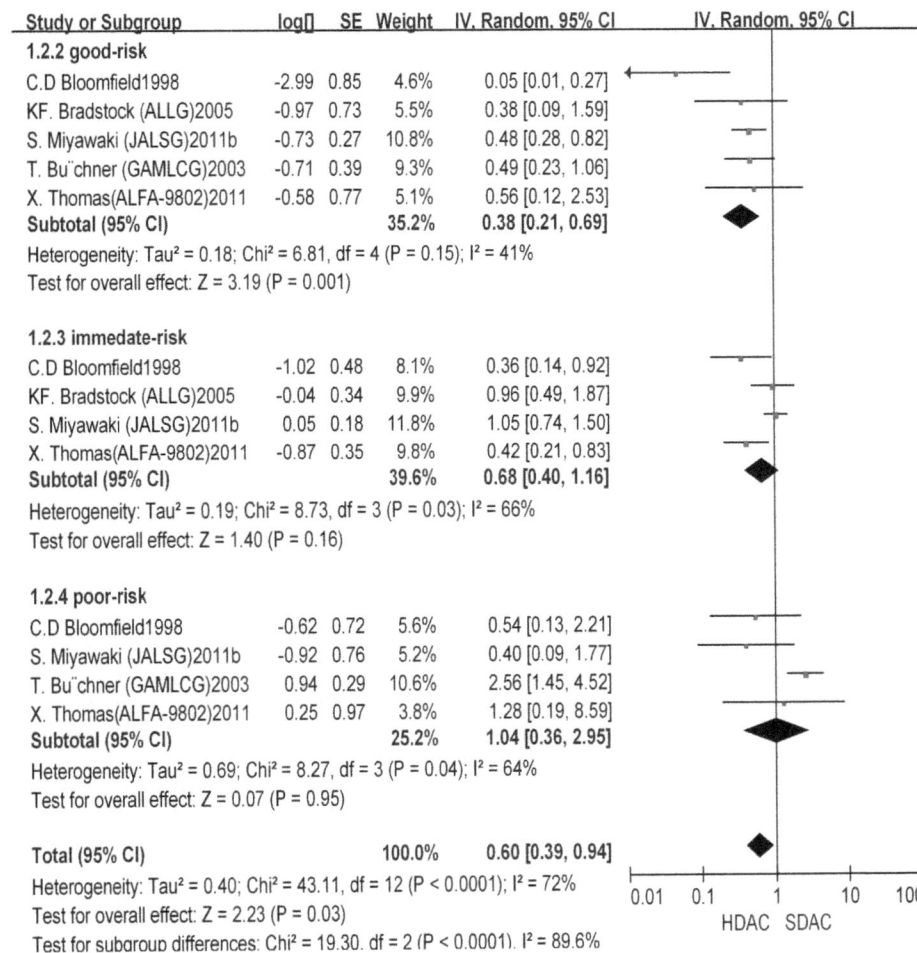

Study or Subgroup	log[]	SE	Weight	IV, Random, 95% CI
1.2.2 good-risk				
C.D Bloomfield1998	-2.99	0.85	4.6%	0.05 [0.01, 0.27]
KF. Bradstock (ALLG)2005	-0.97	0.73	5.5%	0.38 [0.09, 1.59]
S. Miyawaki (JALSG)2011b	-0.73	0.27	10.8%	0.48 [0.28, 0.82]
T. Bu¨chner (GAMLCG)2003	-0.71	0.39	9.3%	0.49 [0.23, 1.06]
X. Thomas(ALFA-9802)2011	-0.58	0.77	5.1%	0.56 [0.12, 2.53]
Subtotal (95% CI)			35.2%	0.38 [0.21, 0.69]

Heterogeneity: Tau² = 0.18; Chi² = 6.81, df = 4 (P = 0.15); I² = 41%
Test for overall effect: Z = 3.19 (P = 0.001)

1.2.3 immedate-risk				
C.D Bloomfield1998	-1.02	0.48	8.1%	0.36 [0.14, 0.92]
KF. Bradstock (ALLG)2005	-0.04	0.34	9.9%	0.96 [0.49, 1.87]
S. Miyawaki (JALSG)2011b	0.05	0.18	11.8%	1.05 [0.74, 1.50]
X. Thomas(ALFA-9802)2011	-0.87	0.35	9.8%	0.42 [0.21, 0.83]
Subtotal (95% CI)			39.6%	0.68 [0.40, 1.16]

Heterogeneity: Tau² = 0.19; Chi² = 8.73, df = 3 (P = 0.03); I² = 66%
Test for overall effect: Z = 1.40 (P = 0.16)

1.2.4 poor-risk				
C.D Bloomfield1998	-0.62	0.72	5.6%	0.54 [0.13, 2.21]
S. Miyawaki (JALSG)2011b	-0.92	0.76	5.2%	0.40 [0.09, 1.77]
T. Bu¨chner (GAMLCG)2003	0.94	0.29	10.6%	2.56 [1.45, 4.52]
X. Thomas(ALFA-9802)2011	0.25	0.97	3.8%	1.28 [0.19, 8.59]
Subtotal (95% CI)			25.2%	1.04 [0.36, 2.95]

Heterogeneity: Tau² = 0.69; Chi² = 8.27, df = 3 (P = 0.04); I² = 64%
Test for overall effect: Z = 0.07 (P = 0.95)

Total (95% CI)			100.0%	0.60 [0.39, 0.94]

Heterogeneity: Tau² = 0.40; Chi² = 43.11, df = 12 (P < 0.0001); I² = 72%
Test for overall effect: Z = 2.23 (P = 0.03)
Test for subgroup differences: Chi² = 19.30, df = 2 (P < 0.0001), I² = 89.6%

Figure 4. Relapse free survival benefit of HDAC in consolidation therapy. A: Total relapse free survival benefit of HDAC in consolidation therapy. **B:** Relapse free survival benefit of different subgroups of HDAC in consolidation therapy.

OS and RFS. The 4-year OS rate in the HDAC group ranged from 32%–71%. No significant differences in OS were observed between the HDAC and SDAC groups (HR = 0.84; 95% CI, 0.55–1.27; P = 0.41) [Figure 3]. However, patients that used HDAC in consolidation therapy showed longer RFS than those used SDAC (HR = 0.67; 95% CI, 0.49–0.9; P = 0.008) [Figure 4]. Therefore, HDAC improved RFS but did not affect OS in consolidation therapy.

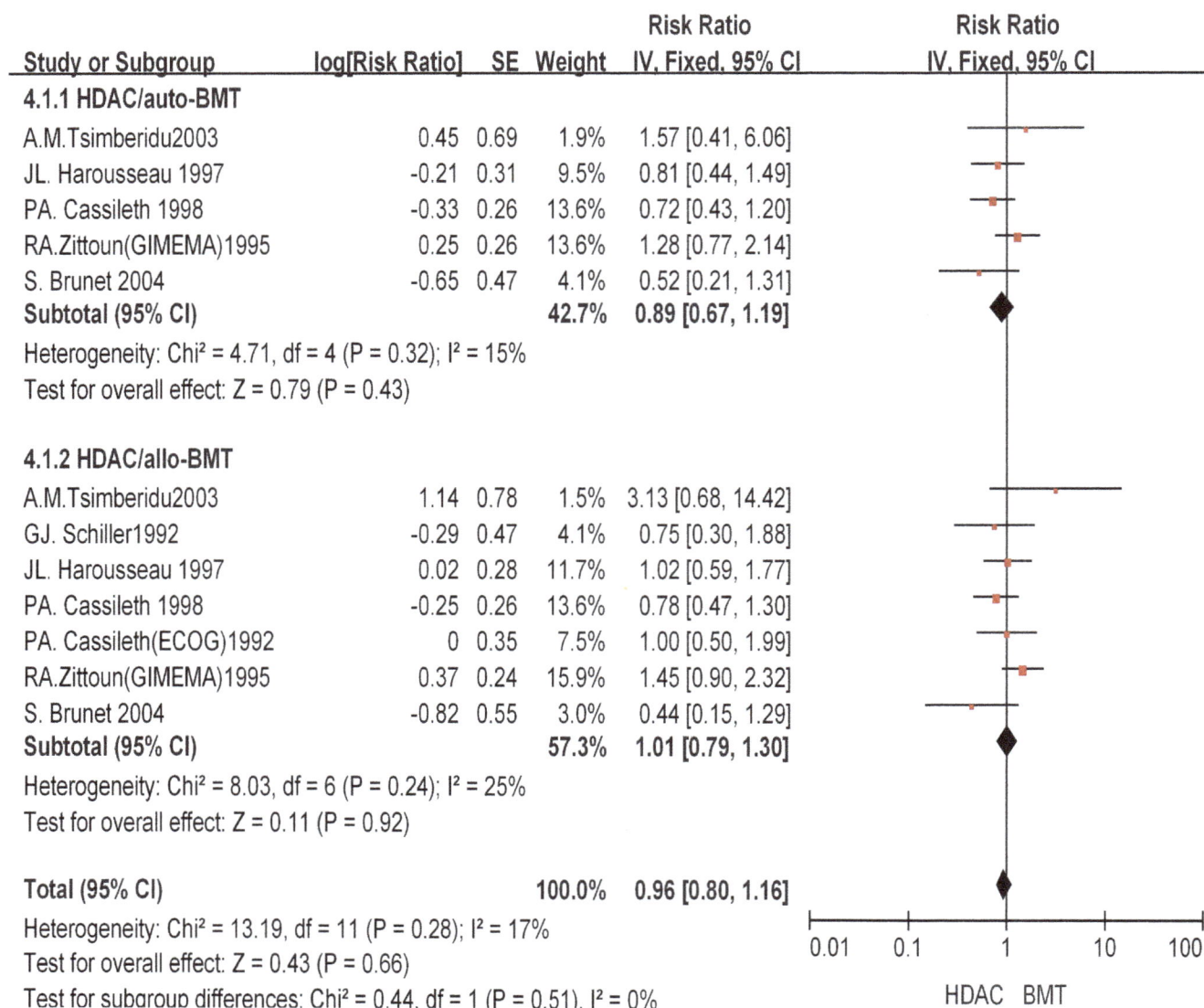

Study or Subgroup	log[Risk Ratio]	SE	Weight	Risk Ratio IV, Fixed, 95% CI
4.1.1 HDAC/auto-BMT				
A.M.Tsimberidu2003	0.45	0.69	1.9%	1.57 [0.41, 6.06]
JL. Harousseau 1997	-0.21	0.31	9.5%	0.81 [0.44, 1.49]
PA. Cassileth 1998	-0.33	0.26	13.6%	0.72 [0.43, 1.20]
RA.Zittoun(GIMEMA)1995	0.25	0.26	13.6%	1.28 [0.77, 2.14]
S. Brunet 2004	-0.65	0.47	4.1%	0.52 [0.21, 1.31]
Subtotal (95% CI)			**42.7%**	**0.89 [0.67, 1.19]**
Heterogeneity: Chi² = 4.71, df = 4 (P = 0.32); I² = 15%				
Test for overall effect: Z = 0.79 (P = 0.43)				
4.1.2 HDAC/allo-BMT				
A.M.Tsimberidu2003	1.14	0.78	1.5%	3.13 [0.68, 14.42]
GJ. Schiller1992	-0.29	0.47	4.1%	0.75 [0.30, 1.88]
JL. Harousseau 1997	0.02	0.28	11.7%	1.02 [0.59, 1.77]
PA. Cassileth 1998	-0.25	0.26	13.6%	0.78 [0.47, 1.30]
PA. Cassileth(ECOG)1992	0	0.35	7.5%	1.00 [0.50, 1.99]
RA.Zittoun(GIMEMA)1995	0.37	0.24	15.9%	1.45 [0.90, 2.32]
S. Brunet 2004	-0.82	0.55	3.0%	0.44 [0.15, 1.29]
Subtotal (95% CI)			**57.3%**	**1.01 [0.79, 1.30]**
Heterogeneity: Chi² = 8.03, df = 6 (P = 0.24); I² = 25%				
Test for overall effect: Z = 0.11 (P = 0.92)				
Total (95% CI)			**100.0%**	**0.96 [0.80, 1.16]**
Heterogeneity: Chi² = 13.19, df = 11 (P = 0.28); I² = 17%				
Test for overall effect: Z = 0.43 (P = 0.66)				
Test for subgroup differences: Chi² = 0.44, df = 1 (P = 0.51), I² = 0%				

Figure 5. Effect of HDAC versus BMT on overall survival.

We further performed stratified analysis for different subgroups. We restricted the stratification for cytogenetic risk (SWOG/ECOG, NCCN, and MRC) (Table S1). Five trials were included in the stratified analysis. A significant RFS benefit was observed with HDAC treatment (HR = 0.38; 95% CI, 0.21–0.69; P = 0.001) in the favorable-risk group [Figure 4]. However, no significant RFS benefit was shown with HDAC treatment in the immediate-risk and poor-risk groups (HR = 0.68; 95% CI, 0.4–1.16; P = 0.16; HR = 1.04; 95% CI, 0.36–2.95; P = 0.95). On the contrary, HDAC did not show any significant effects on OS as compared to SDAC. The OS with HDAC was not significantly different from that with SDAC treatment in all 3 stratified risk groups (HR = 0.81; 95% CI, 0.49–1.35; P = 0.43; HR = 1.09; 95% CI, 0.79–1.49; P = 0.6; HR = 1.01; 95% CI, 0.47–2.14; P = 0.99) [Figure 3].

HDAC versus BMT in consolidation therapy

Nine trials containing the comparison of the effect of HDAC treatment with that of auto-SCT/all-BMT were included in the analysis. They included 5 randomized trials and 4 observational trials. Randomized trials were defined as those in which patients who did not have donors would be randomly allocated into the HDAC and auto-SCT groups. Only 2 trials were multicentre trials. End points of OS and RFS were reported across all cytogenetic risk groups in all 9 trials, so we were not able to perform stratified analysis for different cytogenetic risk groups when evaluating OS and RFS outcomes. A total of 3,128 *de novo* AML patients enrolled from 1986 to 2000 were included. The longest follow-up period of each trial was 8.5 years [Table 2]. Of them, 29.8% patients received auto-SCT; 30.8% received allo-BMT; and 39.4% received HDAC. No imbalance in preparative regimen was observed between trials. The data were highly homogeneous in different studies concerning RFS endpoint ($I^2 = 0\%$). Only patients younger than 65 year-old were enrolled in the analysis considering the risk of transplantation.

This analysis revealed that the combined HR was 0.89 (95% CI, 0.67–1.19; P = 0.43), 1.01 (95% CI, 0.79–1.3; P = 0.92), and that patients received HDAC had an OS similar to that of patients received auto-SCT/allo-BMT in consolidation therapy [Figure 5].

Study or Subgroup	log[Risk Ratio]	SE	Weight	Risk Ratio IV, Random, 95% CI	Risk Ratio IV, Random, 95% CI
5.2.1 HDAC/auto-BMT					
A.M.Tsimberidu2003	0.37	0.72	2.7%	1.45 [0.35, 5.94]	
JL. Harousseau 1997	0.18	0.32	8.8%	1.20 [0.64, 2.24]	
PA. Cassileth 1998	0.5	0.27	10.5%	1.65 [0.97, 2.80]	
R.Bassan 1998	-0.02	0.51	4.8%	0.98 [0.36, 2.66]	
RA.Zittoun(GIMEMA)1995	0.59	0.26	10.9%	1.80 [1.08, 3.00]	
S. Brunet 2004	-0.29	0.47	5.4%	0.75 [0.30, 1.88]	
Subtotal (95% CI)			**43.1%**	**1.41 [1.06, 1.87]**	

Heterogeneity: Tau² = 0.00; Chi² = 3.82, df = 5 (P = 0.58); I² = 0%
Test for overall effect: Z = 2.39 (P = 0.02)

5.2.2 HDAC/allo-BMT					
A.M.Tsimberidu2003	1.7	0.8	2.2%	5.47 [1.14, 26.26]	
GJ. Schiller1992	0.31	0.47	5.4%	1.36 [0.54, 3.43]	
J.L. Harousseau 1991	0.03	0.57	4.0%	1.03 [0.34, 3.15]	
JL. Harousseau 1997	0.22	0.28	10.2%	1.25 [0.72, 2.16]	
PA. Cassileth 1998	1.32	0.28	10.2%	3.74 [2.16, 6.48]	
PA. Cassileth(ECOG)1992	0.55	0.36	7.7%	1.73 [0.86, 3.51]	
R.Bassan 1998	1.63	1.15	1.2%	5.10 [0.54, 48.62]	
RA.Zittoun(GIMEMA)1995	0.92	0.24	11.7%	2.51 [1.57, 4.02]	
S. Brunet 2004	0.03	0.54	4.4%	1.03 [0.36, 2.97]	
Subtotal (95% CI)			**56.9%**	**1.95 [1.35, 2.81]**	

Heterogeneity: Tau² = 0.13; Chi² = 14.68, df = 8 (P = 0.07); I² = 45%
Test for overall effect: Z = 3.56 (P = 0.0004)

Total (95% CI)			**100.0%**	**1.66 [1.30, 2.14]**	

Heterogeneity: Tau² = 0.08; Chi² = 22.20, df = 14 (P = 0.07); I² = 37%
Test for overall effect: Z = 4.00 (P < 0.0001)
Test for subgroup differences: Chi² = 3.70. df = 1 (P = 0.05). I² = 73.0%

0.01   0.1   1   10   100

HDAC   BMT

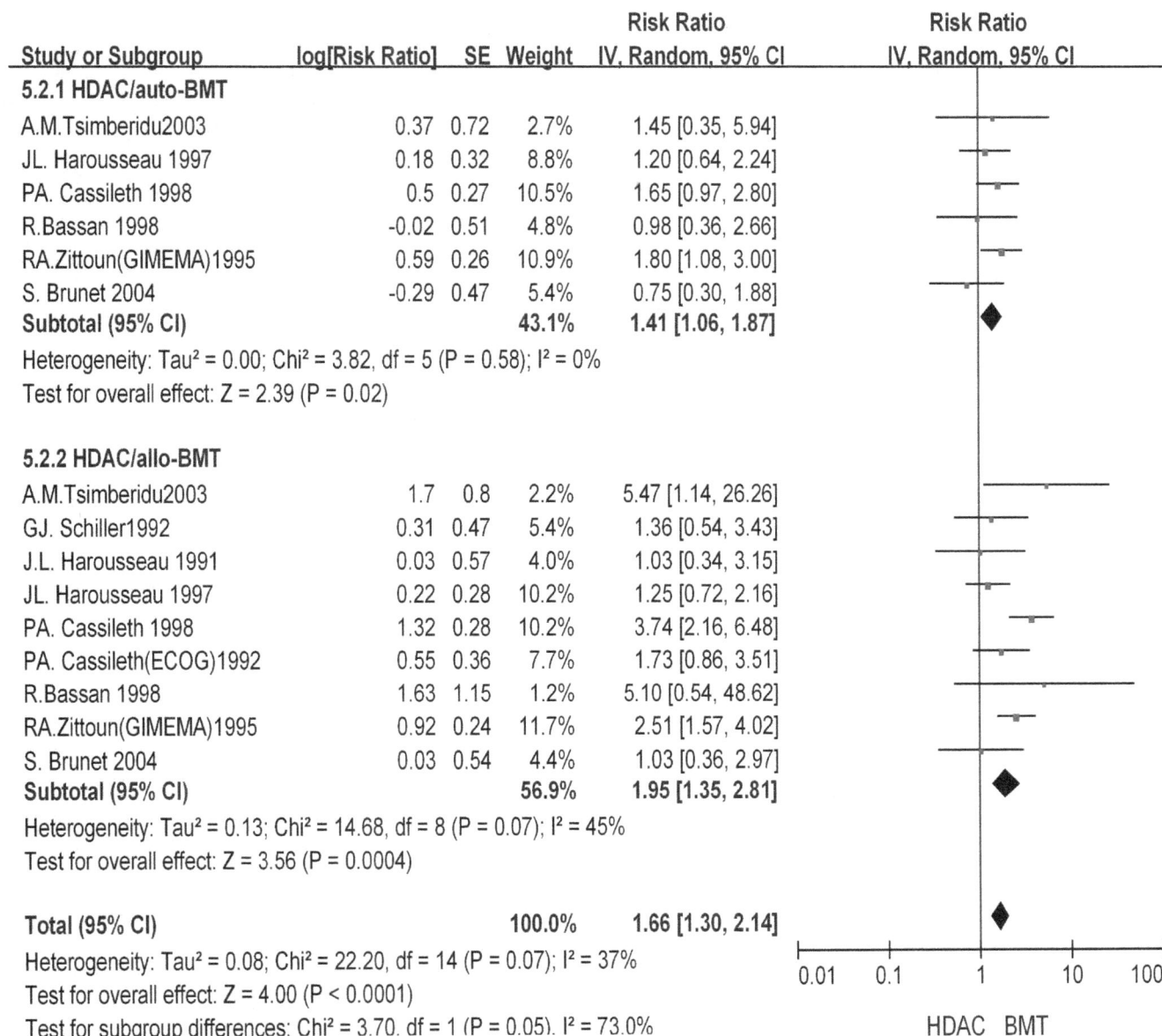

Figure 6. Effect of HDAC versus BMT on relapse free survival.

On the other hand, the RFS was significantly different between the auto-SCT/allo-BMT group and the HDAC group [Figure 6]. Auto-SCT had a combined HR of 1.41 (95% CI, 1.06–1.87; $P = 0.02$), while allo-BMT had a combined HR of 1.95 (95% CI, 1.35–2.81; $P = 0.0004$), indicating a significant RFS benefit of auto-SCT/allo-BMT over HDAC. Overall, the results indicated that auto-SCT/allo-BMT significantly reduced the hazard rate of relapse but failed to improve overall survival.

Discussion

In the past 20 years, Ara-C has been widely used in the induction and consolidation therapy for AML. Multiple prospective studies on Ara-C have been reported, and the application of HDAC has been tested extensively beyond first-line therapy and is considered a standard therapy. However, HDAC started to be questioned in recent studies with larger patient numbers. In this study, we performed a meta-analysis to address whether HDAC application in the induction and consolidation therapy prolongs RFS and decreases AML recurrence comparing with SDAC.

In a recent meta-analysis, 3 trials were analyzed, which discovered no differences in CR rates between HDAC and SDAC treatments. HDAC in induction therapy improved long-term disease control and OS in adults <60 years of age with *de novo* AML [29]. However, the effect of HDAC remains unclear in consolidation therapy, especially that for patients younger than 60 years. Therefore, we systematically collected all trials that used HDAC in both induction therapy and consolidation therapy from Jan. 1990 to Mar. 2013. The regimen of induction and consolidation therapy was restricted, which led to the exclusion of 20 articles containing different regimens of induction and consolidation therapy in HDAC and SDAC groups. All trials we identified were reported on an intent-to-treat basis and included a complete description of withdrawals and drop-outs. Some degrees of heterogeneity still existed in the age inclusion criterion. In one article, patients older than 60 years of age were not analyzed separately from patients younger than 60 years. However, this article was still included because the proportion of patients older than 60 years was very low. Based on the current data, we cannot conclude whether HDAC has the same effects on older patients. The dose of HDAC has also been questioned. In HOVON/SAKK study [30], Ara-C was used at 1.0 g/m^2 q12 h×6 days. In this meta-analysis, we limited HDAC at the dose level of 2.0–3.0 g/m^2 q12 h×3–5 days for the majority of trials.

Overall, endpoint heterogeneity within trials was limited. No evidence was found to support the notion that HDAC improves CR rate as compared to SDAC in induction therapy. However, our analysis revealed that HDAC had a clear benefit on RFS in induction therapy, consistent to the findings from ALSG and CAMLCG [8,10]. A retrospective analysis of CALGB and ECOG studies [14,15,31] discovered a survival advantage of HDAC in consolidation therapy over SDAC. However, our analysis failed to reach this conclusion. Data from the risk group stratified analysis demonstrated that HDAC significantly improved RFS in the favorable-risk group but no significant benefits in the intermediate and poor-risk groups. We also discussed the advantage of using BMT in consolidation therapy and discovered that auto-BMT/allo-BMT improved RFS, but not OS, as compared to HDAC.

In conclusion, this meta-analysis demonstrated that HDAC improved RFS in induction therapy while reducing the relapse rate in consolidation therapy, as compared with SDAC, especially for the favorable-risk group. Auto-BMT/Allo-BMT had a more beneficial effect in prolonging RFS as compared with HDAC. The analysis also posed some challenges to previous trial results. Overall, treatment with HDAC regimen did show some advantages for some outcome endpoints, especially in certain risk groups. However, it failed to show predominant advantages in all cases. Considering its high toxicity, caution should be taken when HDAC treatment regimen is chosen for patients. We also discovered varied degrees of heterogeneity within trials in our meta-analysis, which may interfere with the interpretation of results and limit the validity of the findings. In the future, more comprehensive clinical trails with improved study designs are needed to help elucidate the advantages and drawbacks of each treatment regimen in order to identify the optimal dose and treatment schedule for AML patients.

Acknowledgments

We thank Professor Taixiang Wu (Head of Chinese Clinical Trial Registry; Head of Research Manager. e-mail: txwutx@hotmail.com) for his technical support and careful reading.

Author Contributions

Conceived and designed the experiments: JW. Performed the experiments: WL XG. Analyzed the data: MS XZ. Contributed reagents/materials/analysis tools: BG. Contributed to the writing of the manuscript: YM HW.

References

1. Löwenberg B, Downing JR, Burnett A (1999) Acute myeloid leukemia. N Engl J Med. 341(14): 1051–1062.
2. Bishop JF, Matthews JP, Young GA, Szer J, Gillett A, et al. (1996) A randomized study of high-dose cytarabine in induction in acute myeloid leukemia. Blood. 87: 1710–1717.
3. Moore JO, George SL, Dodge RK, Amrein PC, Powell BL, et al. (2005) Sequential multiagent chemo- therapy is not superior to high-dose cytarabine alone as postremission intensification therapy for acute myeloid leukemia in adults under 60 years of age: Cancer and Leukemia Group B Study 9222. Blood. 105(9): 3420–7.
4. Miyawaki S, Ohtake S, Fujisawa S, Kivoi H, Shinaqawak K, et al. (2011) A randomized comparison of 4 courses of standard-dose multiagent chemotherapy versus 3 courses of high-dose cytarabine alone in post remission therapy for acute myeloid leukemia in adults: the JALSG AML201 Study. Blood. 117(8): 2366–72.
5. Löwenberg B (2013) Sense and nonsense of high-dose cytarabine for acute myeloid leukemia. Blood. 121(1): 26–28.
6. Parmar MK, Torri V, Stewart L (1998) Extracting summary statistics to perform meta-analyses of the published literature for survival endpoints. Stat Med. 17(24): 2815–2834.
7. Matthews JP, Bishop JF, Young GA, Juneia SK, Lowenthal RM, et al. (2001) Patterns of failure with increasing intensification of induction chemotherapy for acute myeloid leukaemia. Br J Haematol. 113(3): 727–36.
8. Weick JK, Kopecky KJ, Appelbaum FR, Head DR, Kingsbury LL, et al. (1996) A randomized investig- ation of high-dose versus standard-dose cytosine arabinoside with daunorubicin inpatients with previously untreated acute myeloid leukemia: a Southwest Oncology Group study. Blood. 88(8): 2841–51.
9. Büchner T, Berdel WE, Schoch C, Haferlach T, Serve HL, et al. (2006) Double induction containing either two courses or one course of high–dose cytarabine plus mitoxantrone and post remission therapy by either autologous stem-cell transplantation or by prolonged maintenance for acute myeloid leukemia. J Clin Oncol. 24(16): 2480–9.
10. Büchner T, Hiddemann W, Wörmann B, Löffler H, Gassmann W, et al. (1999) Double induction strategy for acute myeloid leukemia: the effect of high-dose cytarabine with mitoxantrone instead of standard-dose cytarabine with daunorubicin and 6-thioguanine: a randomized trial by the German AML Cooperative Group. Blood. 15; 93(12): 4116–24.
11. Büchner T, Berdel WE, Haferlach C, Haferlach T, Schnittger S, et al. (2009) Age-related risk profile and chemotherapy dose response in acute myeloid leukemia: a study by the German Acute Mye- loid Leukemia Coo-perative Group. J Clin Oncol. 27(1): 61–9.
12. Bradstock KF, Matthews JP, Lowenthal RM, Baxter H, Catalano J, et al. (2005) A randomized trial of high-versus conventional-dose cytarabine in consolidation chemotherapy for adult de novo acute myeloid leukemia in first remission after induction therapy containing high-dose cytarabine. Blood. 105(2): 481–8.
13. Fopp M, Fey MF, Bacchi M, Cavalli F, Gmuer J, et al. (1997) Post-remission therapy of adult acute myeloid leukaemia: one cycle of high-dose versus standard-dose cytarabine. Leukaemia Project Group of the Swiss Group for Clinical Cancer Research (SAKK). Ann Oncol. 8(3): 251–7.
14. Cassileth PA, Lynch E, Hines JD, Oken MM, Mazza JJ, et al. (1992) Varying intensity of post- remission therapy in acute myeloid leukemia. Blood. 79(8): 1924–30.
15. Mayer RJ, Davis RB, Schiffer CA, Berq DT, Powell BL, et al. (1994) Intensive postremission chemotherapy in adults with acute myeloid leukemia. Cancer and Leukemia Group B. N Engl J Med. 331(14): 896–903.
16. Ohtake S, Miyawaki S, Fujita H, Kiyoi H, Shinaqawa K, et al. (2011) Randomized study of induction therapy comparing standard-dose idarubicin with high-dose daunorubicin in adult patients with previously untreated acute myeloid leukemia: the JALSG AML201 Study. Blood. 117(8): 2358–65.
17. Büchner T, Hiddemann W, Berdel WE, Wörmann B, Schoch C, et al. (2003) 6-Thioguanine, cytarabine, and daunorubicin (TAD) and high–dose cytarabine and mitoxantrone (HAM) for induction, TAD for consolidation, and either prolonged maintenance by reduced monthly TAD or TAD-HAM-TAD and one course of intensive consolidation by sequential HAM in adult patients at all ages with de novo acute myeloid leukemia (AML): a randomized trial of the German AML Cooperative Group. J Clin Oncol. 21(24): 4496–504.
18. Schoch C, Haferlach T, Haase D, Fonatsch C, Löffler H, et al. (2001) Patients with de novo acute myeloid leukaemia and complex karyotype aberrations show a poor prognosis despite intensive treatment: a study of 90 patients. Br J Haematol. 112(1): 118–26.
19. Bloomfield CD, Lawrence D, Byrd JC, Carroll A, Pettenati MJ, et al. (1998) frequency of prolonged remission duration after high-dose cytarabine intensi-fication in acute myeloid leukemia varies by cytogenetic subtype. Cancer Res. Sep 15; 58(18): 4173–9.
20. Thomas X, Elhamri M, Raffoux E, Renneville A, Pautas C, et al. (2011) Comparison of high-dose cytarabine and timed-sequential chemotherapy as consolidation for younger adults with AML in first remission: the ALFA-9802 study. Blood. 118(7): 1754–1762.

21. Tsimberidu AM, Stavroyianni N, Viniou N, Papaioannou M, Tiniakou M, et al. (2003) Comparison of Allogeneic Stem Cell Transplantation, High-Dose Cytarabine, and Autologous Peripheral Stem Cell Transplantation as Post-remission Treatment in Patients with De Novo Acute Myelogenous Leukemia. Cancer. 97(7): 1721–1731.

22. Harousseau JL, Cahn JY, Pignon B, Witz F, Milpied N, et al. (1997) Chemotherapy as Postremission Therapy in Adult Acute Myeloid Leukemia Comparison of Autologous Bone Marrow Transplant- ation and Intensive. Blood. 90(8): 2978–2986.

23. Cassileth PA, Arington DP, Appelbaum FR, Lazarus HM, Rowe JM, et al. (1998) Chemotherapy compared with autologous or allogeneic bone marrow transplantation in the management of acute myeloid leukemia in first remission. N Engl J Med. 339: 1649–56.

24. Zittoun RA, Mandelli F, Willemze R, de Witte T, Labar B, et al. (1995) autologous or allogeneic bone marrow transplantion compared with intensive chemotherapy in acute myelogenous leukemia. N Engl J Med. 332: 217–23.

25. Brunet S, Esteve J, Berlanga J, Ribera JM, Bueno J, et al. (2004) Treatment of primary acute myeloid leukemia: results of a prospective multicenter trial including high-dose cytarabine or stem cell transplantation as post-remission strategy. Haematologica. 89: 940–949.

26. Bassan R, Raimondi R, Lerede T, D'emilio A, Buelli M, et al. (1998) Outcome assessment of age group-specific ($\pm$50 years) post-remission consolidation with high-dose cytarabine or bone marrow autograft for adult acute myelogenous leukemia. Haematologica. 83: 627–635.

27. Schiller GJ, Nimer SD, Territo MC, Ho WG, Champlin RE, et al. (1992) Bone Marrow Transplant- ation Versus High-Dose Cytarabine-based consolidation chemotherapy for acute myelogenous leukemia in First Remission. J Clin Oncol. 10(1): 41–46.

28. Harousseau JL, Milpied N, Briere J, Desablens B, Leprise PY, et al. (1991) Double Intensive Consolid -ation Chemotherapy in Adult Acute Myeloid Leukemia. J Clin Oncol. 9: 1432–1437.

29. Kern W, Estey EH (2006) High-dose cytosine arabinoside in the treatment of acute myeloid leukemia. Cancer. 107: 116–24.

30. Löwenberg B, Pabst T, Vellenga E, van Putten W, Schouten HC, et al. (2011) Cytarabine dose for acute myeloid leukemia. N Engl J Med. 364: 1027–1036.

31. Farag SS, Ruppert AS, Mrózek K, Mayer RJ, Stone RM, et al. (2005) Outcome of induction and postremission therapy in younger adults with acute myeloid leukemia with normal karyotype: a cancer and leukemia group B study. J Clin Oncol. 23(3): 482–93.

20

GroupRank: Rank Candidate Genes in PPI Network by Differentially Expressed Gene Groups

Qing Wang[1], Siyi Zhang[1], Shichao Pang[1], Menghuan Zhang[1], Bo Wang[1], Qi Liu[1,2,3]*, Jing Li[1,4]*

1 Department of Bioinformatics & Biostatistics, School of Life Science and Biotechnology, Shanghai Jiao Tong University, Shanghai, China, 2 Department of Biomedical Informatics, Vanderbilt University School of Medicine, Nashville, Tennessee, United States of America, 3 Center for Quantitative Sciences, Vanderbilt University School of Medicine, Nashville, Tennessee, United States of America, 4 Shanghai Center for Bioinformation Technology, Shanghai, China

Abstract

Many cell activities are organized as a network, and genes are clustered into co-expressed groups if they have the same or closely related biological function or they are co-regulated. In this study, based on an assumption that a strong candidate disease gene is more likely close to gene groups in which all members coordinately differentially express than individual genes with differential expression, we developed a novel disease gene prioritization method GroupRank by integrating gene co-expression and differential expression information generated from microarray data as well as PPI network. A candidate gene is ranked high using GroupRank if it is differentially expressed in disease and control or is close to differentially co-expressed groups in PPI network. We tested our method on data sets of lung, kidney, leukemia and breast cancer. The results revealed GroupRank could efficiently prioritize disease genes with significantly improved AUC value in comparison to the previous method with no consideration of co-exprssed gene groups in PPI network. Moreover, the functional analyses of the major contributing gene group in gene prioritization of kidney cancer verified that our algorithm GroupRank not only ranks disease genes efficiently but also could help us identify and understand possible mechanisms in important physiological and pathological processes of disease.

Editor: Raya Khanin, Memorial Sloan Kettering Cancer Center, United States of America

Funding: The authors acknowledge the support by National Natural Science Foundation of China (31271416, 31000582, J1210047), National Key Basic Research Program (2011CB910204). Additional support from Pujiang Talent Program (12PJ1406600) and Program for "Chen Xing" Young Scholars, Shanghai Jiao Tong University. The funders had no role in study design, data collection and analysis, decision to publish, or preparation of the manuscript.

Competing Interests: The authors have declared that no competing interests exist.

* Email: qi.liu@vanderbilt.edu (QL); jing.li@sjtu.edu.cn (JL)

Background

It remains a big challenge to detect associations between diseases and genes although many disease candidate genes haven been reported through genetic studies such as linkage analysis [1] and association studies [2]. Prioritizing genes according to their likelihood of being disease genes using computational methods can help biologists find the most promising candidate genes for further downstream verification. Many tools have been developed, most of which use a guilt-by-association concept that ranks highest candidate genes similar to known disease genes.

Among them, Endeavour is a well-developed tool that ranks the candidates against the profile of the training set of genes known to be involved in a biological process or a disease of interest, combining 20 data sources such as functional annotations, expression data, regulatory information, literature, pathways, interactions, sequence, and disease probabilities [3,4]. In a variety of data sources, fast accumulating protein-protein interaction (PPI) data is a valuable resource for gene prioritization because the genes tend to be highly connected in the protein-protein interaction network when they are related to a specific biological function or similar disease phenotype [5]. Some tools have been developed to perform gene prioritization using this network and have performed well, including CGI [6], GeneWanderer [7], and DIR [8]. For example, comprising the interactions from HPRD [9], BIND [10], BioGrid [11], IntAct [12] and DIP [13],

GeneWanderer ranks candidate genes using a global network distance measure and random walk analysis for the definition of similarities to known disease genes in protein-protein interaction networks.

But the gene prioritization methods that measure the similarities to known disease genes by guilt-by-association or network distance cannot be applied accurately for a rare or even unknown disease gene. Recently, some efforts have been made to combine PPI network and global gene expression to conduct gene prioritization, the assumption of which is that nodes neighboring to differentially expressed genes are disease gene candidates [14,15]. The advantage of this kind of methods is that no prior knowledge about the biological process or disease genes is needed as a training set. However, we found that there is a risk of high false positive rates and low robustness when candidate genes are close to only a single gene with dramatic change in expression.

Genes usually show co-expression if they have the same or a closely related biological function or are co-regulated by the same transcript factor. In order to prioritize disease genes more precisely and robustly, we proposed a new algorithm called GroupRank to rank disease genes by integrating PPI network and gene groups clustered by coordinately differential expression. Our assumption is that, as well as differentially expressing in cases and controls, a strong disease gene candidate is more likely close to gene groups in which all members coordinately differentially express than to individual ones. To verify this assumption and evaluate the

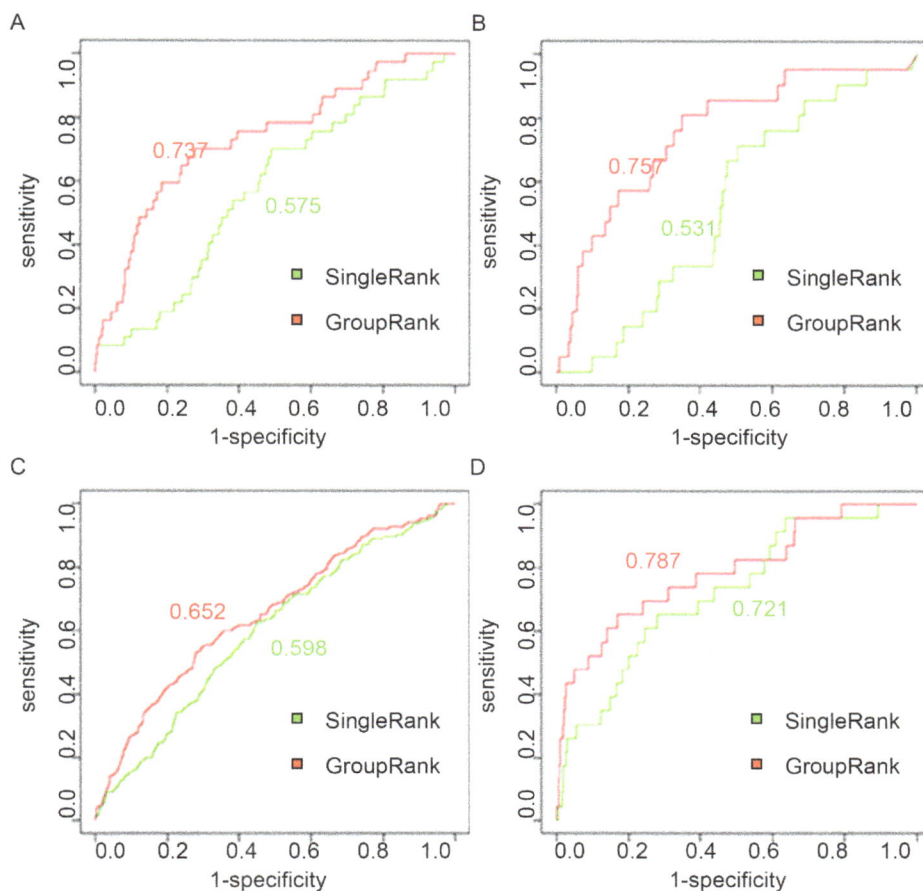

Figure 1. Mean rank ratio of GroupRank using different distance thresholds. The gene groups in GroupRank are partitioned based on a distance threshold with a gradient from 0.1 to 0.9. From A to D, the cancer types are lung cancer, kidney cancer, leukemia and breast cancer.

performance of our method, we applied GroupRank into the gene expression datasets of four cancer types including lung, kidney, leukemia and breast cancer.

Materials and Methods

Gene expression data collection

Four microarray gene expression datasets of humans in case-control design were downloaded from the NCBI Gene Expression Omnibus (GEO) [16] for lung cancer (GSE12428), kidney cancer (GSE6344), leukemia (GSE10631), and breast cancer (GSE29270). All these datasets were curated and reported in the GEO Datasets (GDS). More details about these datasets were summarized in Table S1.

Cancer gene list

We collected disease genes of lung, kidney, leukemia, and breast cancer respectively from OMIM [17] and Cancer Gene Census [18] (see Table S2). The OMIM database provides the connections between genes and lots of diseases. Cancer Gene Census is an ongoing effort to catalogue those genes for which mutations have been causally implicated in cancer.

PPI network

We used HINT as a protein-protein interaction network that is a database of high-quality protein-protein interactions in different organisms (http://hint.yulab.org/) [19]. These PPI links have been compiled from different sources and then filtered both systematically and manually to remove erroneous and low-quality interactions. There are 27493 binary and 7629 co-complex interactions in HINT for *H.sapiens*.

Differential expression analysis

The statistical analysis of gene differential expression was computed by Student t-test and Bonferroni correction was applied. Only the genes having a corrected p-value less than 0.05 remained in the following gene grouping.

Gene grouping

In GroupRank, we first clustered the differentially expressed genes into the co-expressed groups. We defined the distance between two genes by $d = 1 - |Cor_{ij}|$. Here Cor_{ij} represents the Pearson correlation coefficient of the expression of gene i and gene j. Then, hierarchical clustering was applied to partition the differentially expressed genes into groups. The sizes and the number of groups are changed by adjusting the threshed of gene distance d within a group from 0 to 1.

Performance measurement

We measured the performance of ranking algorithms using the method described by Zhao *et al* (2011) [15]. Briefly, for a known disease gene in a candidate gene set of size N, if the predicted ranking position is r, then the rank ratio r/N may reflect how well this gene is ranked as a disease gene by our algorithm. Lower rank ratio represents better predictive performance. Optimized parameters could be determined through minimizing the average rank ratio of all known disease genes. In addition, we applied the receiver operating characteristics (ROC) analysis [18] [20] to evaluate the overall performance.

Algorithm of GroupRank

First, we defined the similarity matrix of genes by adopting *discrete diffusion kernel* from the Diffusion Rank algorithm reported by Yang et al. [21].

As described in Pinta [14], the transition probability matrix W of a random walk on a given graph G is defined as $W = D^{-1}A$. A is the adjacency matrix and D is the diagonal matrix of G. Consider $L = I - W$, and then we obtain the similarity matrix of genes

$$S = (I + \frac{-\alpha}{N}L)^N \qquad (1)$$

where parameter α is the diffusion rate, and N is the number of iterations. In this paper, we set $\alpha = 0.5$ and $N = 3$ as the previous studies found that few iterations is sufficient to reach a considerably good performance [14,22].

Then, from the genes differentially expressed in cancer and normal control, we classify them into co-expressed gene groups by hierarchical clustering. When ranking a candidate gene using a gene group G_i in the PPI network, we define the rank score of a candidate gene obtained from group G_i as

$$r_i = e * s^{(1/log_2^{(1+n)})} \qquad (2)$$

where s is the similarity score between the candidate gene and group G_i, which is measured with the geometric mean of the values in the similarity matrix S between the candidate gene and each member in group G_i. Parameter e represents the differential expression level of the gene group, which is computed by the geometric mean of log2 ratio (cancer/control) of each gene within the group G. n is the group size.

In the analysis of the active gene subnetwork of disease, highly connected nodes are often penalized and the size of the subnetwork is controlled [23]. To avoid bias and control possible false positives in the gene ranking that result from either the super group containing large numbers of gene members or the extremely high degree of the candidate gene itself as a hub in the PPI network, we adopted the method of Gaire et al [23] and added adjustable penalization parameters n_0 and k_0 into the following modified formula (3):

$$r_i = \frac{e * s^{(1/log_2^{(1+n)})}}{1 + log_{n_0}^n * log_{k_0}^k} \qquad (3)$$

k is the degree of the candidate gene in network HINT. The smaller n_0 and k_0 are, the more stringent penalization is carried to the hub genes and the co-expressed group with super-size. Since the mean degree of network HINT is 6.7, we set $k_0 = 15$, and $n_0 = 20$ as default values in this paper.

Finally, the integrated ranking score of a candidate gene contributed by all gene groups is calculated as

$$r = \sum r_i \qquad (4)$$

Results and Discussion

Performance evaluation

We tested GroupRank in four cancer related microarray datasets (lung, kidney, leukemia, and breast cancer) individually. Mean rank ratio (MRR) of known disease genes predicted by our algorithm was used to evaluate its overall performance. By adjusting the threshold of distance d from 0 to 1 with the gradient of 0.01 in defining a gene group, the best MRR was obtained when an optimized threshold was chosen (Table 1). In the results, the best thresholds of distance for different cancer types fell into 0.2–0.6 (Figure 1). A possible explanation is that using a more rigorous threshold, there are not enough effective groups that can be formed, while all genes are possibly classified into very few super groups with poor correlations if a more relaxed threshold is applied.

We compared the performance of GroupRank with the previous similar method that ranks candidate genes based on individual expressed genes in the PPI network [14]. To distinguish from GroupRank, we called this method SingleRank. As the results show in Figure2, the MRR of known disease genes predicted using GroupRank was lower than SingleRank in each testing dataset when a fixed distance threshold of 0.5 was used. We ran a paired Wilcoxon test and revealed that the improvement of MRR brought by GroupRank algorithm was significant (p-value< 0.001).

Additionally we plotted ROC curves to compare GroupRank and SingleRank. Figure 3 shows that GroupRank achieved AUC values from 0.65 to 0.80 in four cancers, which were higher than the values from SingleRank. The results suggest that GroupRank using co-expressed gene groups is a more efficient approach than the method simply using the individual genes in disease gene ranking. It implies that gene prioritization by gene groups could reduce noise and achieve better accuracy.

Table 1. MRR of GroupRank in four cancer types.

Cancer type	Lung cancer	Kidney cancer	Leukemia	Breast cancer
MRR	0.257	0.227	0.298	0.192
Optimized distance	0.42	0.60	0.52	0.24

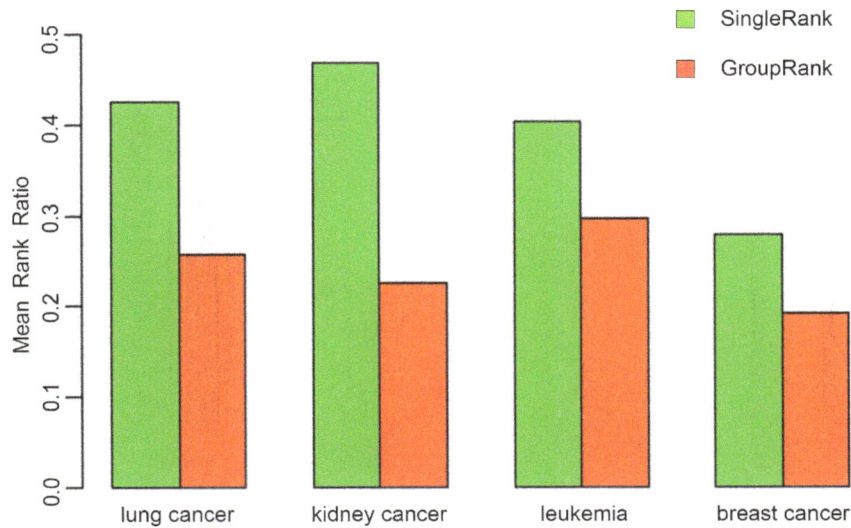

Figure 2. MRR comparisons of GroupRank and SingleRank. The colored bar chart shows the mean rank ratio (MRR) in disease gene ranking using GroupRank (red) and SingleRank (green). It indicates that GroupRank performs better with a lower MRR (p-value<0.001).

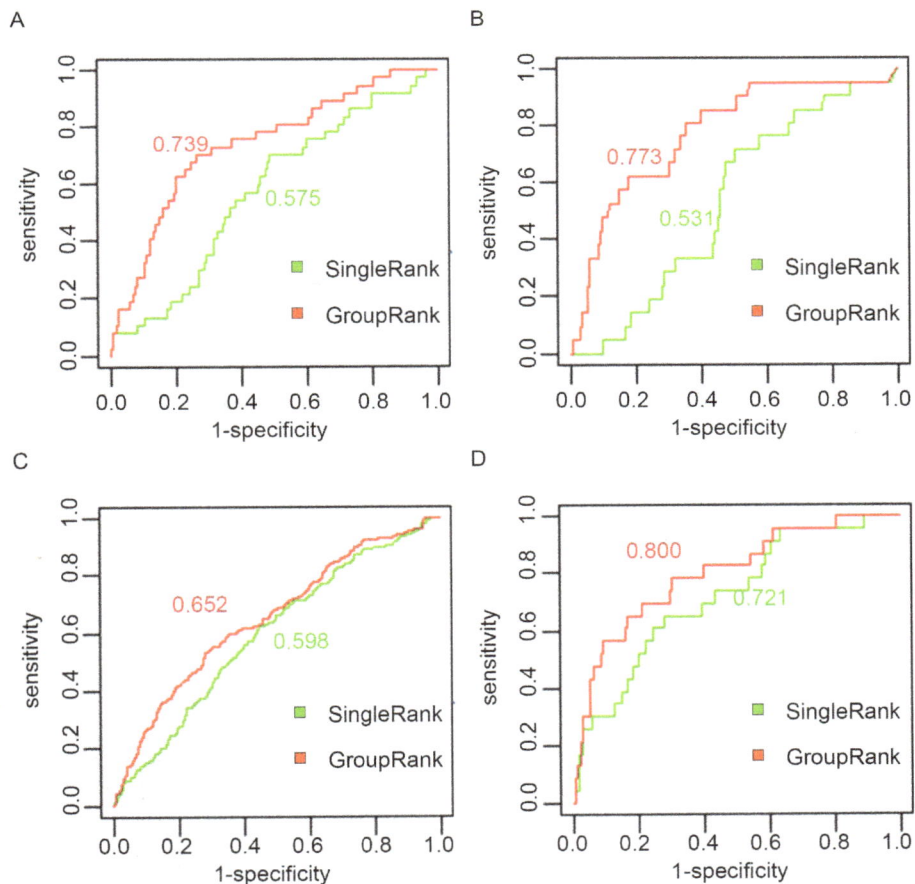

Figure 3. ROC curves of GroupRank and SingleRank. Performance validation using ROC curves. The AUC values of GroupRank and SingleRank achieved in each cancer type are labeled. From A to D, the cancer types are lung cancer, kidney cancer, leukemia and breast cancer.

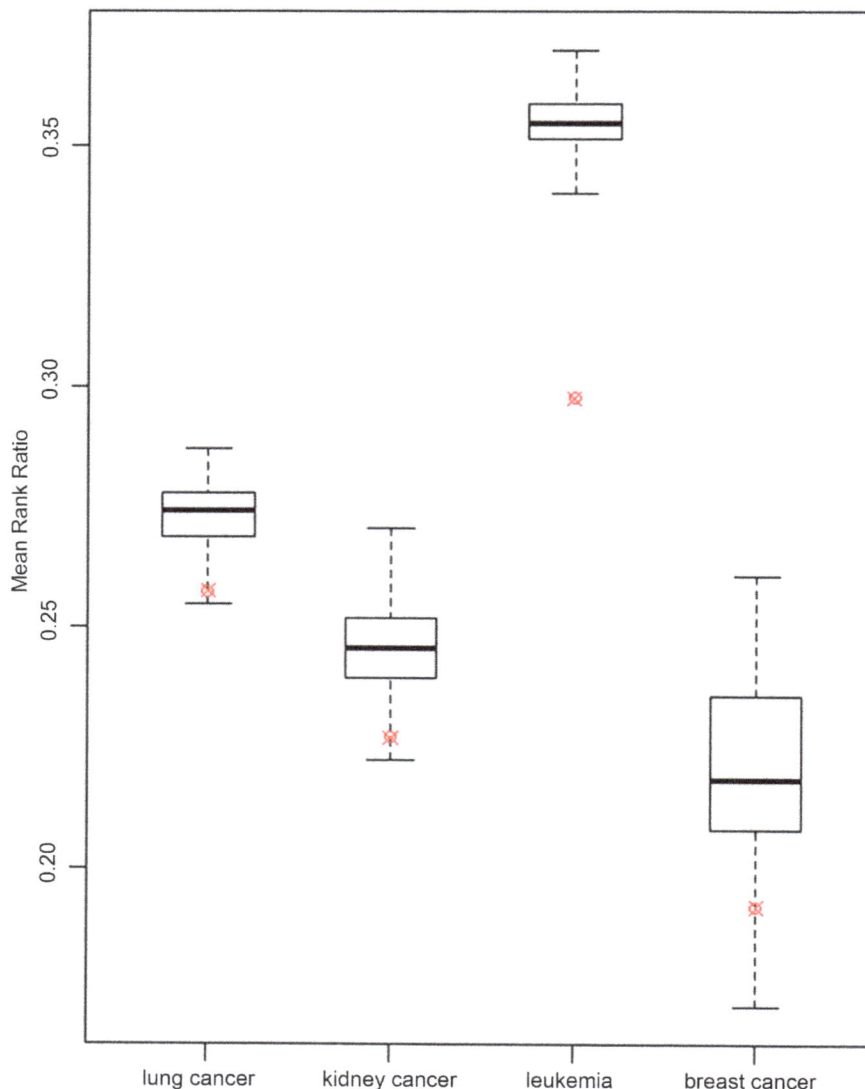

Figure 4. MRR Comparisons of GroupRank using co-expressed and random groups. The red sign represents MRR of GroupRank using co-expressed gene groups in four cancers. Boxplots show the distributions of MRRs using random groups of the same size. The random sampling was repeated 1000 times in each cancer type.

Grouping Efficiency by co-expression

In the GroupRank algorithm, we assumed that the differentially co-expressed gene groups are surrounding a good disease gene and thus are effective to rank disease gene candidates. In order to validate this assumption, we compared the ranking performance using co-expressed and random gene groups. The random groups having the same size were generated by randomly sampling from the PPI network. We repeated the sampling 1000 times. The results indicate that, in all four cancers we studied, the mean rank ratios using co-expressed groups are significantly better than using random gene groups (p-value<0.05) (see Figure 4). It suggested that the downstream genes of a strong disease gene tend to be co-expressed into a number of groups.

Major contributing groups in gene ranking

In the GroupRank algorithm, the co-expressed gene groups comprising the most significantly changed gene members in

cancers and normal controls must play major roles in cancer. Looking at it from another angle, further study on those major contributing groups can help us to explore and understand why a candidate gene is listed in the top rank and which pathway or biological process is influenced by this disease gene candidate in the disease condition. In this paper, kidney cancer was taken as an example, and we investigated the gene groups, especially the major contributing groups in the ranking of the top 20 gene candidates and 21 known kidney cancer genes. As illustrated in Figure 5, based on the accumulated contributions in ranking scores of known tumor genes using GroupRank, four gene groups emerged by explaining 64.7% of the ranking scores of all 21 known kidney cancer genes. We found that the top 20 ranked genes also had strong connections with those four groups. That indicates that these four gene groups are closely related with kidney cancer. We did GO enrichment analysis of these groups using WebGestalt [24] and found that these gene groups, which were differentially expressed in kidney cancer, are involved in cell proliferation,

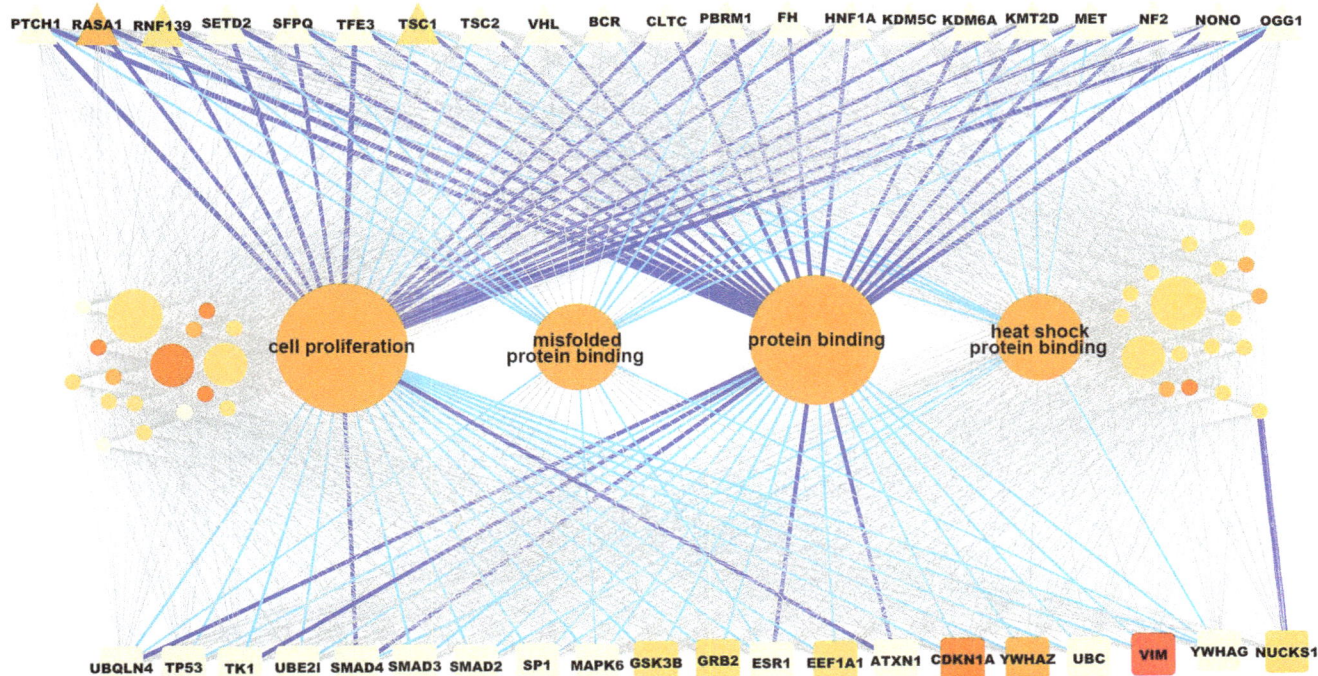

Figure 5. Schematic graph of gene ranking of kidney cancer using GroupRank. The graph illustrates gene ranking of kidney cancer using the algorithm GroupRank. The triangle nodes at the top represent known kidney cancer genes and the square nodes at the bottom represent the top 20 ranked genes of kidney cancer using GroupRank. The circle nodes in middle represent the co-expressed gene groups used to rank disease gene candidates. A known or putative cancer gene is connected with a gene group if it contributes more than 5% of the summed ranking score of this cancer gene. The width of the edge linked to a disease gene is proportional to the scoring contribution obtained from the corresponding gene group. The edges explaining more than 20% of the ranking score of the cancer gene candidate are highlighted in dark blue. The edge is colored in light blue if the scoring contribution of the gene group is from 15% to 20%. The darker node color indicates higher fold change at expression level in cancer and normal control. The size of the circle node representing gene group was proportional to its accumulated contribution in ranking scores of all known kidney cancer genes. The enriched functional annotation is labeled on each of the four major contributing gene groups.

protein binding, misfolded protein binding, and heat shock protein binding respectively (p-value<0.05, bonferroni multiple testing adjustment). It was reported by Short *et al.* (1993) that enhanced cell proliferation occurs at several stages of renal tumorigenesis [25]. Heat shock proteins (Hsps) are overexpressed in a wide range of human cancers and are implicated in tumor cell proliferation, differentiation, invasion, metastasis, death, and recognition by the immune system [26]. Misfolded proteins were also reported in the study of cancer, and targeted degradation of misfolded proteins has become one of the promising new therapeutic approaches in the treatment of cancer [27].

contributing groups in ranking may not only help us predict disease gene candidates but also improve the biological interpretation of data.

Conclusion

In this study, by combining PPI network and gene differential expression and co-expression data, we proposed a new algorithm GroupRank, in which disease candidate genes were ranked by the surrounding differentially co-expressed gene groups in PPI network. The results demonstrated that GroupRank could improve the accuracy of disease gene prioritization significantly. Furthermore, the further functional analysis of the major

Acknowledgments

The authors wish to thank Margot Bjoring for editorial work on this Manuscript.

Author Contributions

Conceived and designed the experiments: QW QL JL. Performed the experiments: QW SZ SP BW. Analyzed the data: QW BW MZ. Wrote the paper: QW QL JL.

References

1. Kruglyak L, Daly MJ, Reeve-Daly MP, Lander ES (1996) Parametric and nonparametric linkage analysis: a unified multipoint approach. Am J Hum Genet 58: 1347–1363.

2. Klein RJ, Zeiss C, Chew EY, Tsai JY, Sackler RS, et al. (2005) Complement factor H polymorphism in age-related macular degeneration. Science 308: 385–389.

3. Aerts S, Lambrechts D, Maity S, Van Loo P, Coessens B, et al. (2006) Gene prioritization through genomic data fusion. Nat Biotechnol 24: 537–544.

4. Tranchevent LC, Barriot R, Yu S, Van Vooren S, Van Loo P, et al. (2008) ENDEAVOUR update: a web resource for gene prioritization in multiple species. Nucleic Acids Res 36: W377–384.

5. Gandhi TK, Zhong J, Mathivanan S, Karthick L, Chandrika KN, et al. (2006) Analysis of the human protein interactome and comparison with yeast, worm and fly interaction datasets. Nat Genet 38: 285–293.

6. Ma X, Lee H, Wang L, Sun F (2007) CGI: a new approach for prioritizing genes by combining gene expression and protein-protein interaction data. Bioinformatics 23: 215–221.

7. Kohler S, Bauer S, Horn D, Robinson PN (2008) Walking the interactome for prioritization of candidate disease genes. Am J Hum Genet 82: 949–958.

8. Chen Y, Wang W, Zhou Y, Shields R, Chanda SK, et al. (2011) In silico gene prioritization by integrating multiple data sources. PLoS One 6: e21137.

9. Peri S, Navarro JD, Kristiansen TZ, Amanchy R, Surendranath V, et al. (2004) Human protein reference database as a discovery resource for proteomics. Nucleic Acids Res 32: D497–501.

10. Bader GD, Betel D, Hogue CW (2003) BIND: the Biomolecular Interaction Network Database. Nucleic Acids Res 31: 248–250.

11. Stark C, Breitkreutz BJ, Reguly T, Boucher L, Breitkreutz A, et al. (2006) BioGRID: a general repository for interaction datasets. Nucleic Acids Res 34: D535–539.

12. Hermjakob H, Montecchi-Palazzi L, Lewington C, Mudali S, Kerrien S, et al. (2004) IntAct: an open source molecular interaction database. Nucleic Acids Res 32: D452–455.

13. Xenarios I, Rice DW, Salwinski L, Baron MK, Marcotte EM, et al. (2000) DIP: the database of interacting proteins. Nucleic Acids Res 28: 289–291.

14. Nitsch D, Tranchevent LC, Goncalves JP, Vogt JK, Madeira SC, et al. (2011) PINTA: a web server for network-based gene prioritization from expression data. Nucleic Acids Res 39: W334–338.

15. Zhao J, Yang TH, Huang Y, Holme P (2011) Ranking candidate disease genes from gene expression and protein interaction: a Katz-centrality based approach. PLoS One 6: e24306.

16. Edgar R, Domrachev M, Lash AE (2002) Gene Expression Omnibus: NCBI gene expression and hybridization array data repository. Nucleic Acids Res 30: 207–210.

17. Hamosh A, Scott AF, Amberger JS, Bocchini CA, McKusick VA (2005) Online Mendelian Inheritance in Man (OMIM), a knowledgebase of human genes and genetic disorders. Nucleic Acids Res 33: D514–517.

18. Futreal PA, Coin L, Marshall M, Down T, Hubbard T, et al. (2004) A census of human cancer genes. Nat Rev Cancer 4: 177–183.

19. Das J, Yu H (2012) HINT: High-quality protein interactomes and their applications in understanding human disease. BMC Syst Biol 6: 92.

20. Fawcett T (2006) An introduction to ROC analysis. Pattern Recognition Letters 27: 861–874.

21. Yang H, King I, Lyu MR (2007) DiffusionRank: a possible penicillin for web spamming. Proceedings of the 30th annual international ACM SIGIR conference on Research and development in information retrieval. Amsterdam, The Netherlands: ACM. 431–438.

22. Francisco AP, Goncalves JP, Madeira SC, Oliveira AL. Using personalized ranking to unravel relevant regulations in the saccharomyces cerevisiae regulatory network; 2009. 3–6.

23. Gaire RK, Smith L, Humbert P, Bailey J, Stuckery PJ, Haviv I (2013). Discovery and analysis of consistent active subnetworks in cancers. BMC Bioinformatics 2013, (Suppl 2): S7.

24. Zhang B, Kirov S, Snoddy J (2005) WebGestalt: an integrated system for exploring gene sets in various biological contexts. Nucleic Acids Res 33: W741–748.

25. Short BG (1993) Cell proliferation and renal carcinogenesis. Environ Health Perspect 101 Suppl 5: 115–120.

26. Ciocca DR, Calderwood SK (2005) Heat shock proteins in cancer: diagnostic, prognostic, predictive, and treatment implications. Cell Stress Chaperones 10: 86–103.

27. Kirkin V, McEwan DG, Novak I, Dikic I (2009) A role for ubiquitin in selective autophagy. Mol Cell 34: 259–269.

21

Tobacco Smoke and Risk of Childhood Acute Non-Lymphocytic Leukemia: Findings from the SETIL Study

Stefano Mattioli[1]*, Andrea Farioli[1], Patrizia Legittimo[2,3], Lucia Miligi[4], Alessandra Benvenuti[4], Alessandra Ranucci[5], Alberto Salvan[6], Roberto Rondelli[7], Corrado Magnani[5] on behalf of the SETIL Study Group[¶]

1 Department of Medical and Surgical Sciences (DIMEC), University of Bologna, Bologna, Italy, **2** Unit of Occupational Medicine, S.Orsola-Malpighi University Hospital, Bologna, Italy, **3** Occupational and Environmental Epidemiology Unit, ISPO Cancer Prevention and Research Institute, Florence, Italy, **4** Occupational and Environmental Epidemiology Unit, ISPO Cancer Prevention and Research Institute, Florence, Italy, **5** Cancer Epidemiology Unit - Department of Translational Medicine, CPO Piemonte and University of Eastern Piedmont, Novara, Italy, **6** Currently retired, IASI-CNR, Rome, Italy, **7** Paediatric Oncology-Haematology "Lalla Seràgnoli", Policlinico S.Orsola-Malpighi, Bologna, Italy

Abstract

Background: Parental smoking and exposure of the mother or the child to environmental tobacco smoke (ETS) as risk factors for Acute non-Lymphocytic Leukemia (AnLL) were investigated.

Methods: Incident cases of childhood AnLL were enrolled in 14 Italian Regions during 1998–2001. We estimated odds ratios (OR) and 95% confidence intervals (95%CI) conducting logistic regression models including 82 cases of AnLL and 1,044 controls. Inverse probability weighting was applied adjusting for: age; sex; provenience; birth order; birth weight; breastfeeding; parental educational level age, birth year, and occupational exposure to benzene.

Results: Paternal smoke in the conception period was associated with AnLL (OR for ≥11 cigarettes/day = 1.79, 95% CI 1.01–3.15; P trend 0.05). An apparent effect modification by maternal age was identified: only children of mothers aged below 30 presented increased risks. We found weak statistical evidence of an association of AnLL with maternal exposure to ETS (OR for exposure>3 hours/day = 1.85, 95%CI 0.97–3.52; P trend 0.07). No association was observed between AnLL and either maternal smoking during pregnancy or child exposure to ETS.

Conclusions: This study is consistent with the hypothesis that paternal smoke is associated with AnLL. We observed statistical evidence of an association between maternal exposure to ETS and AnLL, but believe bias might have inflated our estimates.

Editor: Pal Bela Szecsi, Gentofte University Hospital, Denmark

Funding: The SETIL study was financially supported by research grants received by AIRC (Italian Association on Research on Cancer), MIUR (Ministry for Instruction, University and Research, PRIN Program), Ministry of Health (Ricerca Sanitaria Finalizzata Program), Ministry of Labour and Welfare, Associazione Neuroblastoma, Piemonte Region (Ricerca Sanitaria Finalizzata Regione Piemonte Program), Liguria Region, Comitato per la vita "Daniele Chianelli"- Associazione per la Ricerca e la Cura delle Leucemie, Linfomi e Tumori di Adulti e Bambini, (Perugia). The funders had no role in study design, data collection and analysis, decision to publish, or preparation of the manuscript.

Competing Interests: The authors have declared that no competing interests exist.

* Email: s.mattioli@unibo.it

¶ Membership of the SETIL Study Group is provided in the Acknowledgments.

Introduction

Acute leukemia is the most common childhood cancer; acute lymphoblastic leukemia (ALL) accounts for 75–80% of total cases of childhood leukemia, acute non-lymphocytic leukemia (AnLL) for about 20%. [1] Established risk factors, such as exposure to ionizing radiations and genetic syndromes, explain no more than 10% of cases; [2] Suggested risk factors include: car exhaust fumes, pesticides, non-ionizing radiation, pets, antiepileptic drugs, maternal alcohol consumption, maternal illicit drug use (*cannabis sativa*), maternal age, paternal age, breast feeding, birth order, chemical contamination in drinking water, both viral and bacterial infections, and parental cigarette smoking. [3–5] Alongside occupational exposure to benzene, [6] active tobacco smoking is

an established risk for adult myeloid leukemia. [7] According to the International Agency for Research on Cancer (IARC), the available body of evidence suggests a consistent association of childhood leukemia with preconception and with combined paternal and maternal smoking. [7] Conversely, studies on maternal tobacco smoking often showed modest increases in risk, or null or inverse associations. [7] Only one study was included on second hand smoke and leukemia (namely chronic lymphocytic leukemia) reporting a positive association. [7] Most of the evidence on the relationship between cigarette smoking and childhood leukemia regards ALL, [8], while there is scant evidence for AnLL. [7,9] As shown in supplemental Table S1, several studies highlighted that paternal smoking around the time of conception is a risk factor for childhood ALL. A meta-analysis of heavy paternal smoking (20+ cigarettes/day) highlighted a substantial increase in the risk of childhood leukemia (OR 1.44, 95%CI 1.24–1.68) [8].

Our aim was to investigate parental cigarette consumption and second-hand smoke exposure as risk factors for childhood AnLL, using data collected in a large case-control study primarily designed to evaluate the role of physical agents (including electromagnetic fields), parental occupation and environmental exposure in childhood hematopoietic malignancies. [10–11]

Methods

Study population

SETIL (*Studio sulla Eziologia dei Tumori Infantili Linfoemopoietici*, study on the etiology of childhood lympho-hematopoietic malignancies) is a population-based case-control study conducted in Italy between 1998 and 2003. Details of the study have been given elsewhere. [10–11] Thanks to the support of the Italian Association of Pediatric Hematology and Oncology almost all incident cases of childhood acute leukemia (aged between 0 and 10) in 14 Italian Regions were collected; [12] second primary neoplasms were excluded. Cases were individually matched for date of birth, sex and residence area with 2 population controls randomly drawn from Local Health Authority registries. Parents of eligible cases were contacted through the pediatric oncologist, parents of controls through their general practitioner; eligible subjects were asked to participate in a direct interview (non responders were 8% among cases and 29% among controls). During the study period 82 cases of AnLL, 601 cases of ALL and 1,044 controls (128 matched to AnLL cases and 916 matched to ALL cases) were enrolled.

Information was collected from parents of cases and controls in a direct interview using a standardized questionnaire that was constructed to collect data on many putative causes of childhood leukemia, including personal characteristics and exposure to physical, chemical and biological agents. For practical reasons, interviewers were not blinded to the case or control status of the child.

In the present analysis of AnLL, we broke the individual matching, and included the 82 cases of AnLL and all 1,044 sampled controls (irrespectively of individual matching with AnLL or ALL cases). Matching was retained in additional sensitivity analyses.

The SETIL study was conceived to investigate the etiology of hematopoietic malignancies. Findings on the association between tobacco smoke and risk of childhood acute lymphoblastic leukemia have been recently reported. [13] Queries about collaborations and access to the data can be addressed to the principal investigator of the SETIL Study (Prof. Corrado Magnani; email: magnani@med.unipmn.it). The SETIL study participated in the Childhood Leukemia International Consortium (CLIC, https://clic.berkeley.edu/about). [14]

The SETIL study was authorized by the ethics committee for the Piedmont Region (authorization n.2886, on 15/2/1999; letter n. 1852/28.3 on 17/2/1999) and later by the corresponding board of each participating research unit. Written informed consent was obtained from all participating subjects. The ethics committee approved the consent procedure.

Exposure variables and covariates

An English language translation of the smoking sections of the SETIL questionnaire is presented in appendix S1. Available information on paternal smoking status in the period of conception enabled us to classify fathers in four categories: never a smoker;

former smoker; smoker, 1 to 10 cigarettes per day; and smoker, 11 or more cigarettes per day. Based on preliminary analyses, never smokers and former smokers were merged, creating the category of non-smokers with reference to the period of conception. Information on the smoking status of fathers (smoker or non-smoker) was also available for the pregnancy and the period between birth and diagnosis. As expected, an excellent agreement (Cohen's kappa = 0.96) was found between paternal smoking status in the conception period and smoking status after the child's birth.

For maternal smoking, information was available separately for each trimester of pregnancy. Since the consumption of cigarettes tended to be stable across the pregnancy (Cohen's kappa between first and third trimester = 0.92), smoking status was classified according to the first trimester of pregnancy. After a preliminary analysis and considering the small numbers of active smokers — only three mothers of cases declared they had smoked more than 10 cigarettes/day — a dichotomous variable was created: non-smoker (never a smoker or former smoker); smoker. Mothers were asked to declare how many hours per day they had been exposed to Environmental Tobacco Smoking (ETS) during pregnancy. A three-level variable was created using the collected information: never exposed to passive smoking, and two levels of exposure based on the median of exposure to passive smoking among controls' mothers.

Exposure of children to ETS, measured in cigarettes per day, was collected for every year of life; Hence, we created a cumulative exposure index equal to the number of cigarettes to which the children had been exposed (ETS). Again, a three-level variable was created: never exposed to ETS, and two levels of exposure based on the median of exposure to passive smoking among controls.

Possible confounders were selected *a-priori* and included: sex, age group (less than two years; between two and four years; between four and six years; more than six years), residence area (part of Italy: North, except Lombardy; Lombardy; center; South and islands), birth order; birth weight; duration of breastfeeding; maternal and paternal age at child's birth; maternal and paternal education level; and parental occupational exposure to benzene. Exposure to benzene was assessed by industrial hygienists on the basis of information gathered with a job specific questionnaire. Detailed methods for the evaluation of exposure to benzene were presented in Miligi et al. [10]

Statistical Analysis

Unmatched analyses were performed in order to avoid the loss of cases (9 cases in matching strata without controls). To increase statistical power, considering that the sampling procedure and collection of information were the same for controls matched to AnLL and to ALL cases, we included all the 1,044 enrolled controls in the analysis and not only the 128 individually matched with AnLL cases. Unmatched analyses models always included age, gender and residence area. Matching was retained in additional sensitivity analyses.

In contingency tables, statistical independence of variables was tested using $\chi 2$ test or Fisher exact test, according to Cochran rule. [15] We examined associations between AnLL and each of the aforementioned sources of exposure to tobacco smoke. Odds Ratios (OR) and relative 95% Confidence Intervals (95% CI) were obtained with unconditional logistic regression models. Linear trends for ordinal exposure variables were evaluated using the Wald test, treating the variable as a continuous variable (introduced in the model with 1 degree of freedom). To test for possible interactions on a multiplicative scale, product terms for the interaction between the exposure variable and the proposed effect modifier were created and likelihood ratio tests were used to compare models with and without the interaction terms.

The limited number of cases (n = 82) did not allow the direct inclusion of all covariates in multivariate logistic regression models. To deal with the small number of events per parameter, we performed two separate sets of analyses. Firstly, we adjusted for putative confounders (parameterized as presented in Table 1) via inverse probability weighting (IPW). [16] Then the conditional probability of being exposed given the individual covariates were estimated by fitting probit (for dichotomous exposure) or multinomial probit (for categorical exposure) regression models and we calculated robust standard error for the inference. [16–18]. A second set of regression models including covariates selected based on the change-in-estimates methods were fitted, using a threshold for inclusion of a 10% change in the odds ratios of interest [19]. All analyses were performed using Stata 12.1 SE (Stata corporation, Texas, TX) and all tests were 2 sided. A p-value of 0.05 or less was considered statistically significant.

Results

Characteristics of study participants by case-control status are reported in Table 1. The entire sample of controls, mainly consisting of subjects matched to ALL cases, has a different age distribution compared to AnLL cases and their matched controls. The duration of breastfeeding was comparable in AnLL cases and their matched controls; conversely, long breastfeeding periods were more frequent in the control sample. Parents of cases usually had a lower educational level than controls' parents. All other considered characteristics seemed to have comparable distribution among cases and controls.

The ORs for the association between exposures to tobacco smoke and risk of AnLL are presented in Table 2. Estimates for both the matched and unmatched analyses are reported. In the unmatched analysis, ORs were estimated with reference to the subpopulation with complete data on putative confounders. Depending on the studied exposure, this restriction determined the exclusion of 33–39 controls and, only for paternal smoking in the conception period, of one case. Estimates based on the entire sample were consistent with those presented in Table 2.

As shown in table 2, in matched analysis, paternal smoking in the conception period presented signs of association with the risk of AnLL (OR of smokers, 1–10 cigarettes/day = 1.95, 95%CI 0.76–5.04; OR of smokers, 11 or more cigarettes/day = 1.76, 95%CI 0.91, 3.41; P for trend 0.09). Unmatched analysis of paternal smoking produced similar estimates (adjusted OR of smokers, 1–10 cigarettes/day = 1.34, 95%CI 0.65–2.76; OR of smokers, 11 or more cigarettes/day = 1.79, 95%CI 1.01, 3.15; P for trend 0.05). Although supported by very weak statistical evidence (P = 0.18), the study of the interaction between paternal smoking and maternal age at child's birth showed interesting estimates (Figure 1). Apparently, paternal smoking affected the risk of childhood AnLL only among children born from mothers aged below 30 years, a cut-off selected a priori based on median maternal age. In the multivariable model selected with the change-in-estimate method and including age at diagnosis and maternal educational level, the adjusted OR for moderate smokers (1–10 cigarettes/day) was 2.61 (95%CI0.92–7.36), while the OR for heavy-smoker fathers (11 or more cigarettes/day) was 2.99 (95%CI1.40–6.37). Estimates for children born from mothers aged above 30 years were close to the unit (adjusted OR of smokers, 1–10 cigarettes/day = 1.13, 95%CI0.44–2.92, OR of smokers, 11 or more cigarettes/day = 1.16, 95%CI0.53–2.53). Of note, almost no evidence was found of an interaction between

paternal age and paternal smoking during the conception period (at multivariate analysis p interaction = 0.40, data not shown).

Maternal smoking during the first trimester of pregnancy did not show clear signs of association with the risk of childhood AnLL (Table 2). However, in unmatched analysis, marginal evidence of an association of AnLL with high levels of maternal exposure to ETS during the pregnancy (adjusted OR of mothers exposed more than 3 hours/day = 1.85, 95%CI 0.97–3.52; P for trend = 0.07) were observed. However, the exclusion of active-smoker mothers (n = 117) from the analysis determined a decrease of the estimates (adjusted OR of mothers exposed more than 3 hours/day = 1.42, 95%CI 0.69–2.95). The further adjustment by paternal smoking (an exposure that is likely to be associated with maternal exposure to ETS) caused a modest increase of the estimates (adjusted OR of mothers exposed more than 3 hours/day = 1.61, 95%CI 0.73–3.53).

As shown in Table 2, no evidence supported an association between the exposure of the child to ETS and the risk of AnLL (for children exposed to 4,000 or more cigarettes, OR adjusted through IPW = 1.15, 95%CI 0.45–2.95; P for trend = 0.77).

Discussion

In this analysis of data from a population-based case-control study moderate evidence supporting the hypothesis that children of fathers who smoked in the period of conception have an increased risk of AnLL was found. Interestingly, an apparent effect modification by maternal age was also identified. Indeed, only children of mothers aged below 30 years at the delivery presented an increased risk. We also found weak signs of an association between maternal exposure to second-hand smoke and risk of childhood AnLL. No sign of association was found for maternal smoking during pregnancy. Finally, we did not find any evidence supporting an association between child exposure to second-hand smoke and risk of AnLL.

Plausibility of the results and evidence from previous studies

An association between paternal smoking before the pregnancy and risk of childhood leukemia has already been reported. [7–9,20] However, most of the positive findings regarded ALL, while only limited evidence supports the association between AnLL and paternal smoking. [7] It should be considered that studies on AnLL and paternal smoking are all case-control studies and they are often underpowered, due to the rarity of the disease. Since tobacco smoke is an established leukemogenic in adults, [7] the biological plausibility of an association with childhood AnLL is high. Furthermore, the possible effect of exposure to tobacco smoke of the gametes or the embryo/fetus in utero on the risk of childhood AnLL is in line with the "two hits" model proposed by Greaves. [21] Moderate/weak evidence of a possible interaction between paternal smoking and maternal age at delivery was observed. Possible explanations of the observed interaction could be chance or a strong pattern of confounders differentially acting in the two maternal age strata. However, further investigations should be carried out before excluding causality, since during pre-implantation embryogenesis complex interactions exist between paternal and maternal factors and the biochemical environment. [22]

Our analysis did not produce evidence supporting an association between maternal tobacco smoking and risk of childhood AnLL. Results were broadly in line with those of previous studies. [7] However, one should consider our sample only included 19 women (3 cases and 16 controls) who declared having smoked

Table 1. Characteristics of Acute Non-Lymphocytic Leukemia Cases and Controls in the SETIL Case-Control Study, Italy, 1998-2003.

	AnLL cases		Controls matched to AnLL cases		All sampled controls		P value[a]
	No.	%	No.	%	No.	%	
Gender[d]							
Female	39	47.6	62	48.4	482	46.2	
Male	43	52.4	66	51.6	562	52.8	Na
Age at study reference date (years)[d]							
≤1	21	25.6	35	27.3	156	14.9	
2–3	13	15.9	18	14.1	351	33.6	
4–5	13	15.9	15	11.7	233	22.3	
≥6	35	42.7	60	46.9	304	29.1	Na
Residence area (part of Italy)[d]							
North (except Lombardy)	22	26.8	33	25.8	250	24.0	
Lombardy	16	19.5	32	25.0	260	24.9	
Center	17	20.7	23	18.0	257	24.6	
South and islands	27	32.9	40	31.2	277	26.5	Na
Birth order							
First born	39	47.6	68	53.1	551	52.8	
Second born	31	37.8	39	30.5	379	36.3	
Third born and others	12	14.6	21	16.4	113	10.8	0.49[b]
Birth weight (g)							
<3,000	19	23.2	31	24.2	239	22.9	
3,000–3,299	18	22.0	28	21.9	246	23.6	
3,300–3,599	23	28.0	29	22.7	254	24.4	
≥3,600	22	26.8	40	31.2	304	29.2	0.89[b]
Duration of breastfeeding (months)							
0	12	14.6	26	20.5	232	22.3	
1–3	32	39.0	32	25.2	267	25.7	
4–6	19	23.2	37	29.1	233	22.4	
>6	19	23.2	32	25.2	308	29.6	0.04[b]
Maternal age at child's birth (years)							
≤24	14	17.1	23	18.1	140	13.4	
25–29	25	30.5	41	32.3	382	36.7	
30–34	30	36.6	44	34.6	359	34.5	
≥35	13	15.8	19	15.0	160	15.4	0.65[b]
Birth year of the mother							
<1960	15	18.3	22	17.3	145	13.9	

Table 1. Cont.

	AnLL cases		Controls matched to AnLL cases		All sampled controls		P value[a]
	No.	%	No.	%	No.	%	
1960–1964	27	32.9	32	25.2	328	31.5	
1965–1969	22	26.8	53	31.7	373	35.8	
≥1970	18	22.0	20	15.8	195	18.7	0.36[b]
Maternal educational level							
Less than high school	46	56.1	45	35.2	400	38.4	
High school	26	31.7	64	50.0	503	48.3	
University	10	12.2	19	14.8	139	13.3	<0.01[b]
Paternal age at child's birth (years)							
≤24	3	3.7	6	4.7	33	3.3	
25–29	18	22.2	29	22.8	241	23.8	
30–34	33	40.7	45	35.4	385	38.0	
≥35	27	33.3	47	37.0	353	34.9	0.96[b]
Paternal educational level							
Less than high school	47	58.0	54	42.2	463	44.6	
High school	24	29.6	59	46.1	424	40.9	
University	10	12.4	15	11.7	151	14.6	0.06[b]
Parental occupational exposure to benzene							
Absent	80	97.6	126	98.4	1,009	96.7	
Present	2	2.4	2	1.6	35	3.3	0.65[c]

Abbreviations: AnLL, acute non-lymphocytic leukemia; NA, not appropriate.
[a]Comparison between cases and all controls sampled in the SETIL study (AnLL controls + ALL controls).
[b]P values from χ2 test.
[c]P values from Fisher exact test.
[d]Matching variables.

Table 2. Association Between Acute non-Lymphocytic Leukemia and Sources of Exposure to Tobacco Smoke. The SETIL Study, Italy, 1998–2003.

Exposure	Matched analysis[a]				Unmatched analysis									
					Crude estimates				Models adjusted by sex, age and residence area		Models selected through change-in-estimates strategy		Models weighted by the inverse probability of exposure[f]	
	Ca	Co	OR	95%CI	Ca	Co	OR	95%CI	OR	95%CI	OR	95%CI	OR	95%CI
Paternal smoking in the conception period														
Non smoker	38	80	1.00	Ref.	38	612	1.00	Ref.	1.00	Ref.	1.00[b]	Ref.[b]	1.00	Ref.
Smoker, 1–10 cigs/day	12	15	1.95	0.76–5.04	12	123	1.57	0.80–3.09	1.74	0.87–3.48	1.59[b]	0.80–3.18[b]	1.34	0.65–2.76
Smoker, ≥11 cigs/day	30	33	1.76	0.91–3.41	30	264	1.83	1.11–3.02	1.90	1.14–3.17	1.79[b]	1.07–3.00[b]	1.79	1.01–3.15
P_{trend}				0.09				0.02		0.01		0.02		0.05
Maternal smoking in the 1st trimester of pregnancy														
Non smoker	71	115	1.00	Ref.	70	893	1.00	Ref.	1.00	Ref.	1.00[c]	Ref.[c]	1.00	Ref.
Smoker	11	14	1.22	0.47–3.12	11	111	1.26	0.65–2.46	1.35	0.68–2.66	1.30[c]	0.66–2.56[c]	0.83	0.38–1.81
P_{trend}				0.23				0.02		0.06		0.03		0.07
Maternal exposure to ETS during the pregnancy														
Not exposed	49	84	1.00	Ref.	48	692	1.00	Ref.	1.00	Ref.	1.00[d]	Ref.[d]	1.00	Ref.
≤3 hours/day	15	22	0.99	0.43–2.29	15	188	1.15	0.63–2.10	1.03	0.55–1.92	1.04[d]	0.56–1.92[d]	0.89	0.46–1.72
>3 hours/day	17	19	1.69	0.78–3.64	17	115	2.13	1.18–3.83	1.94	1.06–3.54	2.12[d]	1.16–3.86[d]	1.85	0.97–3.52
P_{trend}				0.29				0.15		0.18		0.39		0.77
Cumulative exposure of child to ETS														
Not exposed	52	89	1.00	Ref.	52	718	1.00	Ref.	1.00	Ref.	1.00[e]	Ref.[e]	1.00	Ref.
<4000 cigs	15	20	1.33	0.57–3.07	15	151	1.37	0.75–2.50	1.27	0.69–2.36	1.18[e]	0.64–2.18[e]	1.25	0.63–2.48
≥4000 cigs	15	20	1.59	0.65–3.87	14	130	1.49	0.80–2.76	1.51	0.78–2.92	1.33[e]	0.69–2.57[e]	1.15	0.45–2.95
P_{trend}														

Abbreviations: 95%CI, 95% confidence interval; cigs, cigarettes; ETS, environmental tobacco smoke; OR, odds ratio; Ref, reference category.
[a] Logistic regression models conditioned on matching variables (date of birth, sex, residence area of the child).
[b] Logistic regression model adjusted by age class and maternal educational level.
[c] Logistic regression model adjusted by age class and maternal educational level.
[d] Logistic regression model adjusted by duration of breastfeeding and paternal educational level.
[e] Logistic regression model adjusted by age class, maternal and paternal educational level.
[f] Logistic regression model adjusted sex, age class, residence area, birth order, birth weight, duration of breastfeeding, maternal and paternal age at child birth, maternal and paternal educational level, birth year of the mother, and parental occupational exposure to benzene (inverse probability weighting).

Risk of acute non–lymphocytic leukemia
Interaction between paternal smoking and maternal age

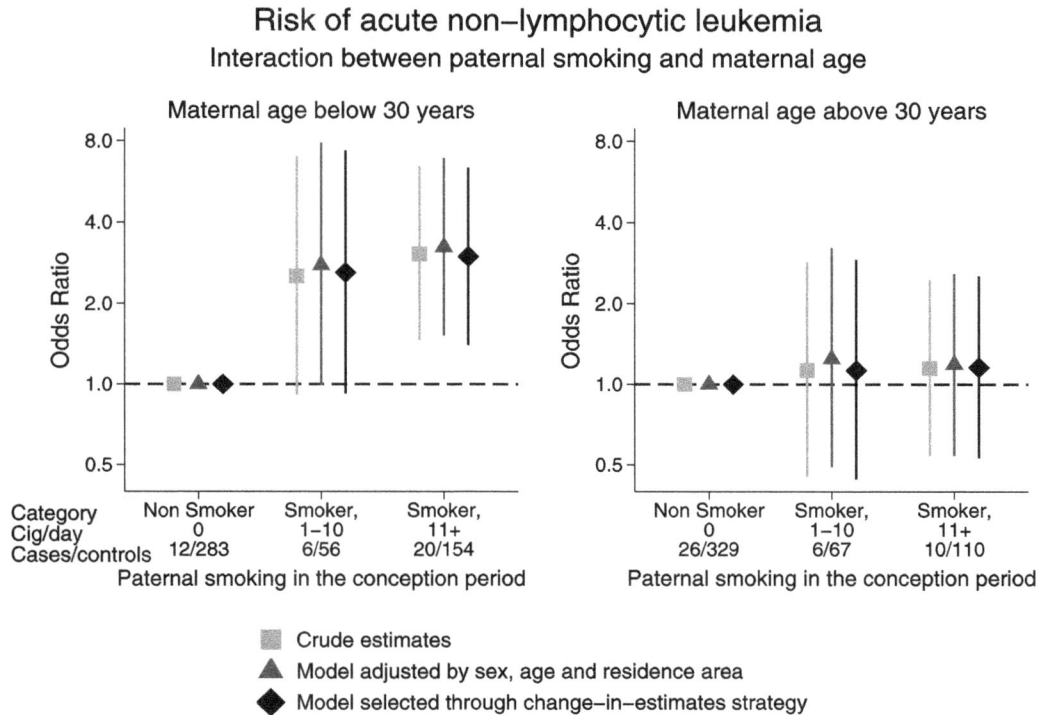

Figure 1. Association Between Paternal Smoking Status During the Period of Conception and Risk of Childhood Acute Non-Lymphocytic Leukemia, According to Maternal Age at Delivery. The SETIL Study, Italy, 1998–2003.

more than 10 cigarettes/day during the first trimester of pregnancy.

Results for maternal exposure to second-hand smoke suggest a possible association with AnLL: to the best of our knowledge, this finding is the first supporting this association [23,24] which makes us cautious in interpreting this apparent association as causal since we consider the self-assessment of second-hand smoke to be a measure prone to misclassification and recall bias. In fact, the presence of a raised risk only for maternal exposure to ETS and not for maternal active smoking is difficult to explain from a biological point of view. Furthermore, evidence suggesting a strong recall bias for maternal exposure to ETS emerged from a former study of ALL performed data from the SETIL study [13].

In most past studies on exposure of children to second-hand smoke and risk of AnLL authors used parental smoking status after pregnancy as a proxy of exposure, and most findings were negative. [25] In the SETIL study, a quantification of child exposure was attempted with direct questions in the questionnaire, but we failed to find any sign of an association between second-hand smoke and AnLL risk.

Strengths and limitations

One strength of this study is the population based design: the identification of incident cases in participating Regions proved to be very accurate [12] and information on exposures was collected by trained interviewers.

Conversely, several limitations should be considered: the response rate of controls was 0.71 and we cannot exclude a selection bias. Recall bias is always a concern when investigating self-reported exposures. Nevertheless, a Swedish study highlighted that retrospective recall of pregnancy smoking is fairly stable over time. [26] Also, interviewed subjects and interviewers were

unaware of the hypothesis investigated in the present report since studying the association between smoking and childhood ALL was not one of the main purposes of the SETIL study; furthermore, the sections aimed at collecting information on smoking were only a small part of the entire questionnaire. On the balance, we do not believe that recall bias is a serious limitation for the study of parental active smoking; on the contrary, recall bias could affect the study of ETS. As the SETIL study was not primarily designed to study the effect of tobacco smoking, misclassification of exposure could be an issue, particularly for ETS exposure.

In the present analysis we were unable to consider the effect of residential and domestic exposure to benzene, possible confounders of the relationship between exposure to cigarette smoke and risk of childhood AnLL.

We decided to break the matching in order to avoid loss of cases and expand the control group. Therefore, we should consider a possible bias due to the use of unconditional logistic regression in analysis that involved both matched and unmatched controls, with respect to AnLL cases. Of note, estimates from conditional logistic regression models (matched analysis) were consistent with the results from unmatched analysis.

The use of a propensity score or inverse probability weighting in case-control studies has been reported to be more problematic than in cohort studies, since estimates might be affected by an artefactual effect modification and residual confounding [27]. To assess whether this sort of bias might influence our estimates a supplemental set of analyses where covariates were selected based on the change-in-estimates method was performed. It is noteworthy to observe that figures from the two sets of analyses were consistent.

Conclusions

Our study supports the hypothesis that paternal smoking is associated with the risk of childhood AnLL; we also found signs of a possible effect modification due to maternal age at delivery that should be considered in future investigations. We found weak evidence of a possible effect of maternal exposure to second-hand smoke on the risk of childhood AnLL. This finding has to be consider with a degree of caution since recall bias is likely. No evidence at all emerged in our analysis for maternal smoking and exposure of the child to second-hand smoke; these results are broadly in line with knowledge from previous researches, but we should underline that the power of our study to detect an association for these exposures was low.

Acknowledgments

The members of the SETIL Study Group (Principal Investigator: Prof. Corrado Magnani, email: magnani@med.unipmn.it) are:

Aricò Maurizio, AOU Meyer, Firenze, Italia;
Assennato Giorgio, ARPA Puglia, Bari, Italy;
Bernini Gabriella, Dipartimento di Oncoematologia, Azienda Ospedaliera Universitaria Meyer, Firenze, Italy (retired);
Biddau Pierfranco, Ospedale Microcitemico, Cagliari, Italia;
Bisanti Luigi, ASL di Milano, Milano, Italia;
Bochicchio Francesco, Istituto Superiore di Sanità, Roma, Italia;
Bocchini Vittorio, Istituto Nazionale per la Ricerca sul Cancro, Genova, Italia;
Cannizzaro Santina, Lega Italiana per la Lotta contro i Tumori Onlus, Ragusa, Italia;
Casotto Veronica, IRCCS Burlo Garofolo, Trieste, Italia;
Celentano Egidio, ARSAN - Agenzia Regionale Sanitaria della Campania, Napoli, Italia;
Chiavarini Manuela, Dipartimento di Specialità Medico Chirurgiche e Sanità Pubblica – Sezione di Sanità Pubblica, Facoltà di Medicina e Chirurgia, Università degli Studi di Perugia, Perugia, Italia;
Cocco Pierluigi, Università di Cagliari, Cagliari, Italia;
Cuttini Marina, Ospedale Pediatrico Bambino Gesù, Roma, Italia;
de Nichilo Gigliola, SPESAL, Barletta, Italia;
De Salvo Gian Luigi, Istituto Oncologico Veneto IRCCS, Padova, Italia;
Forastiere Francesco, Department of Epidemiology, Regional Health Authority - Lazio Region, Rome, Italy;
Gafà Lorenzo, Lega Italiana per la Lotta contro i Tumori Onlus, Ragusa Ibla, Italia;
Galassi Claudia, AOU S.Giovanni Battista e CPO Piemonte, Torino, Italia;
Greco Alessandra, Istituto Oncologico Veneto—IRCCS Padova, Padova, Italia;
Guarino Erni, Istituto Nazionale Tumori, Napoli, Italia
Haupt Riccardo, Istituto Giannina Gaslini, Genova, Italia;
Lagorio Susanna, National Institute of Health, Rome, Italia;
Locatelli Franco, Università di Pavia, Pavia, Italia;
Luzzatto Lia Lidia, ASL 1, Torino, Italy;
Kirchmayer Ursula, Dipartimento Epidemiologia Regione Lazio, Roma, Italia;
Masera Giuseppe, Università Milano Bicocca, Monza, Italia;
Massaglia Pia, Neuropsichiatria Infantile, Torino, Italia;
Merlo Domenico Franco, IRCCS Azienda Ospedaliera Universitaria San Martino- IST Istituto Nazionale per Minelli Liliana, Università degli Studi di Perugia, Perugia, Italia;
Monetti Daniele, Istituto Oncologico Veneto IRCCS, Padova, Italia;
Mosciatti Paola, Università di Camerino, Camerino, Italia;
la Ricerca sul Cancro, Genova, Italia;
Michelozzi Paola, Department of Epidemiology, Regional Health Authority – Lazio – Region, Rome, Italy;
Nuccetelli Cristina, Istituto Superiore di Sanità, Roma, Italia;
Pannelli Franco, Università di Camerino, Dipartimento di Medicina Sperimentale e di Sanità Pubblica, Camerino, Italy;
Pession Andrea, University of Bologna, Bologna, Italia;
Polichetti Alessandro, National Institute of Health, Roma, Italia;
Poggi Vincenzo, A.O.R.N. Santobono – Pausilipon, Napoli, Italia;
Pulsoni Alessandro, La Sapienza, Università di Roma, Roma, Italia;
Sampietro Giuseppe, ASL Città di Milano, Milano, Italia;
Schilirò Gino, Università di Catania, Catania, Italia;
Risica Serena, Istituto Superiore di Sanità, Roma, Italia;
Rizzari Carmelo, A.O. San Gerardo, Fondazione MBBM, Monza, Italia;
Targhetta Roberto, Servizio di Oncoematologia Pediatrica, Ospedale Microcitemico, Cagliari, Italia;
Torregrossa Maria Valeria, Università degli Studi di Palermo; Palermo, Italia;
Valenti Rosaria Maria, Università degli Studi di Palermo, Palermo, Italia;
Varotto Stefania, Dipartimento di Pediatria, Università di Padova, Italia;
Zambon Paola, Registro Tumori del Veneto, Università di Padova, Padova, Italia;

Andrea Farioli's work on this paper was supported by the Master's Degree in Epidemiology, University of Turin.

A special thank to Ms. Victoria Franzinetti for her careful revision of the text.

The SETIL study was financially supported by research grants received by AIRC (Italian Association on Research on Cancer), MIUR (Ministry for Instruction, University and Research, PRIN Program), Ministry of Health (Ricerca Sanitaria Finalizzata Program), Ministry of Labour and Welfare, Associazione Neuroblastoma, Piemonte Region (Ricerca Sanitaria Finalizzata Regione Piemonte Program), Liguria Region, ONLUS Comitato per la vita "Daniele Chianelli"- Associazione per la Ricerca e la Cura delle Leucemie, Linfomi e Tumori di Adulti e Bambini, (Perugia).

Author Contributions

Conceived and designed the experiments: SM LM AS RR CM. Performed the experiments: AF PL AB AR. Analyzed the data: AF SM PL CM. Contributed reagents/materials/analysis tools: AB AR AS. Wrote the paper: AF SM CM.

References

1. Pui CH (2006) Childhood Leukemia. 2nd ed. Cambridge University Press: New York.
2. Greaves MF, Alexander FE (1993) An infectious etiology for common acute lymphoblastic leukemia in childhood? Leukemia 7: 349–360.
3. Belson M, Kingsley B, Holmes A (2007) Risk factors for acute leukemia in children: a review. Environ Health Perspect 115: 138–145.
4. Eden T (2010) Aetiology of childhood leukaemia. Cancer Treat Rev 36: 286–297, doi: 10.1016/j.ctrv.2010.02.004
5. Greaves M (2006) Infection, immune responses and the aetiology of childhood leukaemia. Nat Rev Cancer 6: 193–203, doi: 10.1038/nrc1816
6. Schnatter AR, Rosamilia K, Wojcik NC (2005) Review of the literature on benzene exposure and leukemia subtypes. Chem Biol Interact 153–154: 9–21, doi: 10.1016/j.cbi.2005.03.039
7. WHO-IARC (2009) IARC Monographs on the Evaluation of Carcinogenic Risks to Humans. Volume 100. A Review of Human Carcinogens. Part E: Personal Habits and Indoor Combustions. Lyon: WHO Press.
8. Milne E, Greenop KR, Scott RJ, Bailey HD, Attia J, et al. (2012) Parental prenatal smoking and risk of childhood acute lymphoblastic leukemia. Am J Epidemiol 175: 43–53, doi: 10.1093/aje/kwr275
9. Chang JS (2009) Parental smoking and childhood leukemia. Methods Mol Biol 472: 10–37, doi: 10.1007/978-1-60327-492-0_5

10. Miligi L, Benvenuti A, Mattioli S, Salvan A, Tozzi GA, et al. (2013) Risk of childhood leukaemia and non-Hodgkin's lymphoma after parental occupational exposure to solvents and other agents: the SETIL Study. Occup Environ Med 70: 648–655, doi: 10.1136/oemed-2012-100951

11. Badaloni C, Ranucci A, Cesaroni G, Zanini G, Vienneau D, et al. (2013) Air pollution and childhood leukaemia: a nationwide case-control study in Italy. Occup Environ Med 70: 876–883, doi: 10.1136/oemed-2013-101604

12. AIRTUM Working Group (2008) Italian cancer figures-report 2008. 1. Childhood cancer. (In Italian) Epidemiol Prev 32: 1, 5–13, 16–35.

13. Farioli A, Legittimo P, Mattioli S, Miligi L, Benvenuti A el al. (2014) Tobacco smoke and risk of childhood acute lymphoblastic leukemia: findings from the SETIL case-control study. Cancer Causes Control, doi:10.1007/s10552-014-0371-9

14. Metayer C, Milne E, Clavel J, Infante-Rivard C, Petridou E, et al. (2013) The Childhood Leukemia International Consortium. Cancer Epidemiol 37: 336–47.

15. Cochran WG (1954) Some methods for strengthening the common $\chi 2$ tests. Biometrics 10: 417–451.

16. Robins JM, Hernán MA, Brumback B (2000) Marginal structural models and causal inference in epidemiology. Epidemiology 11: 550–560.

17. Tchernis R, Horvitz-Lennon M, Normand SL (2005) On the use of discrete choice models for causal inference. Stat Med 24: 2197–2212, doi: 10.1002/sim.2095

18. Hernan MA, Brumback BA, Robins JM (2000) Marginal Structural Models to Estimate the Causal Effect of Zidovudine on the Survival of HIV-Positive Men. Epidemiology 11: 561–570.

19. Maldonado G, Greenland S (1993) Simulation study of confounder-selection strategies. Am J Epidemiol 138: 923–36.

20. Lee KM, Ward MH, Han S, Ahn HS, Kang HJ, et al. (2009) Paternal smoking, genetic polymorphisms in CYP1A1 and childhood leukemia risk. Leuk Res 33: 250–258, doi: 10.1016/j.leukres.2008.06.031

21. Greaves M (2005) In utero origins of childhood leukaemia. Early Hum Dev 81: 123–129, doi: 10.1016/j.earlhumdev.2004.10.004

22. Ménézo YJ (2006) Paternal and maternal factors in preimplantation embryogenesis: interaction with the biochemical environment. Reprod Biomed Online 12: 616–621, doi:10.1016/S1472-6483(10)61188-1

23. Trédaniel J, Boffetta P, Little J, Saracci R, Hirsch A (1994) Exposure to passive smoking during pregnancy and childhood, and cancer risk: the epidemiological evidence. Paediatr Perinat Epidemiol 8: 233–255, doi: 10.1111/j.1365-3016.1994.tb00455.x

24. Sasco AJ, Vainio H (1999) From in utero and childhood exposure to parental smoking to childhood cancer: a possible link and the need for action. Hum Exp Toxicol 18: 192–201, doi: 10.1191/096032799678839905

25. Boffetta P, Trédaniel J, Greco A (2000) Risk of childhood cancer and adult lung cancer after childhood exposure to passive smoke: A meta-analysis. Environ Health Perspect 108: 73–82.

26. Post A, Gilljam H, Bremberg S, Galanti MR (2008) Maternal smoking during pregnancy: a comparison between concurrent and retrospective self-reports. Paediatr Perinat Epidemiol 22: 155–161, doi: 10.1111/j.1365-3016.2007.00917.x

27. Månsson R, Joffe MM, Sun W, Hennessy S (2007) On the estimation and use of propensity scores in case-control and case-cohort studies. Am J Epidemiol 166: 332–9.

22

Enhanced Cytotoxicity of Natural Killer Cells following the Acquisition of Chimeric Antigen Receptors through Trogocytosis

Fu-Nan Cho[1,9], Tsung-Hsien Chang[2,9], Chih-Wen Shu[2], Ming-Chin Ko[3], Shuen-Kuei Liao[4], Kang-Hsi Wu[5], Ming-Sun Yu[6], Shyh-Jer Lin[6], Ying-Chung Hong[6], Chien-Hsun Chen[7], Chien-Hui Hung[3], Yu-Hsiang Chang[3,8,9]*

1 Department of Obstetrics and Gynecology, Kaohsiung Veterans General Hospital, Kaohsiung, Taiwan, 2 Department of Medical Education and Research, Kaohsiung Veterans General Hospital, Kaohsiung, Taiwan, 3 Department of Pediatrics, Kaohsiung Veterans General Hospital, Kaohsiung, Taiwan, 4 Graduate Institute of Cancer Biology and Drug Discovery and Center of Excellence for Cancer Research, Taipei Medical University, Taipei, Taiwan, 5 Department of Pediatrics, Children's Hospital and School of Chinese Medicine, China Medical University Hospitals, Taichung, Taiwan, 6 Haematology-Oncology Section, Department of Medicine, Kaohsiung Veterans General Hospital, Kaohsiung, Taiwan, 7 Department of Radiation Oncology, Kaohsiung Veterans General Hospital, Kaohsiung, Taiwan, 8 Faculty of Medicine, National Yang-Ming University, Taipei, Taiwan, 9 Department of Nursing, Tajen University, Yanpu Township, Pingtung County, Taiwan

Abstract

Natural killer (NK) cells have the capacity to target tumors and are ideal candidates for immunotherapy. Viral vectors have been used to genetically modify *in vitro* expanded NK cells to express chimeric antigen receptors (CARs), which confer cytotoxicity against tumors. However, use of viral transduction methods raises the safety concern of viral integration into the NK cell genome. In this study, we used trogocytosis as a non-viral method to modify NK cells for immunotherapy. A K562 cell line expressing high levels of anti-CD19 CARs was generated as a donor cell to transfer the anti-CD19 CARs onto NK cells via trogocytosis. Anti-CD19 CAR expression was observed in expanded NK cells after these cells were co-cultured for one hour with freeze/thaw-treated donor cells expressing anti-CD19 CARs. Immunofluorescence analysis confirmed the localization of the anti-CD19 CARs on the NK cell surface. Acquisition of anti-CD19 CARs via trogocytosis enhanced NK cell-mediated cytotoxicity against the B-cell acute lymphoblastic leukemia (B-ALL) cell lines and primary B-ALL cells derived from patients. To our knowledge, this is the first report that describes the increased cytotoxicity of NK cells following the acquisition of CARs via trogocytosis. This novel strategy could be a potential valuable therapeutic approach for the treatment of B-cell tumors.

Editor: Jacques Zimmer, Centre de Recherche Public de la Santé (CRP-Santé), Luxembourg

Funding: This study was supported by grants from National Health Research Institutes (PS9808, http://english.nhri.org.tw/NHRI_WEB/nhriw001Action.do), and Kaohsiung Veterans General Hospital (VGHKS 102-104 and 103-123, http://www.vghks.gov.tw/English/) to YHC. This work is also supported in part by the Ministry of Health and Welfare of Taiwan (MOHW103-TD-B-111-01), http://www.mohw.gov.tw/EN/Ministry/Index.aspx) to SKL. The funders had no role in study design, data collection and analysis, decision to publish, or preparation of the manuscript.

Competing Interests: The authors have declared that no competing interests exist.

* Email: yhchang@vghks.gov.tw

9 These authors contributed equally to this work.

Introduction

Natural killer (NK) cells have the ability to recognize and eliminate tumor cells, making them ideal candidates for tumor immunotherapy [1,2]. NK cell activity is regulated by the cumulative effects of multiple activating and inhibitory signals that are transmitted through the receptors on the NK cell surface. We have previously genetically modified *in vitro* expanded NK cells to express DAP10 and the chimeric NKG2D receptor containing the CD3ζ signal domain, which altered the balance between the activating and inhibitory signals of NK cells and enhanced the cytotoxicity against NKG2D ligand-bearing tumors [3]. Further, expression of anti-CD19 chimeric antigen receptors (CARs) containing 41BB and CD3ζ signal domains on NK cells enhanced the activating signals originating from CD19 antigen

engagement, leading to cytotoxicity specifically against B-cell leukemia [4].

Trogocytosis is a process in which membrane patches are exchanged between target and immune cells [5–7]. When an NK cell interacts with a target cell, an immune synapse, which is strong enough to allow the transfer of small membrane patches from one cell to its partner cell, is formed [8,9]. Therefore, target cell surface molecules can be found on the surface of NK cells. The chemokine receptor CCR7 has been shown to be transferred from donor cells onto the surface of NK cells via trogocytosis, and this transfer stimulated NK cell migration, leading to enhanced lymph node homing [10,11]. Similarly, T cells captured NKG2D and NKp46 ligands on tumor cells through trogocytosis and promoted NK cell activity [12].

Enhanced Cytotoxicity of Natural Killer Cells following the Acquisition of Chimeric Antigen Receptors through...

209

CD19 is an ideal target antigen for immunotherapy because it is expressed on nearly all leukemia cells in most patients with B-cell acute lymphoblastic leukemia (ALL) and chronic lymphoblastic leukemia (CLL) [13,14]. T cells expressing anti-CD19 CARs containing 41BB and CD3ζ signaling domains have shown remarkable antileukemic effects, leading to prolonged survival [15,16]. Autologous T cells transduced with anti-CD19 CARs have been reported to induce complete remission in patients with chronic lymphoblastic leukemia (CLL) and acute lymphoblastic leukemia (ALL) [17–20].

In this study, we sought to express anti-CD19 CARs on expanded NK cells to enhance their cytotoxicity against B-ALL cells. Viral vectors have been used to genetically modify expanded NK cells to express CARs [4,21]. Because of the safety concerns regarding viral integration into the NK cell genome, non-viral mRNA electroporation methods have been developed to modify NK cells and induce NK cell-mediated killing of leukemia cells [22,23]. Although viral gene transduction and mRNA electroporation are feasible methods, their application is limited because of the high costs and complexity. Therefore, we developed a fast, easy, and low-cost method to modify NK cells via trogocytosis. To the best of our knowledge, this is the first report that describes the use of trogocytosis as a tool to modify NK cells with chimeric antigen receptors to enhance their cytotoxicity against B-cell leukemia cells.

Materials and Methods

Cell lines and B-ALL cells from patients

The human B-lineage ALL cell line OP-1 [t(9;22) (q34;q11)/BCR-ABL] was a generous gift from Dario Campana (St. Jude Children's Research Hospital) [24]. The human B-ALL cell lines RS4;11 and SUP-B15 and the non-B leukemia cell line U937 were obtained from American Type Culture Collection (ATCC; Rockville, MD). The K562 cell line was purchased from Bioresource Collection and Research Center (BCRC; Hsinchu, Taiwan). RPMI-1640 (Invitrogen, Carlsbad, CA) supplemented with 10% fetal bovine serum (FBS; Gibco, Carlsbad, CA) and 100 mg/mL penicillin/streptomycin (Invitrogen) was used to maintain K562, OP-1, and RS4;11 cells. The SupB15 cells were maintained in Iscove's Modified Dulbecco's Medium (IMDM; Gibco, Carlsbad, CA).

Following the approval of the protocols and the written informed consent form by the Institutional Review Board of Kaohsiung Veterans General Hospital (Protocol number: VGHKS13-CT6-11), the patients' bone marrow samples were collected strictly adhering to the current ethical principles of the Declaration of Helsinki. Bone marrow samples were collected only after receiving written informed consents from all individuals. The acute B-cell lymphoblastic leukemia cells were separated by centrifugation on a Lymphoprep (Nycomed, Oslo, Norway) density step. The NK cells were thawed and cultured overnight in NK cell culture medium. The cytotoxicity of NK cells against the primary B-cell leukemia cells was assessed immediately after sample collection to avoid massive cell death after the freeze/thaw cycle.

Human NK cell expansion

Peripheral blood samples were obtained from healthy adult donors. Mononuclear cells collected from the samples by centrifugation on a Lymphoprep (Nycomed, Oslo, Norway) density step were washed twice using medium. To expand the CD56+CD3- NK cells, we co-cultured the peripheral blood mononuclear cells (PBMCs) and the genetically modified K562-mb15-41BBL cell line [4,25]. PBMCs (3×10^6) were co-cultured in a 6-well tissue culture plate with 2×10^6 irradiated or freeze/thaw-treated K562-mb15-41BBL cells in 5 mL of RPMI-1640 medium containing and 10% FBS and 10 IU/mL human IL-2 (eBioscience, San Diego, CA). Once every 2 days, fresh culture medium containing 10% FBS and 20 IU/mL human IL-2 was added to double the volume, and NK cells were split from one well into two wells. After 7 days of co-culture, the T cells were removed using CD3 Dynabeads (Invitrogen, Carlsbad, CA), which yielded cell populations containing >95% CD56+CD3- NK cells. The purified NK cells were stored in liquid nitrogen for further experiments.

For the freeze/thaw cycle, ethanol contained in a 50-mL tube was chilled in a $-80°C$ freezer. Following this, a suspension of K562-mb15-41BBL cells in RPMI medium (5×10^6/mL) contained in a 1.5-mL tube was rapidly frozen using pre-chilled ethanol for 2 min. The K562-mb15-41BBL cells were then thawed quickly in a water bath at $37°C$ for co-culturing with PBMCs as described earlier.

Plasmids, virus production, and gene transduction

The pMSCV-IRES-GFP, pEQ-PAM3(-E), pRDF, and anti-CD19-BB-ζ were generous gifts from Dario Campana (St. Jude Children's Research Hospital) [15]. To generate the RD144-pseudotyped retrovirus, 2.5×10^6 293T cells maintained in 10-cm tissue culture dishes for 16 h were transfected with 3.5 μg of cDNA encoding anti-CD19-BB-ζ constructs, 3.5 μg of pEQ-PAM3(-E), and 3 μg of pRDF using fuGENE 6 (Roche, Indianapolis, IN) reagent [4,15]. The culture supernatant containing the retrovirus was harvested at 48, 72, and 96 h post-transfection. For gene transduction, the supernatant-containing virus particles were filtered and added to RetroNectin (TakaRa, Otsu, Japan)-coated polypropylene tubes. After centrifugation at $1,400 \times g$ for 10 min, the tubes were incubated at $37°C$ for 4 h. After additional centrifugation and removal of the supernatant, K562 cells (5×10^4) were added to the tubes, and the tubes were incubated at $37°C$ for 24 h. This procedure was repeated for 7 more days. Cells were then maintained in RPMI-1640 supplemented with FBS and antibiotics.

The expression of anti-CD19-BB-ζ on the K562 cell surface was analyzed by flow cytometry on a FACSCalibur instrument using CellQuest software (BD Biosciences, San Jose, CA). Biotin-SP-conjugated AffiniPure goat anti-mouse IgG,F(ab')2 fragment-specific antibody (Jackson ImmunoResearch 115-065-072) and PE-conjugated streptavidin (Jackson ImmunoResearch 016-110-084) were used for labeling the cells. Single K562-anti-CD19-BB-ζ cells with the highest expression of anti-CD19-BB-ζ were sorted with a FACSAria cell sorter (BD Biosciences, San Jose, CA).

Trogocytosis and staining

Immediately before trogocytosis, donor or control cells (5×10^6 cells/mL in culture medium) were rapidly frozen in chilled ethanol ($-80°C$) for 2 min and then thawed in a water bath maintained at $37°C$. Trogocytosis of antiCD19BB-ζ was achieved by co-culturing the NK cells with freeze/thaw-treated K562-antiCD19BBζ cells (donor cells) or K562 cells (control cells) in a 24-well plate as described earlier at an acceptor-to-donor cell ratio of 1:1. The plate was centrifuged for 2 min to increase cell-cell contact and was then incubated at $37°C$. After trogocytosis, the cells were gently pipetted to disrupt cell-cell interaction of the immune synapses. The NK cells were separated from the donor or control cells by density gradient centrifugation on Lymphoprep (Nycomed, Oslo, Norway) at $400 \times g$ for 20 min and were cultured in NK cell medium. For staining, the cells were fixed with 1% para

A

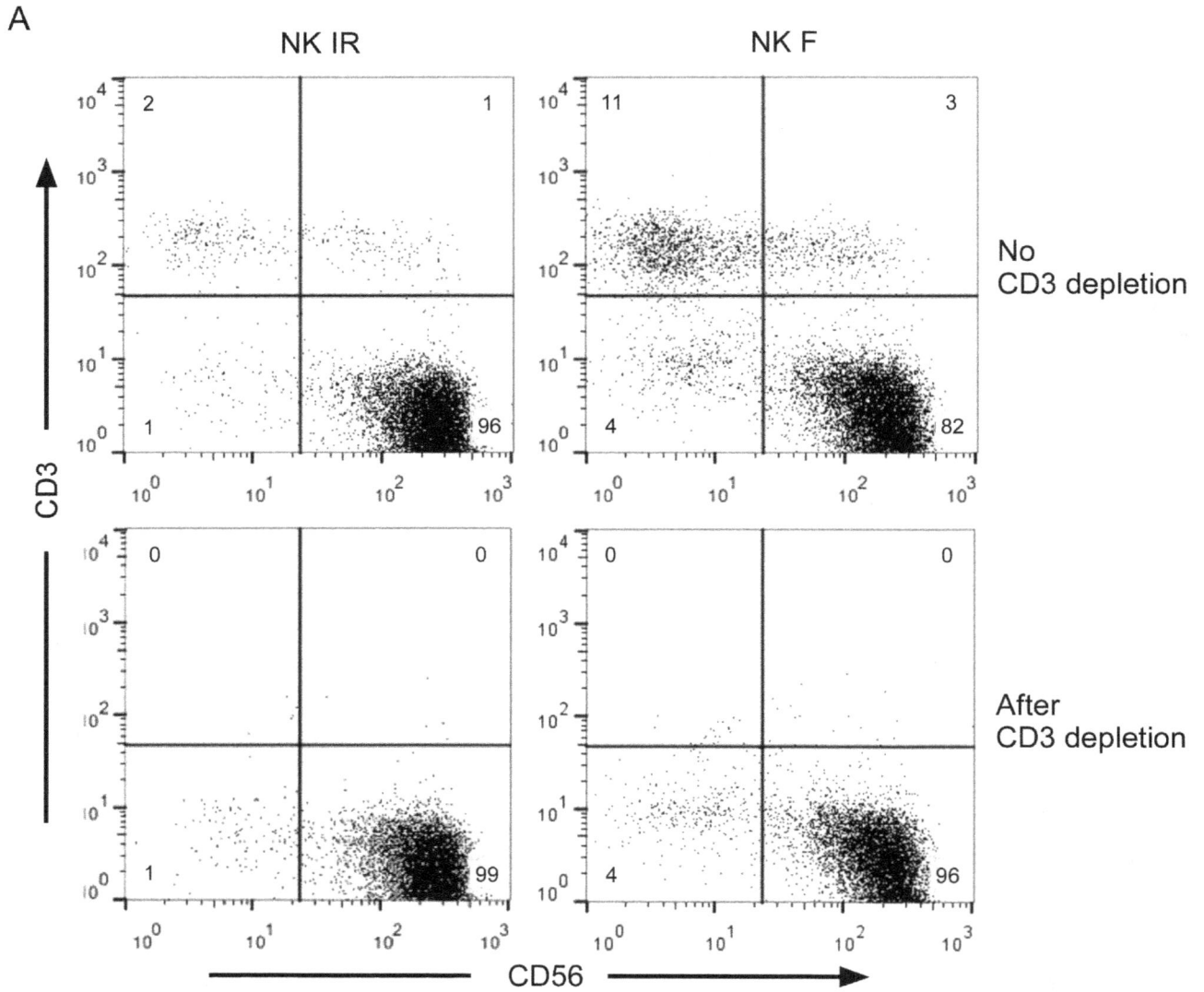

B

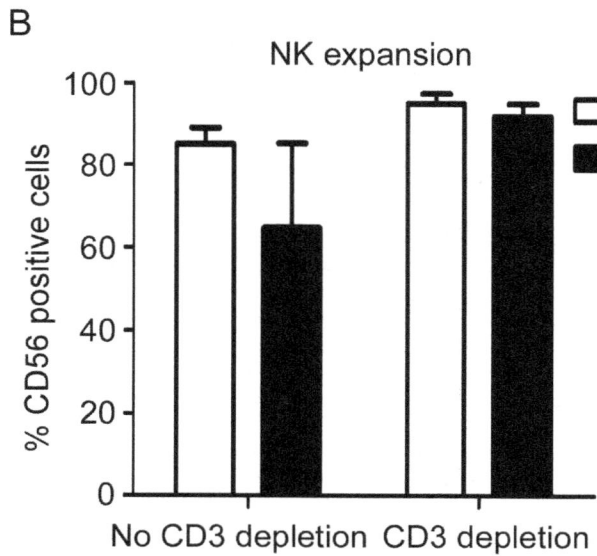

C

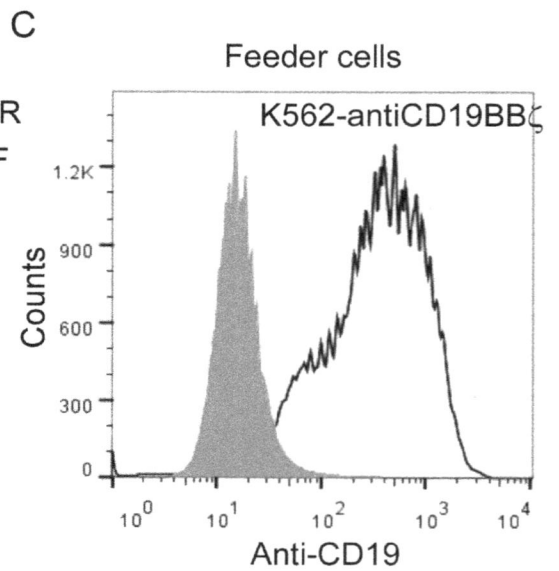

Figure 1. Immunophenotypic features of expanded NK cells (acceptor cells) and K562-antiCD19BBζ cells (feeder cells). A. Expression of CD56 and CD3 on peripheral blood mononuclear cells from a healthy donor was examined after 1 week (top row) of co-culture with irradiated (IR, left column) or freeze/thaw-treated (F, right column) K562-mb15-41BBL cells at a low dose (10 U/mL) of IL-2. The T cells were removed using CD3 Dynabeads, generating cell populations comprising >95% CD56+CD3- NK cells (bottom row). B. Percentage of CD56-positive cells within NK cells expanded by co-culturing with irradiated (IR) or freeze/thaw-treated (F) K562-mb15-41BBL cells prior to and after CD3 depletion on day 7. The data are presented as the mean of values obtained using 3 unrelated NK donors. Error bars represent the SD. C. Histogram illustrating the anti-CD19 expression on K562 cells (control, shaded histogram) and K562-antiCD19BBζ cells (feeder cells, open histogram).

in PBS for 15 min at room temperature. After washing, the cells were stained with biotin-SP-conjugated AffiniPure goat anti-mouse IgG,F(ab')2 fragment-specific antibody (Jackson Immu-noResearch 115-065-072), followed by PE-conjugated streptavidin (Jackson ImmunoResearch 016-110-084) and CD56-FITC. The percentage of the NK cells that acquired anti-CD19-BB-ζ CARs through trogocytosis was determined by flow cytometry.

Immunofluorescence analysis

The NK cells co-cultured with donor cells were fixed using 4% paraformaldehyde in PBS, permeabilized with 0.4% Triton X-100, and blocked with 2% goat serum for 15 min. The cells were then incubated with biotin-SP-conjugated AffiniPure goat anti-mouse IgG,F(ab')2 fragment-specific antibody (Jackson Immu-noResearch 115-065-072) at 4°C overnight. After washing, the cells were incubated with Alexa Fluor 568-conjugated streptavidin (Invitrogen, Carlsbad, CA) and CD56-FITC antibodies (BD Biosciences, San Jose, CA). DAPI was used for staining the nucleus. The localization of fluorescently labeled protein was visualized using a fluorescence microscope (Carl Ziess, Jena, Germany).

Cytotoxicity assay

The target cells were suspended in RPMI-1640 containing 10% FBS, labeled with calcein AM (BD Biosciences, San Jose, CA), and plated onto 96-well flat-bottom plates (Costar, Corning, NY). The NK cells, suspended in RPMI-1640 containing 10% FBS, were then added at various E:T ratios and co-cultured with the target cells for 4 h. Following this, the cells were stained with propidium iodide (Sigma-Aldrich, St. Louis, MO), and the cytotoxicity was assessed by flow cytometry on a FACSCalibur (Becton Dickinson) instrument enumerating the number of viable target cells (calcein AM-positive, propidium-iodide negative, and light scattering properties of viable cells) [3,26].

Degranulation assays

NK cells (1×10^5) were plated in each well of a 96-well flat-bottom plate and incubated with RS4;11 cells at an E:T ratio of 1:4. A phycoerythrin-conjugated anti-human CD107a antibody (BD Biosciences, San Jose, CA) was added at the beginning of the cultures. After 1 h of incubation, GolgiStop (0.15 μL; BD Biosciences, San Jose, CA) was added. The cells were then stained with fluorescein isothiocyanate-conjugated anti-human CD56 antibody (eBiosciences, San Diego, CA) and were analyzed by flow cytometry.

Results

Freeze/thaw treated K562-mbIL15-41BBL cells can be used in NK cell expansion

The NK cells were expanded from PBMCs by co-culturing with irradiated (Figure 1A, left panels) or freeze/thaw-treated (Figure 1A, right panels) K562-mb15-41BBL cells. The freeze/thaw cycle compromised the membrane integrity of K562-mb15-41BBL cells, which allowed trypan blue staining, but intact cell

morphology was maintained. After 7 days of expansion, the PBMCs co-cultured with irradiated K562-mbIL15-41BBL cells produced 95.8% CD56+CD3- NK cells (Figure 1A, left upper panel), whereas K562-mbIL15-41BBL cells subjected to one freeze/thaw cycle yielded 81.8% CD56+CD3- cells (Figure 1A, right upper panel). After CD3 depletion, the percentages of CD56+CD3- NK cells were 98.7% from PBMCs co-cultured with irradiated K562-mbIL15-41BBL cells and 95.5% using a freeze/thawed procedure (Figure 1A, lower panels). The relatively poor expansion of NK cells in co-cultures of PMBCs and freeze/thaw-treated K562-mbIL15-41BBL cells was likely due to the reduced stimulation from mbIL15 and 41BB ligands as a result of freeze/thaw-induced cell damage and lysis.

By day 7 in cultures, approximately 85% (n = 3; Figure 1B, NK IR) of the NK cells expanded from PBMCs co-cultured with irradiated K562-mb15-41BBL cells were CD56-positive, and this number increased to 95% following CD3 depletion. These results were comparable to those of NK cells expanded by co-culturing with freeze/thaw-treated K562-mb15-41BBL cells (Figure 1B, NK F; 92% CD56-positive cells following CD3 depletion). These results indicated that both freeze/thaw-treated and irradiated K562-mbIL15-41BBL cells can be used for NK cell expansion.

To generate donor cells (K562-antiCD19BBζ cells) for trogo-cytosis, K562 cells were transduced with anti-CD19-BB-ζ chimeric antigen receptors (CARs). After single cell sorting, we chose the clone stably expressing high levels of anti-CD19 CARs. The mean fluorescence intensity (MFI) of the K562-antiCD19BBζ cells was 301, which was substantially higher than that (12) of control K562 cells (Figure 1C).

Expanded NK cells acquired anti-CD19 CARs from K562-based donor cells via trogocytosis

To examine whether the NK cells were able to acquire anti-CD19 CARs from donor cells via trogocytosis, we cultured NK cells with live or freeze/thaw-treated donor K562-antiCD19BBζ cells. FACS analysis of NK cells co-cultured with live donor cells revealed that 47.0±16.4% (n = 3, ± s.d.) of the NK cells acquired anti-CD19 CARs (data not shown), and 24.1% of NK cells acquired anti-CD19 CARs from freeze/thawed donor K562-antiCD19BBζ cells (Figure 2A). Although a higher efficiency of trogocytosis was observed in co-cultures with live donor cells, separation of NK cells from live donor cells is challenging. In contrast, donor cells subjected to a freeze/thaw cycle could facilitate the separation of NK cells from nonviable donor cells using Ficoll-Paque centrifugation. Therefore, the NK cells co-cultured with freeze/thaw-treated K562-antiCD19BBζ cells were used for subsequent experiments.

Using these two types of expanded NK cells (Figure 1A, NK IR and NK F), we evaluated the uptake of anti-CD19 CARs by NK cells from donor K562-antiCD19BBζ cells. We found that approximately 19% (n = 3) of the NK F cells expressed anti-CD19 CARs, whereas only 11% (n = 3) of the NK IR cells expressed anti-CD19 CARs (Figure 2B). Therefore, we used NK cells expanded with freeze/thaw-treated K562-mb15-41BBL cells (NK F cells) in subsequent trogocytosis experiments.

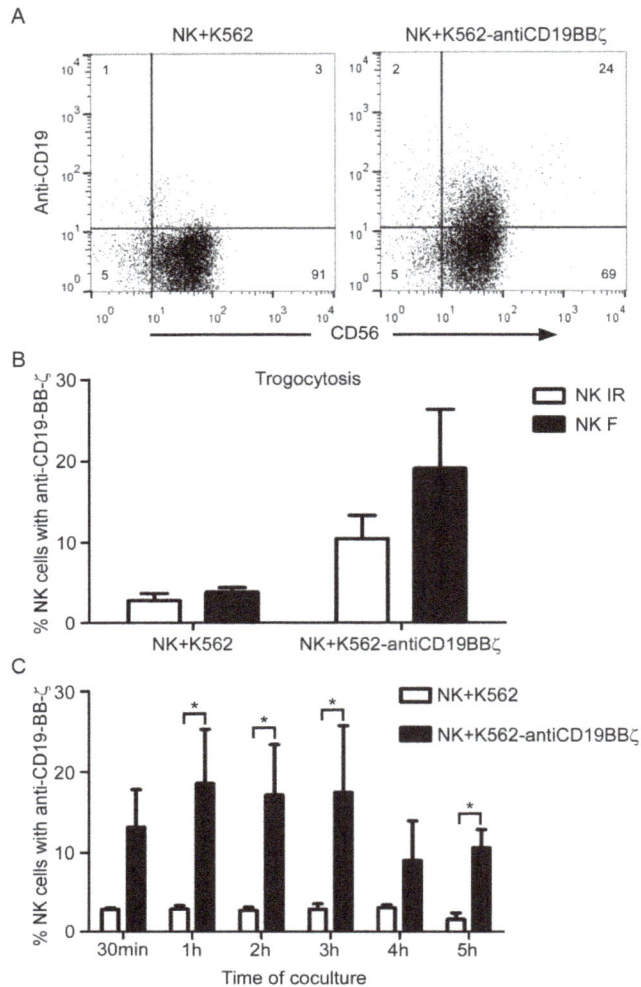

Figure 2. Acquisition of anti-CD19 chimeric antigen receptors (CARs) by NK cells from donor cells via trogocytosis. A. Flow cytometry dot plots illustrating the uptake of anti-CD19 CARs by NK cells via trogocytosis. NK cells co-cultured with K562 cells (control) or K562-antiCD19BBζ cells were stained with an anti-CD56-FITC antibody and a biotin-SP-conjugated AffiniPure goat anti-mouse IgG,F(ab')2 fragment specific antibody, followed by PE-conjugated streptavidin. B. Uptake of anti-CD19 CARs by NK cells expanded by co-culturing with irradiated (IR) or freeze/thaw-treated (F) K562-mb15-41BBL cells. The data are presented as the mean ± SD of values obtained using three unrelated NK donors. C. Kinetics of anti-CD19 CAR uptake by NK cells from K562-antiCD19BBζ cells (black bars) and control K562 cells (white bars). The uptake of anti-CD19 CARs by NK cells was analyzed after co-culturing with feeder cells for the indicated time and was compared with that of NK cells co-cultured with control K562 cells. The data are presented as the mean ± SD of values obtained using 3 unrelated NK cell donors. *: significant increase compared with control cells (p<0.05; two-tailed paired Student's t-tests).

We assessed the optimal duration for the co-culture of NK cells with donor cells. After 1 h of co-culture, approximately 18.6% of the NK cells were anti-CD19-positive (Figure 2C). The uptake of anti-CD19 CARs peaked at 1 h and decreased after 4–5 h of co-culture with K562-antiCD19BBζ cells. These results suggested that the efficiency of NK cell trogocytosis peaked at 1 h of co-culture. Therefore, we used 1 h as the standard duration of co-culture in subsequent experiments.

Immunofluorescence analysis of trogocytosis

To verify that trogocytosis was the mechanism of uptake of anti-CD19 CARs by NK cells, we examined the interaction between NK cells and donor cells during trogocytosis using immunofluorescence microscopy. The NK cells stained positively for CD56 (Figure 3A, green), and the donor cells expressed anti-CD19 CARs (Figure 3B, red). Because the NK cells interacted with donor cells and formed immune synapses over a period of 15 min, these cells were imaged 15 min after co-culture initiation. During trogocytosis, small patches of acquired anti-CD19 CARs were observed on the surface of NK cells (Figure 3C). The NK cells continued to express anti-CD19 CARs (Figure 3D, yellow) on their surfaces after detaching from the donor cells following pipetting and Ficoll-Paque separation.

Acquiring anti-CD19 CARs via trogocytosis enhanced NK cell degranulation and cytotoxicity against B-ALL cell lines

To assess the degranulation of NK cells after stimulating with a B-ALL cell line, NK cells co-cultured with freeze/thaw-treated donor K562-antiCD19BBζ or K562 (control) cells were incubated with RS4;11 cells to induce degranulation. CD107a staining was performed to detect degranulation. The percentage of CD107a-positive NK cells co-cultured with donor K562-antiCD19BBζ cells (9.9±1.2%, n=3) was significantly higher (p<0.05) than that of CD107a-positive NK cells co-cultured with control cells (1.9±0.6%, n=3) (Figure 4A).

To examine whether the gain of anti-CD19 CARs via trogocytosis improved the cytotoxicity of NK cells against B-ALL cells, three B-ALL cell lines (RS4;11, OP-1, and SUP-B15)

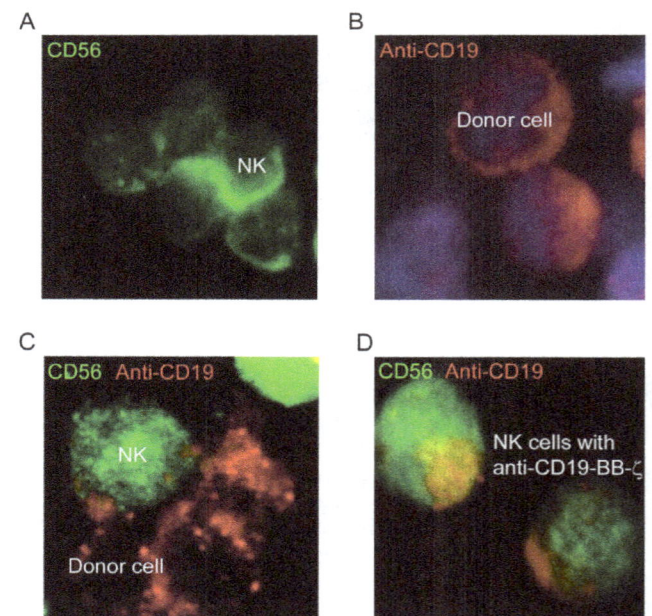

Figure 3. Immunofluorescence analysis for trogocytosis. A. NK cells stained with anti-CD56-FITC antibody. B. K562-antiCD19BBζ cells were stained with a biotin-SP-conjugated AffiniPure goat anti-mouse IgG,F(ab')2 fragment specific antibody, followed by Alexa Fluor 568-conjugated streptavidin. The nucleus was stained with DAPI (blue). C. NK cells co-cultured with K562-antiCD19BBζ cells were stained for CD56 and anti-CD19 CARs, as previously described. D. Acquisition of anti-CD19-BB-ζ by NK cells via trogocytosis was observed.

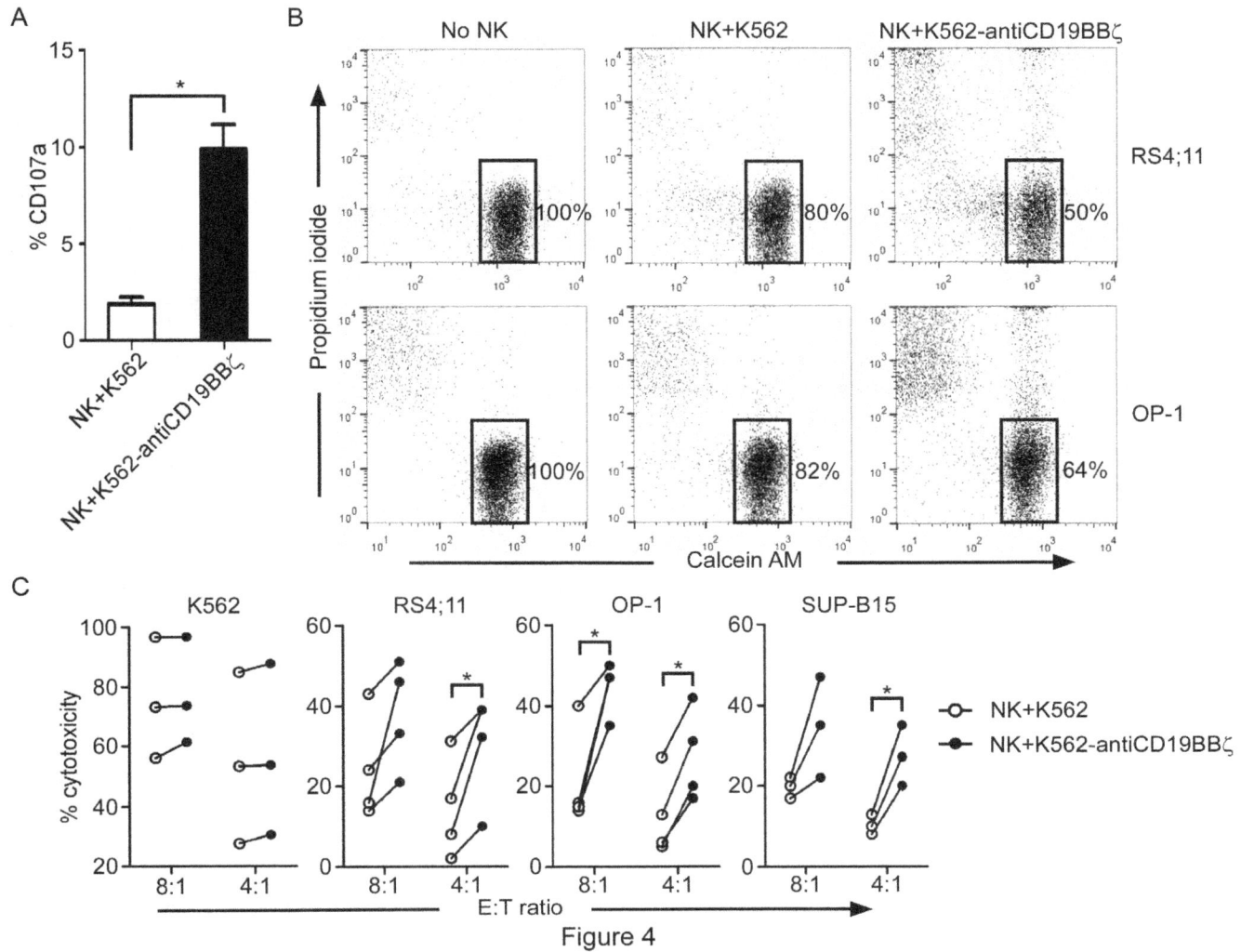

Figure 4

Figure 4. Degranulation and cytotoxicity assays. A. Incubation of NK cells with RS4;11 cells induced degranulation, which was significantly higher in NK cells co-cultured with K562-antiCD19BBζ cells than in NK cells cultured with control K562 cells. Percentages of CD56-positive cells from 3 donors expressing CD107a after a 4-h RS4;11 stimulation are shown. The data are presented as the mean ± SD of values obtained using 3 unrelated NK cell donors. B. Flow cytometric dot plots illustrating the assay used to measure cell killing. Results for RS4;11 and OP-1 cell lines are shown. Tumor cells were either cultured alone (left panel), with NK cells previously co-cultured with K562 cells (middle panel), or with NK cells previously co-cultured with K562-antiCD19BBζ cells (right panel). Residual viable target cells, which were defined as calcein AM-positive and propidium iodide (PI)-negative, are shown in the bottom right corner of each panel, and the percentages of viable cells are shown. C. Cytotoxicity of the non-B leukemia cell line (K562) and B-ALL cell lines (RS4;11, OP1, and SUP-B15) after 4-h co-culture with NK cells previously co-cultured with K562 cells (white circles) and K562-antiCD19BBζ cells (black circles) at the indicated E:T ratios. The equation [(tumor co-culture with NK cells)/(tumor alone)]×100%, represents the quantitative percentage of viable tumor cells. The cytotoxicity was calculated according the following equation: 100% − quantitative percentage of viable tumor cells. Each symbol corresponds to the mean of three values. *: significant increase compared with control cells (p<0.05; two-tailed paired Student's t-tests).

were targeted. We conducted 4-h cytotoxicity assays with NK cells expanded from three donors at effector:target (E:T) ratios of 4:1 and 8:1. As shown in Figure 4B and 4C, the gain of anti-CD19 CARs via trogocytosis significantly increased the cytotoxicity of NK cells against RS4;11, OP-1, and SUP-B15 cells at a 4:1 E:T ratio. Similarly, gains of cytotoxicity were also observed against the three B-ALL cell lines at an 8:1 E:T ratio. In contrast, there was no increase in cytotoxicity against the non-B cell lines, K562 cells (Figure 4C) and U937 cells (data not shown).

Gain of anti-CD19 CARs via trogocytosis increased NK cytotoxicity against primary B-ALL cells from patients

To determine whether the acquisition of anti-CD19 CARs via trogocytosis improved the cytotoxicity of NK cells against the patient-derived primary B-ALL cells, three samples of bone marrow from B-ALL patients were tested. Compared to the mock NK cells, the NK cells that acquired anti-CD19 CARs consistently showed enhanced cytotoxicity against primary B-ALL cells (Figure 5). The p-value was 0.069 (n = 3) at an 8:1 E:T ratio.

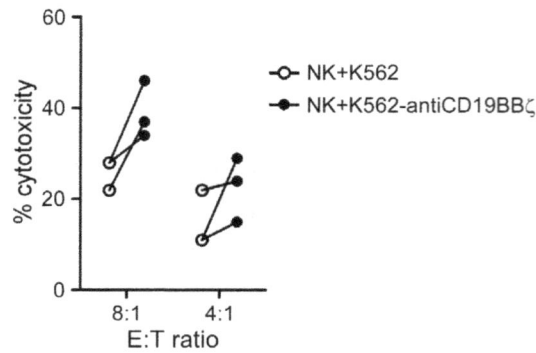

Figure 5. NK cells that acquired anti-CD19 CARs were more cytotoxic against patient-derived primary B-ALL cells. Cytotoxicity against B-ALL cells after 4-h co-culture with NK cells previously co-cultured with K562 cells (white circles) and K562-antiCD19BBζ cells (black circles) at the indicated E:T ratios. Each symbol corresponds to the mean of three values.

Discussion

Because of the safety concerns regarding the use of viral transduction methods, we endeavored to improve the cytotoxicity of adoptively transferred NK cells against B-cell leukemia cells using a simple co-culture method. For NK cell therapy, the clinical protocol required up to 5×10^7 NK cells/kg and CD3 depletion before transfusing into patients, indicating that approximately 10×10^9 NK cells are needed for the treatment of hematological malignancies [27]. If the MSCV retroviral methods were to be used to modify NK cells, a large quantity of viral supernatant would be required to transduce 10×10^9 NK cells [4]. Additionally, there is a safety concern associated with viral integration into the NK cell genome. Further, the application of viral transduction is also very limited because of the complexity of the procedures and high costs. In this study, we evaluated the usefulness of trogocytosis as a relatively simple non-viral method that can be readily scaled up to modify large numbers of NK cells with a single K562-based donor cell line.

The K562 cell line is a typical NK cell target because it lacks major histocompatibility complex class I expression, which triggers inhibitory signals to abolish NK cell activation. Additionally, K562 cells have been genetically modified to express 41BBL and the membrane-bound IL15 or IL21, which allowed the establishment of co-culture methods for the *in vitro* expansion of NK cells [25,28]. Here, we showed that K562 cells were able to donate anti-CD19 CARs to expanded NK cells in co-cultures via trogocytosis. The rapid expression of anti-CD19 CAR on the NK cell surface when co-cultured with donor K562-antiCD19BBζ cells and the lack of expression in NK cells co-cultured with control K562 cells was suggestive of an acquisition from donor cells. This was confirmed by the positive anti-CD19 staining of the NK cell surface (Figure 2A, Figure 4). Previous studies have shown that trogocytosis occurs during cell-cell interactions between target cells and stimulated NK cells [9–11,29,30].

Although the extent of trogocytosis was greater when NK cells were co-cultured with live donor cells (47%, data not shown) than

when cultured with nonviable donor cells (19%), the ease of separating NK cells from nonviable donor cells using Ficoll-Paque centrifugation prompted us to use the latter method. The uptake of CCR7 by NK cells from nonviable donor cells subjected to one freeze/thaw cycle was also lower (50%) than that from live donor cells (80%) [10]. Further, the anti-CD19 CARs acquired by NK cells were rapidly lost, and only less than 20% of the acquired anti-CD19 CARs remained on the NK cell surface after 2 h (data not shown). CCR7 uptake has been reported to decline to baseline levels by 72 h [10]. The rapid loss of the acquired anti-CD19 CARs observed in our study might be due to the degradation of the low amount of anti-CD19 CARs acquired. Fas signaling was reported to promote trogocytosis in T cells [31]. Further studies are needed to improve anti-CD19 CAR uptake and enhance its stability on the NK cell surface.

The CAR, anti-CD19-BB-ζ, comprising an anti-CD19 single-chain variable fragment (scFv), a 41BB signaling domain, and a CD3ζ signaling domain, was transduced into the NK cell genome, inducing powerful anti-leukemic effects [4]. Additionally, expanded NK cells electroporated with anti-CD19-BB-ζ mRNA also exerted significantly higher cytotoxicity against B-cell malignancies than mock NK cells [23]. In this study, we showed enhanced cytotoxicity of NK cells following the acquisition of anti-CD19-BB-ζ protein molecules via trogocytosis.

A reduction in NK cell cytotoxicity was observed after the intercellular transfer of NK Group 2 member D (NKG2D) and MHC class I chain-related molecule (MIC) B proteins at the NK cell immune synapse [32]. The amount of NKG2D, a key activating receptor on NK cell surface, is reduced after trogocytosis because the transfer of NK cell-derived NKG2D to target cells and internalization of NKG2D contribute to receptor down-modulation after interaction, leading to impaired NK cell cytotoxicity [7,32]. In addition, activated NK cells acquired HLA-G, an immunosuppressive molecule, from tumor cells via trogocytosis, leading to impaired cytotoxicity [9]. On the contrary, our study showed enhanced NK cytotoxicity because of expanded NK cells acquiring anti-CD19-BB-ζ from feeder cells via trogocytosis.

To our knowledge, this is the first report that describes the increased cytotoxicity of NK cells following the acquisition of anti-CD19 CARs from donor cells via trogocytosis. Our findings could potentially be extended to develop safer and effective therapeutic strategies for treating B-cell tumors. Our model, which used anti-CD19 CAR for targeting a B-cell tumor, could also be relevant to other tumor types that are targeted by the tumor-directed chimeric antigen receptors [33]. Therefore, further studies are warranted to examine the utility of our method for treating diverse tumor types *in vivo*.

Author Contributions

Conceived and designed the experiments: FNC THC MCK YHC. Performed the experiments: MCK CHC YHC. Analyzed the data: FNC THC CWS MCK SKL CHH YHC. Contributed reagents/materials/analysis tools: KHW MSY SJL YCH. Wrote the paper: FNC THC CWS YHC.

References

1. Ljunggren HG, Malmberg KJ (2007) Prospects for the use of NK cells in immunotherapy of human cancer. Nat Rev Immunol 7: 329–339.
2. Caligiuri MA (2008) Human natural killer cells. Blood 112: 461–469.
3. Chang YH, Connolly J, Shimasaki N, Mimura K, Kono K, et al. (2013) A chimeric receptor with NKG2D specificity enhances natural killer cell activation and killing of tumor cells. Cancer Res 73: 1777–1786.

4. Imai C, Iwamoto S, Campana D (2005) Genetic modification of primary natural killer cells overcomes inhibitory signals and induces specific killing of leukemic cells. Blood 106: 376–383.

5. Rechavi O, Goldstein I, Kloog Y (2009) Intercellular exchange of proteins: the immune cell habit of sharing. FEBS Lett 583: 1792–1799.

6. Caumartin J, Lemaoult J, Carosella ED (2006) Intercellular exchanges of membrane patches (trogocytosis) highlight the next level of immune plasticity. Transpl Immunol 17: 20–22.

7. Roda-Navarro P, Reyburn HT (2007) Intercellular protein transfer at the NK cell immune synapse: mechanisms and physiological significance. FASEB J 21: 1636–1646.

8. Williams GS, Collinson LM, Brzostek J, Eissmann P, Almeida CR, et al. (2007) Membranous structures transfer cell surface proteins across NK cell immune synapses. Traffic 8: 1190–1204.

9. Caumartin J, Favier B, Daouya M, Guillard C, Moreau P, et al. (2007) Trogocytosis-based generation of suppressive NK cells. EMBO J 26: 1423–1433.

10. Somanchi SS, Somanchi A, Cooper LJ, Lee DA (2012) Engineering lymph node homing of ex vivo-expanded human natural killer cells via trogocytosis of the chemokine receptor CCR7. Blood 119: 5164–5172.

11. Marcenaro E, Cantoni C, Pesce S, Prato C, Pende D, et al. (2009) Uptake of CCR7 and acquisition of migratory properties by human KIR+ NK cells interacting with monocyte-derived DC or EBV cell lines: regulation by KIR/HLA-class I interaction. Blood 114: 4108–4116.

12. Domaica CI, Fuertes MB, Rossi LE, Girart MV, Avila DE, et al. (2009) Tumour-experienced T cells promote NK cell activity through trogocytosis of NKG2D and NKp46 ligands. EMBO Rep 10: 908–915.

13. Bene MC, Kaeda JS (2009) How and why minimal residual disease studies are necessary in leukemia: a review from WP10 and WP12 of the European LeukaemiaNet. Haematologica 94: 1135–1150.

14. Rawstron AC, Villamor N, Ritgen M, Bottcher S, Ghia P, et al. (2007) International standardized approach for flow cytometric residual disease monitoring in chronic lymphocytic leukaemia. Leukemia 21: 956–964.

15. Imai C, Mihara K, Andreansky M, Nicholson IC, Pui CH, et al. (2004) Chimeric receptors with 4-1BB signaling capacity provoke potent cytotoxicity against acute lymphoblastic leukemia. Leukemia 18: 676–684.

16. Milone MC, Fish JD, Carpenito C, Carroll RG, Binder GK, et al. (2009) Chimeric receptors containing CD137 signal transduction domains mediate enhanced survival of T cells and increased antileukemic efficacy in vivo. Mol Ther 17: 1453–1464.

17. Porter DL, Levine BL, Kalos M, Bagg A, June CH (2011) Chimeric antigen receptor-modified T cells in chronic lymphoid leukemia. N Engl J Med 365: 725–733.

18. Brentjens RJ, Riviere I, Park JH, Davila ML, Wang X, et al. (2011) Safety and persistence of adoptively transferred autologous CD19-targeted T cells in patients with relapsed or chemotherapy refractory B-cell leukemias. Blood 118: 4817–4828.

19. Grupp SA, Kalos M, Barrett D, Aplenc R, Porter DL, et al. (2013) Chimeric antigen receptor-modified T cells for acute lymphoid leukemia. N Engl J Med 368: 1509–1518.

20. Brentjens RJ, Davila ML, Riviere I, Park J, Wang X, et al. (2013) CD19-targeted T cells rapidly induce molecular remissions in adults with chemotherapy-refractory acute lymphoblastic leukemia. Sci Transl Med 5: 177ra138.

21. Altvater B, Landmeier S, Pscherer S, Temme J, Schweer K, et al. (2009) 2B4 (CD244) signaling by recombinant antigen-specific chimeric receptors costimulates natural killer cell activation to leukemia and neuroblastoma cells. Clin Cancer Res 15: 4857–4866.

22. Li L, Liu LN, Feller S, Allen C, Shivakumar R, et al. (2009) Expression of chimeric antigen receptors in natural killer cells with a regulatory-compliant non-viral method. Cancer Gene Ther.

23. Shimasaki N, Fujisaki H, Cho D, Masselli M, Lockey T, et al. (2012) A clinically adaptable method to enhance the cytotoxicity of natural killer cells against B-cell malignancies. Cytotherapy 14: 830–840.

24. Manabe A, Coustan-Smith E, Kumagai M, Behm FG, Raimondi SC, et al. (1994) Interleukin-4 induces programmed cell death (apoptosis) in cases of high-risk acute lymphoblastic leukemia. Blood 83: 1731–1737.

25. Fujisaki H, Kakuda H, Shimasaki N, Imai C, Ma J, et al. (2009) Expansion of Highly Cytotoxic Human Natural Killer Cells for Cancer Cell Therapy. Cancer Res.

26. Wu KH, Sheu JN, Wu HP, Tsai C, Sieber M, et al. (2013) Cotransplantation of umbilical cord-derived mesenchymal stem cells promote hematopoietic engraftment in cord blood transplantation: a pilot study. Transplantation 95: 773–777.

27. Lapteva N, Durett AG, Sun J, Rollins LA, Huye LL, et al. (2012) Large-scale ex vivo expansion and characterization of natural killer cells for clinical applications. Cytotherapy 14: 1131–1143.

28. Denman CJ, Senyukov VV, Somanchi SS, Phatarpekar PV, Kopp LM, et al. (2012) Membrane-bound IL-21 promotes sustained ex vivo proliferation of human natural killer cells. PLoS One 7: e30264.

29. Carlin LM, Eleme K, McCann FE, Davis DM (2001) Intercellular transfer and supramolecular organization of human leukocyte antigen C at inhibitory natural killer cell immune synapses. J Exp Med 194: 1507–1517.

30. Poupot M, Fournie JJ, Poupot R (2008) Trogocytosis and killing of IL-4-polarized monocytes by autologous NK cells. J Leukoc Biol 84: 1298–1305.

31. Luchetti F, Canonico B, Arcangeletti M, Guescini M, Cesarini E, et al. (2012) Fas signalling promotes intercellular communication in T cells. PLoS One 7: e35766.

32. Roda-Navarro P, Vales-Gomez M, Chisholm SE, Reyburn HT (2006) Transfer of NKG2D and MICB at the cytotoxic NK cell immune synapse correlates with a reduction in NK cell cytotoxic function. Proc Natl Acad Sci U S A 103: 11258–11263.

33. Sadelain M, Brentjens R, Riviere I (2009) The promise and potential pitfalls of chimeric antigen receptors. Curr Opin Immunol 21: 215–223.

23

Regulation of RAB5C Is Important for the Growth Inhibitory Effects of MiR-509 in Human Precursor-B Acute Lymphoblastic Leukemia

Yee Sun Tan[1], MinJung Kim[1,3,4], Tami J. Kingsbury[1,2,3], Curt I. Civin[1,2,3,4], Wen-Chih Cheng[1,4]*

1 Center for Stem Cell Biology & Regenerative Medicine, University of Maryland School of Medicine, Baltimore, Maryland, United States of America, **2** Greenebaum Cancer Center, University of Maryland School of Medicine, Baltimore, Maryland, United States of America, **3** Department of Physiology, University of Maryland School of Medicine, Baltimore, Maryland, United States of America, **4** Department of Pediatrics, University of Maryland School of Medicine, Baltimore, Maryland, United States of America

Abstract

MicroRNAs (miRs) regulate essentially all cellular processes, but few miRs are known to inhibit growth of precursor-B acute lymphoblastic leukemias (B-ALLs). We identified miR-509 via a human genome-wide gain-of-function screen for miRs that inhibit growth of the NALM6 human B-ALL cell line. MiR-509-mediated inhibition of NALM6 growth was confirmed by 3 independent assays. Enforced miR-509 expression inhibited 2 of 2 additional B-ALL cell lines tested, but not 3 non-B-ALL leukemia cell lines. MiR-509-transduced NALM6 cells had reduced numbers of actively proliferating cells and increased numbers of cells undergoing apoptosis. Using miR target prediction algorithms and a filtering strategy, RAB5C was predicted as a potentially relevant target of miR-509. Enforced miR-509 expression in NALM6 cells reduced RAB5C mRNA and protein levels, and RAB5C was demonstrated to be a direct target of miR-509. Knockdown of RAB5C in NALM6 cells recapitulated the growth inhibitory effects of miR-509. Co-expression of the RAB5C open reading frame without its 3′ untranslated region (3′UTR) blocked the growth-inhibitory effect mediated by miR-509. These findings establish RAB5C as a target of miR-509 and an important regulator of B-ALL cell growth with potential as a therapeutic target.

Editor: Linda Bendall, University of Sydney, Australia

Funding: This work was supported by the following grants from National Foundation for Cancer Research (http://www.nfcr.org), the National Institutes of Health (http://www.nih.gov) (PO1CA70970) and Maryland Stem Cell Research Foundation/TEDCO (http://www.mscrf.org) (2007-MSCRFII-0114, 2008-MSCRF-303524 and 2010-MSCRFII-0065-00) to CIC, and Gabrielle's Angel Foundation (http://www.gabriellesangels.org) to WCC. The funders had no role in study design, data collection and analysis, decision to publish, or preparation of the manuscript.

Competing Interests: The authors have declared that no competing interests exist.

* Email: WCheng@som.umaryland.edu

Introduction

More effective and less toxic therapies are needed for precursor-B acute lymphoblastic leukemia (B-ALL), the most common childhood cancer [1–3]. To find novel therapeutic targets, deeper understanding of the mechanisms involved in leukemia cell proliferation and survival is necessary. MicroRNAs (miRs) are short non-coding RNAs which regulate expression of mRNA targets, most commonly by binding to the 3′ untranslated regions (3′UTRs) of mRNAs [4–6]. Each miR has many, often hundreds of predicted mRNA targets, and reciprocally a single mRNA may be targeted by multiple miRs. MiRs are involved in many cellular processes, and dysregulation of miRs has been linked to diseases, prominently including cancer [7]. For instance, overexpression of miR-155 has been detected in certain subtypes of acute myeloid leukemia (AML), chronic lymphoblastic leukemia, and lymphomas [8]. Transplantation of mouse bone marrow cells overexpressing miR-155 resulted in myeloproliferative disorders, and transgenic overexpression of miR-155 resulted in ALL and lymphoma in mice [9,10]. In contrast, miR-34 is a well-studied tumor suppressor miR; its expression is down-regulated in a wide range of solid and hematologic malignancies, and it targets multiple

molecules that promote cancer development and progression, including BCL2 and cyclin D1 [11,12].

Expression profiling studies, such as microarray hybridization, real-time PCR, or sequencing assays of global miR expression in leukemia cells versus normal counterpart cells, are often used to identify miRs associated with acute leukemias [13–15]. In B-ALLs, multiple miRs are known to be dysregulated [16,17], but only a few miRs, including miR-196b [18], miR-124a [19] and miR-143 [20], have been shown to inhibit B-ALL growth. Although expression profiling studies can implicate miRs as biomarkers, it is often difficult to differentiate 'passenger miRs' from 'driver miRs' [21]. As an alternative to expression profiling approaches, functional screens for miRs that drive hallmark cancer properties have successfully identified miRs involved in regulation of cellular processes including growth in melanoma [22], pancreatic cancer [23], and colon cancer [24], as well as metastasis in liver cancer [25]. We previously identified a set of miRs that regulate growth of the human lung fibroblast cell line IMR90 by a miR-high throughput functional screen (miR-HTS) [26]. In this paper, we extended our gain-of-function screening of human miRs to B-ALL cells and identified miR-509 as a novel B-ALL growth-inhibitory miR. MiR-509 inhibited growth of 2 additional B-ALL cell lines.

We went on to determine the cellular mechanism of miR-509-mediated B-ALL growth inhibition and identify RAB5C as a key B-ALL growth-promoting factor targeted by miR-509.

Material and Methods

Functional screen of miRs

Detailed description of the miR-HTS methodology was previously described [26]. Briefly, in each miR-HTS, 1.8 million NALM6 cells were infected at a multiplicity of infection (MOI) = 0.3 with the human Lenti-miR pooled virus library (System Biosciences, Mountain View, CA, USA; Cat# PMIRHPLVA-1) to achieve ~30% transduced cells. 4 μg/ml polybrene (Sigma-Aldrich, St. Louis, MO, USA) was used as the infection vehicle. On days 4, 12, 20 and 28 after infection, a fraction of the infected culture (2 million cells) was harvested and genomic DNA isolated using the DNeasy Blood & Tissue Kit (Qiagen, Valencia, CA, USA). To identify candidate growth-regulatory miRs, nested PCR, customized qPCR assays, and candidate selection were conducted as described [26]. 3 independent miR-HTS was conducted.

Cell lines

NALM6, RCH-ACV, REH, KARPAS-45 were obtained from DSMZ (Braunschweig, Germany). Jurkat and K562 cells were obtained from ATCC (Manassas, VA, USA). All cell lines were maintained according to manufacturer's protocol.

Plasmids and cloning

Overexpression of miRs was achieved by cloning each precursor miR sequence plus ~200 bp of flanking genomic sequence into the pJET1.2 plasmid (Thermo Scientific, Waltham, MA, USA) (Primers listed in Table S1). The genomic sequence of each miR was obtained from the UCSC genome browser. The miR sequences were then subcloned into our pWCC52 lentiviral vector (Empty lentiviral vector #1, EV#1) downstream of GFP driven by human EF1α promoter. MiR-509 was also subcloned into our pWCC72 lentiviral vector (empty lentiviral vector #2, EV#2) downstream of DsRed driven by human EF1α promoter. Both pWCC52 and pWCC72 were generated in our lab based on lentivectors designed to express miRs as described [27].

3 plasmids, each containing a different shRNA targeting RAB5C [shRNA#1 (TRCN0000072935), shRNA#2 (TRCN0000072933), shRNA#3 (TRCN0000072937)], were purchased from Thermo Scientific. The plasmid containing non-targeting scramble control sequence was purchased from Addgene (plasmid 1864) [28]. Next, each of the shRNA plasmids was digested with BamHI and NdeI to subclone the scramble control sequence and the shRNA containing sequences into pLKO.3G lentiviral plasmid (Addgene Plasmid 14748).

For luciferase assays, full length RAB5C 3′UTR was PCR amplified using cDNA of NALM6 as template, and cloned into pmirGLO Dual-Luciferase miRNA Target Expression vector (Promega, Madison, WI, USA). Site directed mutagenesis of RAB5C-3′UTR-luciferase deletion construct 1 (Δ1) was carried out using the QuikChange Lightning Site-Directed Mutagenesis Kit (Agilent Technologies, Santa Clara, CA, USA) according to manufacturer's protocol. For deletion of the second miR-509-3p binding site in Δ2 construct and Δ1Δ2 constructs, standard PCR was performed. Primers used to create the luciferase constructs are listed in Table S2.

A lentivector overexpressing the RAB5C was constructed by PCR amplification of the RAB5C open reading frame from NALM6 cDNA (Primers listed in Table S3). The PCR product was then cloned into the pWCC61 plasmid (Empty lentiviral vector #3; EV#3), a dual-promoter lentiviral vector generated by our lab in which the human EF1α promoter drives RAB5C and the ubiquitin promoter drives DsRed.

Lentivirus production and transduction

Lentivector plasmids were co-transfected with purchased packaging plasmids, pMD2.G (Addgene plasmid 12259) and pCMVR8.74 (Addgene plasmid 22036), using 3 μg of polyethylenimine (Polysciences Inc., Warrington, PA, USA) per μg of DNA. Viruses were then titered in each cell line 3 days after transduction by measuring %GFP+ cells using flow cytometry. Cultures transduced between 30-70% GFP+ were used to calculate lentivirus titer and MOI. To increase transduction efficiency, the following amounts of polybrene was added to each cell line: 0.8 μg/ml polybrene for RCH-ACV and KARPAS-45 cells, 1.6 μg/ml polybrene for Jurkat cells, 4 μg/ml polybrene for NALM6, REH and K562 cells. Mock-transduced cells were cells treated with polybrene but no lentivirus. In all experiments with transduced cells, cells were transduced with each lentivirus to MOI = 2. All transduced cells were washed with phosphate buffered saline (PBS) at 2 days after transduction to remove the polybrene.

GFP competition assay

3 days after transduction, >80% of NALM6 cells were GFP+. 7 days after transduction, the transduced cells were mixed with mock-transduced cells to obtain a cell mixture containing ~50% GFP+ cells, and this time point was set as day 0 for the GFP competition assay. This cell mixture was cultured for 5 weeks, and the %GFP+ cells was measured weekly by flow cytometry (Accuri C6, Becton Dickinson, New Jersey, USA), after gating on only the viable cell population based on the FSC and SSC parameters. Analysis was performed using FlowJo software (Tree Star Inc, Ashland, OR, USA).

Cell growth assays

For alamarBlue (Life Technologies, Grand Island, NY, USA) dye-based cell growth assays, cells were seeded at 5×10^3 cells/100 μl media (NALM6 and RCH-ACV cells) or at 2×10^3 cells/100 μl media (REH cells) in triplicates in 96-well plates at 3 days after transduction. At 7 days after transduction, 10 μl alamarBlue was added to each well and plates incubated (37°C, 4 h) before reading using a VictorX3 (PerkinElmer, Waltham, MA, USA; 530/580 nm excitation/emission filters). For trypan blue exclusion cell counts, 2.5×10^5 cells/ml were seeded in each well of a 96-well plate day on day 3 after transduction. 10 μl of cell suspensions were removed at each time point and counted using a hemocytometer.

RNA isolation and measurement of miR and mRNA expression levels by quantitative real-time reverse-transcription PCR (qRT-PCR)

For qRT-PCR of mature miRs, cell lysates were made using Cell Lysis Buffer (Signosis, Santa Clara, CA, USA) and reverse transcription performed using TaqMan microRNA reverse transcription kit (Life Technologies) according to manufacturer's protocol. For mRNA levels, SYBRGreen qRT-PCR assays were conducted with total RNA isolated using the miRNeasy kit (Qiagen) according to manufacturer's protocol, and reverse transcription performed using the High-capacity-RNA-to-cDNA kit (Life Technologies) according to manufacturer's protocol. Primers for qRT-PCR for genes were obtained from PrimerBank

[29] (Table S4). The TaqMan IDs are listed in Table S5 (Life Technologies). All SYBRGreen and TaqMan qRT-PCR assays were performed using the 7900 HT Real-Time PCR system (Life Technologies). All Ct values >35 were assigned a value of 35 for calculation of fold expression level change. For qRT-PCR of mature miRs, U18 was used as endogenous control. For SYBR-Green qRT-PCR of mRNA genes, GAPDH was used as endogenous control. DNA oligonucleotides (synthesized by Integrated DNA Technologies, Coralville, IA, USA) of mature miR sequences (miRBase.org) were used to create standard curves for absolute qRT-PCR miR quantitation, which was performed as described previously [30,31].

Microarray data

All microarray data has been previously deposited in NCBI Gene Expression Omnibus [32] (GEO Series accession number GSE51908; http://www.ncbi.nlm.nih.gov/geo/query/acc.cgi?acc= GSE51908). Samples used in this analysis include B-ALL cell lines ($n = 27$, replicates of 9 cell lines), primary B-ALL samples ($n = 16$), T-ALL cell lines ($n = 15$, replicates of 5 cell lines), primary T-ALL samples ($n = 8$), AML cell lines ($n = 21$, replicates of 7 cell lines), primary AML samples ($n = 15$), primary blood B lymphocytes ($n = 11$), primary mobilized blood CD34$^+$ hematopoietic stem-progenitor cells (HSPCs) ($n = 4$), primary blood granulocytes ($n = 14$), primary blood monocytes ($n = 5$) and primary blood T lymphocytes ($n = 20$).

Apoptosis and cell cycle analysis

For apoptosis assays, 10^5 NALM6 cells were stained with APC Annexin V and DNA binding dye 7-amino-actinomycin (7-AAD) (Biolegend, San Diego, CA, USA) 4 days after transduction according to manufacturer's protocol and analyzed by flow cytometry (Accuri C6, Becton Dickinson). For cell cycle analysis, at 3 days after transduction, NALM6 cells (0.5×10^6 cells/ml) were cultured for 24 h in fresh medium, then 10^6 cells were labeled with BrdU (Becton Dickinson) for 1 h. Cells were then washed twice in ice cold PBS and the pellet suspended in 500 µl PBS. Cells were fixed in 5 ml ice cold 70% ethanol overnight at −20°C. 2 M hydrochloric acid was then used to denature the DNA for 30 min at room temperature, and the washed pellet resuspended in 1 ml 0.1 M Na$_2$B$_4$O$_7$, pH 8.5 (Sigma-Aldrich) to neutralize the acid for 10 min. Cells were stained with 1 µl APC anti-BrdU antibody (BioLegend) in 20 µl volume for 30 min at room temperature, followed by 20 µl 7-AAD for 15 min at room temperature. APC BrdU and 7-AAD signal was then assessed by flow cytometry (Accuri C6, Becton Dickinson). FlowJo software (Tree Star Inc) was used to determine the cell cycle profile of each sample.

Caspase-3/7 assay

Transduced NALM6 cells were seeded at 500 cells/well in a 384-well plate on day 3 after transduction. On day 7 after transduction, caspase activity was measured using the Apo-ONE homogenous caspase-3/7 assay (Promega) according to manufacturer's instructions at 4 h after addition of reagent to cells, using a VictorX3 (PerkinElmer, 485/535 nm excitation/emission filters).

Luciferase assay

HEK293T cells were cultured overnight at 10^5 cells/450 µl in each well of a 24-well plate. 300 ng of plasmid was co-transfected with 50 nM of miR mimic using 2.5 µl of Lipofectamine2000 (Life Technologies) according to manufacturer's protocol. Lysates were harvested 48 h after transfection and processed using Dual luciferase reporter assay system (Promega) according to manufac-

turer's protocol. Lysates were diluted 400-fold in passive Lysis buffer Assay before plating and read using VictorX3 (PerkinElmer). Renilla luciferase values were used to normalize for transfection efficiency; the ratio of firefly/renilla luciferase is designated as relative luciferase activity.

Western blotting

Lysates of transduced cells were harvested 7 days after transduction and lysed in RIPA buffer (Sigma-Aldrich) containing 1 mM phenylmethanesulfonyl fluoride (Sigma-Aldrich) and 1× complete protease inhibitor cocktail tablet (Roche Applied Science, Indianapolis, USA). Protein concentration was determined by Bio-Rad Protein assay (Bio-Rad, Hercules, CA, USA) according to manufacturer's protocol and lysates containing 30-40 µg protein loaded onto a pre-made 4-12% Bis-Tris NuPAGE gel (Life Technologies) and transferred to a PVDF membrane using an iBlot Dry Blotting system (Life Technologies). RAB5C (ab137919, Abcam, Cambridge, MA, USA) and α-tubulin (T6074, Sigma-Aldrich) antibodies were used according to manufacturer's protocol and signal detected using an ECL detection kit (Thermo Scientific) imaged by the ChemiDOC XRS+ System (Bio-Rad). Bands were analyzed and quantified using ImageLab software (Bio-Rad).

Results

Enforced miR-509 expression inhibited growth of NALM6 cells

We applied our functional miR-HTS to screen a pooled lentivirus library of 578 human miRs or miR clusters for their growth-regulatory properties in human NALM6 B-ALL cells and identified candidate miRs as previously described [26]. 4 miRs (miR-381, miR-509, miR-550a, and miR-873) and 1 miR cluster (miR-432~136) inhibited NALM6 growth in at least 2 of 3 replicate screens performed. In order to confirm the growth inhibitory effects of the candidate miRs identified from the functional screen, each of the 5 miR or miR cluster candidates was cloned into a lentiviral expression vector downstream of green fluorescent protein (GFP) (Figure 1A). We expressed the miR-432~136 cluster as a single unit rather than as 2 individual miRs, to recapitulate the way they were screened and because the 2 miRs may cooperate. The growth inhibitory potential of each candidate miR or miR cluster was then tested, by performing multiple GFP competition assays [33,34]. NALM6 cells were transduced with each of the 5 miR lentiviruses (>80% GFP$^+$ cells), and each culture was then mixed with GFP$^-$ cells to obtain an initial culture with ~50% GFP$^+$ cells. If enforced expression of a given miR or miR cluster inhibited NALM6 growth, the %GFP$^+$ cells in culture would decrease over time. For NALM6 cells transduced with the control empty vector, the %GFP$^+$ cells remained stable at ~50% over the 5-week GFP competition assay (Figure 1B). Similarly, no change in %GFP$^+$ cells was observed over 35 days in the GFP competition assays for miR-381, miR-550a, miR-873 and miR-432~136 (Figure S1A-S1D). In contrast, NALM6 cells transduced with miR-509 lentivirus were out-grown by the GFP$^-$ cells; the %GFP$^+$ cells decreased from 46% at assay day 0 to 10% 35 days later (Figure 1B). ·

As expected, miR-509-5p and miR-509-3p were strongly overexpressed in miR-509-transduced NALM6 cells as assayed by qRT-PCR (Figure 1C). Similarly, overexpression of miR-381, miR-550a, miR-873, and miR-432 was achieved by lentiviral transduction (Figure S1E). These results indicate that miR-381, miR-432, miR-550a, and miR-873 do not inhibit growth of NALM6. However, no expression of miR-136 was detected in

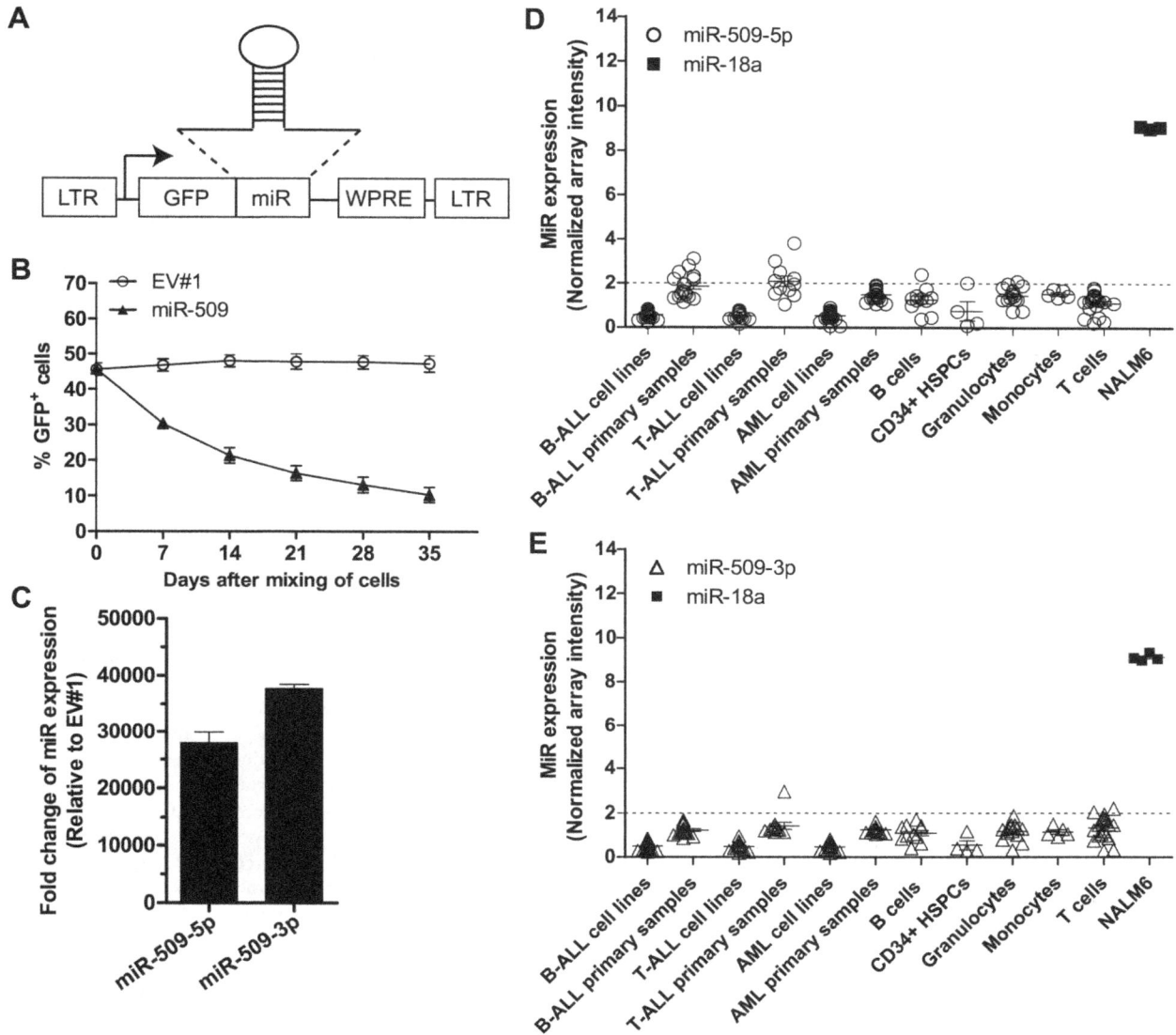

Figure 1. Enforced miR-509 expression inhibits growth of NALM6 cells. (A) Schematic of lentiviral vector used to express miRs. Arrow depicts the direction of human EF1α promoter. LTR: long terminal repeat; GFP: green fluorescent protein; WPRE: woodchuck hepatitis virus post-transcriptional regulatory element. The parental plasmid without miR is denoted as empty vector #1 (EV#1). The miR sequence consists of the native miR hairpin with ~200 bp of its flanking genomic sequences. (B) Assessment of %GFP+ cells by flow cytometry in the GFP competition assay. NALM6 cells were transduced with miR-509 lentivirus or empty vector (EV#1) at MOI = 2, and transduced GFP+ cells were mixed with an equal number of mock-transduced cells (GFP−) 7 days later to achieve an initial culture of ~50%GFP+ cells; this was designated Day 0 and the %GFP+ cells (pre-gated on viable cells) was assessed weekly by flow cytometry. Means ± SEMs are shown for 3 independent experiments. (C) Enforced expression of mature miR-509-5p and miR-509-3p NALM6 cells, as assayed by qRT-PCR. NALM6 cells were transduced with miR-509 lentivirus to MOI = 2, and total RNA was collected at 7 days after transduction. U18 was used as the loading control, and normalized to EV#1-transduced NALM6 cells. Means ± SEMs of 3 independent experiments. (D) Expression of mature miR-509-5p was determined by miR microarray analysis in B-ALL, T-ALL and AML cell lines and primary samples, B cells, CD34+ HSPCs, granulocytes, monocytes and T cells. Dotted line represents normalized microarray intensity of 2 whereby any value <2 denotes undetectable expression. Data points shown are means ± SEMs. Expression data is accessible through GEO Series accession number GSE51908 [32]. (E) Expression of mature miR-509-3p and miR-18a as determined by miR microarray analysis similar to (D). (D, E) Data shown for miR-18a is only for the NALM6 cell line.

miR-432~136 cluster-transduced NALM6 cells. This lack of miR-136 expression could be due to lack of necessary cis-regulatory elements or trans-regulatory factors required for miR-136 biogenesis; we did not investigate the possibility that an alternative approach to successfully express miR-136 in NALM6 would validate a growth inhibitory role for this miR. Instead, we decided to focus on miR-509 for further studies.

Our miR microarray expression analyses [32] (GEO Series accession number GSE51908) revealed undetectable endogenous levels of mature miR-509-5p and miR-509-3p in NALM6 and other acute leukemia cell lines (Figure 1D, 1E), as well as in primary leukemia cases and CD34+ hematopoietic stem-progenitor cells (HSPCs) and blood cell types from normal human donors (Figure 1D, 1E). In absolute qRT-PCR quantifications [30,31], miR-509-transduced NALM6 cells expressed 1,814±95 copies (mean ± SEM) per cell of miR-509-5p (Table 1), comparable to levels of miR-18a, which for reference is expressed at the 70th percentile of all miRs in NALM6 cells based on our miR microarray data (Figure 1D). MiR-509-3p was expressed at $3,656 \pm 117$ copies per cell in miR-509-transduced NALM6 cells, also within the physiological range of miR copy numbers per cell (range: <10 to>30,000 copies per mammalian cell) [30].

MiR-509 reduced NALM6 cell growth by 2 additional independent assays

To further confirm the effect of miR-509 on NALM6 cell growth, we performed trypan blue dye exclusion cell counts and alamarBlue assays. At 8 days after transduction, cultures of miR-509-transduced NALM6 cells contained 43% fewer viable cells than empty vector-transduced cells by trypan blue counts (Figure 2A). Similarly, miR-509-transduced NALM6 cells had 48% reduced ($p < 0.05$) cell growth, as compared to empty vector-transduced cells using the alamarBlue assay (Figure 2B). Since the alamarBlue dye-based assay measures the reducing environment within cells, which is linked to mitochondria metabolism [35], we examined whether miR-509 affected mitochondrial membrane potential. No difference in mitochondrial membrane potential was observed between miR-509-transduced and empty vector-transduced NALM6 cells (data not shown).

MiR-509 inhibited growth of RCH-ACV and REH B-ALL cell lines

We next examined if the growth inhibitory effects of miR-509 extended to other B-ALL (RCH-ACV and REH), T-cell ALL (T-ALL; Jurkat and KARPAS-45) or myeloid leukemia (K562) cell lines. MiR-509-transduced RCH-ACV cells had ~30% reduced growth by trypan blue on day 8 after transduction or alamarBlue assay on day 7 after transduction (Figure 2C, 2D). In addition, miR-509-transduced REH cells had 23% ($p < 0.05$) reduced growth in the alamarBlue assay (Figure 2E). In contrast, no reduction in cell growth was observed in Jurkat, KARPAS-45 or K562 cells transduced with miR-509 as compared to control empty vector using alamarBlue assays (Figure S2A–S2D). This was despite documented overexpression of miR-509 in these transduced cell lines (Figure S3). Thus, miR-509 inhibited the growth of all 3 tested human B-ALL cell lines, NALM6, RCH-ACV and REH.

MiR-509-transduced NALM6 cells had a lower proportion of cells in cell cycle S-phase and increased apoptosis

To investigate the cellular mechanisms by which enforced miR-509 expression inhibits growth, we examined whether miR-509 regulates cell cycle progression by conducting BrdU/7-AAD

staining [36]. 4 days after transduction, miR-509-transduced NALM6 had fewer cells in S-phase than empty vector-transduced cells (Figure 3A), and this was statistically significant (Figure 3B, $p < 0.05$). In addition, there were slightly elevated numbers of cells in the subG$_1$ and G$_2$/M phases, but these differences were not statistically significant. To investigate if miR-509 promotes cell death via apoptosis, Annexin V/7-AAD staining was performed. 4 days after transduction, miR-509-transduced NALM6 cells had 1.5-fold ($p < 0.05$) higher numbers of Annexin V$^+$/7-AAD$^-$ apoptotic cells and 1.4-fold higher numbers of Annexin V$^+$ dying/dead cells ($p < 0.05$), as compared to empty vector-transduced cells (Figure 3C, 3D). Consistent with these findings, we detected a 1.5-fold increase ($p < 0.05$) in activated capase-3/7 activity in miR-509-transduced NALM6 cells as compared to empty vector-transduced cells (Figure 3E).

Informatics prediction of RAB5C as a target of miR-509

To identify targets of miR-509 that might mediate growth of B-ALL cells, we used a filtering strategy to prioritize the many predicted targets of miR-509 (Figure 4A). First, we downloaded the sets of predicted mRNA targets of miR-509-5p and miR-509-3p (Set 1), as well as those of the 4 miRs that we had shown not to inhibit NALM6 growth (i.e. miR-381, miR-432, miR-550a and miR-873; Set 2) from the TargetScan6.2 [37] and/or miRDB [38,39] miR target prediction databases. Since NALM6 cells transduced with miR-432~136 did not result in miR-136 overexpression, we did not include miR-136 targets in Set 2 (Figure 4A). Next, we downloaded the gene expression profile of NALM6, determined by genome-wide microarray profiling as listed in the Cancer Cell Line Encyclopedia (CCLE) [40] and focused on genes which have detectable expression in NALM6 (i.e. annotated as "marginal" or "present" in CCLE; Set 3). Then, we intersected these 3 sets of mRNAs [41] to identify the subset of genes expressed in NALM6 and predictively targeted by miR-509, but not predictively targeted by the 4 miRs that did not inhibit NALM6 growth. This resulted in a set of 395 genes (listed in Table S6). This list was subsequently reduced to 74 genes by selecting for genes known to participate in growth regulation based on annotations at NCBI's "Gene" database, DAVID bioinformatics resources [42,43], as well as our own literature searches. Of these 74 predicted targets of miR-509, 12 genes previously demonstrated in the literature to be either involved in leukemia and oncogenesis (ERLIN2, FLI1, FOXP1, MAML1, RAC1, YWHAB and YWHAG), or predicted as miR-509 targets by both TargetScan6.2 and miRDB (PGRMC1, RAB5C, RAC1, TFDP2, UHMK1, USP9X) were selected for initial qRT-PCR analysis. We used this informatic filtering strategy, as compared to performing global differential gene expression analysis such as microarray analysis, to enable us to rapidly and at low cost identify

Table 1. Absolute copy number of mature miR-509 and miR-18a RNA per NALM6 cell.

| qRT-PCR assay | Copy number per NALM6 cell transduced with | |
	Empty vector #1	miR-509
miR-509-5p	<10	1,814±95
miR-509-3p	<10	3,656±117
miR-18a	1,591±105	1,415±53

RNA was isolated from NALM6 cells on day 7 after transduction with either control empty vector #1 or miR-509, and absolute qRT-PCR quantification was performed for miR-509-5p, miR-509-3p or miR-18a. Copy number per cell was estimated based on standard curves of miR-509-5p, miR-509-3p or miR-18a using DNA oligonucleotides. For reverse transcription, 10 ng RNA (equivalent to 800 cells, i.e. 12.5 pg of total RNA per cell) was used in each reaction. Means ± SEMs of 3 independent experiments.

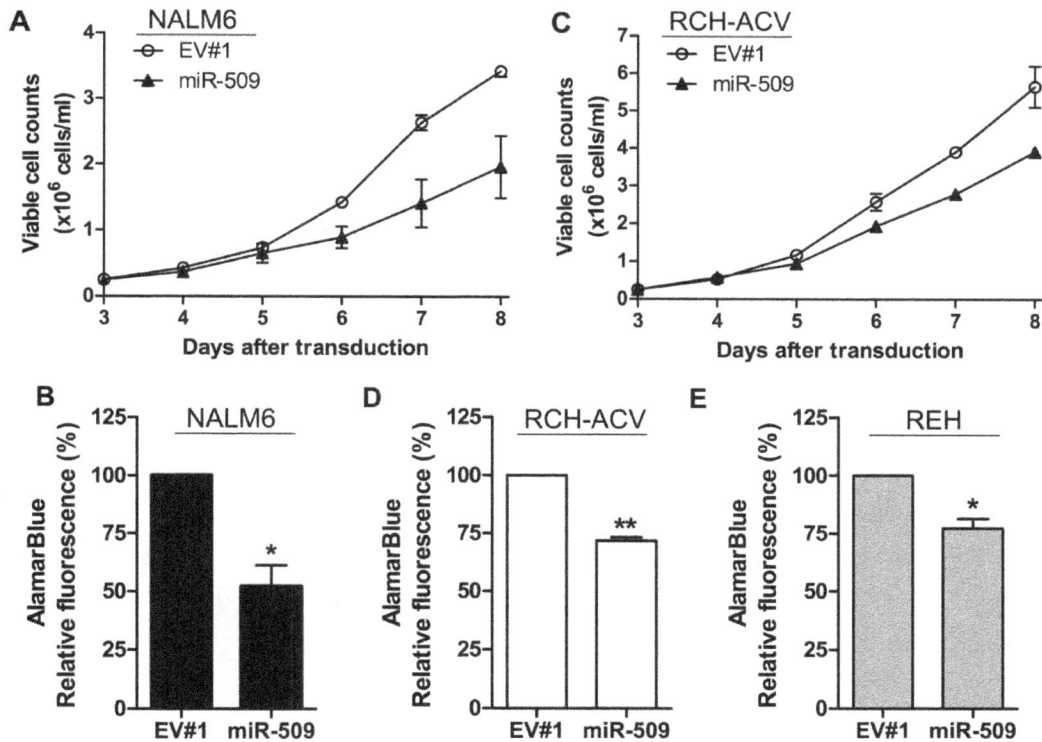

Figure 2. Enforced miR-509 resulted in inhibition of growth of 3 B-ALL cell lines, NALM6, REH and RCH-ACV. (A) Viable cell numbers measured via trypan blue dye exclusion counts of NALM6 cells transduced with either miR-509 lentivirus or empty vector (EV#1); 25,000 cells were plated for each sample starting at 3 days after transduction. (B) AlamarBlue cell growth assay on day 7 after transduction of NALM6 cells transduced with either miR-509 lentivirus or EV#1. Values for miR-509 were normalized to EV#1. (C) Viable cell counts of RCH-ACV cells based on trypan blue exclusion counts, initial plating of 25,000 cells for both samples on 3 days after transduction. Means ± SEMs are plotted, and SEMs for miR-509 were very small. (D) Cell growth of RCH-ACV transduced with either EV#1 or miR-509 overexpressing lentivirus using alamarBlue cell growth assay conducted on day 7 after transduction. Values for miR-509 were normalized to EV#1. (E) MiR-509-transduced REH cells reduced growth compared to EV#1 in an alamarBlue cell growth assay. Cells were transduced 7 days prior to addition of alamarBlue. (A to E) Means ± SEMs, 3 independent experiments done in triplicates. Statistical analysis was done by Student's t test. *p<0.05, **p<0.01.

target genes-of-interest. 3 of these 12 predicted targets (RAB5C, RAC1, and UHMK1) were down-regulated by miR-509 at the mRNA level (Figure 4B). RAB5C mRNA levels showed the greatest reduction, with a 40% lower level (p<0.05) in miR-509-transduced than in empty vector-transduced NALM6 cells (Figure 4B). Correspondingly, RAB5C protein was 85% (p< 0.001) lower in miR-509-transduced cells by western blotting (Figure 4C, 4D). We also observed a ≥86% decrease in RAB5C protein levels in miR-509-transduced RCH-ACV and REH cells as compared to empty vector (Figure S4). Since RAB5 has been implicated in cell cycling [44,45] and is one of the top 3 predicted targets of miR-509-3p by both TargetScan6.2 (Total context+ score = −0.65) and miRDB (Target score = 91), we focused our subsequent studies on RAB5C.

MiR-509 directly targets RAB5C

To examine if miR-509 directly represses RAB5C, we employed RAB5C-3′UTR luciferase reporter assays. There are 2 miR-509-3p binding sequences in the 3′UTR of RAB5C (Figure 5A), as predicted by both miRDB and TargetScan6.2. Both miR-509-3p binding sequences are present in the RAB5C 3′UTR of several species including human, mouse, rat, horse and dog, suggesting that the regulation of RAB5C by miR-509 is also conserved. We cloned the full-length wild type (WT) 3′UTR of RAB5C downstream of firefly luciferase gene (luc2) in the pmirGLO luciferase vector and also generated 3 luciferase constructs

containing 1 (Δ1 or Δ2) or both (Δ1Δ2) deletions of miR-509-3p binding sites (Figure 5B). Co-transfection of miR-509-3p mimic and RAB5C-3′UTR WT luciferase vector resulted in 81% lower (p<0.001) relative luciferase activity than in cells transfected with RAB5C-3′UTR WT luciferase vector alone (Figure 5C). Co-transfection of the non-targeting miR-551b mimic plus the RAB5C-3′UTR WT luciferase vector did not repress luciferase activity. Co-transfection of either RAB5C-3′UTR-luciferase deletion construct, Δ1 or Δ2, plus miR-509-3p mimic resulted in > 50% lower (p<0.01) relative luciferase activity than cells transfected with only the indicated RAB5C-3′UTR deletion constructs. Co-transfection of Δ1Δ2 construct (in which both predicted miR-509-3p binding sites were deleted) with miR-509-3p mimic abolished the reduction in luciferase signal. This indicated that miR-509 directly targets the 3′UTR of RAB5C via both predicted miR-509-3p binding sites.

RAB5C mediates the growth-inhibitory effect of miR-509

We then examined if reduced RAB5C is responsible for the functional effects of miR-509. To determine if repression of RAB5C would phenocopy the growth suppressive effect of miR-509, NALM6 cells were transduced with 3 different lentiviruses, each containing a distinct shRNA against RAB5C. In alamarBlue assays, all 3 shRNAs inhibited NALM6 cell growth by ≥42% (p< 0.01) as compared to cells transduced with the scrambled control (Figure 6A). We verified that all 3 shRNAs resulted in ≥80%

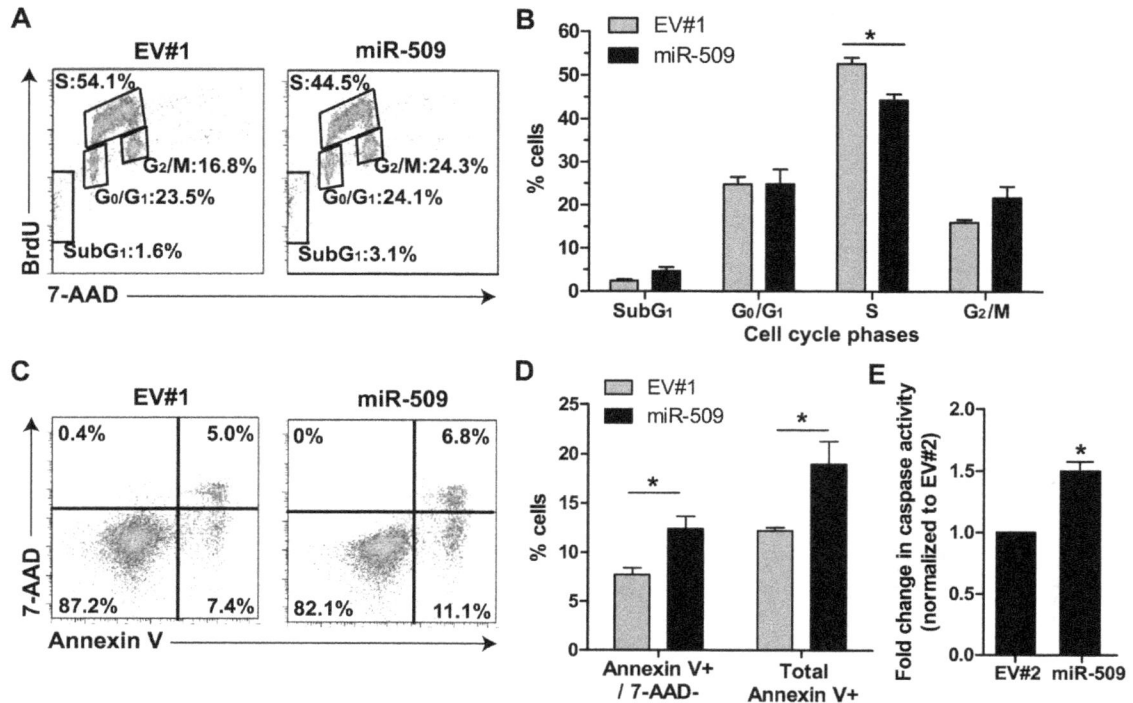

Figure 3. Enforced miR-509 expression in decreased proportion of cells in S-phase, induced apoptosis and activated caspase-3/7. (A) Representative flow cytometric plots showing cell cycle distribution of NALM6 cells transduced with empty vector (EV#1) or miR-509 overexpressing lentivirus. On day 3 after transduction, cells were labeled with BrdU for 1 h. Cells were then fixed overnight and stained on the next day with both BrdU and 7-AAD before analysis by flow cytometry. Percent of cells at each phase of cell cycle are boxed as indicated. (B) Frequencies of cells at the different phases of cell cycle. Means ± SEMs of 3 independent experiments with statistical analysis by Student's t test. *p<0.05. (C) Representative flow cytometric plots of cell death distribution of NALM6 cells transduced with EV#1 or miR-509 overexpressing lentivirus. Cells were stained with both Annexin V and 7-AAD before analysis by flow cytometry on day 4 after transduction. Numbers represent the frequency in each quadrant. (D) Frequencies of apoptotic cells which are Annexin V-positive (Annexin V$^+$) and 7-AAD negative (7-AAD$^-$), as well as total Annexin V$^+$. Means ± SEMs of 3 independent experiments with statistical analysis by Student's t test. *p<0.05. (E) NALM6 cells were transduced with empty vector #2 (EV#2) or miR-509 overexpressing lentivirus, and cells were seeded in 384-well plate on day 3 after transduction. On day 7 after transduction, caspase-3/7 activity was measured and fold-change in caspase activity was normalized to EV#2. Means ± SEMs of 3 independent experiments done in triplicates, with statistical analysis by Student's t test. *p<0.05.

decreased RAB5C protein levels (p<0.01) in NALM6 cells (Figure 6B, 6C) using western blotting.

In order to determine whether RAB5C mediates miR-509 induced growth inhibition in NALM6 cells, we performed a rescue experiment. We cloned the RAB5C open reading frame (ORF) without its 3'UTR into a lentiviral vector. In alamarBlue assays, NALM6 cells co-transduced with miR-509 plus empty vector had 51% lower growth (p<0.001) than cells co-transduced with the 2 control empty lentiviral vectors (Figure 6D). In contrast, NALM6 cells co-transduced with miR-509 plus RAB5C lentiviruses had 36% greater growth than cells co-transduced with miR-509 plus the empty vector (p<0.05). Overexpression of RAB5C ORF in NALM6 cells co-transduced with miR-509 was confirmed by western blotting (Figure 6E, 6F). Thus, RAB5C rescued, in large part, the growth inhibitory effects of miR-509.

Discussion

In this study, we conducted a functional miR-HTS in NALM6 cells and identified miR-509 as a novel inhibitor of human B-ALL cell growth. Using NALM6 B-ALL cell line, enforced expression of miR-509 reduced NALM6 B-ALL cell growth in 3 independent growth assays. MiR-509-mediated growth inhibition was also observed in 2 additional B-ALL cell lines, REH and RCH-ACV. However, miR-509 is not a global inhibitor of cell growth, as

enforced miR-509 expression in 2 T-ALL (Jurkat and KARPAS-45) and 1 myeloid leukemia (K562) cell lines did not inhibit growth. Susceptibility to miR-509 growth inhibition is likely due to differential expression or differential dependence upon miR-509 target genes for cell proliferation and survival [46]. More extensive testing will be necessary to determine if the growth inhibitory effects of miR-509 might be specific to B-ALL cells or some molecularly-defined subset of leukemias or shared with other cancer types. MiR-509 has been reported previously to be down-regulated in renal cell carcinoma as compared to normal tissue counterparts [47,48]. Since miR-509-5p and miR-509-3p are undetectable in normal or leukemic hematopoietic cells, miR-509 does not qualify as a tumor suppressor miR for leukemias. The lack of miR-509 expression in healthy donor blood cell types and CD34$^+$ HSPCs [32] exemplifies the importance of functional screening to identify growth-suppressing miRs, as expression profiling comparing acute leukemia cases versus healthy donor samples would not have identified miR-509 as a miR capable of inhibiting leukemia cell growth.

We further observed that enforced miR-509 expression reduced the number of actively proliferating cells and increased apoptotic and dead NALM6 cells, indicating that miR-509 reduces cell proliferation and survival. Our observations in NALM6 are consistent with previous reports that both miR-509-5p [47] and

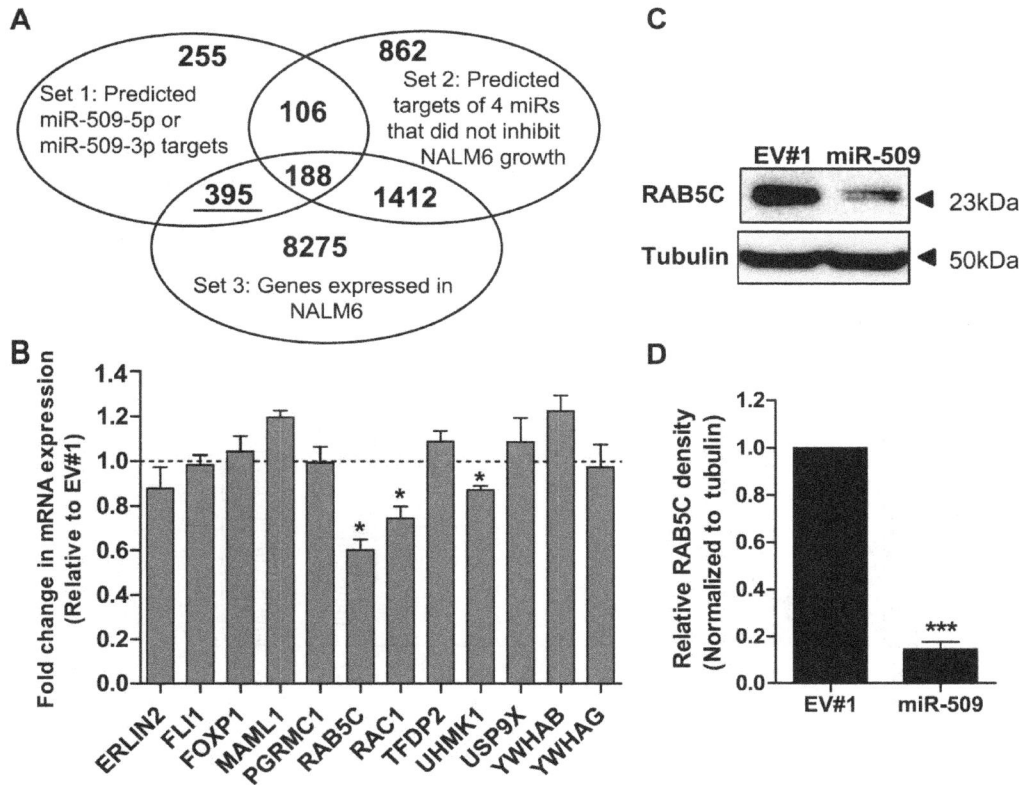

Figure 4. Identifying mRNA targets of miR-509. (A) Venn diagram showing the number of mRNAs that do not overlap, or are shared between each set in our *in silico* strategy to identify relevant targets of miR-509. Set 1 refers to the list of predicted targets of miR-509-5p or miR-509-3p from TargetScan6.2 or miRDB. Set 2 is the list of predicted targets of miRs tested to not inhibit NALM6 growth (i.e. miR-550a, miR-873, miR-381 and miR-432) from TargetScan6.2 or miRDB, while Set 3 is the list of mRNA that is expressed in NALM6, as determined by genome-wide microarray profiling downloaded from the Cancer Cell Line Encyclopedia and its expression levels are denoted in the microarray dataset as "marginal" or "present". (B) Expression levels of 12 putative targets of miR-509 as determined by qRT-PCR. RNA was isolated from NALM6 cells transduced with EV#1 or miR-509 overexpressing lentivirus at 7 days after transduction. All values were normalized to GAPDH and fold-change was calculated relative to EV#1 sample. Data represents means $\pm$ SEMs of 3 independent experiments, with statistical analysis by Student's *t* test. *$p < 0.05$. (C) Representative western blots of RAB5C expression. NALM6 cells were transduced with either EV#1or miR-509 overexpressing lentivirus, and whole cell lysates were harvested at 7 days after transduction. α-tubulin was used for loading control. (D) Densitometry analysis of RAB5C expression of western blot in (C) and 2 other independent experiments. α-tubulin was used for normalization, and relative densitometry was then calculated compared to EV#1. Data shown represent means $\pm$ SEMs, with statistical analysis by Student's *t* test. ***$p < 0.001$.

miR-509-3p [48] suppressed cell growth and induced apoptosis in a human renal cancer cell line.

To identify relevant miR-509 targets, we may in the future employ biochemical or genomic techniques [49,50] to identify all of the targets of miR-509 in NALM6 cells. In the initial study herein, we instead used bioinformatics to define a subset of predicted miR-509 target genes known to be expressed in NALM6 cells but not predicted to be targeted by the miRs that failed to inhibit NALM6 cell growth. We then selected those targets known to be involved in cellular processes that regulate growth (e.g. proliferation, cell cycle, cell death, oncogenes), resulting in a set of 74 growth-related predicted miR-509 targets. Using qRT-PCR to assess levels of 12 of these 74 targets in miR-509-transduced versus empty vector-transduced NALM6 cells, 3 predicted miR-509 targets were reduced in miR-509-transduced NALM6 cells. Although the mRNAs of 9 of the 12 tested predicted miR-509 targets were not reduced in miR-509-transduced NALM6 cells, some of these may still be targets of miR-509 as they might be inhibited at the translational level [51]. However, given that reduction at the mRNA level was observed in $\geq 84\%$ of miR targets with reduced protein levels [52], we decided to focus in the

study herein on predicted targets inhibited by miR-509 at the mRNA level. Moreover, RAB5C mRNA was the target most reduced in response to miR-509 expression, and therefore we focused on RAB5C for further experiments. We showed that miR-509 indeed binds to the 3'UTR of RAB5C via the 2 thermodynamically predicted sites. Upon effective knockdown of RAB5C using each of 3 shRNA constructs, NALM6 cell growth was reduced; thus, RAB5C knockdown phenocopied the growth inhibition observed by enforced miR-509 expression. Our observations that co-transduction of the RAB5C ORF lacking its 3'UTR (therefore no longer regulated by miR-509) rescues miR-509-mediated growth inhibition indicates that reduction of RAB5C is a major mechanism of miR-509-mediated NALM6 growth inhibition. Thus, while future studies may find additional targets of miR-509-5p and/or miR-509-3p that contribute to miR-509-mediated growth inhibition, our current results demonstrate that RAB5C is a novel target of miR-509 and an important driver of the growth of human B-ALL cells.

As members of the Rab family of small monomeric GTPases, RAB5 molecules are central in coordinating vesicle trafficking, particularly in the early stages of endocytosis [53–55]. In addition

A

Position 66-72 of RAB5C 3'UTR 5' ...CUGGAAUCCACUCUA--ACCAAUCG...
                                          | | | | | | | | | | |
hsa-miR-509-3p   3'   GAUGGGUGUCUGCAUGGUUAGU

Position 759-766 of RAB5C 3'UTR 5' ...UUUCUUCAACAUGUA-ACCAAUCAG...
                                           | | | | | | | | | |
hsa-miR-509-3p   3'   GAUGGGUGUCUGCAUGGUUAGU

B

C

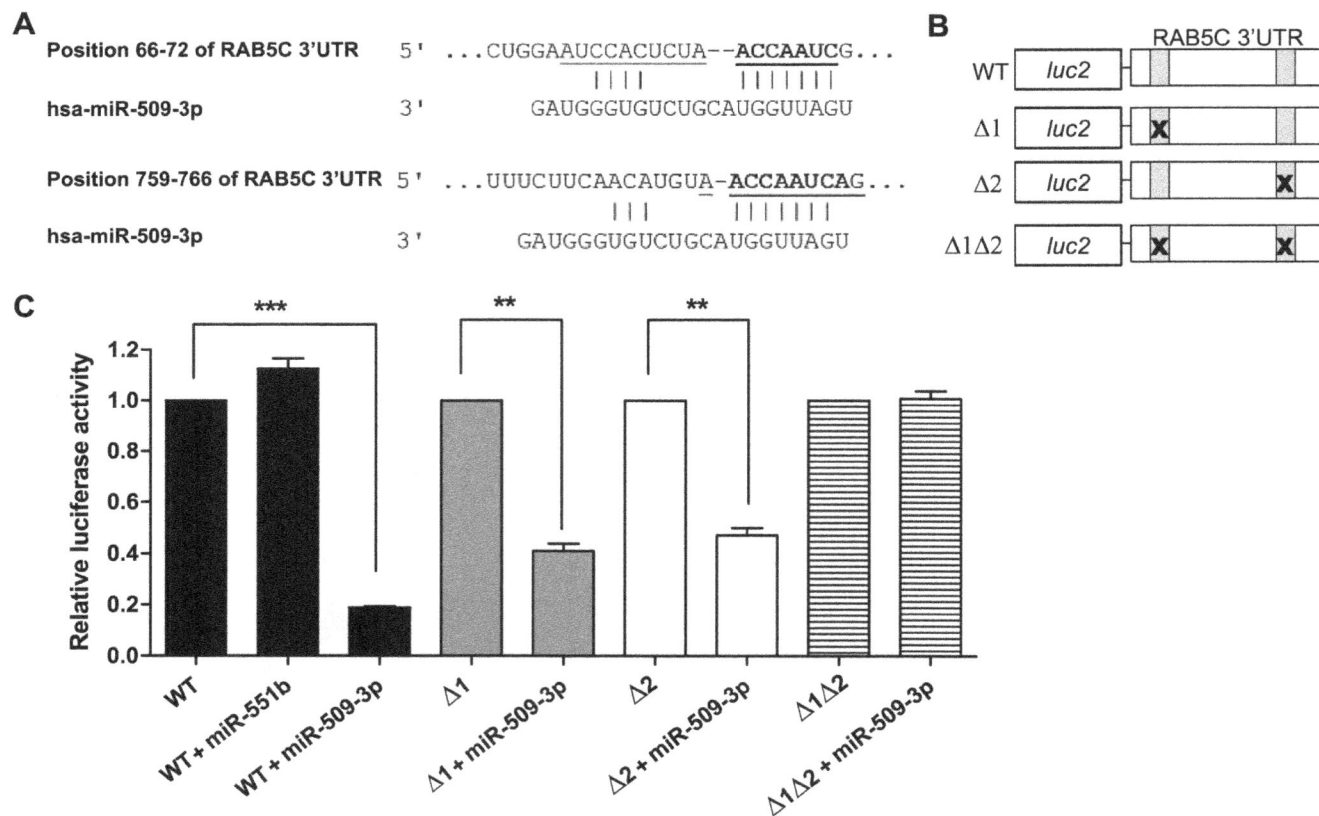

Figure 5. RAB5C is a direct target of miR-509. (A) Sequence alignment of RAB5C to miR-509-3p predicted by TargetScan6.2. The full length 3'UTR of RAB5C is 803 bases. Sequences shown in bold refer to position 66–72 and 759–766 of RAB5C 3'UTR where miR-509-3p is predicted to target. The underlined sequences were deleted in the RAB5C-3'UTR deletion constructs listed in (B) for the luciferase assay. (B) Schematic representation of luciferase vector constructs used in luciferase assay. Full length RAB5C 3'UTR was cloned downstream of the firefly luciferase gene (luc2) in the pmirGLO luciferase vector. Wild type RAB5C 3'UTR is listed as WT. Grey boxes indicate the 2 predicted miR-509-3p target sites (66–72 and 759–766), and the "X" indicates the deletion sites present in the deletion (Δ) constructs. (C) Luciferase assay demonstrates that RAB5C 3'UTR is targeted by miR-509-3p via 2 binding sites. 293T cells were transfected with the 300ng of the indicated luciferase plasmids and 50nM of miR mimics, and harvested for luciferase assay 48 h after transfection. All values were first normalized to Renilla luciferase. Relative luciferase activity was then calculated by normalizing co-transfection of miR mimics plus luciferase constructs to cells transfected with only the respective luciferase construct. MiR-551b was used as a non-targeting miR negative control. Data shown represent means ± SEMs of 3 independent experiments, with statistical analysis by Student's t test. **$p<0.01$, ***$p<0.001$.

to cell cycling [44,45], RAB5 has been reported to play a role in other cellular pathways including autophagy [56,57] and mTOR signaling [58,59]. In humans, the RAB5 subfamily includes 3 isoforms, which may have distinct functions [60–62]. RAB5C isoform has specifically been shown to be involved in cell migration during zebrafish gastrulation [63], cell invasion via regulation of growth factor-stimulated recycling of integrin [64], and cell motility through RAC1 [65]. Protein alignment of RAB5A and RAB5B revealed 83% and 86% sequence similarity to RAB5C protein, respectively [66]. Neither miR-509-5p nor miR-509-3p is predicted to target RAB5A, and we did not detect any change in RAB5A expression in miR-509-transduced NALM6 cells (Figure S5). TargetScan6.2 predicts a miR-509-5p binding site in the 3'UTR of RAB5B (total context+ score = − 0.04). However, using qRT-PCR, we did not detect RAB5B expression in NALM6 cells (Figure S6).

Previously, it has been shown that knockdown of all 3 RAB5 isoforms, but not knockdown of individual isoforms, in human cells resulted in defective alignment of chromosomes, delayed progression though mitosis and defective chromosome segregation [45]. While our BrdU/7-AAD analysis did not detect significantly

elevated numbers of miR-509-transduced NALM6 cells in cell cycle phase G_2/M, this could be due to expression of the compensatory isoform RAB5A. The downstream mechanism by which RAB5C regulates B-ALL cell growth remains unclear. Given that RAB5 is a key regulator of the endosome pathway, the impaired cell growth in miR-509-transduced or RAB5C-knockdown cells might be due to aberrant recycling of surface growth receptors, such as transferrin receptor [53]. In HeLa cells, knockdown of all 3 RAB5 isoforms resulted in delayed internalization of transferrin receptor and reduced uptake of transferrin [62]. Since the transferrin receptor is important in regulation of intracellular iron concentration which in turn affects cell proliferation [67,68], efforts to examine the effects of RAB5C on transferrin receptors and/or other growth-related receptors required for B-ALL growth are ongoing.

Our data indicate that RAB5C is important for B-ALL cell growth. Therefore, we might expect RAB5C to be overexpressed in B-ALL cells as compared to normal counterpart cells. Thus, we queried RAB5C expression in leukemia using the Oncomine cancer microarray database [69], comparing specifically the 'cancer versus normal' analysis with a threshold of p-value ≤

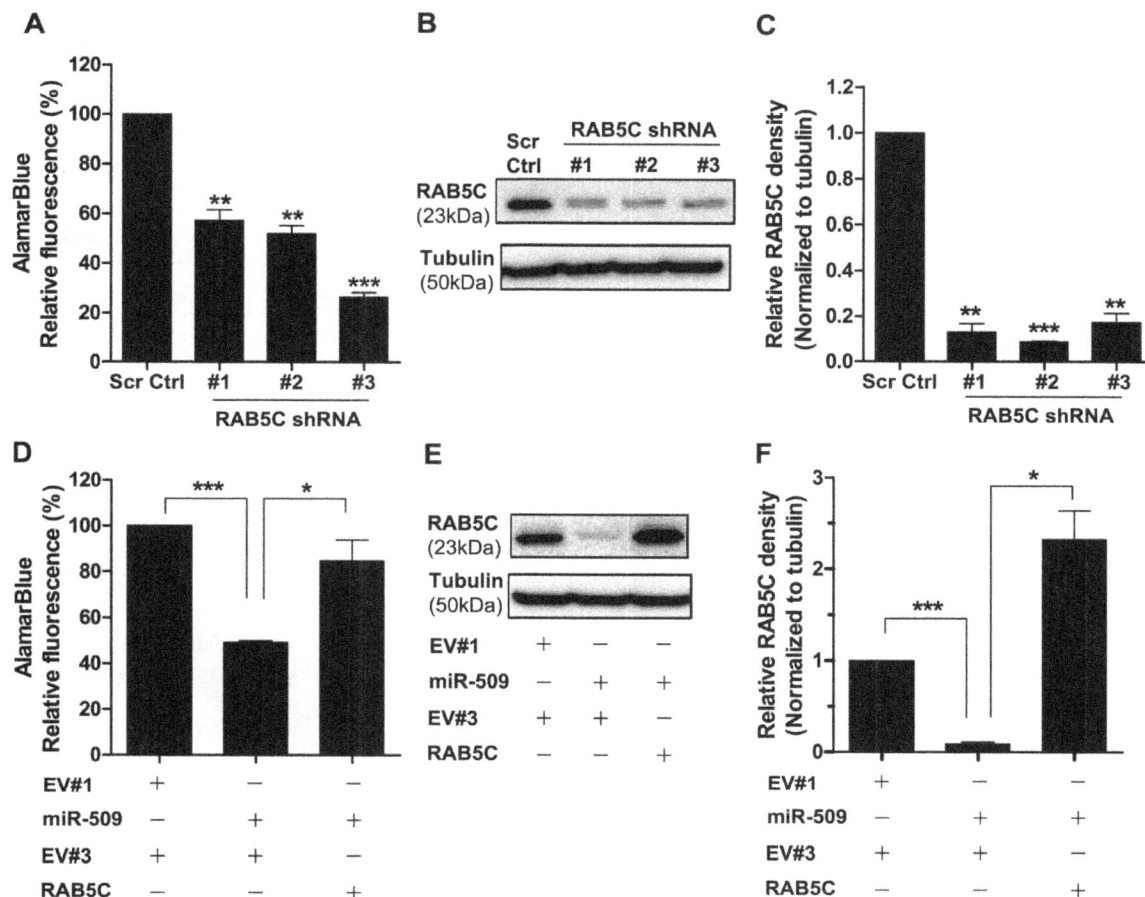

Figure 6. RAB5C mediates the growth-inhibitory effect of miR-509. (A) AlamarBlue assay of NALM6 cells transduced with either lentivirus of scrambled control (Scr Ctrl), shRNA#1, shRNA#2 or shRNA#3 for RAB5C on 7 days after transduction. Data represent means ± SEMs of 3 independent experiments with statistical analysis by Student's t test. **$p<0.01$ and ***$p<0.001$. (B) Representative western blot of NALM6 cells transduced with lentivirus of scrambled control (Scr Ctrl), shRNA#1, shRNA#2 or shRNA#3 for RAB5C. Protein lysates were harvested 7 days after transduction and α-tubulin was used as a loading control. (C) Quantitation of western blots shown in (B) and 2 other independent experiments. Relative densitometry values were calculated relative to Scr Ctrl. Results show means ± SEMs with statistical analysis by Student's t test. **$p<0.01$ and ***$p<0.001$. (D) Enforced expression of RAB5C without its 3′UTR rescues miR-509-mediated growth inhibition. NALM6 cells were co-transduced with the indicated plasmids, and alamarBlue assay was read at 7 days after transduction. The empty lentiviral vector in this experiment is EV#3, which does not have RAB5C cloned in. Results show means ± SEMs of 3 independent experiments, with statistical analysis using Student's t test. *$p<0.05$ and ***$p<0.001$. (E) Representative western blot of NALM6 cells co-transduced with lentivirus of the indicated plasmids. Protein lysates were harvested 7 days after transduction and α-tubulin was used as a loading control. (F) Quantitation of western blots shown in (E) and 2 other independent experiments. Relative densitometry values were calculated relative to EV#1 and EV#3. Results show means ± SEMs with statistical analysis by Student's t test. *$p<0.05$ and ***$p<0.001$.

0.001 and 1.5-fold over-expression. Using these criteria to assess the 14 'cancer versus normal' datasets and focusing solely on leukemia in Oncomine, RAB5C was overexpressed in the dataset of B-ALL patient samples harboring the t(12;21) chromosomal translocation (producing the TEL/AML-1 fusion protein oncogene) as compared to normal B-lymphoid precursors (pro/pre–B cells and immature B cells) from healthy donors [70]. In this TEL/AML-1 B-ALL subset, there was 1.8-fold elevated (average; Student's t test, $p = 3.67^{-6}$) RAB5C expression (Figure S7). The overexpression of RAB5C in this B-ALL subset, along with our findings that RAB5C supports growth of B-ALL cells, suggests that RAB5C may represent a target for treatment of the TEL/AML-1 B-ALL subset, especially if future studies reveal that growth of primary B-ALL cases harboring TEL/AML-1 is highly dependent on RAB5C. In addition, future work may include determining

whether RAB5C overexpression in hematopoietic stem cells can drive B-ALL development.

Despite using the same candidate selection criteria, we were surprised to find that the candidate validation rate (20%) of the miR-HTS conducted in NALM6 cells herein was lower than previously observed for miR-HTS conducted in the IMR90 human lung fibroblast (75% validation rate) [26]. False positives in the miR-HTS may be due to the Monte Carlo effect [71,72], where low template amounts might result in sporadic amplification at the reference time point sample but not the samples at the later time points. Consequently, such a candidate miR will not be validated. Indeed, 2 of the 4 false-positive candidate miRs in this study were detected only at the first or the first 2 time points. Neither of the other 2 false-positive candidates were detected at any of the 4 times points, including the reference time point. We designated these as candidates because we have used the same batch of lenti-miR library to conduct miR-HTS in a total of 4 cell lines (i.e. IMR90, NALM6 and 2 other cell lines) and both of these lenti-miRs were detected at the reference time point in at least one of these 4 cell lines. This suggested to us that the lenti-miR library indeed contained these 2 miR lentiviruses and should have infected the NALM6 as effectively as the other cell lines. Thus, lack of detecting cells containing these 2 lenti-miRs in NALM6 even at the reference time point might be due to a very strong growth-inhibitory effect of these 2 miR candidates. Hence, these 2 miR candidates were included in our validation analyses. However, it is possible that the lenti-miR viruses for these 2 false-positive miR candidates did not actually infect NALM6 cells.

In summary, our findings demonstrate the ability of our miR-HTS platform to identify leukemia cell growth inhibitory miRs and their molecular targets. Our observation that enforced miR-509 expression inhibits growth of B-ALL cell lines provided the clue to identifying the role of RAB5C in the growth of B-ALL cells. To our knowledge, this is the first report of RAB5C as a regulator of B-ALL cell growth. Elucidating the downstream mechanistic roles of RAB5C in growth of human B-ALL cells might suggest novel therapeutic strategies against B-ALL.

Supporting Information

Figure S1 No growth defects were observed for 4 other miR candidates using the GFP competition assay. NALM6 cells were individually transduced with lentivirus of (A) miR-381; (B) miR-550a; (C) miR-873 and (D) miR-432~136 and empty vector (EV#1) to MOI = 2. At 7 days after transduction, cells were mixed with mock-transduced cells to 50% GFP$^+$ cells and this was set as Day 0. The %GFP$^+$ cells (pre-gated on viable cells) of each culture were assessed weekly by flow cytometry for 35 days. Means ± SEMs are shown for three independent experiments. (E) Overexpression of miR candidates in NALM6 cells, as assayed by qRT-PCR. NALM6 cells were transduced with each miR lentivirus to MOI = 2, and total RNA was collected at 7 days after transduction. U18 was used as the loading control. Values shown were calculated as fold overexpression relative to EV#1-transduced NALM6 cells (EV#1). Means ± SEMs are shown for 3 independent experiments.

Figure S2 MiR-509 does not regulate the growth of Jurkat, KARPAS-45 and K562 cells. AlamarBlue cell growth assay was then performed on day 7 after transduction of (A) Jurkat, (B) KARPAS-45 and (C) K562 cells with either miR-509 lentivirus or EV#1. Each cell line was transduced with the indicated lentivirus to MOI = 2. On day 3 after transduction, cells were seeded at the indicated numbers per well/100 μl media: Jurkat (5×10^3 cells), KARPAS-45 (3×10^3 cells) and K562 (1.25×10^3 cells) in triplicates in 96-well plates. Values for miR-509 were normalized to EV#1. Means ± SEMs, ns = no statistical significance was detected by Student's t test.

Figure S3 Enforced expression of miR-509 was detected by qRT-PCR in selected T-ALL and myeloid leukemia cell lines transduced with miR-509 lentivirus. (A) Jurkat, (B) KARPAS-45 and (C) K562 were transduced with miR-509 lentivirus or EV#1. On day 7 after transduction, cells were collected for RNA isolation. U18 was used as the endogenous control. Values shown were calculated as fold overexpression relative to each EV#1-transduced cells. Means ± SEMs are shown for 3 independent experiments.

Figure S4 RAB5C protein levels were decreased in RCH-ACV and REH cells with enforced miR-509 expression. Representative western blot of RAB5C expression in (A) RCH-ACV and (B) REH. Cells were transduced with either EV#1 or miR-509 overexpressing lentivirus, and whole cell lysates were harvested at 7 days after transduction. α-tubulin was used for loading control. The bar graph below represents the densitometry analysis of RAB5C expression of 3 independent experiments, normalized to α-tubulin, and relative densitometry was then calculated compared to EV#1. Data shown represent means ± SEMs, with statistical analysis by Student's t test. **p<0.01, ***p<0.001.

Figure S5 RAB5A mRNA levels show no change in miR-509-transduced NALM6 cells. NALM6 cells were transduced with empty vector #1 (EV#1) to MOI = 2, and RNA was isolated at day 7 after transduction for qRT-PCR. All values were normalized to GAPDH and fold-change was calculated relative to EV#1 sample. Data represents means ± SEMs of 3 independent experiments, with statistical analysis by Student's t test, ns = no statistical significance was detected by Student's t test.

Figure S6 Expression of RAB5A and RAB5C, but not RAB5B, was detected in NALM6 cells using qRT-PCR. NALM6 cells were transduced with empty vector #1 (EV#1) to MOI = 2, and RNA was isolated at day 7 after transduction for qRT-PCR. Ratio to GAPDH (endogenous control) was calculated as 2E[-(RAB5$_{Ct}$ – GAPDH$_{Ct}$)]. Means ± SEMs, n = 3 independent experiments. Value above each bar represents the mean.

Figure S7 Scatter dot plot of RAB5C mRNA expression in B-ALL cells and pre-B lymphocytes based on Oncomine cancer microarray database. RAB5C expression in leukemia was examined using the Oncomine cancer microarray database by comparing specifically the 'cancer versus normal' analysis and setting a threshold of p-value ≤0.001 and 1.5-fold over-expression. 14 'cancer versus normal' datasets were identified and we focused solely on leukemia in Oncomine. RAB5C was overexpressed by 1.8-fold (average; Student's t test, p = 3.67^{-6}) in the dataset of B-ALL patient samples harboring the t(12;21) chromosomal translocation (producing the TEL/AML-1 fusion protein oncogene; n = 17) as compared to normal B-lymphoid precursors (pro/pre–B cells and immature B cells; n = 2) from healthy donors [67]. Error bars represent the mean ± SEM.

Table S1 List of primers used for cloning of miR hairpin with flanking genomic sequences. PCR products were first cloned into pJET1.2 and subcloned into empty lentiviral vector #1 (EV#1; pWCC52) downstream of GFP. MiR-509 was then subcloned from pWCC52-miR-509 into empty lentiviral vector #2 (EV#2; pWCC72) downstream of DsRed.

Table S2 Primers used for PCR of RAB5C-3'UTR and deletion of miR-509-3p binding sites. Full length RAB5C-3'UTR was cloned into pmirGLO Dual-Luciferase miRNA Target Expression vector (Promega). This plasmid was then used as a template for site-directed mutagenesis to delete the first miR-509-3p binding sites in RAB5C-3'UTR-luciferase deletion construct, Δ1 or Δ1Δ2 using primers Del56-72. For the deletion of the second miR-509-3p binding site in RAB5C-3'UTR-luciferase deletion construct, Δ2 or Δ1Δ2, standard PCR was performed using the Del758-767 primers.

Table S3   Primers used in cloning of RAB5C lacking its 3'UTR into pWCC61 lentiviral vector (Empty lentiviral vector #3, EV#3).

Table S4   List of primers used for SYBRGreen qRT-PCR. Primer sequences were obtained from PrimerBank. Fwd: Forward; Rev: Reverse.

Table S5   List of TaqMan microRNA assay ID used for qRT-PCR.

Table S6   List of the 395 predicted targets of miR-509-5p and/or miR-509-3p selected based on filtering strategy shown in Figure 4A. These targets were subjected to a filtering strategy presented in Fig. 4A and meet the following criteria: (i) They are predicted targets of miR-509-5p and/or miR-509-3p

from TargetScan6.2 and/or miRDB. (ii) These targets are not targets of miR-381, miR-550a, miR-873 and miR-432 as predicted by TargetScan6.2 and/or miRDB. (iii) These targets are expressed in NALM6 cells as determined by genome-wide microarray profiling downloaded from the Cancer Cell Line Encyclopedia and its expression levels are denoted in the microarray dataset as "marginal" or "present".

Acknowledgments

We would like to thank all members of the Civin lab and Dr. Marta Lipinski for their helpful suggestions.

Author Contributions

Conceived and designed the experiments: YST WCC. Performed the experiments: YST MK TJK WCC. Analyzed the data: YST MK CIC WCC. Wrote the paper: YST TJK CIC WCC.

References

1. Bassan R, Hoelzer D (2011) Modern therapy of acute lymphoblastic leukemia. J Clin Oncol 29: 532–543. 10.1200/JCO.2010.30.1382.
2. Hunger SP, Raetz EA, Loh ML, Mullighan CG (2011) Improving outcomes for high-risk ALL: Translating new discoveries into clinical care. Pediatr Blood Cancer 56: 984–993. 10.1002/pbc.22996.
3. Raetz EA, Bhatla T (2012) Where do we stand in the treatment of relapsed acute lymphoblastic leukemia? Hematology Am Soc Hematol Educ Program 2012: 129–136. 10.1182/asheducation-2012.1.129.
4. Bartel DP (2009) MicroRNAs: Target recognition and regulatory functions. Cell 136: 215–233. 10.1016/j.cell.2009.01.002.
5. Pasquinelli AE (2012) MicroRNAs and their targets: Recognition, regulation and an emerging reciprocal relationship. Nat Rev Genet 13: 271–282. 10.1038/nrg3162.
6. Ameres SL, Zamore PD (2013) Diversifying microRNA sequence and function. Nat Rev Mol Cell Biol 14: 475–488. 10.1038/nrm3611.
7. Croce CM (2009) Causes and consequences of microRNA dysregulation in cancer. Nat Rev Genet 10: 704–714. 10.1038/nrg2634.
8. Faraoni I, Antonetti FR, Cardone J, Bonmassar E (2009) miR-155 gene: A typical multifunctional microRNA. Biochim Biophys Acta 1792: 497–505. 10.1016/j.bbadis.2009.02.013.
9. O'Connell RM, Rao DS, Chaudhuri AA, Boldin MP, Taganov KD, et al. (2008) Sustained expression of microRNA-155 in hematopoietic stem cells causes a myeloproliferative disorder. J Exp Med 205: 585–594. 10.1084/jem.20072108.
10. Costinean S, Sandhu SK, Pedersen IM, Tili E, Trotta R, et al. (2009) Src homology 2 domain-containing inositol-5-phosphatase and CCAAT enhancer-binding protein beta are targeted by miR-155 in B cells of emicro-MiR-155 transgenic mice. Blood 114: 1374–1382. 10.1182/blood-2009-05-220814.
11. Hermeking H (2010) The miR-34 family in cancer and apoptosis. Cell Death Differ 17: 193–199. 10.1038/cdd.2009.56.
12. Lal A, Thomas MP, Altschuler G, Navarro F, O'Day E, et al. (2011) Capture of microRNA-bound mRNAs identifies the tumor suppressor miR-34a as a regulator of growth factor signaling. PLoS Genet 7: e1002363. 10.1371/journal.pgen.1002363.
13. Garzon R, Volinia S, Liu CG, Fernandez-Cymering C, Palumbo T, et al. (2008) MicroRNA signatures associated with cytogenetics and prognosis in acute myeloid leukemia. Blood 111: 3183–3189. 10.1182/blood-2007-07-098749.
14. Dixon-McIver A, East P, Mein CA, Cazier JB, Molloy G, et al. (2008) Distinctive patterns of microRNA expression associated with karyotype in acute myeloid leukaemia. PLoS One 3: e2141. 10.1371/journal.pone.0002141.
15. Schotte D, De Menezes RX, Akbari Moqadam F, Khankahdani LM, Lange-Turenhout E, et al. (2011) MicroRNA characterize genetic diversity and drug resistance in pediatric acute lymphoblastic leukemia. Haematologica 96: 703–711. 10.3324/haematol.2010.026138.
16. Ju X, Li D, Shi Q, Hou H, Sun N, et al. (2009) Differential microRNA expression in childhood B-cell precursor acute lymphoblastic leukemia. Pediatr Hematol Oncol 26: 1–10. 10.1080/08880010802378338.
17. Schotte D, Pieters R, Den Boer ML (2012) MicroRNAs in acute leukemia: From biological players to clinical contributors. Leukemia 26: 1–12. 10.1038/leu.2011.151.
18. Bhatia S, Kaul D, Varma N (2010) Potential tumor suppressive function of miR-196b in B-cell lineage acute lymphoblastic leukemia. Mol Cell Biochem 340: 97–106. 10.1007/s11010-010-0406-9.
19. Agirre X, Vilas-Zornoza A, Jimenez-Velasco A, Martin-Subero JI, Cordeu L, et al. (2009) Epigenetic silencing of the tumor suppressor microRNA hsa-miR-124a regulates CDK6 expression and confers a poor prognosis in acute lymphoblastic leukemia. Cancer Res 69: 4443–4453. 10.1158/0008-5472.CAN-08-4025.
20. Dou L, Zheng D, Li J, Li Y, Gao L, et al. (2012) Methylation-mediated repression of microRNA-143 enhances MLL-AF4 oncogene expression. Oncogene 31: 507–517. 10.1038/onc.2011.248.
21. Izumiya M, Tsuchiya N, Okamoto K, Nakagama H (2011) Systematic exploration of cancer-associated microRNA through functional screening assays. Cancer Sci 102: 1615–1621. 10.1111/j.1349-7006.2011.02007.x.
22. Poell JB, van Haastert RJ, de Gunst T, Schultz IJ, Gommans WM, et al. (2012) A functional screen identifies specific microRNAs capable of inhibiting human melanoma cell viability. PLoS One 7: e43569. 10.1371/journal.pone.0043569.
23. Izumiya M, Okamoto K, Tsuchiya N, Nakagama H (2010) Functional screening using a microRNA virus library and microarrays: A new high-throughput assay to identify tumor-suppressive microRNAs. Carcinogenesis 31: 1354–1359. 10.1093/carcin/bgq112.
24. Tsuchiya N, Izumiya M, Ogata-Kawata H, Okamoto K, Fujiwara Y, et al. (2011) Tumor suppressor miR-22 determines p53-dependent cellular fate through post-transcriptional regulation of p21. Cancer Res 71: 4628–4639. 10.1158/0008-5472.CAN-10-2475.
25. Okamoto K, Ishiguro T, Midorikawa Y, Ohata H, Izumiya M, et al. (2012) miR-493 induction during carcinogenesis blocks metastatic settlement of colon cancer cells in liver. EMBO J 31: 1752–1763. 10.1038/emboj.2012.25.
26. Cheng WC, Kingsbury TJ, Wheelan SJ, Civin CI (2013) A simple high-throughput screening technology enables gain-of-function screening of human micro-RNAs. BioTechniques 54: 77–86. 10.2144/000113991.
27. Amendola M, Passerini L, Pucci F, Gentner B, Bacchetta R, et al. (2009) Regulated and multiple miRNA and siRNA delivery into primary cells by a lentiviral platform. Mol Ther 17: 1039–1052. 10.1038/mt.2009.48.
28. Sarbassov DD, Guertin DA, Ali SM, Sabatini DM (2005) Phosphorylation and regulation of akt/PKB by the rictor-mTOR complex. Science 307: 1098–1101. 10.1126/science.1106148.
29. Wang X, Spandidos A, Wang H, Seed B (2012) PrimerBank: A PCR primer database for quantitative gene expression analysis, 2012 update. Nucleic Acids Res 40: D1144–9. 10.1093/nar/gkr1013.
30. Chen C, Ridzon DA, Broomer AJ, Zhou Z, Lee DH, et al. (2005) Real-time quantification of microRNAs by stem-loop RT-PCR. Nucleic Acids Res 33: e179. 10.1093/nar/gni178.
31. Heiser D, Tan YS, Kaplan I, Godsey B, Morisot S, et al. (2014) Correlated miR-mRNA expression signatures of mouse hematopoietic stem and progenitor cell subsets predict "stemness" and "myeloid" interaction networks. PLoS One 9: e94852. 10.1371/journal.pone.0094852 [doi].
32. Candia J, Cherukuri S, Doshi KA, Banavar JR, Civin CI, et al. (2014) Uncovering differential multi-microRNA signatures of acute myeloid and lymphoblastic leukemias with a machine-learning-based network approach. In Press.
33. Mavrakis KJ, Wolfe AL, Oricchio E, Palomero T, de Keersmaecker K, et al. (2010) Genome-wide RNA-mediated interference screen identifies miR-19 targets in notch-induced T-cell acute lymphoblastic leukaemia. Nat Cell Biol 12: 372–379. 10.1038/ncb2037.
34. Eekels JJ, Pasternak AO, Schut AM, Geerts D, Jeeninga RE, et al. (2012) A competitive cell growth assay for the detection of subtle effects of gene transduction on cell proliferation. Gene Ther 19: 1058–1064. 10.1038/gt.2011.191.
35. Rampersad SN (2012) Multiple applications of alamar blue as an indicator of metabolic function and cellular health in cell viability bioassays. Sensors (Basel) 12: 12347–12360. 10.3390/s120912347.
36. Kaplan IM, Morisot S, Heiser D, Cheng WC, Kim MJ, et al. (2011) Deletion of tristetraprolin caused spontaneous reactive granulopoiesis by a non-cell-

autonomous mechanism without disturbing long-term hematopoietic stem cell quiescence. J Immunol 186: 2826–2834. 10.4049/jimmunol.1002806.
37. Grimson A, Farh KK, Johnston WK, Garrett-Engele P, Lim LP, et al. (2007) MicroRNA targeting specificity in mammals: Determinants beyond seed pairing. Mol Cell 27: 91–105. 10.1016/j.molcel.2007.06.017.
38. Wang X (2008) miRDB: A microRNA target prediction and functional annotation database with a wiki interface. RNA 14: 1012–1017. 10.1261/rna.965408.
39. Wang X, El Naqa IM (2008) Prediction of both conserved and nonconserved microRNA targets in animals. Bioinformatics 24: 325–332. 10.1093/bioinformatics/btm595.
40. Barretina J, Caponigro G, Stransky N, Venkatesan K, Margolin AA, et al. (2012) The cancer cell line encyclopedia enables predictive modelling of anticancer drug sensitivity. Nature 483: 603–607. 10.1038/nature11003.
41. Hulsen T, de Vlieg J, Alkema W (2008) BioVenn - a web application for the comparison and visualization of biological lists using area-proportional venn diagrams. BMC Genomics 9: 488-2164-9-488. 10.1186/1471-2164-9-488.
42. Huang da W, Sherman BT, Lempicki RA (2009) Systematic and integrative analysis of large gene lists using DAVID bioinformatics resources. Nat Protoc 4: 44–57. 10.1038/nprot.2008.211.
43. Huang da W, Sherman BT, Lempicki RA (2009) Bioinformatics enrichment tools: Paths toward the comprehensive functional analysis of large gene lists. Nucleic Acids Res 37: 1–13. 10.1093/nar/gkn923.
44. Capalbo L, D'Avino PP, Archambault V, Glover DM (2011) Rab5 GTPase controls chromosome alignment through lamin disassembly and relocation of the NuMA-like protein mud to the poles during mitosis. Proc Natl Acad Sci U S A 108: 17343–17348. 10.1073/pnas.1103720108.
45. Serio G, Margaria V, Jensen S, Oldani A, Bartek J, et al. (2011) Small GTPase Rab5 participates in chromosome congression and regulates localization of the centromere-associated protein CENP-F to kinetochores. Proc Natl Acad Sci U S A 108: 17337–17342. 10.1073/pnas.1103516108.
46. Calin GA, Croce CM (2006) MicroRNA signatures in human cancers. Nat Rev Cancer 6: 857–866. 10.1038/nrc1997.
47. Zhang WB, Pan ZQ, Yang QS, Zheng XM (2013) Tumor suppressive miR-509-5p contributes to cell migration, proliferation and antiapoptosis in renal cell carcinoma. Ir J Med Sci 182: 621–627. 10.1007/s11845-013-0941-y.
48. Zhai Q, Zhou L, Zhao C, Wan J, Yu Z, et al. (2012) Identification of miR-508-3p and miR-509-3p that are associated with cell invasion and migration and involved in the apoptosis of renal cell carcinoma. Biochem Biophys Res Commun 419: 621–626. 10.1016/j.bbrc.2012.02.060.
49. Thomas M, Lieberman J, Lal A (2010) Desperately seeking microRNA targets. Nat Struct Mol Biol 17: 1169–1174. 10.1038/nsmb.1921.
50. Thomson DW, Bracken CP, Goodall GJ (2011) Experimental strategies for microRNA target identification. Nucleic Acids Res 39: 6845–6853. 10.1093/nar/gkr330 [doi].
51. Selbach M, Schwanhausser B, Thierfelder N, Fang Z, Khanin R, et al. (2008) Widespread changes in protein synthesis induced by microRNAs. Nature 455: 58–63. 10.1038/nature07228.
52. Guo H, Ingolia NT, Weissman JS, Bartel DP (2010) Mammalian microRNAs predominantly act to decrease target mRNA levels. Nature 466: 835–840. 10.1038/nature09267.
53. Bucci C, Parton RG, Mather IH, Stunnenberg H, Simons K, et al. (1992) The small GTPase rab5 functions as a regulatory factor in the early endocytic pathway. Cell 70: 715–728.
54. Zerial M, McBride H (2001) Rab proteins as membrane organizers. Nat Rev Mol Cell Biol 2: 107–117. 10.1038/35052055.
55. Zeigerer A, Gilleron J, Bogorad RL, Marsico G, Nonaka H, et al. (2012) Rab5 is necessary for the biogenesis of the endolysosomal system in vivo. Nature 485: 465–470. 10.1038/nature11133.
56. Ravikumar B, Imarisio S, Sarkar S, O'Kane CJ, Rubinsztein DC (2008) Rab5 modulates aggregation and toxicity of mutant huntingtin through macroautophagy in cell and fly models of huntington disease. J Cell Sci 121: 1649–1660. 10.1242/jcs.025726.
57. Dou Z, Pan JA, Dbouk HA, Ballou LM, DeLeon JL, et al. (2013) Class IA PI3K p110beta subunit promotes autophagy through Rab5 small GTPase in response to growth factor limitation. Mol Cell 50: 29–42. 10.1016/j.molcel.2013.01.022.
58. Li L, Kim E, Yuan H, Inoki K, Goraksha-Hicks P, et al. (2010) Regulation of mTORC1 by the rab and arf GTPases. J Biol Chem 285: 19705–19709. 10.1074/jbc.C110.102483.
59. Bridges D, Fisher K, Zolov SN, Xiong T, Inoki K, et al. (2012) Rab5 proteins regulate activation and localization of target of rapamycin complex 1. J Biol Chem 287: 20913–20921. 10.1074/jbc.M111.334060.
60. Bucci C, Lutcke A, Steele-Mortimer O, Olkkonen VM, Dupree P, et al. (1995) Co-operative regulation of endocytosis by three Rab5 isoforms. FEBS Lett 366: 65–71.
61. Wainszelbaum MJ, Proctor BM, Pontow SE, Stahl PD, Barbieri MA (2006) IL4/PGE2 induction of an enlarged early endosomal compartment in mouse macrophages is Rab5-dependent. Exp Cell Res 312: 2238–2251. 10.1016/j.yexcr.2006.03.025.
62. Chen PI, Kong C, Su X, Stahl PD (2009) Rab5 isoforms differentially regulate the trafficking and degradation of epidermal growth factor receptors. J Biol Chem 284: 30328–30338. 10.1074/jbc.M109.034546.
63. Ulrich F, Krieg M, Schotz EM, Link V, Castanon I, et al. (2005) Wnt11 functions in gastrulation by controlling cell cohesion through Rab5c and E-cadherin. Dev Cell 9: 555–564. 10.1016/j.devcel.2005.08.011.
64. Onodera Y, Nam JM, Hashimoto A, Norman JC, Shirato H, et al. (2012) Rab5c promotes AMAP1-PRKD2 complex formation to enhance beta1 integrin recycling in EGF-induced cancer invasion. J Cell Biol 197: 983–996. 10.1083/jcb.201201065.
65. Chen PI, Schauer K, Kong C, Harding AR, Goud B, et al. (2014) Rab5 isoforms orchestrate a "division of labor" in the endocytic network; Rab5C modulates rac-mediated cell motility. PLoS One 9: e90384. 10.1371/journal.-pone.0090384; 10.1371/journal.pone.0090384.
66. Sievers F, Wilm A, Dineen D, Gibson TJ, Karplus K, et al. (2011) Fast, scalable generation of high-quality protein multiple sequence alignments using clustal omega. Mol Syst Biol 7: 539. 10.1038/msb.2011.75.
67. May WS Jr, Cuatrecasas P (1985) Transferrin receptor: Its biological significance. J Membr Biol 88: 205–215.
68. O'Donnell KA, Yu D, Zeller KI, Kim JW, Racke F, et al. (2006) Activation of transferrin receptor 1 by c-myc enhances cellular proliferation and tumorigenesis. Mol Cell Biol 26: 2373–2386. 26/6/2373 [pii].
69. Rhodes DR, Yu J, Shanker K, Deshpande N, Varambally R, et al. (2004) ONCOMINE: A cancer microarray database and integrated data-mining platform. Neoplasia 6: 1–6.
70. Maia S, Haining WN, Ansen S, Xia Z, Armstrong SA, et al. (2005) Gene expression profiling identifies BAX-delta as a novel tumor antigen in acute lymphoblastic leukemia. Cancer Res 65: 10050–10058. 10.1158/0008-5472.CAN-05-1574.
71. Karrer EE, Lincoln JE, Hogenhout S, Bennett AB, Bostock RM, et al. (1995) In situ isolation of mRNA from individual plant cells: Creation of cell-specific cDNA libraries. Proc Natl Acad Sci U S A 92: 3814–3818.
72. Bustin SA, Nolan T (2004) Pitfalls of quantitative real-time reverse-transcription polymerase chain reaction. J Biomol Tech 15: 155–166. 15/3/155 [pii].

Permissions

List of Contributors

Sook-Kyoung Heo and Dong-Joon Yoon
Biomedical Research Center, Ulsan University Hospital, University of Ulsan College of Medicine, Ulsan, Republic of Korea

Hawk Kim
Biomedical Research Center, Ulsan University Hospital, University of Ulsan College of Medicine, Ulsan, Republic of Korea
Division of Hematology and Hematological Malignancies, Department of Hematology and Oncology, Ulsan University Hospital, University of Ulsan College of Medicine, Ulsan, Republic of Korea

Eui-Kyu Noh, Jae-Cheol Jo and Jae-Hoo Park
Division of Hematology and Hematological Malignancies, Department of Hematology and Oncology, Ulsan University Hospital, University of Ulsan College of Medicine, Ulsan, Republic of Korea

Julio Finalet Ferreiro, Leila Rouhigharabaei, Helena Urbankova, Jo-Anne van der Krogt, Lucienne Michaux, Peter Vandenberghe and Iwona Wlodarska
Center for Human Genetics, KU Leuven, Leuven, Belgium

Jan Cools
Center for Human Genetics, KU Leuven, Leuven, Belgium
Center for the Biology of Disease, VIB, Leuven, Belgium

Shashirekha Shetty
Molecular Pathology, Cleveland Clinic, Cleveland, Ohio, United States of America

Laszlo Krenacs
Laboratory of Tumor Pathology and Molecular Diagnostics, University of Szeged, Szeged, Hungary

Thomas Tousseyn
Translational Cell and Tissue Research KU Leuven, Department of Pathology UZ Leuven, Leuven, Belgium

Pascale De Paepe
Department of Pathology, AZ St Jan AV, Brugge, Belgium

Anne Uyttebroeck
Department of Pediatrics, UZ Leuven, Leuven, Belgium

Gregor Verhoef
Department of Hematology, UZ Leuven, Leuven, Belgium

Tom Taghon
Department of Clinical Chemistry, Microbiology and Immunology, Ghent University Hospital, Ghent University, Ghent, Belgium

Reuben Thomas, Alan E. Hubbard, Cliona M. McHale, Luoping Zhang, Stephen M. Rappaport and Martyn T. Smith
Superfund Research Program, School of Public Health, University of California, Berkeley, California, United States of America

Qing Lan and Nathaniel Rothman
Division of Cancer Epidemiology and Genetics, National Cancer Institute, National Institutes of Health, Bethesda, Maryland, United States of America

Kathryn Z. Guyton, Jennifer Jinot and Babasaheb R. Sonawane
National Center for Environmental Assessment, Office of Research and Development, US EPA, Washington, DC, United States of America

Roel Vermeulen
Institute of Risk assessment Sciences, Utrecht University, Utrecht, The Netherlands

Kuangguo Zhou, Danmei Xu, Yang Cao, Jue Wang, Yunfan Yang and Mei Huang
Department of Hematology, Tongji Hospital, Tongji Medical College, Huazhong University of Science and Technology, Wuhan, Hubei, P.R.China

Haiwen Ni and Xiangtu Kong
Affiliated Hospital of Nanjing University of TCM, Nanjing, China

Wanzhou Zhao
Sino-EU Biomedical Innovation Center (SEBIC), OG Pharma Corporation, Nanjing, China

Haitao Li
Nanjing University of Chinese Medicine, Nanjing,China

Jian Ouyang
Department of Hematology, Nanjing Drum Tower Hospital, the Affiliated Hospital of Nanjing University Medical School,Nanjing, China

Hemalatha Kuppusamy, Eva Baigorri, Amanda Warkentin, Michael J. Mant, John Mackey, Andrew R. Belch and Linda M. Pilarski
University of Alberta and Cross Cancer Institute, Edmonton, Alberta, Canada

Helga M. Ogmundsdottir
University of Iceland, Reykjavik, Iceland

Hlif Steingrimsdottir and Vilhelmina Haraldsdottir
Landspitali University Hospital, Reykjavik, Iceland

James B. Johnston
Dept.of Hematology, Cancer Care Manitoba and the University of Manitoba, Winnipeg, Manitoba, Canada

Sophia Adamia
Medical Oncology, Dana-Farber Cancer Institute, Harvard Medical School, Boston, Massachusetts, United States of America

Emmelie Björklund, Anders Blomqvist, Joel Hedlin and Christopher J. Fowler
Department of Pharmacology and Clinical Neuroscience, Umeå University, Umeå, Sweden,

Emma Persson
Department of Radiation Sciences, Umeå University, Umeå, Sweden

Xiao Li, Chunkang Chang, Dong Wu, Lingyun Wu, Jiying Su, Xi Zhang, Liyu Zhou, Luxi Song, Zheng Zhang and Feng Xu
Department of Hematology, the Sixth People's Hospital affiliated with Shanghai Jiaotong University, Shanghai, China

Qiang Song and Ming Hou
Department of Hematology, Qilu Hospital affiliated with Shandong University, Jinan, China,

Yu Chen
Department of Hematology, Ruijin Hospital affiliated with Shanghai Jiaotong University School of Medicine, Shanghai, China

Elisa Fueller and Robert K. Slany
Department of Genetics, Friedrich Alexander University, Erlangen, Germany

Daniel Schaefer, Ute Fischer, Pina F. I. Krell and Arndt Borkhardt
Department of Pediatric Oncology, Hematology and Clinical Immunology, University Children's Hospital, Medical Faculty, Heinrich Heine University, Du¨sseldorf, Germany

Martin Stanulla
Department of Pediatric Hematology and Oncology, Hannover Medical School, Hannover, Germany

Wengang Song
Beihua University, Jinlin, China

Yongzhe Liu
Department of Toxicology, School of Public Health, Tianjin Medical University, Tianjin, China

Ying Liu
Department of Toxicology, School of Public Health, Jilin University, Changchun, China

Cong Zhang and Shilong Sun
Ministry of Health, Key Laboratory of Radiobiology, Jilin University, Changchun, China, National Laboratory of Medical Molecular Biology, Tsinghua University, Beijing, PR China

Bao Yuan
College of Animal Sciences, Jilin University, Changchun, China

Lianbo Zhang
Department of Plastic and Reconstructive Surgery, China-Japan Union Hospital of Jilin University, Changchun, China

Velizar Shivarov
Laboratory of Hematopathology and Immunology, National Hematology Hospital, Sofia, Bulgaria

Milena Ivanova and Elissaveta Naumova
Department of Clinical Immunology, Alexandrovska University Hospital, Medical University, Sofia, Bulgaria

Zi-Jie Long, Yuan Hu, Xu-Dong Li, Yi He, Ruo-Zhi Xiao, Zhi-Gang Fang, Dong-Ning Wang, Jia-Jun Liu, Ren-Wei Huang and Dong-Jun Lin
Department of Hematology, Third Affiliated Hospital, Sun Yat-sen University, Sun Yat-sen Institute of Hematology, Sun Yat-sen University, Guangzhou, China

Quentin Liu
Department of Hematology, Third Affiliated Hospital, Sun Yat-sen University, Sun Yat-sen Institute of Hematology, Sun Yat-sen University, Guangzhou, China
Institute of Cancer Stem Cell, Dalian Medical University, Dalian, China

Jin-Song Yan
Department of Hematology, Second Affiliated Hospital, Dalian Medical University, Dalian, China

M. Christina Cox, Caterina Tatarelli and Bruno Monarca
Hematology Unit, Sant'Andrea Hospital,
Department of Clinical and Molecular Medicine
La Sapienza University, Rome, Italy

Arianna Di Napoli, Stefania Scarpino, Caterina Talerico, Mariangela Lombardi and Luigi Ruco
Pathology Unit, Department of Clinical and Molecular Medicine, Sant'Andrea Hospital, La Sapienza University, Rome, Italy

Gerardo Salerno
Clinical Pathology Unit, Department of Clinical and Molecular Medicine Sant'Andrea Hospital, La Sapienza University, Rome, Italy

Sergio Amadori
Hematology Department, Tor Vergata University, Rome, Italy

Yimeng Niu, Rurong Tang and Yan Li
Department of Hematology, The First Affiliated Hospital of China Medical University, Shenyang, Liaoning, P.R.China

Rui Zhang
Department of Hematology, The First Affiliated Hospital of China Medical University, Shenyang, Liaoning, P.R. China
Department of Pediatrics, University of Oklahoma Health Sciences Center, Oklahoma City, Oklahoma, United States of America

Xianfu Wang, Weihong Xu, Xiaoxia Hu, Xianglan Lu and Shibo Li
Department of Pediatrics, University of Oklahoma Health Sciences Center, Oklahoma City, Oklahoma, United States of America

Ji-Yun Lee
Department of Pediatrics, University of Oklahoma Health Sciences Center, Oklahoma City, Oklahoma, United States of America
Department of Pathology, College of Medicine, Korea University, Seoul, South Korea

Minghua Yang, Pei Zeng, Yan Yu, Liangchun Yang and Lizhi Cao
Department of Pediatrics, Xiangya Hospital, Central South University, Changsha Hunan, China

Daolin Tang
Department of Infectious Diseases, Xiangya Hospital, Central South University, Changsha, Hunan, China

Department of Surgery, University of Pittsburgh Cancer Institute, Pittsburgh, Pennsylvania, United States of America

Rui Kang
Department of Surgery, University of Pittsburgh Cancer Institute, Pittsburgh, Pennsylvania, United States of America

Rebeca Manso
Pathology Department, Fundación Jiménez Díaz, Madrid, Spain

Socorro María Rodríguez-Pinilla
Pathology Department, Fundación Jiménez Díaz, Madrid, Spain
Molecular Pathology Programme, Lymphoma Group, CNIO, Madrid, Spain

Gorka Ruiz de Garibay
Molecular Pathology Programme, Lymphoma Group, CNIO, Madrid, Spain
Clinical Immunology Department, Hospital Clínico de San Carlos, Madrid, Spain

Maria del Mar López
Molecular Pathology Programme, Lymphoma Group, CNIO, Madrid, Spain
Biotechnology Programme, Monoclonal Antibodies Unit, CNIO, Madrid, Spain

Margarita Sánchez-Beato
Molecular Pathology Programme, Lymphoma Group, CNIO, Madrid, Spain
Oncology-Haematology Area, Instituto Investigación Sanitaria, Hospital Universitario Puerta de Hierro-Majadahonda, Madrid, Spain

Miguel Ángel Piris
Molecular Pathology Programme, Lymphoma Group, CNIO, Madrid, Spain
Pathology Department, Hospital Universitario Marqués de Valdecilla, Universidad de Cantabria, IFIMAV, Santander, Spain

Luis Lombardia
Clinical Research Programme, Molecular Diagnostics Clinical Research Unit, CNIO, Madrid, Spain

Luis Requena
Dermatology Department, Fundación Jimenez Díaz, Madrid, Spain

Lydia Sánchez
Biotechnology Programme, Immunohistochemistry Unit, CNIO, Madrid, Spain

Corrado Tarella, Angela Gueli, Riccardo Bruna, Marco Ruella and Daniela Gottardi
Department of Biotechnology and Life Sciences, University of Torino, Torino, Italy
Hematology and Cell Therapy Division, Mauriziano Hospital, Torino, Italy

Daniele Caracciolo
Department of Biotechnology and Life Sciences, University of Torino, Torino, Italy
Division of Hematology I, A. O. Citta` della Salute, Torino, Italy

Federica Delaini, Andrea Rossi, Anna Maria Barbui, Giuseppe Gritti and Cristina Boschini
Hematology and Bone Marrow Transplant Units, A. O. Papa Giovanni XXIII, Bergamo, Italy

Alessandro Rambaldi
Division of Hematology I, A. O. Citta` della Salute, Torino, Italy

Roberto Passera
Division of Nuclear Medicine, University of Torino, Torino, Italy

Marta E. Capala, Edo Vellenga and Jan Jacob Schuringa
Department of Experimental Hematology, Cancer Research Center Groningen (CRCG), University Medical Center Groningen, University of Groningen, Groningen, the Netherlands

Wei Li, Xiaoyuan Gong, Mingyuan Sun, Xingli Zhao, Benfa Gong, Hui Wei and Yingchang Mi
Leukemia Diagnosis and Treatment Center, Institute of Hematology and Blood Disease Hospital, Chinese Academy of Medical Sciences and Peking Union of Medical College, Tianjin, China

Jianxiang Wang
Leukemia Diagnosis and Treatment Center, Institute of Hematology and Blood Disease Hospital, Chinese Academy of Medical Sciences and Peking Union of Medical College, Tianjin, China
State Key Laboratory of Experimental Hematology, Institute of Hematology and Blood Disease Hospital, Chinese Academy of Medical Sciences and Peking Union of Medical College, Tianjin, China

Qing Wang, Siyi Zhang, Shichao Pang, Menghuan Zhang and Bo Wang
Department of Bioinformatics & Biostatistics, School of Life Science and Biotechnology, Shanghai Jiao Tong University, Shanghai, China

Qi Liu
Department of Bioinformatics & Biostatistics, School of Life Science and Biotechnology, Shanghai Jiao Tong University, Shanghai, China
Department of Biomedical Informatics, Vanderbilt University School of Medicine, Nashville, Tennessee, United States of America
Center for Quantitative Sciences, Vanderbilt University School of Medicine, Nashville, Tennessee, United States of America

Jing Li
Department of Bioinformatics & Biostatistics, School of Life Science and Biotechnology, Shanghai Jiao Tong University, Shanghai, China
Shanghai Center for Bioinformation Technology, Shanghai, China

Stefano Mattioli and Andrea Farioli
Department of Medical and Surgical Sciences (DIMEC), University of Bologna, Bologna, Italy

Patrizia Legittimo
Unit of Occupational Medicine, S.Orsola-Malpighi University Hospital, Bologna, Italy
Occupational and Environmental Epidemiology Unit, ISPO Cancer Prevention and Research Institute, Florence, Italy

Lucia Miligi and Alessandra Benvenuti
Occupational and Environmental Epidemiology Unit, ISPO Cancer Prevention and Research Institute, Florence, Italy

Alessandra Ranucci and Corrado Magnani
Cancer Epidemiology Unit - Department of Translational Medicine, CPO Piemonte and University of Eastern Piedmont, Novara, Italy

Alberto Salvan
Currently retired, IASI-CNR, Rome, Italy

Roberto Rondelli
Paediatric Oncology-Haematology "Lalla Sera` gnoli", Policlinico S.Orsola-Malpighi, Bologna, Italy

Fu-Nan Cho
Department of Obstetrics and Gynecology, Kaohsiung Veterans General Hospital, Kaohsiung, Taiwan

Tsung-Hsien Chang and Chih-Wen Shu
Department of Medical Education and Research, Kaohsiung Veterans General Hospital, Kaohsiung, Taiwan

Ming-Chin Ko and Chien-Hui Hung
Department of Pediatrics, Kaohsiung Veterans General Hospital, Kaohsiung, Taiwan

Yu-Hsiang Chang
Department of Pediatrics, Kaohsiung Veterans General Hospital, Kaohsiung, Taiwan
Faculty of Medicine, National Yang-Ming University, Taipei, Taiwan
Department of Nursing, Tajen University, Yanpu Township, Pingtung County, Taiwan

Shuen-Kuei Liao
Graduate Institute of Cancer Biology and Drug Discovery and Center of Excellence for Cancer Research, Taipei Medical University, Taipei, Taiwan

Kang-Hsi Wu
Department of Pediatrics, Children's Hospital and School of Chinese Medicine, China Medical University Hospitals, Taichung, Taiwan

Ming-Sun Yu, Shyh-Jer Lin and Ying-Chung Hong
Haematology-Oncology Section, Department of Medicine, Kaohsiung Veterans General Hospital, Kaohsiung, Taiwan

Chien-Hsun Chen
Department of Radiation Oncology, Kaohsiung Veterans General Hospital, Kaohsiung, Taiwan

Yee Sun Tan
Center for Stem Cell Biology & Regenerative Medicine, University of Maryland School of Medicine, Baltimore, Maryland, United States of America

Tami J. Kingsbury
Center for Stem Cell Biology & Regenerative Medicine, University of Maryland School of Medicine, Baltimore, Maryland, United States of America

Greenebaum Cancer Center, University of Maryland School of Medicine, Baltimore, Maryland, United States of America
Department of Physiology, University of Maryland School of Medicine, Baltimore, Maryland, United States of America

Curt I. Civin
Center for Stem Cell Biology & Regenerative Medicine, University of Maryland School of Medicine, Baltimore, Maryland, United States of America
Greenebaum Cancer Center, University of Maryland School of Medicine, Baltimore, Maryland, United States of America
Department of Physiology, University of Maryland School of Medicine, Baltimore, Maryland, United States of America
Department of Pediatrics, University of Maryland School of Medicine, Baltimore, Maryland, United States of America

Min Jung Kim
Center for Stem Cell Biology & Regenerative Medicine, University of Maryland School of Medicine, Baltimore, Maryland, United States of America
Department of Physiology, University of Maryland School of Medicine, Baltimore, Maryland, United States of America
Department of Pediatrics, University of Maryland School of Medicine, Baltimore, Maryland, United States of America

Wen-Chih Cheng
Center for Stem Cell Biology & Regenerative Medicine, University of Maryland School of Medicine, Baltimore, Maryland, United States of America
Department of Pediatrics, University of Maryland School of Medicine, Baltimore, Maryland, United States of America

Index

www.ingramcontent.com/pod-product-compliance
Lightning Source LLC
Chambersburg PA
CBHW080516200326
41458CB00012B/4235